VOLUME **6**

DISEASE CONTROL PRIORITIES • THIRD EDITION

Major Infectious Diseases

DISEASE CONTROL PRIORITIES • THIRD EDITION

Series Editors

Dean T. Jamison

Rachel Nugent

Hellen Gelband

Susan Horton

Prabhat Jha

Ramanan Laxminarayan

Charles N. Mock

Volumes in the Series

Essential Surgery

Reproductive, Maternal, Newborn, and Child Health

Cancer

Mental, Neurological, and Substance Use Disorders

Cardiovascular, Respiratory, and Related Disorders

Major Infectious Diseases

Injury Prevention and Environmental Health

Child and Adolescent Health and Development

Disease Control Priorities: Improving Health and Reducing Poverty

DISEASE CONTROL PRIORITIES

Budgets constrain choices. Policy analysis helps decision makers achieve the greatest value from limited available resources. In 1993, the World Bank published *Disease Control Priorities in Developing Countries* (*DCP1*), an attempt to systematically assess the cost-effectiveness (value for money) of interventions that would address the major sources of disease burden in low- and middle-income countries. The World Bank's 1993 *World Development Report* on health drew heavily on *DCP1*'s findings to conclude that specific interventions against noncommunicable diseases were cost-effective, even in environments in which substantial burdens of infection and undernutrition persisted.

DCP2, published in 2006, updated and extended *DCP1* in several aspects, including explicit consideration of the implications for health systems of expanded intervention coverage. One way that health systems expand intervention coverage is through selected platforms that deliver interventions that require similar logistics but deliver interventions from different packages of conceptually related interventions, for example, against cardiovascular disease. Platforms often provide a more natural unit for investment than do individual interventions. Analysis of the costs of packages and platforms—and of the health improvements they can generate in given epidemiological environments—can help to guide health system investments and development.

DCP3 differs importantly from *DCP1* and *DCP2* by extending and consolidating the concepts of platforms and packages and by offering explicit consideration of the financial risk protection objective of health systems. In populations lacking access to health insurance or prepaid care, medical expenses that are high relative to income can be impoverishing. Where incomes are low, seemingly inexpensive medical procedures can have catastrophic financial effects. *DCP3* offers an approach to explicitly include financial protection as well as the distribution across income groups of financial and health outcomes resulting from policies (for example, public finance) to increase intervention uptake. The task in all of the *DCP* volumes has been to combine the available science about interventions implemented in very specific locales and under very specific conditions with informed judgment to reach reasonable conclusions about the impact of intervention mixes in diverse environments. *DCP3*'s broad aim is to delineate essential intervention packages and their related delivery platforms to assist decision makers in allocating often tightly constrained budgets so that health system objectives are maximally achieved.

DCP3's nine volumes are being published throughout 2015–18 in an environment in which serious discussion continues about quantifying the sustainable development goal (SDG) for health. *DCP3*'s analyses are well-placed to assist in choosing the means to attain the health SDG and assessing the related costs. Only when these volumes, and the analytic efforts on which they are based, are completed will we be able to explore SDG-related and other broad policy conclusions and generalizations. The final *DCP3* volume will report those conclusions. Each individual volume will provide valuable, specific policy analyses on the full range of interventions, packages, and policies relevant to its health topic.

More than 500 individuals and multiple institutions have contributed to *DCP3*. We convey our acknowledgments elsewhere in this volume. Here we express our particular gratitude to the Bill & Melinda Gates Foundation for its sustained financial support, to the InterAcademy Medical Panel (and its U.S. affiliate, the Institute of Medicine of the National Academy of Sciences), and to World Bank Publications. Each played a critical role in this effort.

Dean T. Jamison
Rachel Nugent
Hellen Gelband
Susan Horton
Prabhat Jha
Ramanan Laxminarayan
Charles N. Mock

VOLUME **6**

DISEASE CONTROL PRIORITIES • THIRD EDITION

Major Infectious Diseases

EDITORS

King K. Holmes
Stefano Bertozzi
Barry R. Bloom
Prabhat Jha

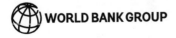 **WORLD BANK GROUP**

ISBNs and DOIs:

Softcover:
ISBN: 978-1-4648-0524-0
ISBN (electronic): 978-1-4648-0525-7
DOI: 10.1596/978-1-4648-0524-0

Hardcover:
ISBN: 978-1-4648-0526-4

DOI: 10.1596/978-1-4648-0526-4

Cover photo: © Jim Pridgeon/University of Washington. Used with the permission of Jim Pridgeon/University of Washington. Further permission required for reuse.

Cover design: Debra Naylor, Naylor Design, Washington, DC

Chapter opener photos: **chapter 1:** © European Union/ECHO/Isabel Coello. Used via a Creative Commons license (https://creativecommons.org/licenses/by/2.0/). Original photo was cropped to fit template; **chapter 2:** © Joerg Boethling/Alamy Stock Photo. Used with permission; further permission required for reuse; **chapter 3:** © Joerg Boethling/Alamy Stock Photo. Used with permission; further permission required for reuse; **chapter 4:** © Joerg Boethling/Alamy Stock Photo. Used with permission; further permission required for reuse; **chapter 5:** © Joerg Boethling/Alamy Stock Photo. Used with permission; further permission required for reuse; **chapter 6:** © Charles Pieters. Used via a Creative Commons license (https://creativecommons.org/licenses/by/2.0/). Original photo was cropped to fit template; **chapter 7:** © International Women's Health Coalition. Used via a Creative Commons license (https://creativecommons.org/licenses/by/2.0/). Original photo was cropped to fit template; **chapter 8:** © Joerg Boethling/Alamy Stock Photo. Used with permission; further permission required for reuse; **chapter 9:** © Joerg Boethling/Alamy Stock Photo. Used with permission; further permission required for reuse; **chapter 10:** © International Women's Health Coalition. Used via a Creative Commons license (https://creativecommons.org/licenses/by/2.0/). Original photo was cropped to fit template; **chapter 11:** © Bhopal Medical Appeal. Used via a Creative Commons license (https://creativecommons.org/licenses/by/2.0/). Original photo was cropped to fit template; **chapter 12:** © European Commission DG ECHO. Used via a Creative Commons license (https://creativecommons.org/licenses/by/2.0/). Original photo was cropped to fit template; **chapter 13:** © European Commission DG ECHO. Used via a Creative Commons license (https://creativecommons.org/licenses/by/2.0/). Original photo was cropped to fit template; **chapter 14:** © Albert González Farran, UNAMID. Used via a Creative Commons license (https://creativecommons.org/licenses/by/2.0/). Original photo was cropped to fit template; **chapter 15:** © Md. Khalid Rayhan Shawon. Used with permission; further permission required for reuse; **chapter 16:** © Penny Tweedie/Alamy Stock Photo. Used with permission; further permission required for reuse; **chapter 17:** © Knut-Erik Helle. Used via a Creative Commons license (https://creativecommons.org/licenses/by/2.0/). Original photo was cropped to fit template; **chapter 18:** © European Commission DG ECHO. Used via a Creative Commons license (https://creativecommons.org/licenses/by/2.0/). Original photo was cropped to fit template.

Library of Congress Cataloging-in-Publication Data has been requested.

Contents

Foreword

Since the publication of the second edition *of Disease Control Priorities* in 2006, we have experienced some of the most substantial progress in infectious disease–caused mortality and morbidity. The number of annual deaths attributable to human immunodeficiency virus/acquired immune deficiency syndrome (HIV/AIDS) declined 50 percent between 2004 and 2015, thanks to an unprecedented expansion of life-saving antiretroviral therapy to over 18 million people (UNAIDS 2016); since 2006, mother-to-child transmission of HIV has been reduced to low levels, even in generalized epidemic settings (AVERT 2017). Similarly, fewer children and adults die from malaria, diarrheal diseases, and lower respiratory infections. Two infectious diseases are close to eradication: polio and dracunculiasis (Guinea worm disease).

This third edition of the *Disease Control Priorities* (*DCP3*) comes at a pivotal moment for infectious disease control and research. Its chapters clearly demonstrate that, despite the remarkable progress, infectious diseases remain a major threat to health worldwide—particularly in South Asia and Sub-Saharan Africa—but that an increasing range of highly cost-effective interventions is available.

As this volume amply illustrates, innovations in the prevention, diagnosis, and treatment of infectious diseases have been impressive. They include preexposure prophylaxis (PrEP) to prevent HIV infection, new forms of computer-based education for clinicians to manage sexually transmitted infections, HPV vaccines to prevent cervical cancer, and a cure for hepatitis C. The new attention to viral hepatitis in this volume is most welcome, as greatly improved control is now technically feasible—although the history of tuberculosis illustrates that a cure alone is insufficient to bring a disease under control. Much of the progress is due to political and technical leadership, greatly increased funding,

and improved delivery of interventions through health systems and other sectors. Community engagement is the key to success in many cases; a community buy-in to very simple, non-technological prevention mechanisms was instrumental in the sharp decline in dracunculiasis cases, from 130,000 in 2000 to only 22 in 2015 and 0 cases at the time of writing in 2017. However, dogs, which act as alternative hosts for the worm, present a threat to total eradication and remind us of the importance of a "One Health" approach.

At the same time, several epidemics and new pathogens have emerged, including the swine flu (H1N1) pandemic; the Middle East Respiratory Syndrome (MERS); the largest Ebola outbreak ever known in the West African region where it had never caused an outbreak; and an epidemic of Zika and associated neurological disorders. In particular, the collective failure to respond to the Ebola outbreak in a timely and coordinated fashion before it spiraled out of control—infecting over 28,000 people and causing over 11,000 deaths—was a wake-up call for the world. The disastrous impact of the Ebola epidemic prompted an urgent rethinking of how governments, nongovernmental organizations, and international organizations can better work to contain emerging disease threats in an increasingly interconnected world.

It is, however, noteworthy that almost as many people in the three Ebola-affected West African countries died from the disease's disruption on increasing mortality from HIV/AIDS, tuberculosis, and malaria as from Ebola itself (Parpia and others 2016). These three diseases, as well as diarrheal diseases and lower respiratory infections, continue to exact a heavy burden, particularly in Sub-Saharan Africa, where infectious diseases remain the leading cause of death. In 2015, over 1.8 million people worldwide died from tuberculosis (including

0.4 million among people with HIV) (WHO 2017); 1.1 million people from AIDS (UNAIDS 2016); and an estimated 429,000 people died from malaria (WHO 2016). In spite of real achievements in improved access to HIV treatment, over 2 million new infections occur each year, with hardly any decline in new infections over the past five years, and several subpopulations continue to be heavily affected. A critical review of current HIV strategies may be needed to achieve the United Nations goals of ending the AIDS epidemic. Lower respiratory infections remain a major persistent cause of death in children.

Many of these infectious diseases have sophisticated vaccines, diagnostics, and therapeutics available, but political, economic, and social factors limit the extent to which populations can benefit. Furthermore, in a world of growing resistance to antimicrobials and drug-resistant infections, we need to continue to develop innovations in biomedicine. We also need to improve incentives for rational antibiotic use, antimicrobial stewardship, and increased acceptance of the importance of prevention to avoid infection.

The global health agenda is an increasingly crowded space, and the cost-effectiveness of interventions is under growing scrutiny. While there is more information than ever regarding the cost-effectiveness of different interventions in a growing spectrum of contexts, hard choices remain in terms of allocating scarce funding to infectious diseases, especially in light of the complexities of fragile health systems, comorbidities with other infections and NCDs, structural factors that can undermine disease prevention, and treatment programs. One particularly valuable facet of *DCP3* is that it demonstrates that some of the most effective steps we can take to reduce the burden of infections are not necessarily expensive, as exemplified by the low cost per disability-adjusted life year averted of condoms for female sex workers or insecticide-treated bednets. Often, the key is not just more, but smarter, investment, for example, better integration of services, strong community engagement, and targeted interventions based on the population most in need in specific locations. In addition to cost-effectiveness, key questions are whether people will accept and use the interventions, whether the interventions are affordable and work in various parts of the real world, and what the best way is to deliver them.

If we are to reach the ambitious targets under the Sustainable Development Goals, we must focus not only on delivery of innovation but also on "innovation of delivery." One example might be new systems of community-based treatment for tuberculosis to minimize transmission in health care settings. *DCP3* helps us to think about improving health care delivery models through its unique focus on packages of interventions, and on the interrelationships among different kinds of interventions, at both the policy level and in terms of the outcomes across populations.

DCP3 is to be lauded for its focus on equity, recognizing that cost-effective intervention is not cost-effective if the financial burden falls on the poor. With this *DCP3* volume on major infectious diseases, we have a highly pragmatic addition to the literature that will help policy makers across the world make smarter decisions to improve health sustainably and equitably in the ongoing fight against infectious disease threats, old and new.

Peter Piot, MD, PhD
Director, London School of Hygiene & Tropical Medicine
London, United Kingdom

REFERENCES

AVERT. 2017. "Prevention of Mother-to-Child Transmission (Pmtct) of HIV." AVERT. https://www.avert.org/professionals/hiv-programming/prevention/prevention-mother-child.

Parpia, A. S., M. L. Ndeffo-Mbah, N.S. Wenzel, and A. P. Galvani. 2016. "Effects of Response to 2014–2015 Ebola Outbreak on Deaths from Malaria, HIV/AIDS, and Tuberculosis, West Africa." *Emerging Infectious Diseases* 22 (3): 433–41.

UNAIDS. 2016. "AIDS by the Numbers." UNAIDS, Geneva.

WHO (World Health Organization). 2016. "10 Facts on Malaria." WHO, Geneva. http://www.who.int/features/factfiles/malaria/en/.

———. 2017. "Tuberculosis: Fact Sheet." WHO, Geneva. http://www.who.int/mediacentre/factsheets/fs104/en/.

Abbreviations

ACTs	artemisinin-combination therapies
ADCs	AIDS-defining cancers
AEM	AIDS Epidemic Model
AIDS	acquired immune deficiency syndrome
AIM	AIDS Impact Model
ANC	antenatal clinic
ART	antiretroviral treatment
BCC	behavior change communication
CBT	community-based testing
CDC	Centers for Disease Control and Prevention (U.S.)
CHMI	controlled human malaria infection
CHW	community health worker
CI	confidence interval
CQ	chloroquine
CRP	C-reactive protein
CSF	cerebrospinal fluid
CVD	cardiovascular disease
DAA	direct-acting antiviral
DALYs	disability-adjusted life years
DBS	dried blood spots
DCP2	*Disease Control Priorities in Developing Countries*, second edition
DCP3	*Disease Control Priorities* (third edition)
DDT	dichloro-diphenyl-trichloroethane
DMPPT	Decision Makers' Program Planning Tool
EID	early infant diagnostic
ELISA	enzyme-linked immunosorbent assay
EMOD	Epidemiological Modeling
EMTCT	elimination of mother-to-child transmission
EPP	Epidemic Projection Package
FBC	facility-based care
FI	febrile illness
FSW	female sex worker

G6PD	glucose-6-phosphate dehydrogenase
GBD	Global Burden of Disease
GDP	gross domestic product
GHD	Global Health Decisions
GMAP	Global Malaria Action Plan
GMEP	Global Malaria Eradication Program
GRADE	Grading of Recommendations, Assessment, Development and Evaluation
GRNE	Global Resource Needs Estimates
GTS	Global Technical Strategy
HAI	health care-associated infections
HAT	Human African trypanosomiasis
HBC	home-based care
HBV	hepatitis B virus
HCC	hepatocellular carcinoma
HCV	hepatitis C virus
HDL	high-density lipoprotein cholesterol
HHV-8	human herpes virus 8
HICs	high-income countries
HIV/AIDS	human immunodeficiency virus/acquired immune deficiency syndrome
HIVAM	HIV-associated malignancies
HIV	human immunodeficiency virus
HPV	human papillomavirus
HRQL	health and health-related quality of life
HSV	herpes simplex virus
HTC	HIV testing and counseling
HTS	HIV/AIDS testing service
ICER	incremental cost-effectiveness ratio
IDU	injecting drug user
IMAI	Integrated Management of Adolescent and Adult Illness
IMCI	Integrated Management of Childhood Illness
IRS	indoor residual spraying
ITN	insecticide-treated net
IVM	integrated vector management
JEV	Japanese encephalitis virus
KS	Kaposi sarcoma
LDL	low-density lipoprotein cholesterol
LGBT	lesbian, gay, bisexual, and transgender
LICs	low-income countries
LLIN	long-lasting insecticide-treated nets
LMICs	low- and middle-income countries
LTFU	loss to follow-up
MCH	maternal and child health
MDA	mass drug administration
MDG	Millennium Development Goal
MDR-TB	multidrug-resistant tuberculosis
MMC	medical male circumcision
MERS	Middle East respiratory syndrome
MCC	mobile clinic care

MRSA	Methicillin-resistant *Staphylococcus aureus*
MSM	men who have sex with men
MTCT	mother-to-child transmission
NADCs	non–AIDS-defining cancer
NBS	National Bureau of Statistics
NCC	noncommunicable chronic comorbidities
NCDs	noncommunicable diseases
NECT	nifurtimox-eflornithine combination therapy
NHL	non-Hodgkin lymphoma
NNRTI	non-nucleoside reverse transcriptase inhibitors
NRTI	nucleoside reverse transcriptase inhibitors
NSP	needle and syringe program
NTDs	neglected tropical diseases
NT-NMFI	nontreatable nonmalaria febrile illness
OOP	out of pocket
PCR	polymerase chain reaction
PEPFAR	President's Emergency Plan for AIDS Relief (United States)
PMI	President's Malaria Initiative
PMTCT	prevention of mother-to-child transmission
POC	point-of-care
POCT	point-of-care test
PPT	periodic presumptive treatment
PrEP	preexposure prophylaxis
PROMISE	Promoting Maternal-Infant Survival Everywhere
QALY	quality-adjusted life year
RNM	Resource Needs Model
RBM	Roll Back Malaria (Partnership)
RPR	rapid plasma reagin
RCT	randomized controlled trial
RDTs	rapid diagnostic tests
SAC	school-age children
SARS	severe acute respiratory syndrome
SDG	Sustainable Development Goal
SMART	Strategies for Management of Antiretroviral Therapy
STDs	sexually transmitted diseases
SP	sulfadoxine/pyrimethamine
STIs	sexually transmitted infections
STH	soil-transmitted helminthiases
SW	sex workers
TasP	treatment as prevention
TB	tuberculosis
TCPs	target candidate profiles
T-NMFI	treatable nonmalaria febrile illness
UI	uncertainty interval
UNAIDS	Joint United Nations Programme on HIV/AIDS
UN	United Nations

VCT	voluntary counseling and testing
VIMT	vaccines that interrupt malaria transmission
VMMC	voluntary male medical circumcision
WHO	World Health Organization
WWR	What Works Reviews
YLDs	years lived with disability
YLLs	years of life lost

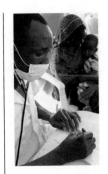

Major Infectious Diseases: Key Messages from *Disease Control Priorities*, Third Edition

King K. Holmes, Stefano Bertozzi, Barry R. Bloom, Prabhat Jha,
Hellen Gelband, Lisa M. DeMaria, and Susan Horton

INTRODUCTION

Infectious diseases were responsible for the largest global burden of premature death and disability until the end of the twentieth century, when that distinction passed to noncommunicable diseases. Over the previous centuries, global pandemics of infectious diseases, such as smallpox, cholera, and influenza, periodically threatened the survival of entire populations. At least as early as the late 1800s, improved living conditions (such as better sanitation and piped water supplies), particularly in high-income countries (HICs), began to drive down the infectious disease burden.

By the mid-twentieth century, safe, effective, and affordable vaccines and the increasing availability of antibiotics had further reduced the toll of infectious diseases in HICs. Not until the second half of the twentieth century did large-scale efforts begin to better control infectious diseases in low- and middle-income countries (LMICs), where the infectious disease burden was greatest and highly varied. These efforts included a global commitment to immunize the world's children against the major infections for which vaccines are available and global campaigns to control malaria and diarrheal disease. The International Health Regulations of the World Health Organization (WHO) represent a key agreement among 196 countries to implement metrics and measures to detect and control outbreaks of infectious diseases and to prevent pandemics (World Health Assembly 2005).

Global under-five mortality fell by almost two-thirds (from 14 percent to 5 percent) between 1970 and 2010 (Norheim and others 2015). In 1980, smallpox, responsible for 300 million–500 million deaths in the twentieth century, was declared to be the first disease eradicated from the planet following a global immunization campaign led by the WHO. Wild Poliovirus has been eliminated from all but three countries (Afghanistan, Nigeria, and Pakistan) and currently is the focus of a major eradication program.

The decline of the vaccine-preventable diseases has contributed to a recognition of the potential for using vaccines to prevent other infectious diseases, including human immunodeficiency virus/acquired immune deficiency syndrome (HIV/AIDS), tuberculosis (TB), malaria, hepatitis C, and a variety of neglected tropical diseases (NTDs). Hepatitis B and C substantially increase the risk of death from cirrhosis and liver cancer. The effect of viral hepatitis is significant. Indeed, an important recent study (Stanaway and others 2015) found that viral hepatitis led to an estimated 0.9 million deaths in 1990 (including hepatitis-caused deaths from cirrhosis and liver cancer). Furthermore, this number has been increasing rapidly—to an estimated 1.5 million deaths in 2013—despite the fact that hepatitis B is a vaccine-preventable disease and that hepatitis B and C are both treatable.

Emerging pandemic viral infections remain a constant threat, many entering the human population from

Corresponding author: King K. Holmes, Departments of Global Health and Medicine, University of Washington, Seattle, Washington, United States; kkh@uw.edu.

contact with animals. The most recent such infections include SARS (severe acute respiratory syndrome), MERS (Middle East respiratory syndrome), and Ebola and Zika viruses (Madhav and others 2018) as well as, perennially, influenza and chikungunya infections. Compared with antibiotics to treat bacterial infections, relatively few antiviral drugs have been developed to treat these emerging viral infections. Therefore, the most important intervention is to break the chain of transmission. A global increase in antibiotic-resistant bacteria includes a small but growing number that are resistant to most or essentially all of the available antimicrobials.

Spectacular progress has been made in reducing mortality from most infectious diseases (table 1.1). For example, in low-income countries (LICs) from 2000 to 2010, the number of deaths before age 70 years from HIV/AIDS, TB, and malaria fell by 46 percent, 35 percent, and 36 percent, respectively (Norheim and others 2015). Rapid progress was also reported in other country income groups. However, table 1.1 shows also that if the death rates of 2010 remain static, about 5.1 million people will still die in 2030 from these three conditions and from other communicable diseases, many of which are concentrated in LMICs. In contrast, mortality in HICs from these conditions (except for HIV/AIDS) will be relatively small, although major pandemics of other pathogens are not predictable. Hence, infectious diseases will remain a major threat to humankind, especially in LMICs, requiring vigilance, surveillance, and new interventions of all types.

APPROACHES TO INFECTIOUS DISEASE CONTROL IN THE TWENTY-FIRST CENTURY

Vaccines and curative treatments for some of the major infectious diseases have existed for decades. Many of them are relatively inexpensive and highly cost-effective, yet many are underused because of cost and lack of access attributed to poorly functioning health care systems. New drugs and vaccines will continue to be the mainstays in preventing and treating infections, but delivery of such interventions will be critical to driving down the burden of infection.

An ultimate goal for selected infections is eradication. To date, only two diseases—smallpox in humans and rinderpest in cattle and other ruminant animals—have been eradicated. Elimination of polio, yaws, and Guinea worm infections is being pursued. This is a more distant but still possible goal for malaria (Shretta and others 2017). A handful of other infections—such as measles, mumps, rubella, lymphatic filariasis, and cysticercosis—are candidates for elimination because of disease characteristics or the available means to control them (CDC 1993). Those infectious diseases that persist require continued effort to develop new drugs and vaccines for treatment and prevention as well as strategies that allow such treatments to be used most effectively across the globe. Despite the development of new drugs to combat infectious diseases, antimicrobial resistance is threatening to remove many of the tools in our current armamentarium.

Table 1.1 Projected 2030 Mortality and 10-Year Trends for Selected Infections, by Country Income Group

Cause	Deaths in 2030 (millions)	Change (% per decade)[a]	Deaths in 2030 (millions)	Change (% per decade)[a]	Deaths in 2030 (millions)	Change (% per decade)[a]	Deaths in 2030 (millions)	Change (% per decade)[a]	Deaths in 2030 (millions)
	Low income		Lower middle income		Upper middle income		High income		Global[c]
HIV/AIDS	0.92	−46	0.76	0	0.41	17	< 0.01	—	2.10
Tuberculosis	0.32	−35	0.65	−43	0.14	−52	< 0.01	—	1.12
Malaria	0.37	−36	0.33	−28	0.02	—	< 0.01	—	0.73
Other communicable diseases[b]	0.35	−23	0.59	−15	0.14	−30	0.05	—	1.13
All causes	8.62	−24	18.11	−16	11.60	−23	3.00	−16	41.33

Source: Norheim and others 2015.

Note: — = not available; HIV/AIDS = human immunodeficiency virus/acquired immune deficiency syndrome. Table estimates the number of deaths before age 70 years (age 0–69 years) that would occur in 2030 if the rate of change (percentage per decade) during 2000–10 were to continue for standardized death rates of those under age 70 years in each country income group (as classified by the World Bank).

a. "Change (% per decade)" = percentage change during 2000–10.

b. "Other communicable diseases" mostly align with other infectious conditions covered in this volume (such as hepatitis, sexually transmitted infections, and neglected tropical diseases) but not completely for some diseases (for example, meningitis).

c. Global totals are by summation of each of the four regions.

Infection Control: Targeting and Integration of Specialized Services

One approach—targeting settings and populations with the highest transmission rates—is being used to improve HIV/AIDS control. The continued emergence of new pandemics, like Ebola, will be addressed with similarly targeted approaches. However, for the ongoing, highly prevalent infections in LMICs—TB, hepatitis, sexually transmitted infections (STIs), malaria, typhoid, and other febrile illnesses—the future lies in improving and integrating services at the primary care level and up the chain to the highest levels of hospital care.

The high incidence of comorbidities—such as TB and viral hepatitis in immunocompromised persons with HIV infection—calls for integration of HIV, TB, and viral hepatitis diagnosis and treatment. Patients who are seen in STI clinics and their sex partners have an elevated risk of having another STI, such as HIV infection. Therefore, integration of HIV testing, care, and evaluation of sex partners into all STI clinic settings offers opportunities for efficiently managing this set of infections. Selected populations for whom specialized services are already the norm (such as pregnant women) can receive additional attention. This may include screening for HIV and syphilis (see chapter 6 of this volume, John-Stewart and others 2017).

Health care service integration at this level requires strategic planning. For example, integration of HIV and TB diagnosis and management must be done in ways that are safe: crowded clinics with long waiting times create a perfect opportunity for TB transmission from someone with active TB to an immunosuppressed HIV patient. Integrated, population-level intervention packages can focus not only on interventions that are financed mainly by the health sector, such as increased immunization and treatment, but also on interventions related to the agriculture or infrastructure sector (and financed mainly by those ministries, not the health ministry), such as the following:

- Improve access to sanitation, clean water, and hygiene.
- Reduce population growth and crowding.
- Decrease day-to-day close contact with animals.
- Change the environments that sustain vectors of important pathogens.

A related cross-sectoral priority is preventing antimicrobial resistance through the development, availability, and use of affordable diagnostics to guide appropriate antimicrobial use in humans, while also enforcing policies to prevent nontherapeutic use of antimicrobials as growth promoters in livestock.

Importance of Rapid Differential Diagnosis in Infection Control

Even for infectious diseases requiring specialized services, many infections will initially be diagnosed or suspected at the primary care level or first-level hospital and then referred to a second- or third-level hospital. Many infectious illnesses are caused by pathogens that can be life threatening. This makes differential diagnosis—based in part on symptom assessment, clinical manifestations, physical exam, medical history, history of exposures, age and gender, laboratory testing where available, and availability of treatment—the key to population infection control (Burnett and others 2016).

The widespread adoption of rapid tests for malaria diagnosis is an example of an easy-to-use diagnostic that has vastly improved malaria treatment in many places. Rapid point-of-care tests are available for HIV, hepatitis C, influenza, and syphilis but are still in development for some other infections. In addition, conventional microbiology is being transformed by molecular testing, which could be available even in LICs within the decade. A series of publications illustrates the significant effect of integrated infectious disease training on diagnosis (in Uganda) and infectious disease management (Imani and others 2015; Weaver and others 2014)

This volume focuses on major infectious diseases that are common in LMICs, particularly among adults (see box 1.1). Unlike most of the serious infections that predominate among children, many of these are long-lived chronic infections (including some acquired as children). The perspective includes an emphasis on what has changed since the first edition of *Disease Control Priorities in Developing Countries* in 1993 (box 1.2). We first review the major interventions for priority infectious diseases, namely HIV/AIDS, other STIs, TB, malaria and other febrile illnesses, hepatitis, and NTDs. We then address the cross-cutting issues of antimicrobial resistance.

Box 1.1

Volume Focus: Infectious Disease Control

This volume focuses on *control* of the major infectious diseases. Infectious disease control involves not only prevention of transmission and spread of infectious disease at the population and individual levels, but also effective treatment and cure of infectious diseases in individuals.

Box 1.2

Comment by the Series Editors of *Disease Control Priorities*, Third Edition

Budgets constrain choices. Policy analysis helps decision makers achieve the greatest value from limited resources. In 1993, the World Bank published the first edition of *Disease Control Priorities in Developing Countries* (*DCP1*), which sought to assess systematically the cost-effectiveness (value for money) of interventions that would address the major sources of disease burden in LMICs (Jamison and others 1993). The World Bank's 1993 *World Development Report* on health drew heavily on the findings in *DCP1* to conclude that specific interventions against noncommunicable diseases were cost-effective, even in environments where substantial burdens of infection and undernutrition persisted (World Bank 1993).

Disease Control Priorities in Developing Countries, second edition (*DCP2*), published in 2006, updated and extended *DCP1* in several respects, explicitly considering the implications for health care systems of expanded intervention coverage (Jamison and others 2006). One way that health care systems can expand coverage of health interventions is through selected delivery platforms for those interventions that require similar logistics but address heterogeneous health problems. Platforms often provide a more natural unit for investment than do individual interventions, but conventional health economics has offered little understanding of how to make choices across platforms. Analysis of the costs of packages and platforms—and of the health improvements they can generate in given epidemiological environments—can help guide health care system investments and development.

This third edition of *Disease Control Priorities* (*DCP3)* introduces the notion of packages of interventions (Jamison and others 2015–18). Whereas "platforms" refer to logistically related sets of interventions, "packages" comprise conceptually related ones. (The 21 packages of interventions developed in the nine volumes of *DCP3* include those targeting surgery and cardiovascular disease, for example.) In addition, *DCP3* explicitly considers the financial risk protection objective of health care systems. In populations lacking access to health insurance or prepaid

care, medical expenses that are high relative to income can be impoverishing. Where incomes are low, seemingly inexpensive medical procedures can have catastrophic financial effects. *DCP3* considers financial protection and the distribution across income groups of the outcomes from policies (for example, public financing of health care) to increase intervention uptake and to improve delivery quality (Verguet, Laxminarayan, and Jamison 2015). All of the volumes seek to combine the available science about interventions implemented in specific locales and conditions with informed judgment to reach reasonable conclusions about the effects of intervention mixes in diverse environments. *DCP3*'s broad aim is to delineate essential intervention packages—such as those, in this volume, for major infectious diseases—and their related delivery platforms. This information will assist decision makers in allocating often tightly constrained budgets and achieving health care system objectives.

Four of *DCP3*'s nine volumes were published in 2015 and 2016, and the remaining five will appear in 2017 and 2018. The volumes appear in an environment in which serious discussion continues about quantifying and achieving the Sustainable Development Goal (SDG) for health (UN 2015b). *DCP3*'s analyses are well placed to assist in choosing the means to attain the health SDG and assessing the related costs. These volumes, and the analytic efforts on which they are based, will enable researchers to explore SDG-related and other broad policy conclusions and generalizations. The final volume will report those conclusions. Each volume will provide specific policy analyses on the full range of interventions, packages, and policies relevant to its health topic.

Dean T. Jamison
Rachel Nugent
Hellen Gelband
Susan Horton
Prabhat Jha
Ramanan Laxminarayan
Charles N. Mock

We provide updated estimates of the cost-effectiveness of the major sets of interventions, recognizing that there are large knowledge gaps concerning the economics of many conditions in LMICs. We conclude by outlining future strategies that are relevant to continued progress against these major infectious diseases.

MAJOR INFECTIOUS DISEASES IN THIS VOLUME

HIV/AIDS and Other Sexually Transmitted Infections

HIV/AIDS, the worst human pandemic since the 1918 influenza epidemic, has accounted for more than 25 million deaths since it was first identified in 1981 and it has hit Sub-Saharan Africa the hardest. However, the tide is beginning to turn as life-extending antiretroviral treatment (ART) and preventive interventions are scaled up and as sexual behaviors may have become less risky in many settings.

Antiretroviral drugs are now widely available in most settings and are highly affordable at US$315 per person per year (UNAIDS 2015). Worldwide, 17 million HIV-infected people are receiving these life-extending drugs—an impressive number given that only 2.2 million people were on ART in 2005. However, this number is still far short of the Joint United Nations Programme on HIV/AIDS (UNAIDS) target to treat the 37 million people currently living with HIV. The estimated number of deaths annually from HIV/AIDS has declined from 2 million in 2005 to 1.1 million in 2015, the lowest number since 1998 (UNAIDS 2015, 2016). Yet AIDS still ranks sixth among the global causes of death—and first in Sub-Saharan Africa.

Building on the progress to date, UNAIDS has set two important goals: (a) a 75 percent reduction in new HIV infections (compared with 2010) by 2030 and (b) successful achievement of the UNAIDS 90-90-90 campaign, which seeks to have 90 percent of all people living with HIV knowing they have HIV, 90 percent of those diagnosed with HIV receiving treatment, and 90 percent of those on treatment having an undetectable viral load (virally suppressed). Furthermore, UNAIDS seeks to eliminate mother-to-child transmission of both HIV and syphilis. We now have the tools to attain these goals, even despite the remaining challenges of needing an HIV vaccine for prevention (as we have vaccines to prevent hepatitis B virus [HBV] and human papillomavirus [HPV] infection); an effective cure for HIV infection (as we have for the hepatitis C virus [HCV] infection); and an effective suppressive therapy for hepatitis B.

In addition to effective medical interventions (table 1.2), national legislative and policy frameworks are needed to enable effective deployment of these interventions. Mother-to-child transmission of HIV will not be eliminated by 2030, the current goalpost, without effective national policies to support prevention. Even more important, laws and policies to protect and reduce

Table 1.2 Essential HIV/AIDS Intervention Package, by Delivery Platform

Intervention type	Delivery platforms[a]				
	Nationwide policies and regulations	Community health post or pharmacy	Primary health center	First-level hospital	Second- and third-level hospitals
Prevention					
Legal and human rights	1. Laws and policies to protect and reduce stigma for key populations, with full decriminalization of LGBT population*	2. Gender-based violence counseling and rape-response referral (medical and justice)			
Structural interventions	3. Universal access to HIV testing, with immediate linkage to care and treatment and intensified outreach to populations at higher risk of infection				
	4. Universal access to drug substitution therapy for addiction				
	5. Brothels: Condoms required*				
	6. Needle exchange encouraged*				

table continues next page

Intervention type	Nationwide policies and regulations	Community health post or pharmacy	Primary health center	First-level hospital	Second- and third-level hospitals
			Delivery platforms[a]		
Direct (biological) prevention			7. PrEP for discordant couples 8. Male circumcision service provision* 9. PMTCT (Option B+)		
Behavioral interventions: Prevention		10. HIV education and counseling for pregnant women, sex workers, IDUs, GBT males, and HIV+ persons and their partners* 11. Access to needle exchange for IDU* 12. Condom distribution* 13. Partner notification* 14. Adherence support for high-risk or failing patients			
Social marketing: Information, education, and communication	15. Promotion of condoms, VMMC, and testing at national and facility-based levels*				
Treatment					
Treatment	16. Policies and guidelines to support all steps of HIV care continuum, including expanded testing through diverse strategies; linkage to care; ART initiation with support for adherence and retention; and performance and efficiency optimization through data-driven management, task shifting, and decentralization, as appropriate for level of epidemic	17. Community-based HIV testing and counseling (for example, through mobile units or venue-based testing)* 18. Household HIV testing and counseling in high-prevalence settings 19. Referral and navigation of HIV+ individuals to HIV care sites to ensure linkage	20. Provider-initiated counseling and HIV testing (as well as TB and STI testing) for all in contact with health care system in high-prevalence settings, including prenatal care* 21. ART initiation 22. Support for adherence and retention 23. Laboratory viral load monitoring		
Behavioral and structural interventions: Care		24. Adherence support including adherence clubs, community-based ART groups, text reminders, and other means 25. Nutrition, transportation, and financial reimbursement	26. Case manager		

Note: Interventions shown in orange indicate areas that are relatively neglected by governments. ART = antiretroviral treatment; GBT = gay, bisexual, or transgender; HIV = human immunodeficiency virus; HIV+ = HIV-positive; IDU = injection drug users; LGBT = lesbian, gay, bisexual, and transgender; Option B+ = a three-drug ART regime in pregnancy and postpartum for HIV-positive mothers; PMTCT = prevention of mother-to-child transmission; PrEP = preexposure prophylaxis; STI = sexually transmitted infection; TB = tuberculosis; VMMC = voluntary male medical circumcision.

a. All interventions listed for lower-level platforms can be provided at higher levels. Similarly, each facility level represents a spectrum and diversity of capabilities. The column in which intervention is listed is the lowest level of the health care system in which it would usually be provided.

Interventions marked with an asterisk (*) should be closely integrated with STI prevention and treatment interventions.

stigma for key populations are urgently needed in many countries. Indeed, in recent years, lesbian, gay, bisexual, and transgender (LGBT) rights have regressed in some settings, and criminalization of these populations has increased. Two chapters in this volume provide useful detail for policy makers who are considering such issues: chapter 8 (Wilson and Taaffe 2017) outlines the factors to consider when tailoring a response to a local epidemic, and chapter 9 (Kahn and others 2017) presents various models that can help guide decisions regarding the cost-effectiveness of the different interventions.

Optimal HIV management requires managing people across the continuum of care, from testing to counseling and from ART to adherence support. Sociocultural barriers in gaining access to care include the following:

- Fear of diagnosis, complicated by a culture of stigma and discrimination in many countries
- Structural barriers such as distance to health clinics
- System-level barriers such as clinic hours, coordination among clinics, and shortages of health care workers

Biomedical interventions that have come to the forefront since the publication of *Disease Control Priorities in Developing Countries*, second edition *(DCP2)* by the World Bank (Jamison and others 2006) and that have proven highly effective at preventing HIV transmission include treatment as prevention (Gomez and others 2013); preexposure prophylaxis (PrEP); male circumcision; and new treatment regimens for prevention of mother-to-child transmission (PMTCT). Furthermore, these interventions can be successfully delivered at first-level care facilities, thereby increasing accessibility.

PrEP—using a once-a-day tablet, the current version of which includes two antiretroviral drugs—provides a method beyond condoms for at-risk people to prevent becoming infected with HIV (Baeten 2016; Jenness and others 2016). PrEP access is still limited in LMICs and does not prevent other STIs.

Voluntary male medical circumcision (VMMC) significantly reduces sexual acquisition of HIV by men and is most cost-effective in settings where HIV is highly prevalent. Recent studies have shown that demand is high for VMMC, which can be offered at some first-level health care facilities and at health centers. In some countries, VMMC has even been delivered effectively in mobile vans.

Advances have increased the effectiveness of PMTCT treatment as well. For an HIV-infected mother not yet receiving ART, the recommendations are to start ART at the first prenatal visit (regardless of the mother's CD4 cell count or WHO clinical stage)[1] and to continue lifelong ART. Use of this protocol could significantly reduce the number of newborns infected during the birth process and the mother-to-child transmission of HIV. Substantial progress has been made in this regard: new pediatric HIV infections declined by 50 percent from 2010 to 2015 (UNAIDS 2016).

Interventions to offer household-based testing in high-prevalence settings will contribute to the first "90" of the UNAIDS 90-90-90 goals (90 percent of all people living with HIV know they have HIV). Interventions to effectively and promptly link newly diagnosed persons living with HIV to services and treatment contribute to the second "90" (90 percent of HIV-diagnosed people receive treatment) and are critical across all settings. Finally, multiple strategies for promoting adherence to treatment and retention in care—ranging from community support groups to mobile health interventions—are critical to ensuring that treatment is effective and continuous, thus achieving the third "90" (90 percent of those being treated have an undetectable viral load).

Burden of STIs other than HIV/AIDS

In addition to HIV, another 40 bacterial, viral, and parasitic pathogens have been identified as primarily sexually transmitted, or as potentially sexually transmissible (see annex 1A). The common curable bacterial STIs include trichomoniasis, chlamydia infection, gonorrhea, and syphilis. In 2012, the WHO estimated the global incidence of these four curable STIs among men and women ages 15–49 years: 131 million new cases of chlamydia infection, 78 million of gonorrhea, 143 million of trichomoniasis, and 6 million of syphilis (WHO 2016b). These estimates mean that approximately 1 million new infections could be cured with existing treatments each day (Newman and others 2015).

Other common sexually transmitted pathogens are herpes simplex virus (HSV-1 and HSV-2, both of which cause genital herpes) and HPV.[2] In 2012, the global prevalence of HSV-2 among men and women ages 15–49 years was 417 million, with higher prevalence in women than in men. An estimated 19.2 million individuals ages 15–34 years were newly infected with HSV-2 in 2012 (Looker and others 2015).

Extensive studies of the prevalence of oncogenic genital HPV infections included a global systematic review of age-specific prevalence of oncogenic types of HPV infection in males (Smith and others 2011) and in females (Winer and others 2012). In general, these studies show high prevalence of oncogenic HPV types among those with new sex partners or a high number of lifetime partners.

Common STIs may cause significant complications to women's reproductive health, including pelvic inflammatory disease, tubal pregnancy infertility, cervical cancer, perinatal and neonatal morbidity, mother-to-child transmission of syphilis or HIV, and a host of other conditions (Chesson, Mayaud, and Aral 2017, chapter 10 in this volume). However, for morbidity and mortality, years of life lost, disability-adjusted life years (DALYs), and costs of medical care, the major STIs are as follows:

- HIV infection
- HBV and HCV infection
- HPV infection, with HPV-related genital, anal, and oropharyngeal cancers
- Syphilis, with its related perinatal and pediatric morbidity and mortality
- HSV-1 and HSV-2 infection, with related central nervous system and pediatric morbidity

In aggregate, these major pathogens cause extensive morbidity and mortality attributable to unsafe sex. Moreover, the consequences of STIs disproportionately affect women and children. STIs, including HIV/AIDS, are one of the leading causes of morbidity and mortality, as measured by DALYs, for reproductive-age women in LMICs (Owusu-Edusei and others 2014).

In addition to the mortality and morbidity attributable to the major STI pathogens listed earlier, other STI pathogens account for severe morbidity, including infertility, ectopic pregnancy, epididymitis, neonatal eye infection, and other common diseases. These other pathogens that can be transmitted sexually include the Zika and Ebola viruses and group C *Neisseria meningitidis*. Sexual transmissions of these pathogens have been documented but are not yet well studied (Hader 2017).

Unsafe Sex as a Global Risk Factor for Death and Disability in Adolescents and Young Adults

The Global Burden of Disease (GBD) study recently reported annual assessments of risk factors for death and DALYs in adolescents and young adults in 188 countries for 2013 (Mokdad and others 2016). Among adolescent males ages 15–19 years, unsafe sex was the second most common risk factor for death. Among adolescent females ages 15–19 years, unsafe sex was the number one risk factor. Among young adults ages 20–24 years (males and females combined), unsafe sex was the second most common risk factor.

As for the risk of disability (as measured by DALYs), unsafe sex was the second most common risk factor in 2013. Important to the global burden, the number and proportion of the worldwide population who are adolescents are also steadily growing (Hader 2017).

Key Populations for STI Control in LMICs

Although adolescents and young adults experience a large proportion of STIs, including HIV infection, the role of key populations in the epidemiology and control of HIV and other STIs in LMICs has become increasingly clear (Baral and others 2007; Baral and others 2012). These key populations include, in particular, female sex workers; men who have sex with men (MSM), who are understudied and underserved in most LMICs; and injection drug users, who are at risk not only for HIV but also for other blood-borne STIs such as syphilis and hepatitis viruses. Patterns of sexual networks linking MSM with heterosexual populations warrant future research.

Until recently, HCV was repeatedly described as *not* sexually transmitted, and its transmission had been associated with injection drug use, blood transfusions, and iatrogenic exposures but not with heterosexual transmission. However, HCV recently has been found in the semen of men with HCV viremia, and rectal HCV shedding was found in 20 of 43 (47 percent) HIV-infected MSM who also had HCV infection. The presence of HCV in rectal fluid was associated with high blood levels of HCV (Foster and others 2017). Most important, co-infections with HCV and HIV have been commonly found in Australia, Europe, and North America. Thus, screening for HCV—a curable infection—is now being recommended for HIV-infected MSM in high-income countries (Harrison and others 2017; Kratz and others 2015; Nanduri and others 2016).

STI Interventions: Prevention, Treatment, and Education

Prevention and treatment are both important to STI control, and the HIV epidemic has influenced changes in the approach to STI prevention in general. During the 1980s and 1990s, behavioral prevention dominated the HIV world and gained prominence in the STI domain. However, since the turn of the century, recognition has grown that behavioral interventions (heavily weighted toward condom use) have not decreased STI incidence sufficiently and sustainably (Aral 2011; Kippax and Stephenson 2012).

STI Prevention

Concurrently, remarkable progress has been made in biomedical approaches to preventing HIV/AIDS, including male circumcision, PrEP, and ART (Baeten and others 2012; Dodd, Garnett, and Hallett 2010; Grant and others 2010; Katz and Wright 2008; Pretorius and others 2010). Given the success of these biomedical approaches, the field of STI prevention is increasingly drawing on them, reinforced by development of effective biomedical interventions for preventing STIs other than HIV. More specifically, these interventions include promotion and provision of the HPV and HBV vaccines to females and males, early detection and curative treatment of HCV infection, point-of-care diagnostic tests for syphilis, dual tests for syphilis and HIV, and an understanding of the effects of male circumcision for preventing certain STIs other than HIV.

In addition, clinical platforms offering STI-related reproductive health services are playing a key role in screening patients for HIV and HCV. They also emphasize outreach to sex partners for HIV and other STI screening. Table 1.3 provides an assessment of the platforms and essential interventions for preventing and treating STIs.

Pharmacy Treatment of STIs and Clinician Online Education

Individual treatment of STIs in LMICs is largely based on syndromic management, which is often provided by pharmacies without clinical examination. Provision of guidelines and training to pharmacy workers can significantly improve STI management by pharmacy workers (García and others 2012).

However, this practice, linked to the increasing availability of new antimicrobials in LMICs, may be contributing to emerging antimicrobial resistance in LMICs (Miller-Petrie, Pant, and Laxminarayan 2017, chapter 18 of this volume). Although the common curable STIs can be managed effectively in LMICs with widely available antibiotics, global development of antibiotic resistance has eroded the success of treatment of some infections, including gonorrhea.

Canchihuaman and others (2011) have also demonstrated the feasibility and effectiveness of using computer-based education to reach out to clinicians and midwives to vastly expand and improve the scope and effect of online continuing education of STI management. This approach is a critical and effective step to guide large groups of clinicians and communities, even in remote rural areas, to better health care in general but especially regarding infectious diseases.

Table 1.3 Essential STI Intervention Package, by Delivery Platform

	Platforms for intervention delivery					
	Nationwide, regional, and local health systems, policies and regulations	Community health post[a]	Pharmacies[b]	Primary health and reproductive health clinics[c]	First-level hospitals	Second-, and third-level hospitals[d]
Structural	1. Organize, coordinate, and where possible, integrate programs for STI and HIV/AIDS into one national center and into regional centers, with essential funding and system support for local programs* 2. National policies to enable prevention and treatment efforts for key populations*	3. Linkages to clinical services for FSW, MSM, sex partners of persons with STI/HIV* 4. Training for police to ensure access to services for key populations, especially needle exchange* 5. Home-based services and Internet use for partner notification, HIV diagnosis, and initiating HIV treatment in patients with HIV infection*	6. Training on syndromic treatment of STIs by pharmacists			
Behavioral prevention	7. Social marketing linked to education on STI/HIV risks, and on sexual health, including condom and safe sex promotion*e 8. National curriculum and policy regarding sexual health education (including online education)*	9. School-based sexual health education (STI/HIV risks, condom use, substance abuse, key vaccines, VMMC)* 10. Condom promotion; Needle exchange for IDU*f				

table continues next page

Table 1.3 Essential STI Intervention Package, by Delivery Platform (continued)

	Platforms for intervention delivery					
	Nationwide, regional, and local health systems, policies and regulations	Community health post[a]	Pharmacies[b]	Primary health and reproductive health clinics[c]	First-level hospitals	Second-, and third-level hospitals[d]
Biomedical prevention	11. Guidelines, funding, and social marketing for HPV and HBV vaccines; and for VMMC (adolescents, adults, infants)	12. School-based and health post provision of HPV and HBV vaccines, and linkage to or provision of VMMC services 13. Access to needle exchange for IDU* 14. Screening and treatment for major STIs among prison populations 15. Preexposure antimicrobial prophylaxis in high risk populations*		16. Vaccine provision (HPV, HBV) (females and males) 17. VMMC* 18. Visual inspection with acetic acid for cervical dysplasia		
Diagnosis and treatment	19. Guidelines for expedited partner therapy via pharmacies		20. Syndromic-based treatment of STIs		21. Diagnosis and treatment of suspected pelvic inflammatory disease; viral hepatitis; ART, plus detection and treatment or referral of comorbidities, and some HIV comorbidities	22. Diagnosis and treatment of anal, oropharyngeal, and liver cancers; and other HIV comorbidities.

Note: Interventions shown in orange indicate areas that are relatively neglected by governments. Interventions marked with an asterisk (*) should be closely integrated with HIV prevention and treatment interventions.

FSW = female sex workers; HBV = hepatitis B virus; HIV/AIDS = human immunodeficiency virus/acquired immune deficiency syndrome; HPV = human papillomavirus; IDU = injection drug users; MSM = men who have sex with men; PrEP = preexposure prophylaxis; STD = sexually transmitted disease; STI = sexually transmitted infection; VMMC = voluntary male medical circumcision.

a. This platform involves extension of health services beyond conventional clinical platforms to reach high-risk populations.

b. Pharmacies are very accessible (proximity, short wait times, low cost) and provide much of the treatment for STI syndromes. Yet, adherence to STD treatment guidelines in pharmacies has been dismal (Chalker and others 2000). However, training of physicians, midwives, and pharmacy workers can lead to greatly improved STD syndromic management (Garcia and others 2012). After training of pharmacy workers, pharmacy-based STD syndromic management was cost-effective, when only program costs are used, and cost saving from the societal perspective (Adams and others 2003).

c. For this volume, we are assuming that most clinical service delivery at the primary care and reproductive health clinics level is provided by nurses. Primary health clinics in LICs and MICs tend to lack diagnostic testing but also have lower costs and are more accessible than hospitals.

d. Service delivery by physicians, physician assistants, or nurses. Specialist expertise includes reproductive health, laboratory capacity, obstetrics and gynecology, and pediatrics.

e. Curricula should include information on condoms, safe-sex promotion and provision, warning signs, and accessing care.

f. Sanchez and others 1998.

Tuberculosis

TB is arguably the world's leading cause of death from an infectious agent.[3] The WHO estimates that 10.4 million new cases and 1.5 million deaths occur from TB each year (WHO 2016a). One-third of TB cases remain unknown to the health care system. For those accessing treatment, however, prevalence and mortality have declined significantly, and millions of lives have been saved.

TB is caused by the bacterium *Mycobacterium tuberculosis*, which is transmitted between humans through the respiratory route and most commonly affects the lungs but can damage any tissue. Only a minority (approximately 10 percent) of individuals infected with *M. tuberculosis* progress to active TB disease, while the remainder may maintain a latent infection that serves as a reservoir. TB has special challenges, including (a) a substantial number of patients with active disease are asymptomatic, capable of transmitting infection without knowing it; (b) patients must maintain compliance with treatment for six to nine months; and (c) the pathogen persists in many infected individuals in a latent state for many years but can be reactivated over a lifetime to cause disease and become transmissible.

People at every rung of the socioeconomic ladder are at risk, although TB disproportionately affects the poor. Approximately 80 percent of patients reside in 22 high-burden countries. Treatment of TB disease requires multiple drugs for many months. These lengthy drug regimens are challenging for both patients and health care systems—especially in LMICs, where the disease burden often far outstrips local resources. For TB susceptible to first-line drugs (the least expensive), cure rates greater than 90 percent are expected at a cost of US$200 to US$500. The increasing incidence of multidrug-resistant TB (MDR-TB), which requires even longer treatment regimens with expensive and difficult-to-tolerate drugs, represents an emerging threat, not least to hospital and clinic personnel.

The United Nations' (UN) Sustainable Development Goal (SDG) 3 seeks to end the TB epidemic altogether by 2030, but the decline in incidence of TB has been slow, only about 1.5 percent per year.[4] Without new tools, the UN targets are unlikely to be met even by 2050. The current policy of passive case finding (waiting for patients to be ill enough to seek treatment) is suboptimal in high-burden countries. Faster rates of progress on TB will require earlier, more accurate case detection; rapid commencement of and adherence to effective treatment; and, where possible, preventive treatment of latent TB (table 1.4).

Durable control will require new strategies and tools that are more effective than those now in use—for example, new, shorter drug regimens that are effective for both drug-sensitive and drug-resistant TB. These must be not only cost-effective but also affordable and capable of being effective on a large scale. In addition to new tools, effective TB control requires the strengthening of weak health care systems (including improvements in surveillance, information technology, logistics, and drug supply) and strengthening of community health care systems to be more responsive and effective.

Within the context of current knowledge, Bloom and others (2017) in chapter 11 in this volume advocate for optimizing the approaches known to be effective, including the following:

- Identify high-transmission countries and hot spots within countries where targeted efforts can be more effective and cost-effective.
- Increase early TB detection and diagnosis, particularly in selected high-burden countries, by introduction of new tools for active case finding.
- Rapidly provide appropriate and better maintenance for patients diagnosed with either drug-susceptible TB or MDR-TB, enabling higher levels of completion and care.

- Expand preventive therapy to reduce transmission from TB patients to contacts, especially to children and HIV-positive individuals.
- Emphasize community-based delivery of TB treatment and services wherever possible to improve treatment completion, reduce the dangers of hospital transmission, decrease costs, and improve patient quality of life.
- Improve hospital and clinic infection control.
- Enhance drug supply chains for access to TB treatments that have small markets.
- Expand information technology and electronic medical records to enable more effective disease control.

The need is urgent for new tools, including inexpensive and sensitive point-of-care diagnostic tests, rapid tests for drug resistance, new and shorter drug regimens for both drug-susceptible and drug-resistant TB, and a more effective vaccine to prevent the disease.

Malaria and Other Adult Febrile Illnesses

Febrile illnesses are major causes of morbidity and mortality in LMICs for children and adults, and most are largely indistinguishable on clinical presentation. Simple rapid diagnostic tests (RDTs) are lacking for the common, serious causes of fever except malaria, making appropriate treatment uncertain for most febrile patients, only a minority of whom have malaria.

Malaria

The massive investment in malaria control over the past decade has been successful in greatly reducing malaria prevalence, but eliminating malaria is a very distant goal in most of Sub-Saharan Africa and much of Asia. Continued progress depends on maintaining and increasing the use of effective preventive measures (such as insecticide-treated nets, indoor residual spraying, and intermittent preventive therapy for pregnant women and infants); widespread use of RDTs; and treatment with effective artemisinin-combination therapies (ACTs) to bring the countries with the highest endemic rates to preelimination levels (Shretta and others 2017, chapter 12 in this volume). Table 1.5 summarizes the essential interventions for prevention and treatment of malaria.

Continued surveillance and substantial expenditures over many years will be needed to eventually eradicate malaria, and whether it can be done globally without adding at least one more effective tool to the set of interventions in widespread use is unclear. The currently available vaccines may or may not be effective enough to boost results sufficiently. In April 2017, the WHO

Table 1.4 Essential Tuberculosis Intervention Package, by Delivery Platform

Intervention type	Delivery platform				
	Nationwide policies and regulations	Community health post or pharmacy	Primary health center	First-level hospital	Second- and third-level hospitals
Surveillance and disease detection	1. Passive case finding 2. Active case finding in high-burden countries	3. Symptomatic surveillance 4. Active contact tracing of TB-positive patients			
Data collection and patient tracking	5. Information systems				
Diagnosis and drug sensitivity testing Relapse and reinfection diagnosis	6. National guidelines promoting the provision of diagnostic labs; diagnostic technology including GeneXpert or culture for drug-susceptible TB; fixed/mobile X-ray; and training	7. Symptomatic diagnosis, local sputum smears 8. Referral for diagnosis and drug-susceptible TB tests	9. Sputum smears 10. Testing of children and household members and HIV+ individuals for case finding in both drug-susceptible and MDR-TB cases 11. Availability of fixed/mobile X-ray for diagnosis	12. GeneXpert/RIF[a] or culture for diagnosis of drug-susceptible TB	
Treatment of drug-susceptible TB	13. WHO guidelines: four-drug regimen for two months, then two drugs-regimen for four months	14. Provision and observation of treatment after one month at first-level hospital 15. Use of cell-phone SMS to support treatment adherence		16. Treatment of drug-susceptible TB until transmission is reduced (one month), then transfer of treatment to community level	
Treatment of drug-resistant TB	17. WHO guidelines: Multiple-drug regimen after drug-susceptible TB testing for nine months to two years		18. Provision of appropriate second-line drugs, monitoring 19. INH preventive therapy	20. Treatment until sputum is negative or GeneXpert is negative; treatment as outpatients after sputum is negative	21. Specialized treatment for treatment failures, MDR-TB, surgery
Coinfection with HIV		22. Provider incentives to improve quality of TB care	23. Referral or provision of HIV treatment as appropriate 24. Information systems to link diagnostic hospital care to outpatient and community care	25. Separate areas in health facilities for TB to avoid transmission to AIDS patients	

Note: Interventions shown in orange indicate areas that are relatively neglected by governments. HIV = human immunodeficiency virus; HIV+ = HIV-positive; INH = isoniazid; MDR-TB = multidrug-resistant tuberculosis; SMS = short message service (text messaging); TB = tuberculosis; WHO = World Health Organization.
a. GeneXpert/RIF refers to a new test that simultaneously detects *Mycobacterium* TB complex (MTBC) and resistance to rifampin (RIF).

announced that Ghana, Kenya, and Malawi will participate in a pilot malaria vaccine implementation program in select areas, beginning in 2018 (WHO 2017).

Despite global guidelines to the contrary, presumptive treatment of undifferentiated febrile illness as malaria is still appropriate in places where RDTs (or microscopy) cannot be reliably applied and malaria prevalence is high (Babigumira, Gelband, and Garrison 2017, chapter 15 in this volume). When the test for malaria is negative, patients with severe disease should receive an antimicrobial regimen tailored to locally important nonmalarial pathogens (Crump and others 2017, chapter 14 in this volume).

Table 1.5 Essential Malaria Intervention Package, by Delivery Platform

	Delivery platform[a]				
Intervention type	Population-based health interventions	Community	Health center	First-level hospital	Second- and third-level hospitals
All malaria-endemic countries					
Case management: Uncomplicated malaria (or fever)	1. Prophylaxis for travelers	2. Diagnosis with RDTs or microscopy, including parasite species			
		3. Treatment with ACTs (or current first-line combination) for malaria-positive individuals where diagnosis is available			
		4. Where both RDTs and microscopy are unavailable and malaria is common, presumptive treatment with ACTs for nonsevere suspected malaria; if severe, ACTs plus antibiotics			
		5. *Plasmodium vivax.* Chloroquine alone or chloroquine plus 14-day course of primaquine (for G6PD normal individuals)			
		6. Case investigation, reactive case detection, proactive case detection (including mass screening and treatment)			
Case management: Severe malaria		7. Single-dose rectal artesunate, then referral to first-level hospital		8. Parenteral artesunate, then full-course ACTs	
Vector control: ITNs		9. ITNs available in health centers and antenatal clinics and via social marketing			
Malaria elimination countries					
		10. Mass drug administration to high-risk groups in geographic or demographic clusters			
		11. Single low-dose primaquine added to first-line treatment			
Malaria control countries					
Vector control: IRS		12. IRS in selected areas with high transmission and entomologic data on IRS susceptibility			
Vector control: Larviciding and water management		13. Larviciding and water management in specific circumstances where breeding sites can be identified and regularly targeted			
Mass drug administration		14. IPTp, IPTi, and SMC Sahel region			

Note: Interventions shown in orange indicate areas that are relatively neglected by governments. ACTs = artemisinin-combination therapies; G6PD = glucose-6-phosphate-dehydrogenase; IPTi = intermittent preventive treatment in infants; IPTp = intermittent preventive treatment of pregnant women; IRS = indoor residual spraying; ITN = insecticide-treated net; RDT = rapid diagnostic test; SMC = seasonal malaria chemoprevention.
a. All interventions listed for lower-level platforms can be provided at higher levels. Similarly, each facility level represents a spectrum and diversity of capabilities. The column in which an intervention is listed is the lowest level of the health care system in which it would usually be provided.

Where an understanding of locally important bloodstream infections and other pathogens is lacking, standardized fever etiology research is needed to inform management. The development of accurate point-of-care diagnostic or biomarker tests would improve targeting of antimicrobials.

Nonmalarial Fever

A diverse set of pathogens contributes to nonmalarial fever. Prevention efforts may target pathogen reservoirs (for example, by vaccinating livestock for brucellosis); target sources of infection (such as through vector control to reduce arbovirus infections); interrupt transmission (for example, by reducing occupational exposure to *Coxiella burnetii* among abattoir workers); and provide immunologic protection (such as through typhoid vaccines).[5]

A lack of knowledge and a lack of tools hamper progress in combating nonmalarial fevers. The predominant causes of fever in LMICs are largely unknown because research on fever etiology has not been done. National surveillance or sentinel site studies, preferably coordinated globally, are urgently needed to identify major causes of severe febrile illness, especially bloodstream infections and pathogens with specific treatments (for example, brucellosis, rickettsioses, and Q fever)

(Crump and others 2017, chapter 14 in this volume). Concomitantly, research to identify priorities for improvements in management, such as selection of empiric antimicrobial therapies, should be undertaken in the same countries.

The laboratory methods that can be used for research are impractical at the bedside in low-resource settings. For such settings, accurate RDTs are needed—first, to distinguish viral from bacterial (and potentially easily treatable) infections; and second, to provide pathogen-specific tests for major causes of treatable nonmalarial fevers, based on surveillance and other local research.

Finally, cost and outcome data are needed to develop credible estimates of the total burden of nonmalarial febrile illnesses and to enable accurate cost-effectiveness analyses related to fever in order to strengthen resource-stratified approaches to the adoption and integration of interventions (summarized in table 1.6). This information is particularly important because decisions on services to include in universal health coverage are being made.

Viral Hepatitis

Five mostly unrelated viruses—hepatitis A, B, C, D, and E—infect the liver, with varied routes of infection:

Table 1.6 Essential Intervention Package for Adult Febrile Illness, by Delivery Platform

Intervention type	Delivery platform[a]				
	Nationwide policies and regulations	Community health post or pharmacy	Primary health center	First-level hospital	Second- and third-level hospitals
Case management: All fevers	1. Standard practice guidelines 2. Essential medicines, including relevant antibacterials		3. Evaluation for malaria with RDT or microscopy (see malaria interventions) 4. If negative for malaria, referral if fever persists beyond seven days	5. Clinical history and examination to identify source of fever 6. Evaluation for malaria and HIV 7. Treatment for the apparent cause and reevaluation after one week	8. Reference diagnostics for major causes of nonmalarial fever
Case management: Severe febrile illness			9. Prereferral antimicrobial according to standard practice guidelines (for example, extended-spectrum cephalosporin)	10. Emergency management of septic shock with intravenous fluids, supplemental oxygen, and antimicrobial according to standard practice guidelines 11. Clinical history and physical examination to identify source of fever 12. Blood culture before antimicrobial; hemoglobin and glucose measurement 13. Treatment of apparent cause	14. Reference diagnostics for major causes of nonmalarial fever

table continues next page

Table 1.6 Essential Intervention Package for Adult Febrile Illness, by Delivery Platform (continued)

Intervention type	Nationwide policies and regulations	Community health post or pharmacy	Primary health center	First-level hospital	Second- and third-level hospitals
		Delivery platform[a]			
Prevention: Vaccines	15. National policy on typhoid vaccines				
	16. National policy on control of brucellosis and leptospirosis in livestock				
Prevention: Nonvaccine measures	17. National policies on control of sources of nationally important causes of nonmalarial fever (such as vector control for arbovirus infections)				
	18. National policies on interruption of transmission of nationally important causes of nonmalarial fever (for example, management of occupational exposure to *Coxiella burnetii* among abattoir workers)				
Surveillance	19. Nationwide or sentinel site surveillance to identify major causes of severe febrile illness, especially bloodstream infections				
	20. Assurance that national recommendations for antimicrobial management of severe febrile illness match etiologic findings				

Note: HIV = human immunodeficiency virus; RDT = rapid diagnostic test.

a. All interventions listed for lower-level platforms can be provided at higher levels. Similarly, each facility level represents a spectrum and diversity of capabilities. The column in which an intervention is listed is the lowest level of the health care system in which it would usually be provided.

- Hepatitis A and E are transmitted by the fecal-oral route through contaminated water and food; they can also be transmitted sexually.
- Most hepatitis B (HBV) infections occur through mother-to-child and early-life horizontal transmission between family members, among adults through sexual intercourse, and through unsafe injection practices and transfusion of unscreened blood.
- Most hepatitis C (HCV) infections occur through unsafe injections, either in medical settings (from reuse of medical equipment and substandard application of infection control measures) or through unsafe practices among people who inject drugs. Sexual transmission of hepatitis C is rare in heterosexual couples but more common among HIV/AIDS-infected MSM.
- Hepatitis D is transmitted by blood and bodily fluids.

Most hepatitis deaths (96 percent) are caused by HBV and HCV, which cause chronic, lifelong infection resulting in progressive liver damage leading to cirrhosis and hepatocellular carcinoma. Mortality rates from hepatitis are highest in West Africa and parts of Asia; in absolute numbers, East Asia and South Asia account for just over half of hepatitis deaths, which totaled 1.45 million globally in 2013. An estimated 250 million people live with chronic HBV infection; 80 million have chronic HCV infection (Gower and others 2014; Schweitzer and others 2015).

In some West African countries, more than 8 percent of the population is infected with hepatitis. The regions with the highest prevalence of HCV infection are West and Central Africa, Eastern Europe, and Central Asia. Hepatitis C prevalence is extremely high in a few other countries as well, most notably the Arab Republic of Egypt and Pakistan, where high incidence persists largely because of weak preventive measures, such as reuse of syringes and needles in health care settings.

Hepatitis Prevention

Hepatitis A and E infections can be prevented through improved sanitation. Although no reliable estimates are available, the incidence of hepatitis A and E has declined likely as part of the overall reduction in the number of deaths owing to diarrhea. An effective hepatitis A vaccine exists, and 18 countries have introduced universal childhood hepatitis A vaccination.

The most notable achievement in hepatitis prevention is the reduction in incidence of acute and chronic HBV infection as a result of universal childhood hepatitis B vaccination. At the end of 2013, 183 of 194 countries had introduced universal childhood vaccination; global coverage with three doses of hepatitis B vaccine is estimated to be 81 percent effective (WHO 2015). Universal infant vaccination with high coverage levels has led to major reductions in the prevalence of chronic HBV infection among children. In China, the prevalence of chronic HBV infection declined from approximately 8 percent in 1992 to 1 percent in 2006 among children ages one to four years (Liang and others 2009).

However, challenges remain in achieving further reductions in incidence. Full protection for children requires that they receive the first vaccine dose within 24 hours of birth, which is a logistical challenge and a barrier to further progress.

Other proven interventions for hepatitis prevention that have not been fully implemented around the world (for various technical and political reasons) are universal safe injections, blood supply screening for HBV and HCV, and harm reduction for injection drug users (for example, provision of sterile needles and opioid substitutes).

Hepatitis Treatment

Chronic HBV and HCV infections can be treated effectively. The new direct-acting antiviral medicines for hepatitis C can cure more than 90 percent of individuals with chronic infection with a two- to three-month course of treatment, although the current costs of treatment are very high. Hepatitis C treatment could also reduce HCV transmission because people who have been cured do not transmit the infection. There is no cure for chronic hepatitis B, but effective antiviral treatments can suppress viral replication and prevent disease progression. Table 1.7 summarizes both the preventive and the treatment interventions for hepatitis.

Neglected Tropical Diseases

NTDs affect more than 1 billion of the poorest, most marginalized people of the world. These infections are a consequence of the environmental and socioeconomic conditions in which the poor live, and the ill health and disability they cause are a primary factor locking the poor into poverty. At least 18 diseases are recognized as NTDs by World Health Assembly resolutions.[6] Although not covered further here, the WHO has recently added snakebite deaths to the NTD list. Snakebite causes about 50,000 deaths in India per year and an estimated 100,000 deaths globally (Mohapatra and others 2011).

The NTD concept was developed to draw attention to a disease control opportunity that had been overlooked by the Millennium Development Goals. The ending of NTD epidemics is now embedded within the SDGs for 2030, under target 3.3, reflecting the UN's High-Level Political Forum on Sustainable Development 2016 promise of "ensuring that no one is left behind."[7] Chapter 17 of this volume (Fitzpatrick and others 2017) focuses on specific WHO targets for control, elimination, and eradication of a subset of these diseases.

Interventions to End NTDs

Three key interventions address a large share of the burden of disease caused by this set of diseases. In recognition of the increasingly integrated delivery of interventions to the poorest, most remote, and otherwise most marginalized communities of the world, we consider them by intervention rather than by disease, as follows:

- Preventive chemotherapy by mass drug administration
- Innovative and intensified disease management
- Vector ecology and management

Table 1.7 Essential Hepatitis Intervention Package, by Delivery Platform

Intervention type	Delivery platform[a]				
	Nationwide policies and regulations	Community health post or pharmacy	Primary health care	First-level hospital	Second- and third-level hospitals
Hepatitis B vaccination	1. Policy for universal newborn and childhood vaccination		2. Delivery of hepatitis B vaccination including birth dose		
Interventions to reduce hepatitis transmission in health care settings	3. Policy for hepatitis B vaccination of health care workers		4. Vaccination of health care workers		
Harm-reduction services for IDU	5. Policy for the provision of harm-reduction services (including injection equipment and opioid substitution therapy) to IDU; use of this wording for HIV or STI safe injection* 6. Community services: IDU-friendly harm reduction with sufficient coverage				
Hepatitis testing services	7. National testing policy identifying priority groups for testing and setting a testing strategy	8. Hepatitis testing of individuals as identified in the national testing policy	9. Referral of persons with hepatitis infection to care		
Hepatitis treatment	10. Treatment guidelines		11. Referral of persons with hepatitis infection to assessment for treatment eligibility 12. Assuming sufficient training, initiation of hepatitis treatment and follow-up	13. Treatment of hepatitis B and C for eligible persons 14. Mentoring of primary-care personnel involved in treatment initiation and follow-up	
				15. Screening blood transfusion for hepatitis B and C	

Note: Interventions shown in orange indicate areas that are relatively neglected by governments. HIV = human immunodeficiency virus; IDU = injection drug users; STI = sexually transmitted infection. Interventions marked with an asterisk (*) should be closely integrated with HIV/AIDS and STI prevention and treatment interventions.

a. All interventions listed for lower-level platforms can be provided at higher levels. Similarly, each facility level represents a spectrum and diversity of capabilities. The column in which an intervention is listed is the lowest level of the health care system in which it would usually be provided.

The interventions are discussed in detail in chapter 17 in this volume (Fitzpatrick and others 2017) but are summarized as follows:

Preventive chemotherapy by mass drug administration is effective against lymphatic filariasis, onchocerciasis, schistosomiasis, soil-transmitted helminthiases, and trachoma. The specific drugs and regimens vary by disease, and many populations are affected by more than one of these conditions. Mass campaigns can be combined to target several pathogens at once.

Innovative and intensified disease management refers to a shift from passive management to active surveillance, early diagnosis, and treatment, with the aim to eliminate or control, not just to manage. Treatment of Buruli ulcer, for example, has evolved from late-stage surgical removal of infected or dead tissue and correction of deformity to the early-stage use of antibiotics. The gains go beyond health benefits to include reductions in hospitalization costs to health care systems and to individuals.

The NTDs for which the primary intervention is disease management are Buruli ulcer, Chagas disease, human African trypanosomiasis (HAT), leishmaniasis, leprosy, and yaws.

Vector ecology and management aims to control the transmission of the causative pathogens of insect-borne NTDs with proven interventions that are applied in an ecologically friendly manner. The main NTDs for which this is an important strategy are Chagas disease, dengue, chikungunya, visceral leishmaniasis (kala azar), and Zika virus. Table 1.8 summarizes the essential interventions for preventing and treating NTDs.

Recent Progress against NTDs

Since the NTD concept took hold, substantial successes have been recorded, including a reduction in deaths caused by visceral leishmaniasis, rabies, schistosomiasis, HAT, Chagas disease, and soil-transmitted helminthiases (among which, for example, ascariasis is estimated to

Table 1.8 Essential Intervention Package for Neglected Tropical Diseases, by Delivery Platform

Intervention type	Delivery platform[a]				
	Nationwide policies or regulations	Community health post or pharmacy	Primary health care	First-level hospital	Second- and third-level hospitals
Preventive chemotherapy	1. Integrated guidelines and strategy on the coordinated use of preventive chemotherapy for NTDs	2. Mass drug administration for lymphatic filariasis, onchocerciasis, schistosomiasis, soil-transmitted helminthiases, trachoma, and food-borne trematodiases as appropriate			
Innovative and intensified disease management	3. Integrated guidelines and strategy for skin-related NTDs including (in addition to those listed elsewhere in this table) Buruli ulcer and mycetoma	4. Lymphedema management 5. Early detection and treatment of Chagas disease, human African trypanosomiasis, leprosy, and leishmaniases 6. Total community treatment for yaws		7. Hydrocele and trichiasis surgery	
Vector ecology and management	8. Integrated vector management guidelines and strategy	9. Sustained vector management for Chagas disease, dengue, and visceral leishmaniasis			
Veterinary public health services	10. Not covered in *DCP3* chapter; for interventions for the control of echinococcosis and rabies, see World Bank (2012).				
Water, sanitation, and hygiene	11. See interventions in chapter 9 of *DCP3* volume 7 (Hutton and Chase 2017).				

Note: DCP3 = Disease Control Priorities, third edition (Jamison and others 2015–18); NTDs = neglected tropical diseases.

a. All interventions listed for lower-level platforms can be provided at higher levels. Similarly, each facility level represents a spectrum and diversity of capabilities. The column in which an intervention is listed is the lowest level of the health care system in which it would usually be provided.

have caused 142,000 deaths in 2012, down from about 220,000 in 2000) (WHO 2014). In addition, the following results were recorded:

- New HAT cases have fallen by 80 percent between 2000 and 2014, to an estimated total of fewer than 4,000 cases per year.
- The number of cases of visceral leishmaniasis (kala azar) in Bangladesh, India, and Nepal fell by 75 percent between 2005 (when a regional program was launched) and 2014, to a reported 10,209 cases.
- In 2000, more than 130,000 cases of dracunculiasis (Guinea worm disease) were reported; in 2015, only 22 cases were reported, reflecting near eradication.

Much of the burden of NTDs occurs with morbidity rather than mortality—and here, too, the progress has been good, albeit somewhat less dramatic: the total number of DALYs decreased by 19 percent between 2000 and 2012, from 1.0 percent of the GBD to 0.8 percent (WHO 2014).

ANTIMICROBIAL RESISTANCE

Every use of an antibiotic, whether appropriate or inappropriate, exerts selection pressure, giving resistant bacteria an advantage and accelerating the development of resistance. Bacterial resistance to first-line, second-line, and last-resort antibiotics is growing wherever it has been monitored (CDDEP 2016). Increased travel, trade, and migration mean that resistant bacteria can spread faster than ever (Du and others 2016; Johnson and Woodford 2013).

The burden of antimicrobial resistance falls heavily on LMICs. They typically have high burdens and rapid spread of infectious disease, poor nutrition, and increasing rates of antibiotic consumption in humans and animals, in addition to weaker health care systems and sparse standards and regulations governing access, use, and quality of antibiotics (Okeke and others 2005).

Drivers of Increased Antibiotic Use

The increase in antibiotic use is driven by the burden of infectious disease as well as by economic, behavioral, environmental, and structural factors. For instance, expanded insurance coverage and increased physician density intensify the consumption of antibiotics (Klein and others 2015; Zhang, Lee, and Donohue 2010). Decision fatigue and patient demand also increase antibiotic prescribing.

Antibiotic consumption increased by an estimated 30 percent or more in 71 countries between 2000 and 2010, reaching approximately 70 billion standard units (single-dose units) in 2010 (Van Boeckel and others 2014). This increase was primarily in first-line classes of antibiotics, including penicillins and cephalosporins, which together make up more than half of global consumption. Use of last-resort antibiotic classes, especially carbapenems and polymyxins, also increased.

Despite the recent increases in antibiotic consumption worldwide, with few exceptions, per capita consumption in LMICs is much lower than in HICs. Alongside increasing consumption and rising rates of antibiotic resistance, lack of access to antibiotics is still a serious concern for most LMICs. Each year, pneumonia kills approximately 1 million children under age five years, and an estimated 445,000 could be saved with the universal provision of antibiotics for community-acquired pneumococcal infections (Miller-Petrie, Pant, and Laxminarayan 2017, chapter 18 in this volume). When they are available, first-line antibiotic treatments are still relatively affordable, but newer antibiotics needed to treat resistant infections may be out of reach for LMICs (Miller-Petrie, Pant, and Laxminarayan 2017, chapter 18 in this volume).[8]

Interventions to Ensure Appropriate Antibiotic Use

Certain interventions are effective at reducing antibiotic use or increasing appropriate use, but their effects on antibiotic resistance rates are difficult to determine because of the long timeline for effects to become apparent. Therefore, recommendations are based largely on success in changing patterns of use. Interventions aim to both reduce the *need* for antibiotics by preventing infections and reduce the inappropriate or unnecessary *use* of antibiotics (in both humans and animals). The broad categories of interventions are as follows (summarized from Miller-Petrie, Pant, and Laxminarayan 2017, chapter 18 of this volume):

- *Reduce and eventually phase out subtherapeutic antibiotic use in agriculture.* Improved sanitation and hygiene at the farm level would reduce the need for prophylactic antibiotics. Antibiotic use in animal agriculture should be reduced, focusing on the involvement of farmers and the agricultural industry in carefully phasing out the use of growth promoters and premixed animal feeds (Laxminarayan, Van Boeckel, and Teillant 2015).
- *Adopt incentives that encourage antibiotic stewardship and discourage overuse.* Ensuring that payments are not linked to prescribing and introducing rewards for compliance may improve prescribing patterns.

- *Improve hospital infection control and antibiotic stewardship.* Antibiotic stewardship programs, infection prevention and control, and especially handwashing with soap can reduce infections, antibiotic use, and resistance while also improving patient outcomes.
- *Educate health care professionals, policy makers, and the public about sustainable antibiotic use.* Although public awareness is growing that antibiotic resistance presents a threat, there is little awareness of individual actions to reduce antibiotic use. Patients, parents, health care providers, stakeholders, and hospital heads all need to be aware of what they can do to reduce unnecessary use.
- *Reduce the need for antibiotics through improved water, sanitation, and immunization.* Disease prevention achieves the dual purposes of keeping people healthy and saving antibiotic doses. Water, sanitation, hygiene, and vaccination should be core components of any response, with financing from infrastructure and health sectors.
- *Ensure political commitment to meet the threat of antibiotic resistance.* Without national commitment in the form of implemented action plans, the long-term sustainability of efforts to curb antibiotic resistance will be weakened. Although international efforts to curb antibiotic resistance have focused largely on national action, international support is also needed.

COST-EFFECTIVENESS OF INTERVENTIONS FOR ADULT INFECTIOUS DISEASE

The substantial mobilization of donor resources by organizations including The Global Fund to Fight AIDS, Tuberculosis, and Malaria; The President's Emergency Plan for AIDS Relief; and the President's Malaria Initiative has been accompanied by efforts to ensure value for money, which has led to a substantial literature on the costs and cost-effectiveness of interventions to combat some major infectious diseases (but little beyond these diseases).

Figure 1.1 summarizes various estimates of cost-effectiveness, measured per DALY prevented—the metric most commonly used in economic studies to compare cost-effectiveness across different health interventions. The estimates are summarized from expert searches of the literature undertaken for the chapters in this volume. For full details of the individual studies used, along with bibliographic references, see annex 1B. All cost-effectiveness results have been translated into 2012 U.S. dollars for comparability. A few studies (particularly publications from the WHO-CHOICE (CHOsing Interventions that are Cost-Effective) project, which provides results in international dollars of a WHO region)[9] could not be converted and were omitted.

Cost-effectiveness results depend on context. The cost-effectiveness of the same intervention in two different countries may vary depending on local costs; health interventions, on average, cost more in countries with higher income because of higher salaries. Vaccines generally cost more in countries not eligible for bulk purchasing discounts (such as prices of Gavi, the Vaccine Alliance).[10] In addition, the cost-effectiveness of vaccination and screening programs (and some other interventions) vary according to prevalence of the condition; prevention programs are often more cost-effective where prevalence is higher. Cost-effectiveness may vary with comorbidities and with opportunities to deliver the intervention synergistically with other interventions (and therefore at lower cost). *Usual care* (the usual comparator of cost-effectiveness) may also vary.

In some cases, the interventions are subdivided by study location (for example, southern Africa or Southeast Asia) or by low-income or middle-income country designation. Where neither is specified, the results apply to low- and lower-middle-income countries, which are the main emphases of this third edition of *Disease Control Priorities* (Jamison and others 2015–18). Fewer results for upper-middle-income countries are included. HIV/AIDS interventions account for almost half of the interventions and studies, consistent with its share of funding relative to other health conditions.

Figure 1.1 represents a reductionist view of the large literature on cost-effectiveness of infectious disease interventions and should be interpreted with caution, especially when comparing results of two different studies that rely on inconsistent underlying assumptions. However, more than half of the interventions listed in figure 1.1 cost less than US$100 per DALY prevented, suggesting that they could be cost-effective even in the poorest countries. These interventions include some that are preventive, such as providing female condoms to sex workers in South Africa (although in practice, widespread use has been difficult to achieve); undertaking voluntary male circumcision in high-incidence African countries; and supplying insecticide-treated nets in Africa to prevent malaria. Biomedical treatment interventions costing less than US$100 per DALY prevented include treating severe malaria with artesunate; screening and treating pregnant women for syphilis; treating malaria (with ACTs); treating TB (with first-line drugs); and, for various NTDs, providing detection and treatment and preventive biomedical therapy for some conditions in endemic areas.

Figure 1.1 Estimated Costs of Selected Infectious Disease Interventions

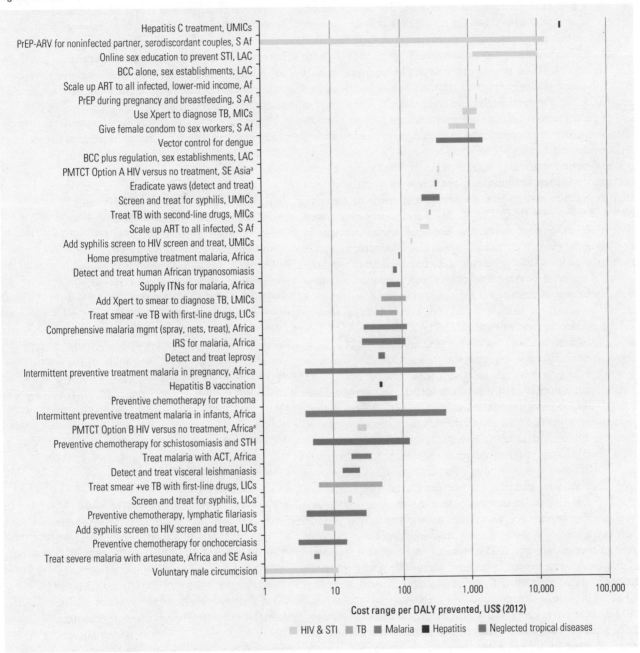

Sources: Estimates based on sources listed by subject in annex 1B of this chapter.

Note: ACT = artemisinin-combination therapy; ART = antiretroviral treatment; ARV = antiretroviral; BCC = behavior change communications; DALY = disability-adjusted life year; HIV = human immunodeficiency virus; IRS = indoor residual spraying; ITNs = insecticide-treated nets; LAC = Latin America and the Caribbean; LICs = low-income countries; LMICs = low- and middle-income countries; MICs = middle-income countries; PrEP = preexposure prophylaxis (provision of ART to noninfected individuals at risk); PMTCT = prevention of mother-to-child transmission; S Af = southern Africa; SE Asia = Southeast Asia; STH = soil-transmitted helminthiases; STI = sexually transmitted infection; TB = tuberculosis; UMICs = upper-middle-income countries.

a. "Option A" is a two-drug ART regimen in pregnancy and postpartum for HIV-positive mothers. "Option B" is a three-drug ART regime in pregnancy and postpartum for HIV-positive mothers.

Another group of interventions costs US$100–US$399 per DALY prevented and thus would be considered cost-effective (less than the per capita annual income) of all but the poorest four to five countries. This second group includes providing ART for people with HIV/AIDS, with pregnant women being a particularly high priority (to prevent transmission to their children while also treating HIV in the mother). This group of interventions also includes intermittent preventive treatment of malaria in infants and pregnant women as well as treatment of MDR-TB with second-line (more expensive) drugs.

Some interventions, such as those requiring behavioral change or those being implemented in Latin America, cost more than US$400 per DALY prevented. These include programs aiming to change sexual behavior as well as vector control interventions for dengue. PrEP, which includes provision of ART to the uninfected partner in an HIV-serodiscordant couple, varies considerably in cost-effectiveness, ranging from being cost saving to costing more than US$5,000 per DALY prevented, depending on the context.

Interventions can be cost-effective according to global norms but still too expensive for most LICs to provide to everyone in need, especially where prevalence of the condition is high. Examples include the provision of ART in low-income African countries (Alistar, Grant, and Bendavid 2014) and the treatment of drug-resistant TB (Fitzpatrick and Floyd 2012).

Certain other interventions are likely to be cost-effective, but no studies could be identified for the context. For example, needle exchange programs for injection drug users are expected to be cost-effective given that HIV prevalence among this group worldwide is 19 percent; such programs could also prevent hepatitis B and C (Wilson and others 2015). However, cost-effectiveness estimates for needle exchange programs were not identified for low- or lower-middle-income countries.

In yet other cases, studies evaluated interventions that have been superseded by more effective measures, or several studies of the same intervention had widely divergent results. These have not been included among studies used for the cost-effectiveness analysis of infectious disease interventions (for example, PMTCT Option A has now been supplanted by Option B/B+).

CONCLUSIONS

The variety and distribution of infectious diseases have evolved over time, and they will continue to challenge the global community—as the Zika and Ebola virus outbreaks have reminded us over the past couple of years. Through basic and translational research, some of the most devastating diseases of humankind—polio, diphtheria, measles, and tetanus—have been dramatically reduced, and smallpox has been eradicated. Meanwhile, new pathogens emerge, and newly drug-resistant organisms represent continuing and unpredictable threats.

Four main challenges will need to be met to achieve meaningful progress in the fight against the diseases addressed in this volume.

1. Focusing and Targeting of Intervention Strategies

If we have relearned something in the decade since *DCP2*, it is that infectious diseases are not distributed uniformly—not across continents, not across countries, not even in communities. Strategies should be designed to understand and respond appropriately to disease hot spots and key populations, thus ensuring access to the most effective interventions for the right populations in the right places at the right time, especially in LMICs, where the disease burden is greatest. Given the prodigious heterogeneity in the distribution of diseases (both geographically and across population subgroups) and the scarcity of resources, efficiency is increased by matching those resources to the populations that would benefit the most. Globally, infectious diseases disproportionately affect people in LMICs, which, at current rates of progress, will bear the bulk of premature deaths from infectious disease in 2030. In LMICs, the poorer, more marginalized, and often stigmatized populations are most at risk and the hardest to reach. Whereas the need for *treatment* may become obvious as it is demanded by the sick, the need and demand for *prevention* are often poorly matched. Prevention efforts can track incidence only if we know where the incidence is highest, which requires purposeful, population-based surveillance. Reaching marginalized populations will require not only dedicating resources to them but also working to remove the stigma, discrimination, and taboos that hamper effective prevention and treatment.

2. Scale-Up of Interventions against Major Infectious Diseases

Although we have evidence of interventions that work to prevent and treat disease, in many cases, those services have not been implemented at the scale necessary to sufficiently reduce incidence and the resulting morbidity and mortality. Scaling up these interventions requires that they be tailored for distribution at the lowest appropriate level of health care service delivery and that staff is adequately trained and supervised. Areas ripe for this approach include training of pharmacists in syndromic treatment of STIs and malaria RDTs at the lowest health care level. However, scale-up will not be possible unless we address the next challenge: integration.

3. Integration of Services More Effectively across Disease Areas

Reaching the world's poor with an entire arsenal of specialized clinics is impossible. People are frequently affected by more than one condition: those who are at risk for one NTD are also likely at risk for a number of others; sex workers are at risk for multiple STIs, and HIV patients are especially susceptible to TB infection. Moreover, treatment of infectious disease has grown increasingly complex (for example, ART and TB treatment) as well as costly (as evidenced by the new hepatitis C treatment). Consequently, efforts to combat certain major diseases that have similar modes of transmission (such as HIV, STIs, and hepatitis) would benefit from shared strategies for their prevention and diagnosis. Although specialized care is clearly needed for especially rare or difficult-to-treat conditions, standardizing prevention and treatment protocols and making information and communication technologies available enable care to be pushed out to integrated service points close to where patients live, study, and work. Proximity and integration of services help ensure continuity of care from prevention or diagnosis through treatment and follow-up care. Addressing each of these challenges requires strengthening of health care systems, including communication; information technology; logistics, drug and vaccine supplies; and training of health care providers, which includes community health workers in LMICs. Additionally, improving health care systems for infectious diseases, particularly those such as HIV, TB, and hepatitis that require extended medical treatment and monitoring, provides a basis and could serve as a model for improving care and treatment for noncommunicable diseases.

4. Development of New Technologies—Drugs, Vaccines, Diagnostics, Behavioral Interventions, and Delivery Methods—to Prevent and Treat These Diseases

Most urgent is the need for the global community to invest in developing new antimicrobials. This approach includes rethinking global development assistance to focus not only on providing services and key inputs (drugs, diagnostics, and vaccines) but also on financing research and development and operational research to create new tools or to make far better use of existing tools (Hecht and others 2012). In particular, as antimicrobial resistance continues to increase, diseases once thought to be highly treatable could, without significant investment in development of new drugs, pose a much more serious threat to global health.

A generation ago, as antibiotics were cheating death and vaccines were clearing diseases from entire continents, the world's population believed that it was moving into the postinfectious disease era. HIV seemed to be the exception that proved the rule and, at any rate, would quickly be tamed with a vaccine. Instead, these genetically facile microorganisms, which have survival as their evolutionary goal, have taught us humility. We will still be struggling against infectious diseases in future generations, but the struggle will be far less costly in lives and resources if we invest today in their control.

ANNEXES

The following annexes to this chapter are available at http://www.dcp-3.org/infectiousdiseases:

- Annex 1A: Forty Sexually Transmitted and Sexually Transmissible Pathogens
- Annex 1B: Sources of Cost-Effectiveness Analysis for Selected Infectious Disease Interventions

ACKNOWLEDGMENTS

The editors of this volume wish to thank Desiree Bernard, Elisabeth Gunningham, Varsha Malhotra, and Alicair Peltonen for their valuable assistance on this effort. They especially thank Brianne Adderley for her hard work keeping this large endeavor well organized.

NOTES

World Bank Income Classifications as of July 2014 are as follows, based on estimates of gross national income (GNI) per capita for 2013:

- Low-income countries (LICs) = US$1,045 or less
- Middle-income countries (MICs) are subdivided:
  (a) lower-middle-income = US$1,046 to US$4,125
  (b) upper-middle-income (UMICs) = US$4,126 to US$12,745
- High-income countries (HICs) = US$12,746 or more.

1. The U.S. Centers for Disease Control and Prevention (CDC) assesses the severity of HIV disease by cluster of differentiation 4 (CD4) cell counts and the presence of specific HIV-related conditions. The WHO Clinical Staging and Disease Classification System—which can be used readily in resource-constrained settings without access to CD4 cell count measurements or other diagnostic or laboratory testing methods—classifies HIV disease on the basis of clinical manifestations that clinicians can recognize and treat (U.S. Department of Health and Human Services 2014).

2. For a comprehensive list of sexually transmitted and sexually transmissible pathogens, see annex 1A at http://www.dcp-3.org/infectiousdiseases.

3. Whether TB or HIV causes more deaths depends on how one allocates the deaths in coinfected individuals. There is no clear, correct answer.

4. SDG 3, titled "Good Health and Well-Being," aims to "Ensure healthy lives and promote well-being for all at all ages." It sets nine primary targets, including target 3.3: "By 2030, end the epidemics of AIDS, tuberculosis, malaria and neglected tropical diseases and combat hepatitis, water-borne diseases and other communicable diseases."

5. See table 14.2. "Nonmalarial Febrile Diseases: Exposure, Diagnosis, Prevention, and Treatment" (Crump and others 2017, chapter 14 in this volume).

6. The 18th World Health Assembly–recognized NTDs are Buruli ulcer, Chagas disease, dengue and chikungunya, dracunculiasis (Guinea worm disease), echinococcosis, food-borne trematodiases, human African trypanosomiasis (sleeping sickness), leishmaniasis, leprosy (Hansen's disease), lymphatic filariasis, mycetoma, onchocerciasis (river blindness), rabies, schistosomiasis, soil-transmitted helminthiases, taeniasis/cysticercosis, trachoma, and yaws (endemic treponematosis) ("Neglected Tropical Diseases," WHO website, http://www.who.int/neglected_diseases/diseases/en/).

7. The High-Level Political Forum on Sustainable Development is the UN's central platform for the follow-up and review of the 2030 Agenda for Sustainable Development (UN 2015a), adopted at the United Nations Sustainable Development Summit on September 25, 2015 ("High-Level Political Forum on Sustainable Development 2016: Ensuring that No One Is Left Behind," UN Sustainable Development Knowledge Platform, https://sustainabledevelopment.un.org/hlpf/2016).

8. As is represented by the photo on the cover of this volume, the high global burden of infectious diseases (both in humans and in animals), combined with the increasing availability, use, and dispensing of antimicrobials (often based upon syndromic diagnosis rather than on diagnostic tests), contribute to the global acceleration of antimicrobial resistance.

9. The CHOICE (CHOosing Interventions that are Cost-Effective) project is a WHO initiative developed in 1998 to provide policy makers with evidence for deciding on interventions and programs that maximize health for the available resources ("Cost-Effectiveness and Strategic Planning (WHO-CHOICE)," WHO website, http://www.who.int/choice//en/). "An international dollar would buy in the cited country a comparable amount of goods and services a U.S. dollar would buy in the United States ("What Is an 'International Dollar'?" World Bank Knowledge Base, https://datahelpdesk.worldbank.org/knowledgebase/).

10. Gavi, the Vaccine Alliance is an international organization established in 2000 to bring together the public and private sectors with the shared goal of creating equal access to new and underused vaccines for children living in the poorest countries. For more information about Gavi's vaccine pricing strategy, see Gavi, the Vaccine Alliance (2011).

REFERENCES

Adams, E. J., P. J. García, G. P. Garnett, W. J. Edmunds, and K. K. Holmes. 2003. "The Cost-Effectiveness of Syndromic Management in Pharmacies in Lima, Peru." *Sexually Transmitted Diseases* 30 (5): 379–87.

Alistar, S. S., P. M. Grant, and E. Bendavid. 2014. "Comparative Effectiveness and Cost-Effectiveness of Antiretroviral Therapy and Pre-Exposure Prophylaxis for HIV Prevention in South Africa." *BMC Medicine* 12 (1): 46.

Aral, S. O. 2011. "Utility and Delivery of Behavioural Interventions to Prevent Sexually Transmitted Infections." *Sexually Transmitted Infections* 87 (Suppl 2): ii31–33.

Babigumira, J., H. Gelband, and L. P. Garrison Jr. 2017. "Cost-Effectiveness of Strategies for the Diagnosis and Treatment of Febrile Illness in Children." In *Disease Control Priorities* (third edition): Volume 6, *Major Infectious Diseases*, edited by K. K. Holmes, S. Bertozzi, B. R. Bloom, and P. Jha. Washington, DC: World Bank.

Baeten, J. M. 2016. "Making an Impact with Preexposure Prophylaxis for Prevention of HIV Infection." *Journal of Infectious Diseases* 214 (12): 1787–89.

Baeten, J. M., D. Donnell, P. Ndase, N. R. Mugo, J. D. Campbell, and others. 2012. "Antiretroviral Prophylaxis for HIV Prevention in Heterosexual Men and Women." *New England Journal of Medicine* 367 (5): 399–410.

Baral, S., C. Beyrer, K. Muessig, T. Poteat, A. L. Wirtz, and others. 2012. "Burden of HIV among Female Sex Workers in Low-Income and Middle-Income Countries: A Systematic Review and Meta-Analysis." *The Lancet Infectious Diseases* 12 (7): 538–49.

Baral, S., F. Sifakis, F. Cleghorn, and C. Beyrer. 2007. "Elevated Risk for HIV Infection among Men Who Have Sex with Men in Low- and Middle-Income Countries 2000–2006: A Systematic Review." *PLoS Medicine* 4 (12): e339.

Bloom, B. R., R. Atun, T. Cohen, C. Dye, H. Fraser, and others. 2017. "Tuberculosis." In *Disease Control Priorities* (third edition): Volume 6, *Major Infectious Diseases*, edited by K. K. Holmes, S. Bertozzi, B. R. Bloom, and P. Jha. Washington, DC: World Bank.

Burnett, S. M., M. K. Mbonye, R. Martin, A. Ronald, S. Zawedd-Muyania, and others. 2016. "Effect of On-Site Support on Laboratory Practice for Human Immunodeficiency Virus, Tuberculosis, and Malaria Testing." *American Journal of Clinical Pathology* 146 (4): 469–77.

Canchihuaman, F. A., P. J. García, S. S. Gloyd, and K. K. Holmes. 2011. "An Interactive Internet-Based Continuing Education Course on Sexually Transmitted Diseases for Physicians and Midwives in Peru." *PLoS One* 6 (5): e19318.

CDC (U.S. Centers for Disease Control and Prevention). 1993. "Recommendations of the International Task Force for Disease Eradication." *Morbidity and Mortality Weekly Report* 42 (RR-16): 8.

CDDEP (Center for Disease Dynamics, Economics and Policy). 2016. "Resistance Map." CDDEP, Washington, DC. http://www.cddep.org/projects/resistance-map.

Chalker, J., N. T. K. Chuc, T. Falkenberg, N. T. Do, and G. Tomson. 2000. "STD Management by Private Pharmacies in Hanoi: Practice and Knowledge of Drug Sellers." *Sexually Transmitted Infections* 76 (4): 299–302.

Chesson, H. W., P. Mayaud, and S. O. Aral. 2017. "Sexually Transmitted Infections: Impact and Cost-Effectiveness of Prevention." In *Disease Control Priorities* (third edition): Volume 6, *Major Infectious Diseases*, edited by K. K. Holmes, S. Bertozzi, B. R. Bloom, and P. Jha. Washington, DC: World Bank.

Crump, J., P. N. Newton, S. J. Baird, and Y. Lubell. 2017. "Febrile Illness in Adolescents and Adults." In *Disease Control Priorities* (third edition): Volume 6, *Major Infectious Diseases*, edited by K. K. Holmes, S. Bertozzi, B. R. Bloom, and P. Jha. Washington, DC: World Bank.

Dodd, P. J., G. P. Garnett, and T. B. Hallett. 2010. "Examining the Promise of HIV Elimination by 'Test and Treat' in Hyper-Endemic Settings." *AIDS* 24 (5): 729–35.

Du, L., J. You, K. M. Nicholas, and R. H. Cichewicz. 2016. "Chemoreactive Natural Products that Afford Resistance against Disparate Antibiotics and Toxins." *Angewandte Chemie International Edition* 18 (55): 4220–25.

Fitzpatrick, C., U. Nwankwo, E. Lenk, S. de Vlas, and D. Bundy. 2017. "An Investment Case for Ending Neglected Tropical Diseases." In *Disease Control Priorities* (third edition): Volume 6, *Major Infectious Diseases*, edited by K. K. Holmes, S. Bertozzi, B. R. Bloom, and P. Jha. Washington, DC: World Bank.

Fitzpatrick, M. C., and K. Floyd. 2012. "A Systematic Review of the Cost and Cost-Effectiveness of Treatment for Multidrug-Resistant Tuberculosis." *Pharmacoeconomics* 30 (1): 63–80.

Foster, A. L., M. M. Gaisa, R. M. Hijdra, S. S. Turner, T. J. Morey, and others. 2017. "Shedding of Hepatitis C Virus into the Rectum of HIV-Infected Men Who Have Sex with Men." *Clinical Infectious Diseases* 64 (3): 284–88.

García, P. J., C. P. Carcamo, G. P. Garnett, P. E. Campos, and K. K. Holmes. 2012. "Improved STD Syndrome Management by a Network of Clinicians and Pharmacy Workers in Peru: The PREVEN Network." *PLoS One* 7 (10): e47750.

Gavi, the Vaccine Alliance. 2011. "Market Shaping: Access to Low and Sustainable Vaccine Prices." Document 6a for the Gavi Pledging Conference, London, June 13. http://www.gavialliance.org/library/publications/pledging-conference-for-immunisation/6a--market-shaping--access-to-low-and-sustainable-vaccine-prices/.

Gomez, G. B., A. Borquez, K. K. Case, A. Wheelock, A. Vassall, and C. Hankins. 2013. "The Cost and Impact of Scaling Up Pre-Exposure Prophylaxis for HIV Prevention: A Systematic Review of Cost-Effectiveness Modelling Studies." *PLoS Medicine* 10 (3): e1001401.

Gower, E., C. Estes, S. Blach, K. Razavi-Shearer, and H. Razavi. 2014. "Global Epidemiology and Genotype Distribution of the Hepatitis C Virus Infection." *Journal of Hepatology* 61 (1): S45–57.

Grant, R. M., J. R. Lama, P. L. Anderson, V. McMahan, A. Y. Liu, and others. 2010. "Preexposure Chemoprophylaxis for HIV Prevention in Men Who Have Sex with Men." *New England Journal of Medicine* 363 (27): 2587–99.

Hader, S. 2017. "(Preventing) the Coming Epidemic: HIV in Youth." Presentation to the annual Conference on Retroviruses and Opportunistic Infections (CROI), Seattle, WA, February 15.

Harrison, O. B., K. Cole, J. Peters, F. Cresswell, G. Dean, and others. 2017. "Genomic Analysis of Urogenital and Rectal *Neisseria Meningitidis* Isolates Reveals Encapsulated Hyperinvasive Meningococci and Coincident Multidrug-Resistant Gonococci." *Sexually Transmitted Infections* 2017 (January): 1–7. doi:10.1136/sextrans-2016-052781.

Hecht, R., D. T. Jamison, J. Augenstein, G. Partridge, and K. Thorien. 2012. "Vaccine Research and Development." In *Rethink HIV: Smarter Ways to Invest in Ending HIV in Sub-Saharan Africa*, edited by B. Lomborg, 299–320. New York: Cambridge University Press.

Hutton, G., and C. Chase. 2017. "Water Supply, Sanitation, and Hygiene." In *Disease Control Priorities* (third edition): Volume 7, *Injury Prevention and Environmental Health*, edited by C. N. Mock, O. Kobusingye, R. Nugent, and K. R. Smith. Washington, DC: World Bank.

Imani, P. 2015. "Effect of Integrated Infectious Disease Training and On-Site Support on the Management of Childhood Illnesses in Uganda: A Cluster Randomized Trial." *BMC Pediatrics* 5 (13).

Jamison, D. T., J. G. Breman, A. R. Measham, G. Alleyne, M. Claeson, D. B. Evans, and P. Musgrove, eds. 2006. *Disease Control Priorities in Developing Countries*, second edition. Washington, DC: World Bank and Oxford University Press.

Jamison, D. T., W. H. Mosley, A. R. Measham, and J. L. Bobadilla, eds. 1993. *Disease Control Priorities in Developing Countries*. Washington, DC: World Bank and Oxford University Press.

Jamison, D. T., R. Nugent, H. Gelband, S. Horton, P. Jha, R. Laxminarayan, and C. N. Mock, eds. 2015–18. *Disease Control Priorities*. Third edition. 9 volumes. Washington, DC: World Bank.

Jenness, S. M., S. M. Goodreau, E. Rosenberg, E. N. Beylerian, K. W. Hoover, and others. 2016. "Impact of the Centers for Disease Control's HIV Preexposure Prophylaxis Guidelines for Men Who Have Sex with Men in the United States." *The Journal of Infectious Diseases* 214 (12): 1800–07.

Johnson, A. P., and N. Woodford. 2013. "Global Spread of Antibiotic Resistance: The Example of New Delhi Metallo-β-Lactamase (NDM)-Mediated Carbapenem Resistance." *Journal of Medical Microbiology* 62 (Pt 4): 499–513.

John-Stewart, G., R. W. Peeling, C. Levin, P. J. Garcia, D. Mabey, and J. Kinuthia. 2017. "Prevention of Mother-to-Child Transmission of HIV and Syphilis." In *Disease Control Priorities* (third edition): Volume 6, *Major Infectious Diseases*, edited by K. K. Holmes, S. Bertozzi, B. R. Bloom, and P. Jha. Washington, DC: World Bank.

Kahn, J. G., L. Bollinger, J. Stover, and E. Marseille. 2017. "Improving the Efficiency of the HIV/AIDS Policy Response: A Guide to Resource Allocation Modeling." In *Disease Control Priorities* (third edition): Volume 6, *Major Infectious Diseases*, edited by K. K. Holmes, S. Bertozzi, B. R. Bloom, and P. Jha. Washington, DC: World Bank.

Katz, I. T., and A. A. Wright. 2008. "Circumcision—A Surgical Strategy for HIV Prevention in Africa." *New England Journal of Medicine* 359 (23): 2412–15.

Kippax, S., and N. Stephenson. 2012. "Beyond the Distinction between Biomedical and Social Dimensions of HIV Prevention through the Lens of a Social Public Health." *American Journal of Public Health* 102 (5): 789–99.

Klein, E. Y., M. Makowsky, M. Orlando, E. Hatna, N. P. Braykov, and others. 2015. "Influence of Provider and Urgent Care Density across Different Socioeconomic Strata on Outpatient Antibiotic Prescribing in the USA." *Journal of Antimicrobial Chemotherapy* 70 (5): 1580–87.

Kratz, M. M, D. Weiss, A. Ridpath, J. R. Zucker, A. Geevarughese, and others. 2015. "Community-Based Outbreak of *Neisseria meningitidis* Serogroup C Infection in Men Who Have Sex with Men, New York City, New York, USA 2010–2013." *Emerging Infectious Disease* 21 (8): 1379–86.

Laxminarayan, R., T. Van Boeckel, and A. Teillant. 2015. "The Economic Costs of Withdrawing Antimicrobial Growth Promoters from the Livestock Sector." Food, Agriculture, and Fisheries Papers 78, Organisation for Economic Co-operation and Development, Paris.

Liang, X., S. Bi, W. Yang, L. Wang, G. Cui, and others 2009. "Evaluation of the Impact of Hepatitis B Vaccination among Children Born during 1992–2005 in China." *Journal of Infectious Diseases* 200 (1): 39–47.

Looker, K. J., A. S. Magaret, K. M. E. Turner, P. Vickerman, S. L. Gottliev, and others. 2015. "Global Estimates of Prevalent and Incident Herpes Simplex Virus Type 2 Infections in 2012." *PLoS One* 10 (10): e0140765.

Madhav, N., B. Oppenheim, M. Galivan, P. Mulembakani, E. Rubin, and N. Wolfe. 2018. "Pandemics: Risks, Impacts, and Mitigation." In *Disease Control Priorities* (third edition): Volume 9, *Disease Control Priorities: Improving Health and Reducing Poverty*, edited by D. T. Jamison, R. Nugent, H. Gelband, S. Horton, P. Jha, R. Laxminarayan, and C. N. Mock. Washington, DC: World Bank.

Miller-Petrie, M., S. Pant, and R. Laxminarayan. 2017. "Drug-Resistant Infections." In *Disease Control Priorities* (third edition): Volume 6, *Major Infectious Diseases*, edited by K. K. Holmes, S. Bertozzi, B. R. Bloom, and P. Jha. Washington, DC: World Bank.

Mohapatra, B., D. A. Warrell, W. Suraweera, P. Bhatia, N. Dhingra, and others. 2011. "Snakebite Mortality in India: A Nationally Representative Mortality Survey." *PLoS Neglected Tropical Diseases* 5 (4): e1018.

Mokdad, A. H., M. H. Forouzanfar, F. Daoud, A. A. Mokdad, C. El Bcheraoui, and others. 2016. "Global Burden of Diseases, Injury, and Risk Factors for Young People's Health during 1990–2013: A Systematic Analysis for the Global Burden of Disease Study 2013." *The Lancet* 387 (10036): 2383–401.

Nanduri, S., C. Foo, V. Ngo, C. Jarashow, R. Civen, and others. 2016. "Outbreak of Serogroup C Meningococcal Disease Primarily Affecting Men Who Have Sex with Men—Southern California." *Morbidity and Mortality Weekly Report* 65 (35): 939–40.

Newman, L., J. Rowley, S. Vander Hoorn, N. S. Wijesooriya, M. Unemo, and others. 2015. "Global Estimates of the Prevalence and Incidence of Four Curable Sexually Transmitted Infections in 2012 Based on Systematic Review and Global Reporting." *PLoS One* 10 (12): e0143304.

Norheim, O., P. Jha, K. Admasu, T. Godal, R. Hum, and others. 2015. "Avoiding 40% of the Premature Deaths in Each Country, 2010–30: Review of National Mortality Trends to Help Quantify the UN Sustainable Development Goal for Health." *The Lancet* 385 (9964): 239–52.

Okeke, I. N., K. P. Klugman, Z. A. Bhutta, A. G. Duse, P. Jenkins, and others. 2005. "Antimicrobial Resistance in Developing Countries. Part II: Strategies for Containment." *The Lancet Infectious Diseases* 5 (9): 568–80.

Owusu-Edusei, K., Jr., G. Tao, T. L. Gift, A. Wang, L. Wang, and others. 2014. "Cost-Effectiveness of Integrated Routine Offering of Prenatal HIV and Syphilis Screening in China." *Sexually Transmitted Diseases* 41 (2): 103–10.

Pretorius, C., J. Stover, L. Bollinger, N. Bacaer, and B. Williams. 2010. "Evaluating the Cost-Effectiveness of Pre-Exposure Prophylaxis (PrEP) and Its Impact on HIV-1 Transmission in South Africa." PLOS ONE 5(11).

Sánchez, J., E. Gotuzzo, J. Escamilla, C. Carrillo, L. Moreyra, and others. 1998. "Sexually Transmitted Infections in Female Sex Workers: Reduced by Condom Use but Not by a Limited Periodic Examination Program." *Sexually Transmitted Diseases* 25 (2): 82–89.

Schweitzer, A., J. Horn, R. T. Mikolajczyk, G. Krause, and J. J. Ott. 2015. "Estimations of Worldwide Prevalence of Chronic Hepatitis B Virus Infection: A Systematic Review of Data Published Between 1965 and 2013." *The Lancet* 386 (10003): 1546–55.

Shretta, R., J. Liu, C. Cotter, J. Cohen, C. Dolenz, and others. 2017. "Malaria Elimination and Eradication." In *Disease Control Priorities* (third edition): Volume 6, *Major Infectious Diseases*, edited by K. K. Holmes, S. Bertozzi, B. R. Bloom, and P. Jha. Washington, DC: World Bank.

Smith J. S., P. A. Gilbert, A. Melendy, R. K. Rana, and J. M. Pimenta. 2011. "Age-Specific Prevalence of Human Papillomavirus Infection in Males: A Global Review." *Journal of Adolescent Health* 48 (6): 540–52.

Stanaway, J. D., A. D. Flaxman, M. Naghavi, C. Fitzmaurice, T. Vos, and others. 2015. "The Global Burden of Viral Hepatitis from 1990 to 2013: Findings from the Global Burden of Disease Study 2013." *The Lancet* 388 (10049): 1081–88.

UN (United Nations). 2015a. *Resolution Adopted by the General Assembly on 25 September 2015. Transforming Our World: The 2030 Agenda for Sustainable Development.* Resolution A/RES/70/1, United Nations General Assembly, New York.

———. 2015b. *The Millennium Development Goals Report 2015.* New York: UN.

UNAIDS (Joint United Nations Programme on HIV/AIDS). 2015. *AIDS by the Numbers 2015.* Booklet, UNAIDS, Geneva.

———. 2016. "Global HIV Statistics." Fact sheet, November, UNAIDS, Geneva.

U.S. Department of Health and Human Services. 2014. *Guide for HIV/AIDS Clinical Care.* Clinical reference guide, HIV/AIDS Bureau, Health Resources and Services Administration, U.S. Department of Health and Human Services, Rockville, MD.

Van Boeckel, T. P., S. Gandra, A. Ashok, Q. Caudron, B. T. Grenfall, and others. 2014. "Global Antibiotic Consumption 2000 to 2010: An Analysis of National Pharmaceutical Sales Data." *The Lancet Infectious Diseases* 114 (8): 742–50.

Verguet, S., R. Laxminarayan, and D. T. Jamison. 2015. "Universal Public Finance of Tuberculosis Treatment in India: An Extended Cost-Effectiveness Analysis." *Health Economics* 24 (3): 318–32.

Weaver, M.R., S.M. Burnett, I. Crozier, S.N. Kinoti, I. Kirunda, and others. 2014. "Improving Facility Performance in Infectious Disease Care in Uganda: A Mixed Design Study with Pre/Post and Cluster Randomized Trial Components." *PLoS One.* 9(8).

WHO (World Health Organization). 2014. "Global Health Estimates 2014 Summary Tables: DALY by Cause, Age, Sex by World Bank Income Category, 2000–2012." WHO, Geneva. http://www.who.int/healthinfo/global_burden_disease/en.

———. 2015. *Investing to Overcome the Global Impact of Neglected Tropical Diseases: Third WHO Report on Neglected Tropical Diseases.* Geneva: WHO.

———. 2016a. *Global Tuberculosis Report 2016.* Geneva: WHO.

———. 2016b. "Sexually Transmitted Infections (STIs)." Fact sheet, WHO, Geneva.

———. 2017. "Ghana, Kenya and Malawi to Take Part in WHO Malaria Vaccine Pilot Programme." News Release, WHO, Geneva, April 24.

Wilson, D. P., B. Donald, A. J. Shattock, D. Wilson, and N. Fraser-Hurt. 2015. "The Cost-Effectiveness of Harm Reduction." *International Journal of Drug Policy* 26 (Suppl 1): S5–11.

Wilson, D. P., and J. Taaffe. 2017. "Tailoring the Local HIV/AIDS Response to Local HIV/AIDS Epidemic." In *Disease Control Priorities* (third edition): Volume 6, *Major Infectious Diseases*, edited by K. K. Holmes, S. Bertozzi, B. R. Bloom, and P. Jha. Washington, DC: World Bank.

Winer, R. L., J. P. Hughes, Q. Feng, L. F. Xi, S. K. Lee, and others. 2012. "Prevalence and Risk Factors for Oncogenic Human Papillomavirus Infections in High-Risk Mid-Adult Women." *Sexually Transmitted Diseases* 39 (11): 848–56.

World Bank. 1993. *World Development Report 1993: Investing in Health.* Washington, DC: World Bank and Oxford University Press.

———. 2012. *People, Pathogens and Our Planet: Volume 2, The Economics of One Health.* Economic and Sector Work, Report 69145-GLB. Washington, DC: World Bank.

World Health Assembly. 2005. *International Health Regulations (2005).* Geneva: World Health Organization.

Zhang, Y., B. Y. Lee, and J. M. Donohue. 2010. "Ambulatory Antibiotic Use and Prescription Drug Coverage in Older Adults." *Archives of Internal Medicine* 170 (15): 1308–14.

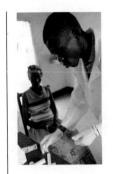

Chapter 2

Global Mortality and Morbidity of HIV/AIDS

Kristen Danforth, Reuben Granich, Danielle Wiedeman,
Sanjiv Baxi, and Nancy Padian

INTRODUCTION

The HIV/AIDS epidemic has seen dramatic shifts since the first cases were described in 1981. Initially perceived as a disease among gay men or Haitians in Western countries, HIV transmission has been reported in virtually all parts of the world. Prevalence levels in the 1990s reached more than 30 percent among adults in many Sub-Saharan African cities, and no accessible, effective treatment was available. Although treatment was available for a limited number of people in wealthier settings shortly after the studies on triple therapy in 1996, mortality nevertheless soared, particularly in Sub-Saharan Africa, slashing the hard-won gains in life expectancy resulting from social and economic development and advances in medical technology and nutrition (United Nations Population Division 2004) by more than a decade within a few years.

Since 2000, remarkable progress has been made in the diagnosis and treatment of persons living with HIV/AIDS. With medications now affordable at a cost of approximately US$129–$568 per person per year even in the hardest hit countries (Bendavid and others 2010; Menzies, Berruti, and Blandford 2012; PEPFAR 2013; UNAIDS 2015a; Walensky and others 2013), 17 million people were receiving antiretroviral therapy (ART) in 2015. The international targets are to treat nearly three-quarters of those living with HIV/AIDS by 2030 (UNAIDS 2012, 2014b, 2015b, 2016b; WHO 2013c).

ART has reduced HIV/AIDS morbidity and mortality significantly (Cohen and others 2011; Danel and others

2015; INSIGHT START Study Group 2015; Kitahata and others 2009; Lopez-Cortes, Gutierrez-Valencia, and Ben-Marzouk-Hidalgo 2016; Lundgren, Babiker, and Neaton 2016; Médecins Sans Frontières 2013; Montaner and others 2006; SMART Study Group and others 2006; Sterne and others 2009; Violari and others 2008). In high-income countries (HICs), access to early treatment has led to near-normal life expectancy for persons living with HIV/AIDS (Johnson and others 2013; May and others 2014; Rodger and others 2013; Samji and others 2013). As a result, the focus of clinical care of HIV/AIDS in these settings has shifted from treatment of a usually fatal infectious disease with multiple comorbidities (see chapter 4 [Harripersaud and others 2017] and chapter 11 [Bloom and others 2017] of this volume) to management of a chronic condition and prevention of illness, death, and transmission for individuals who remain adherent to treatment (Attia and others 2009; Cohen and others 2011; Das and others 2010; Fang and others 2004; Montaner and others 2010).

New Focus on Treatment and Care

Treatment access and care recommendations have dramatically changed all over the world since the second edition of *Disease Control Priorities in Developing Countries* (Jamison and others 2006) (Bertozzi and others 2006; WHO 2010, 2013a, 2015b). Accumulating evidence definitively demonstrates that treatment reduces morbidity and mortality, irrespective of disease stage or

Corresponding author: Kristen Danforth, School of Public Health, University of Washington, Seattle, Washington, United States; danfortk@uw.edu.

immunological competence, for example, CD4 level (Danel and others 2015; INSIGHT START Study Group 2015; Kitahata and others 2009). Treatment simultaneously prevents onward transmission (chapter 5 in this volume, Holmes and others 2017; Attia and others 2009). Accordingly, the dream of ending the epidemic as a public health threat by 2030 (UNAIDS 2015d) no longer seems impossible.

Expanded Surveillance

The drive to end the epidemic has resulted in the expansion of surveillance. In addition to tracking the burden of incidence, prevalence, and mortality, programs now track success in meeting the 90-90-90 targets as part of their efforts to monitor and evaluate the continuum of care (IAPAC 2016; UNAIDS 2014e, 2015c, 2016b).

The new focus on care in treatment is reflected in the recent changes in the World Health Organization's (WHO) guidelines (2015b) and demonstrated by the 90-90-90 campaign of the Joint United Nations Programme on HIV/AIDS (UNAIDS), which recommend treating infected individuals as soon as possible. These 90-90-90 targets propose achievement of the following by 2020:

- Ninety percent of all people living with HIV/AIDS will know their HIV/AIDS status
- Ninety percent of people with diagnosed HIV/AIDS infection (or 81 percent of all people living with HIV) will receive sustained ART
- Ninety percent of all people receiving ART will be virally suppressed—that is, will achieve 73 percent population-based suppression in people living with HIV (UNAIDS 2014a). Achieving 90-90-90 is the first step to ensuring access to treatment for nearly everyone by 2030, which could lead to ending AIDS as a public threat, as well as the virtual elimination of HIV transmission in many settings (Granich 2016).

The UNAIDS Fast-Track Targets for 2020 (Stover and others 2016) include reducing by 75 percent the number of people newly infected annually (compared with 2010), with zero new infections among children, and reducing the annual number of people dying from HIV/AIDS-related causes to fewer than 500,000. These targets are the next steps to the even more challenging yet achievable 95-95-95 goals for 2030, when annual deaths related to HIV/AIDS should be fewer than 200,000 and incidence should be reduced by 90 percent (compared with 2010).

Some may argue that this is an aspirational slogan, but assessing accomplishments in care is consistent with recent recommendations by the U.S. Centers for Disease Control (CDC) (AIDS.gov 2017). In addition, these targets are subject to meaurement challenges (many of which are described subsequently); however, they are critical to address success in epidemic control. Although measurement of disease burden is informative, it falls short of meeting needs in public health for which the influences of positive health—such as successes in care and treatment—must also be tracked (Thacker and others 2006).

In addition to monitoring regional burdens, more precise surveillance tools, including geospatial mapping and targeted surveillance, have uncovered microepidemics concentrated in small regions and in key, vulnerable populations, which heretofore might have been missed. The availability of such detailed surveillance data at subnational and smaller local levels has revealed the microepidemics defined by locality or risk group that fuel generalized epidemics in Sub-Saharan Africa (Tanser and others 2014). Although we address this phenomenon in this chapter, more extensive detail about the concentration of infection among key populations and risk groups is provided in chapter 8 of this volume (Wilson and Taaffe 2017).

Chapter Content

This chapter is divided into two sections. The first describes the distribution of surveillance indicators for effective monitoring of national HIV/AIDS programs. These indicators include the conventional, key outcomes of mortality and morbidity—incidence, prevalence, and disability-adjusted life years (DALYs)—as well as more recent indicators that reflect the pivot to ending the epidemic: tracking 90-90-90 targets and examining surveillance in smaller units of analysis, including microepidemics and key populations. The second part of the chapter addresses challenges in the measurement of all of these indicators.

Subsequent chapters in this volume address current cost-effective approaches for treatment (chapter 5, Holmes and others 2017), prevention of mother-to-child transmission (chapter 6, John-Stewart and others 2017), and combination prevention (chapter 7, Garnett and others 2017). The burden, prevention, and management of HIV/AIDS-related comorbidities, including other sexually transmitted infections and tuberculosis, are discussed in chapter 10 (Chesson and others 2017) and chapter 11 (Bloom and others 2017) of this volume. The goal of this chapter is not to provide a complete review of available data on burden, but rather to situate this volume—volume 6, *Major Infectious Diseases*—of the third edition of *Disease Control Priorities* (*DCP3*) in the context of an HIV/AIDS epidemic and response that is at a turning point.

DISTRIBUTION OF KEY EPIDEMIC MEASURES: MORTALITY, INCIDENCE, PREVALENCE, AND DALYS

Given the outsized importance of HIV/AIDS among donors and global health organizations, a variety of sources for burden of disease estimates at global and national levels exist, such as UNAIDS, the WHO, and the Institute for Health Metrics and Evaluation (UNAIDS 2016a; Wang and others 2016; WHO 2013b). To maintain consistency with the other volumes in the *DCP3* series and the chapters that follow in this volume, we focus primarily on data from two sources, UNAIDS and the WHO's Global Health Estimates, supplemented with country-specific studies, where relevant, for illustrative purposes. No estimate is without limitations, and the UNAIDS and WHO figures are no exception. These limitations are discussed in a later section, titled "Measurement: Challenges in Surveillance."

Global and Regional Trends in Mortality

Global trends in AIDS-related mortality reveal the remarkable success of HIV treatment and other prevention. Deaths peaked at just more than 2 million per year from 2004 to 2005 (figure 2.1) and have been steadily declining since, driven primarily by gains in Sub-Saharan Africa. The 1.1 million individuals who lost their lives to AIDS in 2015 represent the lowest number since 1998, and this number was 45 percent lower than at the peak of the epidemic (UNAIDS 2016a, 2016b). Despite this progress, high-burden countries will need to accelerate access to ART treatment to avert millions of premature AIDS deaths and new HIV infections (Granich and others 2015).

Despite these gains, AIDS remains a significant cause of death, and global trends mask persistent regional and subregional variation. AIDS is the sixth-leading cause of death globally and the leading cause in Sub-Saharan Africa, a fact that has not changed since 2000, despite the 41 percent decline in the region's AIDS-related mortality rate. AIDS was responsible for one in nine deaths in the WHO's African region in 2012 (WHO 2013b). In contrast to declining rates in Sub-Saharan Africa, AIDS-related mortality rates per 100,000 population from 2000 to 2012 increased from 3.6 to 10.2 in Europe, from 2.7 to 5.6 in the Eastern Mediterranean Region, and from 1.6 to 3.2 in the

Figure 2.1 Number of Deaths Related to AIDS, 1990–2015

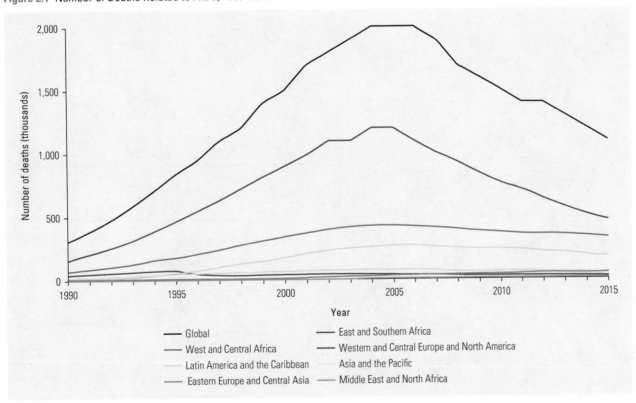

Source: Based on UNAIDS 2016a.
Note: AIDS = acquired immune deficiency syndrome.

Western Pacific Region. The numbers of AIDS-related deaths in Europe and the Eastern Mediterranean Region have also been steadily increasing and have tripled since 2000 (WHO 2013b).

Morbidity: Incidence and Prevalence

Trends in HIV/AIDS prevalence are similar to those of mortality, although one must note that by definition, increased treatment results in increased prevalence. In the current era of massive global antiretroviral scale up, with plans for reaching millions more (UNAIDS 2012, 2014b; WHO 2013c), there are critical drivers of changing morbidity in persons living with the disease. Most important, with earlier initiation of ART and improved access to care, persons with HIV are living longer (Kitahata and others 2009; Sterne and others 2009; SMART Study Group and others 2006; U.S. National Institutes of Health 2015; Violari and others 2008) and therefore are experiencing the health consequences of aging. This is an outcome of improved treatment options and increased access to interventions that lead to longer lives. Global prevalence rates peaked in

2001, three years earlier than AIDS-related mortality peaked, and they have been slowly declining or have plateaued over the past decade in most regions (figure 2.2). The trends in prevalence reveal that HIV/AIDS remains a predominantly East and Southern Africa health challenge, with a 2014 prevalence of 7.4 percent, more than triple that of the western and central part of the continent. However, low prevalence rates in low disease burden settings still present major challenges, even, for example, in the United States (Del Rio 2015). More to the point, although prevalence rates are currently low in Eastern Europe and Central Asia, they are the only regions where prevalence rates are still rising, with rates increasing from 0.1 percent in 1990 to 0.8 percent in 2014.

A central focus of the new UNAIDS goals is a 75 percent reduction in new infections (compared with 2010) by 2030. Models of incidence suffer from significant methodological limitations, which are discussed later in this chapter in the section on measurement challenges. Incident infections have fallen substantially since their peak of an estimated 3.5 million per year in 1997 to 2.1 million in 2015. However, current projections from UNAIDS and the Institute of Health Metrics and

Figure 2.2 Trends in HIV Prevalence, by Region, 1990–2015

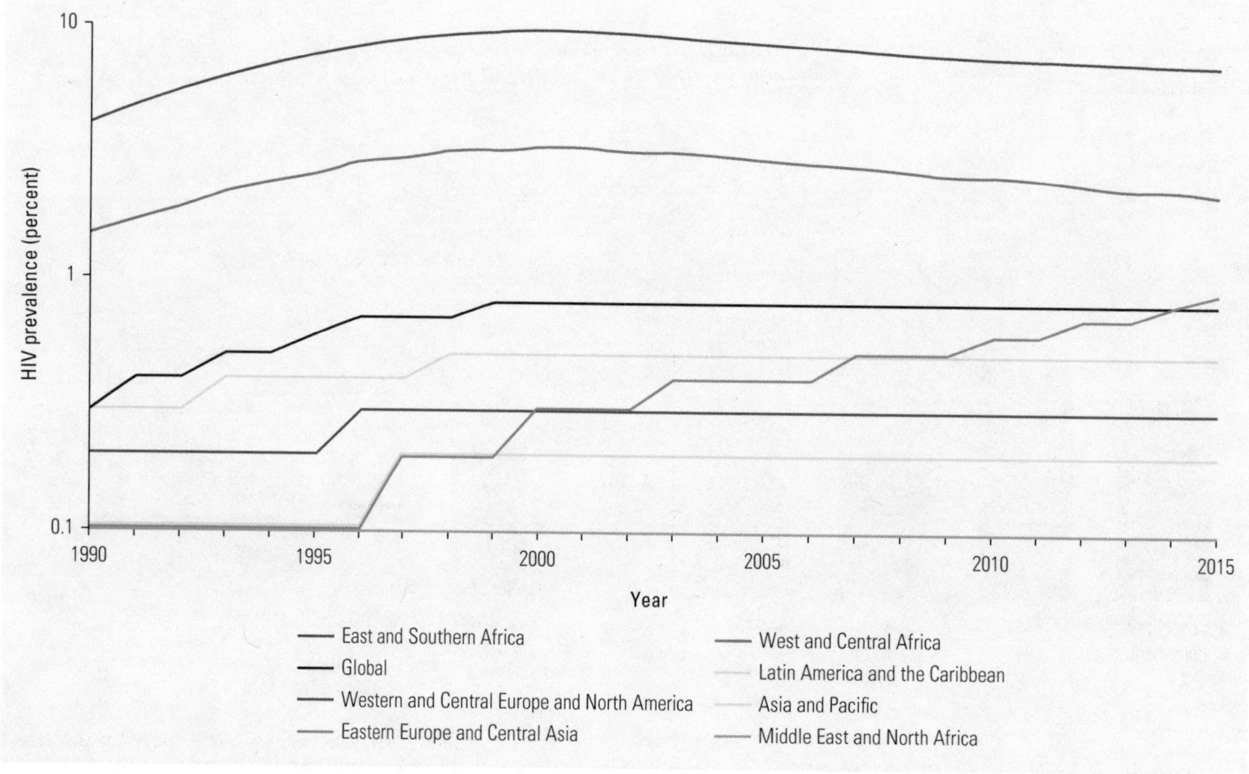

Source: Based on UNAIDS 2016a.
Note: HIV = human immunodeficiency virus.

Evaluation indicate that, in general, the world is not yet on track to meet the UNAIDS goal (UNAIDS 2016a; Wang and others 2016); new infections declined 14 percent globally between 2010 and 2014 (UNAIDS 2016a). Although HIV prevalence remains heavily concentrated in Africa, other regions have also emerged as important sources of new infections (figure 2.3). Between 1990 and 2015, the proportion of incident infections in East and Southern Africa steadily declined from 59 percent to 46 percent, and those in Eastern Europe and Central Asia and Asia and the Pacific steadily increased from 1 percent to 9 percent and from 10 percent to 15 percent, respectively. While these relative relationships are informative, the assumptions underlying incidence models, and thus current and future projections, are likely to be revised as new empirical data improve our knowledge about the effect of ART scale-up on HIV-transmission rates in these regions.

Morbidity: Disability-Adjusted Life Years

In 2012, 91.9 million DALYs were lost worldwide because of HIV/AIDS, second only to diarrhea in terms of morbidity from infectious disease and seventh overall, but

nevertheless representing a 9.6 percent decrease from 2000. In 2012, by region, Africa accounted for 66.8 million DALYs lost (72.7 percent); South-East Asia, 11.8 million (12.8 percent); Europe, 4.5 million (4.9 percent); Eastern Mediterranean, 2.0 million (2.2 percent); Western Pacific, 3.3 million (3.6 percent); and the Americas, 3.5 million (3.8 percent). HIV/AIDS is still the leading cause of morbidity in Africa, but DALYs lost declined 19.2 percent since 2000 (WHO 2013b). The Global Burden of Disease data present lower absolute values for DALYs (69.4 million in 2013), but show a similar decline from 2000 to 2013 (IHME 2016b).

As with mortality and incidence, these regional numbers mask significant subregional variation. In the African region, 31 percent of all DALYS lost in Botswana were due to HIV/AIDS (324,000), compared to 6.9 percent of DALYs in Ethiopia (3,353,000) and 4.3 percent of DALYs in Eritrea (126,000) (WHO 2013b).

The trends in global DALYs show both the promise of ART and the gap that remains in getting effective treatment to all who need it and ensuring adherence among those receiving it. The decline in DALYs is driven largely by reductions in AIDS deaths, and thus the pattern of DALYs lost because of HIV/AIDS parallels that for

Figure 2.3 Proportion of Incident HIV Infections, by Region, 1990 and 2015
thousands

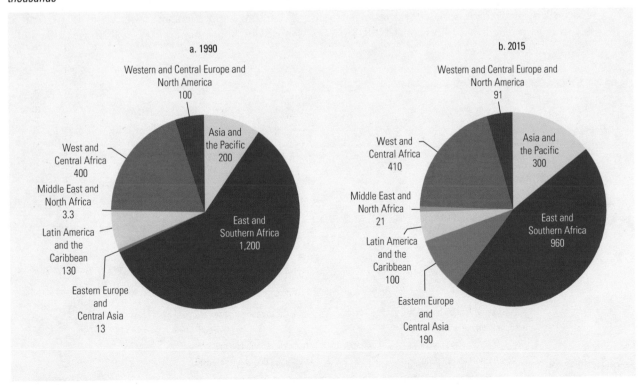

Source: Based on UNAIDS 2016a.
Note: HIV = human immunodeficiency virus.

mortality (Wang and others 2016). Although deaths decreased 18 percent between 2000 and 2012, morbidity declined by only 9.6 percent (UNAIDS 2016a; WHO 2013b). One contributing factor is that a small but important portion of morbidity is due to years lived with disability, which has plateaued since 2005, driven in part by the estimated 46 percent of HIV-positive individuals globally who are not currently on ART (IHME 2016a; UNAIDS 2016b; Wang and others 2016). Among those who are, fewer than half remain virally suppressed three years after initiating treatment (UNAIDS 2015b; WHO 2015a). A better understanding of the structure and composition of epidemics, including global resource allocation for AIDS (Granich and others 2016) within countries, is an essential next step as the world shifts from trying to manage the epidemic to trying to end it.

REACHING THE 90-90-90 TARGETS

Tracking progress toward the achievement of the 90-90-90 targets is a central challenge for surveillance efforts, particularly in measurement, given the lack of individual cohort data from most regions. Moreover, the methods used to determine the national cascades included in estimating regional cascades often vary and often do not follow the WHO recommendations. The lack of viral load data necessary for estimating the final component of the cascade is particularly problematic because the data are not available to most people living with HIV (UNAIDS 2014e).

As such, regional cascade results should be viewed with considerable caution. Nevertheless, even these suboptimal estimates reveal critical trends. Perhaps more important, especially with regard to comparative estimates across countries or regions or over time, the data enforce the value of monitoring the health outcomes that are essential for epidemic control.

Preliminary estimates from Levi and others (2016), based on data from 69 countries for which data were available, show that progress is uneven.

Progress in achieving the first 90 percent in predominantly high-income regions is encouraging; in six out of nine countries across North America, Australasia, and Western Europe, 80 percent or more of individuals know their HIV status. In the majority of these countries, the most significant gap is the proportion of HIV-positive individuals who currently receive ART. Conversely, in lower-income regions, the need for scaled-up testing services coupled with demand creation to meet the first 90 percent target is great. For example, data from Levi and others (2015) for countries where full treatment cascades were available in the African and Asian regions suggest that fewer than half of all HIV-positive individuals are aware of their status (figure 2.4). In Sub-Saharan Africa, the majority of those who know they are HIV-positive are successfully initiated on ART, and roughly 75 percent achieve viral suppression. For the Kyrgyz Republic, the Russian Federation, and Vietnam, fewer than 35 percent of those who know they are HIV-positive are successfully

Figure 2.4 Cascade of HIV Care in Africa and Asia

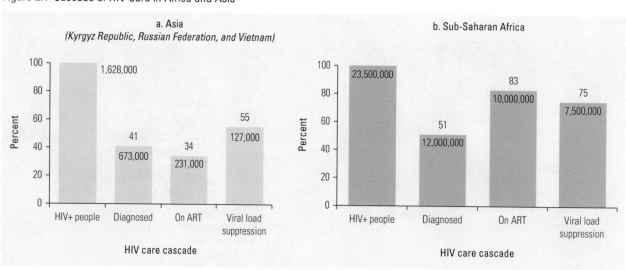

Sources: Adapted from data from Levi and others 2015; UNAIDS 2015e.
Note: ART = antiretroviral therapy; HIV = human immunodeficiency virus. The numbers above each bar represent the number of individuals at that stage as a proportion of the number of individuals at the preceding stage. Sub-Saharan Africa viral load data from Botswana, Burkina Faso, Cameroon, Côte d'Ivoire, Kenya, Malawi, Mali, Mozambique, Nigeria, Senegal, South Africa, Tanzania, Uganda, Zambia, and Zimbabwe.

initiated on ART, and among these, only about half are virally suppressed. Data such as these, which are essential to inform program planners where to effectively invest resources, illustrate the uneven progress of regions toward achievement of the 90-90-90 targets. These data also reinforce how success cannot be realized without consideration of the complete cascade. Although rates of viral suppression among those on ART in the 15 Sub-Saharan African countries with data available are high, the very low rates of diagnosis mean that, overall, fewer than 32 percent of HIV-positive individuals in those countries are virally suppressed.

REGIONAL MICROEPIDEMICS AND KEY POPULATIONS

Regional Microepidemics

Global and regional estimates conceal significant country-level heterogeneity and within-country variability that is characterized by microepidemics—pockets of illness concentrated among specific populations and smaller subnational geographic regions. In Brazil, most AIDS cases and HIV infections occur in fewer than 10 percent of the country's 5,570 municipalities (UNAIDS 2014c). In India, national prevalence was only 0.4 percent in 2011, but 71 of 672 districts had a prevalence of ≥ 1.0 percent. Three-quarters of these 71 districts are located in the southern and northeastern parts of the country (National AIDS Control Organisation 2012).

Similarly, although the epidemic is disproportionately concentrated in countries of East and Southern Africa, pockets of high rates of transmission within countries are driving the spread of the disease. Data from 1,724 sites supported by the President's Emergency Plan for AIDS Relief (PEPFAR) and community-based services in Zimbabwe show that from October 2013 to September 2014, approximately 80 percent of all newly diagnosed people living with HIV/AIDS were identified by only 30 percent of sites (figure 2.5).

One of the earliest studies to investigate subnational analyses examined geospatial data on HIV/AIDS in KwaZulu-Natal, South Africa (MEASURE Evaluation 2016; Tanser and others 2009). Within a relatively homogeneous population, where age-adjusted prevalence was 27 percent for women and 14 percent for men, local prevalence had notable spatial variation, with three very-high-prevalence clusters (approximately 36 percent) along the main national road and three relatively low-prevalence clusters (6 percent) (Tanser and others 2009). In another study, Magadi (2013) examined spatial distribution of HIV/AIDS infection in relation to various demographic factors. She found that the urban poor in Sub-Saharan Africa had significantly higher rates of infection than did their urban nonpoor counterparts and that the well-documented higher risk among women was amplified among the urban poor.

Anderson and others (2014) modeled and demonstrated the importance of targeting prevention services, including early treatment, to microepidemics. For example, in Kenya, just 9 of 47 counties represented an

Figure 2.5 HIV Diagnoses Yield from PEPFAR-Supported Testing Sites, Zimbabwe, 2013–14

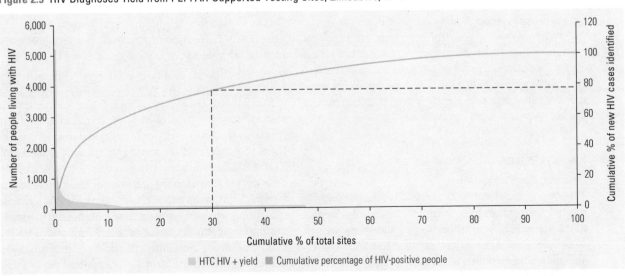

Source: UNAIDS 2015d.

Note: HIV = human immunodeficiency virus; HTC = HIV testing and counseling; PEPFAR = President's Emergency Plan for AIDS Relief.

Map 2.1 Estimated New Infections in Kenya, 2014

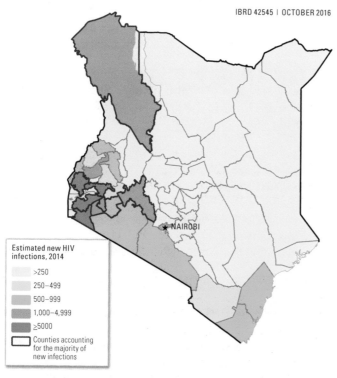

IBRD 42545 | OCTOBER 2016

Estimated new HIV
infections, 2014

- >250
- 250–499
- 500–999
- 1,000–4,999
- ≥5000
- Counties accounting
  for the majority of
  new infections

Source: UNAIDS 2015d.

estimated 65 percent of all new infections, and HIV prevalence varied substantially across counties, from less than 1 percent to 22 percent in 2014 (map 2.1) (UNAIDS 2015d). Similar uneven regional variation can also be seen in the United States (map 2.2) and in many other countries. Using these data to model the rollout of prevention programs, Anderson and others (2014) demonstrated that a focused approach using local epidemiologic data to direct prevention programs would achieve greater effect than would a uniform approach for the same amount of investment. Such focused surveillance is necessary for a more targeted response to the epidemic and is the hallmark of PEPFAR 3.0 and the pivot to a data-driven approach that strategically targets microepidemics, hot spots, and key populations.

Key Populations

Defining Key Populations

The emergence of smaller, subnational regions as substantial contributors to incident infections is due in part to the presence of key populations, traditionally defined as people who inject drugs, commercial sex workers, and men who have sex with men (MSM), (addressed more fully in chapter 8 of this volume [Wilson and Taaffe 2017]), and more recently, young women and

mobile migrant populations in Sub-Saharan Africa. Given that issues related to stigma, discrimination, and punitive legislations make tracking these groups extremely challenging, some patterns are clear. High rates of transmission among people who inject drugs and among sex workers are the main drivers of new infections in the Middle East and North Africa, and MSM is the main contributor in Latin America and the Caribbean. In Pakistan, transmission to female spouses of HIV-positive injection drug users and bisexual men, and subsequently to children through mother-to-child transmission, is a critical source of new infections in these regions. Patterns vary substantially across countries in Eastern Europe and Central Asia with respect to the relative contribution of such key populations (Gouws and Cuchi, on behalf of the International Collaboration on Estimating HIV Incidence by Modes of Transmission 2012), which is limited by the severe lack of data and signficant issues in surveillance discussed subsequently. Similarly, the pattern within Africa is mixed. In Kenya, HIV/AIDS overall prevalence among key populations is extremely high at 5.3 percent: 29 percent among sex workers, 18 percent among MSM, and 18 percent among people who inject drugs (UNAIDS 2015d, 2016a).

Other key populations include prisoners and individuals in the military, for whom regional statistics are sorely lacking. The risk of infection among transgender people has recently emerged as a public health emergency. Although the global picture of HIV/AIDS among transgender people is varied—with HIV prevalence ranging from 8 percent to 68 percent—transgender people are among the groups most affected by HIV/AIDS, particularly in the Latin America and the Caribbean and Asia and the Pacific regions (WHO 2011).

These studies highlight the assumption that significant proportions of new HIV infections, even in Sub-Saharan Africa, may occur among key populations (Hirnschall 2015). This means that no way exists to fully end the epidemic without addressing infections in these key populations, even though stigma, social norms, and legal restrictions present formidable challenges to identifying and engaging them in programs for prevention or care (Wilson and Taaffe 2017).

A deeper dive into the statistics in the United States reveals that minority race, especially African Americans, constitutes another key population. African Americans are overrepresented among people living with HIV in every region in the United States. In contrast, Asians and Caucasians constitute the proportion of the population with the lowest infection rates. Notably, adjusting for poverty reduces the magnitude of these differences,

Map 2.2 Rates of Persons Ages 25–34 Years Living with HIV/AIDS Diagnosis, by County, United States, 2013

IBRD 42546 | OCTOBER 2016

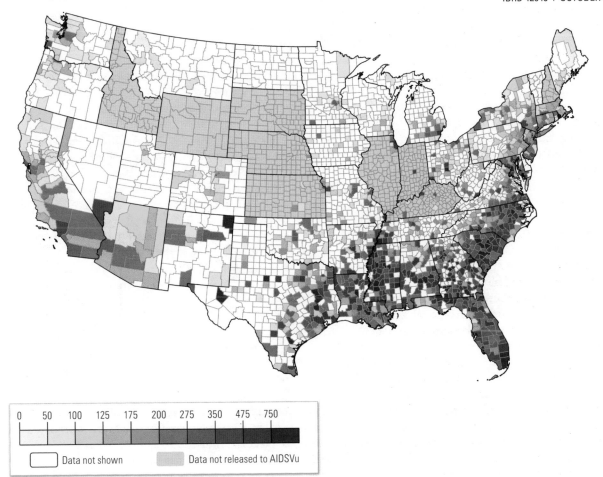

0   50   100   125   175   200   275   350   475   750

Data not shown   Data not released to AIDSVu

Source: AIDSVu 2016.
Note: AIDS = acquired immune deficiency syndrome; HIV = human immunodeficiency virus.

but it did not change the trends based on race and ethnicity (Del Rio 2015). These same trends are mirrored in AIDS cases and in access to HIV-specific health services (Del Rio 2015) and show that many of the challenges and surveillance needs in LMICs discussed in this chapter are also relevant to HICs, and substantial opportunities exist for cross-learning.

Reaching 90-90-90 Targets among Key Populations

Not surprisingly, the success in meeting 90-90-90 targets also varies by key populations; factors such as stigma and discrimination present even greater obstacles to linking these populations to care. One study of people living with HIV/AIDS in the United States found that only 59 percent of transgender participants, compared to 82 percent of participants with a birth-assigned gender, were accessing ART (Melendez and others 2006). HIV/AIDS-related stigma also creates a barrier to getting tested for many key

populations. In one study in the United States, 73 percent of transgender women who tested HIV-positive were previously unaware of their status (U.S. CDC 2011), a figure that can be far greater in other parts of the world. Similarly, in the Asia and Pacific region, fewer than half of the key populations know their HIV status (figure 2.6).

MEASUREMENT: CHALLENGES IN SURVEILLANCE

Prevalence and Incidence

Any summary report of morbidity and mortality is only as good as available data and the methodologies used for collection. The accuracy of estimates of prevalence, incidence, and disease-specific mortality are challenging for any health outcome, especially in low-income, high-mortality countries where vital registration and

Figure 2.6 HIV Testing Coverage among Key Populations, Asia and Pacific Region, 2007–12

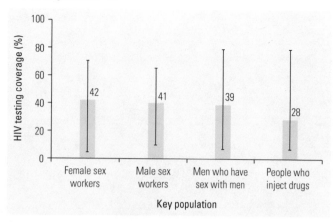

Source: UNAIDS 2014a.
Note: HIV = human immunodeficiency virus.

cause-of-death data may be lacking or incomplete (Lopman and others 2006; Mathers and others 2005; Murray and Lopez 2013). As a result, almost all global or large regional estimates of morbidity and mortality require some modeling, the results of which can vary depending on assumptions and sources of data (Flaxman, Vos, and Murray 2015; UNAIDS 2014d). For example, for generalized epidemics, UNAIDS estimates are based on routine surveillance of antenatal clinics, augmented with results from population-based household surveys, where available (UNAIDS 2013). These estimates can lead to oversampling of urban populations and provide no direct information on HIV/AIDS prevalence rates in men. These data are supplemented by models of transmission from Spectrum (UNAIDS 2016c) and models of progression from the International Epidemiologic Databases to Evaluate AIDS. These data sources tend to underrepresent high-risk groups within the general population, and UNAIDS estimates for concentrated epidemics rely on extrapolating from individual studies of key populations (Mahy 2016; UNAIDS 2013).

A salient example of the limitations and fragility of these surveillance methods is the revised estimate by UNAIDS of infection and mortality among adolescents presented at the 2016 meeting of the International AIDS Society (Mahy 2016). On the basis of more robust empirical data on the relative demographic growth of adolescents, the effect of prevention of mother-to-child transmission programs, and ART coverage among adolescents, estimates of adolescent HIV/AIDS-related mortality were revised. Significantly, HIV/AIDS-specific causes of death are now ranked eighth in the leading causes of death in this age group, down from second before these revisions.

Moreover, regardless of the accuracy of surveillance tools, population-based prevalence estimates invariably suffer from survey methodological limitations, such as representativeness and potential nonresponse bias (Flaxman, Vos, and Murray 2015). These challenges can be particularly salient for HIV/AIDS because of social reasons, such as the persistent stigma and discrimination that come with a diagnosis (Tanser and others 2014) or with identification as a person in a key population that is at exceptionally high-risk (see chapter 8 in this volume [Wilson and Taaffe 2017]) and with the methodological challenges of assessing an asymptomatic infection for which representative sampling is imperative.

Most surveillance is primarily designed to assess mortality and prevalence. However, epidemics change; although incidence is associated with prevalence, other factors, such as migration, mortality, survival rates, and the inherent epidemic trajectory, attenuate the legitimacy of using prevalence as a measure of incidence (Brookmeyer 2010). Incidence rates modeled from prevalence are also constrained by the time between surveys, as well as in-and-out population mobility and migration that is especially critical for men in Sub-Saharan Africa who often migrate for work (Brookmeyer 2010; Busch and others 2010; Hallett and others 2008; Marston, Harriss, and Slaymaker 2008). Although incidence rates obtained from prospective data are most robust, these rates are subject to the potential for nonrandom loss to follow-up where sicker individuals are more likely to be lost. Newer surveillance methods using a geospatial approach to monitoring, combined with more reliable incidence assays, can provide more robust estimates to identify weaker performance sites or regions where enhanced efforts are warranted. Data from PEPFAR-supported, ongoing, population-based HIV/AIDS impact assessments—a multicountry initiative to measure the reach and impact of programs in PEPFAR-supported countries through population-based surveys to estimate incidence, prevalence, and viral load suppression among adults and children in Malawi, Uganda, Zambia, and Zimbabwe—should be well-suited to this purpose (ICAP 2016).

Loss to Follow-Up

Loss to follow-up also affects facility-based HIV/AIDS surveillance estimates. Even at care and treatment clinics that have individual-level patient data, high rates of loss to follow-up undermine estimates of facility-based survival and mortality (Egger and others 2011; Geng, Bangsberg, and others 2010; Geng, Glidden, and others 2010; Geng, Nash, and others 2010; Geng and others 2008; Geng and others 2012; Geng and others 2013). Attempts to validate HIV/AIDS-related mortality have been attempted through verbal autopsies (Lopman and others 2006) and actual autopsies (Coulibaly and others 1994; Domoua and others 1995; Greenberg and others 1995; Lucas, Diomande, and others 1994; Lucas, Hounnou, and others 1994). However, verbal autopsies lack external validity and must be tailored to specific context, and actual autopsies present a major challenge to scale-up. Unfortunately, the costs and efforts required to intensively track all missing patients is likely to be prohibitive in most settings.

Geng and others (2015) offer a viable alternative: intensively trace a manageable *random* sample of the individuals lost to follow-up and incorporate their weighted outcomes into the available clinic sample. The power of this approach is evident in a review they conducted of mortality from 14 clinics in Eastern Africa. Sample-corrected estimates of three-year mortality in each clinic ranged from 2 times to more than 10 times higher compared to the naïve (that is, unadjusted) estimates (Geng, Odeny, and Lyamuya 2016; Geng and others 2015). Similar results are apparent from additional analyses in the same clinics also by Geng, Odeny, and Lyamuya (2016) examining retention in care. Using only routine clinic data without supplementation by tracing, after two years of ART, they found 26 percent of patients were reported as lost to follow-up; sampled corrected estimates revealed that 14 percent of the clinic population who were presumed lost had actually transferred their care elsewhere. Although such data can be used to correct facility or regional estimates, they require individual data collection.

Cohort approaches allow for accountability for each patient started on treatment, and with the push toward 90-90-90, programs that use unique identifiers for those diagnosed with HIV coupled with a national cohort will be able to better account for retention—including transfers from clinic to clinic and other outcomes, regardless of geographic location. As in other transmissible infectious diseases programs that are responsible for providing access to successful treatment, this approach will ensure access to life-saving treatment, prevent transmission, and allow follow-up for everyone on ART.

Surveillance at Smaller Units of Analysis: Microepidemics and Key Populations

Regional and subnational variation discussed throughout this chapter is in addition to mapping infection by key populations (Wilson and Taaffe 2017). The principle of "knowing your epidemic" (UNAIDS 2008) has shifted to "know your local epidemics," and the practice of monitoring data at the country or province level has shifted to collecting data at the community and facility levels (UNAIDS 2014c). These more precise pictures of the epidemic permit local governments to set priorities,

devote resources, and design programs that clearly match local epidemic realities and to determine whether HIV/AIDS services are appropriately matched, sufficient, and best packaged.

To facilitate these kinds of analyses, the UNAIDS Reference Group on Estimates, Modelling and Projections is reconsidering assumptions underlying the Spectrum model that drives surveillance estimates. The group is working toward standardizing the data collection that underlies spatial analysis, as well as the optimal methods and the frequency of use of such methods, recognizing the need for user-friendly programs to make these estimates possible (UNAIDS Reference Group on Estimates, Modelling and Projections 2013). Other modeling efforts will also be helpful to provide a critique of the standard approaches as we learn more about the effect on incidence and prevalence of key interventions such as treatment, circumcision, and other prevention methods. Supplemental phylogenetic studies assess the contribution of high-risk groups and provide critical knowledge about transmission dynamics and the accuracy of targeting those at risk. However, the cost and technical capacity for such studies currently prohibit their widespread use. A related ongoing challenge is the best method for empirical estimation of population sizes of hidden high-risk groups (Tanser and others 2014). In settings nearing HIV elimination, future efforts will likely rely on the most current phylogentic studies to identify new cases in clusters combined with traditional public health outbreak control methods to end ongoing transmission.

MEASUREMENT: CHALLENGES IN ASSESSING THE 90-90-90 TARGETS

The tremendous benefits in early treatment and viral suppression, both for improving individual health and stemming transmission, have led to the 90-90-90 framing of the HIV/AIDS response, led by UNAIDS, PEPFAR, and other organizations. Surveillance efforts now aim to track the success in meeting these targets; methodologies for doing so have been standardized to the extent possible to permit regional and national comparisons using numerous population-based household surveys—primarily the Demographic and Health Surveys for 24 countries conducted between 2007 and 2013 and for the first 90 percent.

- Given the methodological issues and potential biases related to survey data, getting a robust estimate of the true percentage of people in a population who are infected remains a challenge, although the use of biologic sampling and careful attention to regional variations have improved newer surveys.

- The first 90 percent, HIV diagnosis, is estimated using the number of people diagnosed with HIV divided by the estimate of people living with HIV. UNAIDS produces annual estimates for the denominator (number of people living with HIV).
- The second 90 percent, treatment coverage, is estimated using the annual country figure for the number of people on treatment (N) divided by the number of people diagnosed with HIV. UNAIDS produces annual and midyear estimates for treatment coverage (Stover and others 2014; UNAIDS 2016c).
- The third 90 percent is derived from the universal viral load indicator that is defined in the Global AIDS Response Progress reports and is the percentage of people on ART who are virally suppressed, but it is the estimate for which the data are weakest. Viral load data are often not available for everyone on treatment, and surrogate measures such as the proportion of samples in the national lab that meet viral suppression criteria are often used for estimates (UNAIDS 2015c).

As noted previously, accurate estimates can only be derived using a cohort approach. Valid measurement of these targets requires that individuals be followed longitudinally from the time they are tested until the time they are virally suppressed. This level of granularity would also provide more robust estimates of microepidemics and key populations in both prevalence and incidence. This level is essential for monitoring long-term follow-up.

CONCLUSIONS

As HIV/AIDS programmatic efforts transition to a unified focus on ending the epidemic by 2030 (UNAIDS 2015d), new demands, including accurate monitoring of 90-90-90 goals, are being placed on monitoring and surveillance strategies. Broad measures of national prevalence and mortality are no longer sufficient to guide interventions that will need to increase in efficiency to effectively target hard-to-reach populations. Data needed to target key populations and microepidemics will need to be collected through subnational surveillance methods, which have both time and budget implications. Expanding resources for surveillance and monitoring of a disease that is already one of the best documented in history may not be appealing in an era of ever-increasing competing priorities, but it will be necessary if programs are to be targeted in order to maximize their effect. Improved surveillance systems and techniques must be responsive to and informed by effective interventions for treatment and other prevention interventions.

Notably, however, the critical nature of this approach is not new. It parallels the need for targeted active case-finding, long recognized as a critical aspect of epidemic control for diseases such as smallpox (Kerrod and others 2005), severe acute respiratory syndrome (Cheng and others 2013), Ebola virus (Tom-Aba and others 2015), and tuberculosis (Yuen and others 2015). The ability to accomplish disease control is a global good and requires an ongoing international effort; neither risk nor infection respects political boundaries, and our ability to improve public health is directly dependent on the weakest link in the chain.

NOTE

World Bank Income Classifications as of July 2014 are as follows, based on estimates of gross national income (GNI) per capita for 2013:

- Low-income countries (LICs) = US$1,045 or less
- Middle-income countries (MICs) are subdivided:
  (a) lower-middle-income = US$1,046 to US$4,125
  (b) upper-middle-income (UMICs) = US$4,126 to US$12,745
- High-income countries (HICs) = US$12,746 or more.

REFERENCES

AIDS.gov. 2017. "National HIV/AIDS Strategy: Overview." https://www.aids.gov/federal-resources/national-hiv-aids -strategy/overview/.

AIDSVu. 2016. "Maps—AIDSVu." Rollins School of Public Health, Emory University. http://aidsvu.org/map/.

Anderson, S. J., P. Cherutich, N. Kilonzo, I. Cremin, D. Fecht, and others. 2014. "Maximising the Effect of Combination HIV Prevention through Prioritisation of the People and Places in Greatest Need: A Modelling Study." *The Lancet* 384 (9939): 249–56.

Attia, S., M. Egger, M. Muller, M. Zwahlen, and N. Low. 2009. "Sexual Transmission of HIV According to Viral Load and Antiretroviral Therapy: Systematic Review and Meta-Analysis." *AIDS* 23 (11): 1397–404.

Bendavid, E., E. Leroux, J. Bhattacharya, N. Smith, and G. Miller. 2010. "The Relation of Price of Antiretroviral Drugs and Foreign Assistance with Coverage of HIV Treatment in Africa: Retrospective Study." *BMJ* 341: C6218.

Bertozzi, S., N. S. Padian, J. Wegbreit, L. M. Demaria, B. Feldman, and others. 2006. "HIV/AIDS Prevention and Treatment." In *Disease Control Priorities in Developing Countries* (second edition), edited by D. T. Jamison, J. G. Breman, A. R. Measham, G. Alleyne, M. Claeson, D. B. Evans, P. Jha, A. Mills, and P. Musgrove. Washington, DC: Oxford University Press and World Bank.

Bloom, B. R., R. Atun, T. Cohen, C. Dye, H. Fraser, and others. 2017. "Tuberculosis." In *Disease Control Priorities* (third edition): Volume 6, *Major Infectious Diseases*, edited by K. K. Holmes, S. Bertozzi, B. R. Bloom, and P. Jha. Washington, DC: World Bank.

Brookmeyer, R. 2010. "Measuring the HIV/AIDS Epidemic: Approaches and Challenges." *Epidemiologic Reviews* 32: 26–37.

Busch, M. P., C. D. Pilcher, T. D. Mastro, J. Kaldor, G. Vercauteren, and others. 2010. "Beyond Detuning: 10 Years of Progress and New Challenges in the Development and Application of Assays for HIV Incidence Estimation." *AIDS* 24 (18): 2763–71.

Cheng, V. C., J. F. Chan, K. K. To, and K. Y. Yuen. 2013. "Clinical Management and Infection Control of SARS: Lessons Learned." *Antiviral Research* 100 (2): 407–19.

Chesson, H. W., S. O. Aral, and P. Mayaud. 2017. "Sexually Transmitted Infections: Impact and Cost-Effectiveness of Prevention." In *Disease Control Priorities* (third edition): Volume 6, *Major Infectious Diseases*, edited by K.K. Holmes, S. Bertozzi, B. R. Bloom, and P. Jha. Washington, DC: World Bank.

Cohen, M. S., Y. Q. Chen, M. Mccauley, T. Gamble, M. C. Hosseinipour, and others. 2011. "Prevention of HIV-1 Infection with Early Antiretroviral Therapy." *New England Journal of Medicine* 365 (6): 493–505.

Coulibaly, G., M. N'Dhatz, K. Domoua, E. Aka-Danguy, F. Traore, and others. 1994. "[Prevalence of Pneumocystosis in HIV-Infected Patients in a Pneumology Unit. Autopsy Study Performed in Abidjan (Côte d'Ivoire)]." *Revue de Pneumologie Clinique* 50 (3): 116–20.

Danel, C., R. Moh, D. Gabillard, A. Badje, J. Le Carrou, and others. 2015. "A Trial of Early Antiretrovirals and Isoniazid Preventive Therapy in Africa." *New England Journal of Medicine* 373 (9): 808–22.

Das, M., P. L. Chu, G. M. Santos, S. Scheer, E. Vittinghoff, and others. 2010. "Decreases in Community Viral Load Are Accompanied by Reductions in New HIV Infections in San Francisco." *PLoS One* 5 (6): e11068.

Del Rio, C. 2015. "Health Disparities: What Do They Have to Do with CFAR?" 19th Annual CFAR Meeting, Center for Applied Rationality, Seattle, WA, November 4–6.

Domoua, K., M. N'Dhatz, G. Coulibaly, F. Traore, J. B. Konan, and others. 1995. "[Autopsy Findings in 70 AIDS Patients Who Died in a Department of Pneumology in Ivory Coast: Impact of Tuberculosis]." *Medecine Tropicale: Revue du Corps de Sante Colonial* 55 (3): 252–54.

Egger, M., B. D. Spycher, J. Sidle, R. Weigel, E. H. Geng, and others. 2011. "Correcting Mortality for Loss to Follow-Up: A Nomogram Applied to Antiretroviral Treatment Programmes in Sub-Saharan Africa." *PLoS Medicine* 8 (1): e1000390.

Fang, C. T., H. M. Hsu, S. J. Twu, M. Y. Chen, Y. Y. Chang, and others. 2004. "Decreased HIV Transmission after a Policy of Providing Free Access to Highly Active Antiretroviral Therapy in Taiwan." *Journal of Infectious Diseases* 190 (5): 879–85.

Flaxman, A. D., T. Vos, and C. J. Murray. 2015. *An Integrative Metaregression Framework for Descriptive Epidemiology.* Publications on Global Health, Institute for Health Metrics and Evaluation. Seattle, WA: University of Washington Press.

Garnett, G. P., S. Krishnaratne, K. Harris, T. B. Hallett, M. Santos, and others. 2017. "Cost-Effectiveness of Interventions to Prevent HIV Acquisition." In *Disease Control Priorities* (third edition): Volume 6, *Major Infectious Diseases*, edited by K. K. Holmes, S. Bertozzi, B. R. Bloom, and P. Jha. Washington, DC: World Bank.

Geng, E. H., D. R. Bangsberg, N. Musinguzi, N. Emenyonu, M. B. Bwana, and others. 2010. "Understanding Reasons for and Outcomes of Patients Lost to Follow-Up in Antiretroviral Therapy Programs in Africa Through a Sampling-Based Approach." *Journal of Acquired Immune Deficiency Syndromes* 53 (3): 405–11.

Geng, E. H., M. B. Bwana, W. Muyindike, D. V. Glidden, D. R. Bangsberg, and others. 2013. "Failure to Initiate Antiretroviral Therapy, Loss to Follow-Up and Mortality among HIV-Infected Patients during the Pre-ART Period in Uganda." *Journal of Acquired Immune Deficiency Syndromes* 63 (2): e64–71.

Geng, E. H., N. Emenyonu, M. B. Bwana, D. V. Glidden, and J. N. Martin. 2008. "Sampling-Based Approach to Determining Outcomes of Patients Lost to Follow-Up in Antiretroviral Therapy Scale-Up Programs in Africa." *Journal of the American Medical Association* 300 (5): 506–7.

Geng, E. H., D. V. Glidden, D. R. Bangsberg, M. B. Bwana, N. Musinguzi, and others. 2012. "A Causal Framework for Understanding the Effect of Losses to Follow-Up on Epidemiologic Analyses in Clinic-Based Cohorts: The Case of HIV-Infected Patients on Antiretroviral Therapy in Africa." *American Journal of Epidemiology* 175 (10): 1080–87.

Geng, E. H., D. V. Glidden, N. Emenyonu, N. Musinguzi, M. B. Bwana, and others. 2010. "Tracking a Sample of Patients Lost to Follow-Up Has a Major Impact on Understanding Determinants of Survival in HIV-Infected Patients on Antiretroviral Therapy in Africa." *Tropical Medicine and International Health* 15 (Suppl 1): 63–69.

Geng, E. H., D. Nash, A. Kambugu, Y. Zhang, P. Braitstein, and others. 2010. "Retention in Care among HIV-Infected Patients in Resource-Limited Settings: Emerging Insights and New Directions." *Current HIV/AIDS Reports* 7 (4): 234–44.

Geng, E. H., T. A. Odeny, and R. E. Lyamuya. 2016. "Retention in Care and Patient-Reported Reasons for Undocumented Transfer or Stopping Care among HIV-Infected Patients on Antiretroviral Therapy in Eastern Africa: Application of a Sampling-Based Approach." *Clinical Infectious Diseases* 62 (7): 935–44.

Geng, E. H., T. A. Odeny, R. E. Lyamuya, A. Nakiwogga-Muwanga, L. Diero, and others. 2015. "Estimation of Mortality among HIV-Infected People on Antiretroviral Treatment in East Africa: A Sampling Based Approach in an Observational, Multisite, Cohort Study." *The Lancet HIV* 2 (3): e107–16.

Gouws, E., and P. Cuchi, on behalf of the International Collaboration on Estimating HIV Incidence by Modes of Transmission. 2012. "Focusing the HIV Response Through Estimating the Major Modes of HIV Transmission: A Multi-Country Analysis." *Sexually Transmitted Infections* 88 (Suppl 2): i76–85.

Granich, R. 2016. "Adoption of New Guidelines: A Work In Progress." Presentation at the UN 90-90-90 Target Workshop, Durban, South Africa, July 17.

Granich, R., S. Gupta, B. Hersh, B. Williams, J. Montaner, and others. 2015. "Trends in AIDS Deaths, New Infections and ART Coverage in the Top 30 Countries with the Highest AIDS Mortality Burden; 1990–2013." *PLoS One* 10 (7): e0131353.

Granich, R., S. Gupta, J. Montaner, B. Williams, and J. M. Zuniga. 2016. "Pattern, Determinants, and Impact of HIV Spending on Care and Treatment in 38 High-Burden Low- and Middle-Income Countries." *Journal of the International Association of Providers of AIDS Care* 15 (2): 91–100.

Greenberg, A. E., S. Lucas, O. Tossou, I. M. Coulibaly, D. Coulibaly, and others. 1995. "Autopsy-Proven Causes of Death in HIV-Infected Patients Treated for Tuberculosis in Abidjan, Côte d'Ivoire." *AIDS* 9 (11): 1251–54.

Hallett, T. B., B. Zaba, J. Todd, B. Lopman, W. Mwita, and others. 2008. "Estimating Incidence from Prevalence in Generalised HIV Epidemics: Methods and Validation." *PLoS Medicine* 5 (4): e80.

Harripersaud, K., M. McNairy, S. Ahmed, E. J. Abrams, H. Thirumurthy, and W. M. El-Sadr. 2017. "Management of HIV/AIDS and Co-Morbidities in Children and Adults: Cost-Effectiveness Considerations." In *Disease Control Priorities* (third edition): Volume 6, *Major Infectious Diseases*, edited by K. K. Holmes, S. Bertozzi, B. R. Bloom, and P. Jha. Washington, DC: World Bank.

Hirnschall, G. 2015. "Key Populations: Demographics, Epidemiology, Epidemic Drivers." Presentation given at the IAS-ILF Thematic Roundtable on Key Populations, Seattle, WA, February 24.

Holmes, C. B., T. Hallett, R. P. Walensky, T. Bärnighausen, Y. Pillay, and others. 2017. "Effectiveness and Cost-Effectiveness of Treatment as Prevention for HIV/AIDS." In *Disease Control Priorities* (third edition): Volume 6, *Major Infectious Diseases*, edited by K. K. Holmes, S. Bertozzi, B. R. Bloom, and P. Jha. Washington, DC: World Bank.

IAPAC (International Association of Providers of AIDS Care.) 2016. "Global HIV 90-90-90 Watch." http://www.hiv90-90 -90watch.org/.

ICAP (International Center for AIDS Care and Treatment Program). 2016. "Population-Based HIV Impact Assessments." Columbia Mailman School of Public Health, Columbia University, New York. http://icap.columbia.edu /global-initatives/the-phia-project/.

IHME (Institute for Health Metrics and Evaluation). 2016a. "GBD Compare." http://vizhub.healthdata.org/gbd -compare/.

———. 2016b. "Data and Tools." IHME, University of Washington, Seattle. http://www.healthdata.org/data-tools.

INSIGHT START Study Group. 2015. "Initiation of Antiretroviral Therapy in Early Asymptomatic HIV Infection." *New England Journal of Medicine* 373 (9): 795–807.

Jamison, D. T., J. G. Breman, A. R. Measham, G. Alleyne, M. Claeson, D. B. Evans, P. Jha, A. Mills, and P. Musgrove, editors. 2006. *Disease Control Priorities in Developing Countries* (second edition). Washington, DC: Oxford University Press and World Bank.

Johnson, L. F., J. Mossong, R. E. Dorrington, M. Schomaker, C. J. Hoffmann, and others. 2013. "Life Expectancies of South African Adults Starting Antiretroviral Treatment: Collaborative Analysis of Cohort Studies." *PLoS Medicine* 10 (4): e1001418.

John-Stewart, G., R. Peeling, C. Levin, P. Garcia, D. Mabey, and J. Kinuthia. 2017. "Prevention of Mother-to-Child Transmission of HIV and Syphilis." In *Disease Control Priorities* (third edition): Volume 6, *Major Infectious Diseases*, edited by K. K. Holmes, S. Bertozzi, B. R. Bloom, and P. Jha. Washington, DC: World Bank.

Kerrod, E., A. M. Geddes, M. Regan, and S. Leach. 2005. "Surveillance and Control Measures during Smallpox Outbreaks." *Emerging Infectious Diseases* 11 (2): 291–97.

Kitahata, M. M., S. J. Gange, A. G. Abraham, B. Merriman, M. S. Saag, and others. 2009. "Effect of Early versus Deferred Antiretroviral Therapy for HIV on Survival." *New England Journal of Medicine* 360 (18): 1815–26.

Levi, J., A. Raymond, A. Pozniak, P. Vernazza, P. Kohler, and others. 2015. "Can the UNAIDS 90–90–90 Target Be Reached? Analysis of 12 National Level HIV Treatment Cascades." *Journal of the International AIDS Society* 18 (5 Suppl 4).

Levi, J., A. Raymond, A. Pozniak, P. Vernazza, P. Kohler, and others. 2016. "Can the UNAIDS 90-90-90 Target Be Achieved? A Systematic Analysis of National HIV Treatment Cascades." *BMJ Global Health* 1 (2).

Lopez-Cortes, L. F., A. Gutierrez-Valencia, and O. J. Ben-Marzouk-Hidalgo. 2016. "Antiretroviral Therapy in Early HIV Infection." *New England Journal of Medicine* 374 (4): 393.

Lopman, B. A., R. V. Barnabas, J. T. Boerma, G. Chawira, K. Gaitskell, and others. 2006. "Creating and Validating an Algorithm to Measure AIDS Mortality in the Adult Population Using Verbal Autopsy." *PLoS Medicine* 3 (8): e312.

Lucas, S. B., M. Diomande, A. Hounnou, A. Beaumel, C. Giordano, and others. 1994. "HIV-Associated Lymphoma in Africa: An Autopsy Study in Côte d'Ivoire." *International Journal of Cancer* 59 (1): 20–24.

Lucas, S. B., A. Hounnou, C. Peacock, A. Beaumel, A. Kadio, and others. 1994. "Nocardiosis in HIV-Positive Patients: An Autopsy Study in West Africa." *International Journal of Tuberculosis and Lung Disease* 75 (4): 301–7.

Lundgren, J., A. G. Babiker, and J. D. Neaton. 2016. "Antiretroviral Therapy in Early HIV Infection." *New England Journal of Medicine* 374 (4): 394.

Magadi, M. A. 2013. "The Disproportionate High Risk of HIV Infection among the Urban Poor in Sub-Saharan Africa." *AIDS and Behavior* 17 (5): 1645–54.

Mahy, M. 2016. "Global Adolescent Mortality Data: Where Do the Numbers Come from and How Can We Improve Them?" Powerpoint presentation at AIDS 2016: 21st International AIDS Conference, Durban, South Africa, July.

Marston, M., K. Harriss, and E. Slaymaker. 2008. "Non-Response Bias in Estimates of HIV Prevalence Due to the Mobility of Absentees in National Population-Based Surveys: A Study of Nine National Surveys." *Sexually Transmitted Infections* 84 (Suppl 1): i71–77.

Mathers, C. D., D. M. Fat, M. Inoue, C. Rao, and A. D. Lopez. 2005. "Counting the Dead and What They Died from: An Assessment of the Global Status of Cause of Death Data." *Bulletin of the World Health Organization* 83 (3): 171–77.

May, M. T., M. Gompels, V. Delpech, K. Porter, C. Orkin, and others. 2014. "Impact on Life Expectancy of HIV-1 Positive Individuals of CD4+ Cell Count and Viral Load Response to Antiretroviral Therapy." *AIDS* 28 (8): 1193–202.

MEASURE Evaluation. 2016. *PLACE: Priorities for Local AIDS Control Efforts.* Chapel Hill, NC: University of North Carolina. http://www.cpc.unc.edu/measure/resources/tools /hiv-aids/place.

Médecins Sans Frontières. 2013. *Untangling the Web of Antiretroviral Price Reductions,* 16th ed. Geneva: Médecins Sans Frontières.

Melendez, R. M., T. A. Exner, A. A. Ehrhardt, B. Dodge, R. H. Remien, and others. 2006. "Health and Health Care among Male-to-Female Transgender Persons Who Are HIV Positive." *American Journal of Public Health* 96 (6): 1034–37.

Menzies, N. A., A. Berruti, and J. M. Blandford. 2012. "The Determinants of HIV Treatment Costs in Resource Limited Settings." *PLoS ONE* 8 (5): http://dx.doi.org/10.1371 /journal.pone.0048726.

Montaner, J. S., R. Hogg, E. Wood, T. Kerr, M. Tyndall, and others. 2006. "The Case for Expanding Access to Highly Active Antiretroviral Therapy to Curb the Growth of the HIV Epidemic." *The Lancet* 368 (9534): 531–36.

Montaner, J. S., V. D. Lima, R. Barrios, B. Yip, E. Wood, and others. 2010. "Association of Highly Active Antiretroviral Therapy Coverage, Population Viral Load, and Yearly New HIV Diagnoses in British Columbia, Canada: A Population-Based Study." *The Lancet* 376 (9740): 532–39.

Murray, C. J., and A. D. Lopez. 2013. "Measuring the Global Burden of Disease." *New England Journal of Medicine* 369 (5): 448–57.

National AIDS Control Organisation. 2012. *HIV Sentinel Surveillance 2010–2011: A Technical Brief.* New Delhi: Department of AIDS Control, Ministry of Health and Family Welfare, Government of India.

PEPFAR (President's Emergency Plan for AIDS Relief). 2013. "2013 Report on Costs of Treatment in the President's Emergency Plan for AIDS Relief (PEPFAR)." PEPFAR, Washington, DC.

Rodger, A. J., R. Lodwick, M. Schechter, S. Deeks, J. Amin, and others. 2013. "Mortality in Well Controlled HIV in the Continuous Antiretroviral Therapy Arms of the SMART and ESPRIT Trials Compared with the General Population." *AIDS* 27 (6): 973–79.

Samji, H., A. Cescon, R. S. Hogg, S. P. Modur, K. N. Althoff, and others. 2013. "Closing the Gap: Increases in Life Expectancy among Treated HIV-Positive Individuals in the United States and Canada." *PLoS One* 8 (12): e81355.

SMART (Strategies for Management of Antiretroviral Therapy) Study Group, W. M. El-Sadr, J. Lundgren, J. D. Neaton, F. Gordin, and others. 2006. "CD4+ Count-Guided Interruption of Antiretroviral Treatment." *New England Journal of Medicine* 355 (22): 2283–96.

Sterne, J. A., M. May, D. Costagliola, F. de Wolf, A. N. Phillips, and others. 2009. "Timing of Initiation of Antiretroviral Therapy in AIDS-Free HIV-1-Infected Patients: A Collaborative Analysis of 18 HIV Cohort Studies." *The Lancet* 373 (9672): 1352–63.

Stover, J., K. Andreev, E. Slaymaker, C. Gopalappa, K. Sabin, and others. 2014. "Updates to the Spectrum Model to Estimate Key HIV Indicators for Adults and Children." *AIDS* 28 (Suppl 4): S427–34.

Stover, J., L. Bollinger, J. A. Izazola, L. Loures, P. DeLay, and others. 2016. "What Is Required to End the AIDS Epidemic as a Public Health Threat by 2030? The Cost and Impact of the Fast-Track Approach." *PLoS One* 11 (5): e0154893.

Tanser, F., T. Bärnighausen, G. S. Cooke, and M. L. Newell. 2009. "Localized Spatial Clustering of HIV Infections in a Widely Disseminated Rural South African Epidemic." *International Journal of Epidemiology* 38 (4): 1008–16.

Tanser, F., T. de Oliveira, M. Maheu-Giroux, and T. Bärnighausen. 2014. "Concentrated HIV Subepidemics in Generalized Epidemic Settings." *Current Opinion in HIV and AIDS* 9 (2): 115–25.

Thacker, S. B., D. F. Stroup, V. Carande-Kulis, J. S. Marks, K. Roy, and others. 2006. "Measuring the Public's Health." *Public Health Reports* 121 (1): 14–22.

Tom-Aba, D., A. Olaleye, A. T. Olayinka, P. Nguku, N. Waziri, and others. 2015. "Innovative Technological Approach to Ebola Virus Disease Outbreak Response in Nigeria Using the Open Data Kit and Form Hub Technology." *PLoS One* 10 (6): e0131000.

UNAIDS (Joint United Nations Programme on HIV/AIDS). 2008. *UNAIDS Annual Report: Knowing Your Epidemic.* Geneva: UNAIDS.

———. 2012. *UNAIDS Report on the Global AIDS Epidemic 2012.* Geneva: United Nations.

———. 2013. "Methodology: Understanding the HIV Estimates." UNAIDS, Geneva.

———. 2014a. *90–90–90—An Ambitious Treatment Target to Help End the AIDS Epidemic.* Geneva: UNAIDS.

———. 2014b. *The Gap Report.* Geneva: UNAIDS.

———. 2014c. *Local Epidemics Issues Brief.* Geneva: UNAIDS.

———. 2014d. "Methodology: Understanding the HIV Estimates." UNAIDS, Geneva.

———. 2014e. "Ambitious Treatment Targets: Writing the Final Chapter of the AIDS Epidemic." UNAIDS discussion paper, UNAIDS, Geneva.

———. 2015a. "'15 by 15': A Target Achieved." UNAIDS, Geneva.

———. 2015b. "AIDS by the Numbers 2015." UNAIDS, Geneva.

———. 2015c. *Global AIDS Response Progress Reporting 2015.* Geneva: UNAIDS.

———. 2015d. *On the Fast Track to End AIDS by 2030: Focus on Location and Population.* Geneva: UNAIDS.

———. 2015e. *How AIDS Changed Everything.* Geneva: UNAIDS.

———. 2016a. "AIDSinfo." http://aidsinfo.unaids.org/.

———. 2016b. "Global AIDS Update 2016." UNAIDS, Geneva.

———. 2016c. "Spectrum/EPP." UNAIDS, Geneva. http://www.unaids.org/en/dataanalysis/datatools/spectrumepp.

UNAIDS Reference Group on Estimates, Modelling and Projections. 2013. "Identifying Populations at Greatest Risk of Infection: Geographic Hotspots and Key Populations." UNAIDS, Geneva.

United Nations Population Division. 2014. *World Population Prospects: The 2004 Revision.* New York: United Nations.

U.S. CDC (United States Centers for Disease Control and Prevention). 2011. "HIV among Transgender People." http://www.cdc.gov/hiv/group/gender/transgender/.

U.S. National Institutes of Health. 2015. "Starting Antiretroviral Treatment Early Improves Outcomes for HIV-Infected Individuals." News release, May 27.

Violari, A., M. F. Cotton, D. M. Gibb, A. G. Babiker, J. Steyn, and others. 2008. "Early Antiretroviral Therapy and Mortality among HIV-Infected Infants." *New England Journal of Medicine* 359 (21): 2233–44.

Walensky, R. P., E. L. Ross, N. Kumarasamy, R. Wood, F. Noubary, and others. 2013. "Cost-Effectiveness of HIV Treatment as Prevention in Serodiscordant Couples." *New England Journal of Medicine* 369 (18): 1715–25.

Wang, H., T. M. Wolock, A. Carter, G. Nguyen, H. H. Kyu, and others. 2016. "Estimates of Global, Regional, and National Incidence, Prevalence, and Mortality of HIV, 1980–2015: The Global Burden of Disease Study 2015." *The Lancet HIV* 3 (8): e361–87.

WHO (World Health Organization). 2010. *Antiretroviral Therapy for HIV Infection in Adults and Adolescents: Recommendations for a Public Health Approach.* Geneva: WHO.

———. 2011. *Prevention and Treatment of HIV and Other Sexually Transmitted Infections among Men Who Have Sex with Men and Transgender People: Recommendations for a Public Health Approach.* Geneva: WHO.

———. 2013a. *Consolidated Guidelines on the Use of Antiretroviral Drugs for Treating and Preventing HIV Infection: Recommendations for a Public Health Approach.* Geneva: WHO.

———. 2013b. "Global Health Estimates." http://www.who.int/healthinfo/global_burden_disease/en/.

———. 2013c. *Global Update on HIV Treatment 2013: Results, Impact and Opportunities.* Geneva: WHO.

———. 2013d. "WHO Methods and Data Sources for Global Burden of Disease Estimates 2000–2011." WHO, Geneva.

———. 2015a. *Global Health Sector Response to HIV, 2000–2015: Focus on Innovations in Africa.* Geneva: WHO.

———. 2015b. *Guideline on When to Start Antiretroviral Therapy and on Pre-Exposure Prophylaxis for HIV.* Geneva: WHO.

Wilson, D., and J. Taaffe. 2017. "Tailoring the Local HIV Response to Local HIV Epidemics." In *Disease Control Priorities* (third edition): Volume 6, *Major Infectious Diseases*, edited by K. K. Holmes, S. Bertozzi, B. R. Bloom, and P. Jha. Washington, DC: World Bank.

Yuen, C. M., F. Amanullah, A. Dharmadhikari, E. A. Nardell, J. A. Seddon, and others. 2015. "Turning Off the Tap: Stopping Tuberculosis Transmission through Active Case-Finding and Prompt Effective Treatment." *The Lancet* 386 (10010): 2334–43.

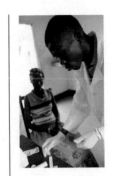

Chapter 3

HIV/AIDS Comorbidities: Impact on Cancer, Noncommunicable Diseases, and Reproductive Health

Corey Casper, Heidi Crane, Manoj Menon, and
Deborah Money

INTRODUCTION

The total number of people living with human immunodeficiency virus (HIV) worldwide continues to grow annually, attributable to both new infections and the increased longevity of infected persons treated with potent antiretroviral therapy (ART). This growing population bears the burden of associated health conditions that complicate long-term HIV infection. Specifically, secondary epidemics of cancer; reproductive ill health; and noncommunicable diseases, such as cardiovascular disease, diabetes, renal dysfunction, and liver damage, have been observed across the globe. This wide spectrum of illnesses complicating ongoing HIV infection is a challenging global health threat and underscores the need for a greater understanding of these comorbidities, broader access to treatment, and increasingly sophisticated treatment to avoid widespread preventable morbidity and death.

This chapter provides an overview of some of the most common, most rapidly increasing, or most morbid complications of persistent HIV infection; it is not meant to be exhaustive. Additionally, many comorbidities of long-term HIV infection are addressed in detail in other chapters of this volume.

The first portrayals of the epidemic in the early 1980s in the United States described a surge of cancer cases among men who have sex with men (MSM). Since the initial reports from the early epidemic, it has become clear that HIV threatens the reproductive health of women across income settings and populations. Paradoxically, in an age of new hope for prolonged lifespan stemming from the success of ART, increased longevity is also bringing a host of noncommunicable chronic comorbidities (NCCs).

Among cancers—the focus of the first section of this chapter—the pandemic initially saw an annual rise through 1996 in what came to be known as acquired immune deficiency syndrome (AIDS)–defining cancers (ADCs), including Kaposi sarcoma (KS), non-Hodgkin lymphoma (NHL), and cervical cancer (CDC 1992). These cancers decreased in incidence with the widespread availability of ART in high-resource settings but never fell to the levels seen before HIV; they continue with little change in incidence in low- and middle-income countries (LMICs). Additionally, a troubling rise in other, non-AIDS defining cancers (NADCs)—such as anal cancer, hepatocellular carcinoma (HCC), and lung cancer—continues to be observed globally despite access to ART.

The next section of the chapter considers the multifaceted impact of HIV on women's reproductive health.

Corresponding author: Corey Casper, Fred Hutchinson Cancer Research Center, Seattle, Washington, United States; ccasper@fredhutch.org.

Girls and women who are at risk of HIV or who are already infected are vulnerable to problems of access to adequate reproductive choice and contraceptive options. Yet, the evidence suggests that preventing mother-to-infant transmission of HIV can effectively be achieved through the prevention of unplanned or unwanted pregnancies. Barrier contraceptive methods, although suboptimal at preventing pregnancy, do protect against HIV. The section also examines the complicated influence of HIV on infertility in women and the transmission of human papillomavirus (HPV), herpes simplex virus (HSV), pelvic inflammatory disease, bacterial vaginosis, and others.

The final section of the chapter highlights the wide range of NCCs associated with long-standing HIV infection, including cardiovascular and metabolic illnesses.

Taken together, the data from many parts of the world clearly show that despite the dramatic decrease in deaths due to HIV with the continued expansion of access to successful treatment, access to ART alone will not prevent, and in some cases may precipitate, a wide spectrum of complications of long-term HIV infection. These challenges require the attention of health care providers, policy makers, and researchers, empowered by access to accurate information on the burden of these diseases and the growing number of potential solutions.

HIV AND CANCER

At the beginning of the global HIV pandemic, an outbreak of cancer among MSM in the United States was described in 1981 (Hymes and others 1981). Since then, the evidence suggests that the risk of cancer is 2–3,000 times higher among people with HIV than those who are not infected (Grulich and others 2007); up to 9 percent of people living with long-term HIV infection will develop cancer over the course of their HIV care (Shiels and others 2011). Cancer is the leading non-AIDS cause of death worldwide among people with HIV (Smith and others 2014).

Epidemiology of Cancer among People with HIV

In high-income countries (HICs), the incidence of cancer in people with HIV rose annually until 1996, when access to potent ART became widely available and observers noted a sharp decline in new cancer cases (Shiels and others 2011).

Since 1998, however, the incidence of cancer among people with HIV has been gradually rising annually in the United States. Initially, the overwhelming number were ADCs (CDC 1992), including KS; NHL; Burkitt, immunoblastic, and primary central nervous system lymphomas;

and cervical cancer. These malignancies, all associated with a viral oncogenic infection, were frequently found in individuals with low CD4 T-cell counts, and therefore common before ART became widely available.

Over time, additional cancers were observed to be more common in people with HIV, but these were not considered to be AIDS defining (Patel and others 2008; Shiels and others 2011; Silverberg and others 2015). These NADCs—which are significantly more common in people with HIV than in peers without it in the same population—include anal cancer, HCC, and lung cancer.

Today, incident cancer cases are roughly equally divided between ADCs and NADCs. In the United States, approximately one person will develop cancer for every 100 people with HIV each year (Riedel and others 2013). One study estimates a similar incidence of cancer among HIV-infected South Africans receiving ART (0.87 cases of cancer developing for every 100 people with HIV followed over a year) (Sengayi and others 2016).

The time that has passed since initial infection with HIV also influences which cancer arises; ADCs are more common soon after diagnosis, and NADCs are more common after five or more years (Robbins and others 2015). Survival after a diagnosis of cancer accompanying HIV appears to be considerably shorter, on average, especially for NADCs, compared with similar cancers in people without HIV (Achenbach and others 2011; Coghill and others 2015).

Less is known about the epidemiology of cancer among people with HIV in LMICs. Cancer registries that cover the entire population are few in these areas and do not routinely capture HIV status of cancer cases. A retrospective analysis from 13 clinical sites in the East Asia and Pacific region, as part of the TREAT Asia HIV Observational Database study, revealed data comparable to that seen among the non-Asian HIV populations. In that analysis, CD4 T-cell counts greater than 200 cells per cubic millimeter (mm^3) were found protective against ADCs; older patients and those not on potent ART were more likely to be diagnosed with an NADC (Petoumenos and others 2010).

Attempts to match cancer registries with data on individual HIV status have been conducted in Uganda (Mbulaiteye and others 2006), Nigeria (Akarolo-Anthony and others 2014), and South Africa (Sengayi 2016), and found the cancers to be more common among people with HIV, similar to the United States. Hospital-based cancer registries in India also show a similar spectrum of cancer in people with HIV, except for a notably lower frequency of KS (Venkatesh and others 2012).

Few studies have assessed survival after diagnosis of HIV-associated malignancies (HIVAMs) in resource-limited settings, but the odds of death appear to be significantly higher among people with HIV (Coghill and others 2013). Cohort studies conducted in high-income regions have found cancer to be among the leading causes of death of people with HIV (Bonnet and others 2004; Kowalska and others 2012; Smith and others 2014).

Pathogenesis of HIV-Associated Malignancies

People with HIV are predisposed to a higher risk of cancer through a variety of mechanisms. First, the immunosuppression that accompanies CD4 T-cell depletion may lead to the development of cancer when the immune system fails to seek out early cancer occurrences and destroy them. This helps explain why the risk for many HIVAMs is inversely related to CD4 T-cell count (Biggar and others 2007).

The observation that some cancers (cervical cancer and Hodgkin lymphoma) in people with HIV were not associated with lower CD4 T-cell counts—coupled with epidemiologic studies suggesting that the risk for cancer was greater among people with HIV than among highly immunosuppressed recipients of organ transplantation (Grulich and others 2007)—led to the exploration of mechanisms beyond CD4 T-cell depletion that could lead to cancer in people with HIV.

HIV replication itself may foster the development of cancer, potentially through the induction of angiogenic, anti-apoptotic, or proliferative signaling. That failure to suppress HIV replication (or time spent with HIV detectable in the plasma) is independently associated with risk of cancer (Bruyand and others 2009) supports this hypothesis. Other mechanisms being explored that cause cancer in persons with HIV include immune activation, immune exhaustion, and HIV integration. The individual components of ART may also reduce cancer risk beyond their effect on immune reconstitution. Gantt, Casper, and Ambinder (2013) found that protease inhibitors have antineoplastic properties, and nucleoside reverse transcriptase inhibitors (NRTIs) suppress viruses that cause cancer in people with HIV.

Specific HIV-Associated Malignancies

Cervical Cancer

Globally, cervical cancer, caused by HPV (Forman and others 2012), is the fourth most common cancer and third leading cause of cancer-related death among women; the incidence in LMICs is second only to breast cancer (De Vuyst and others 2013; Ferlay and others 2013). In Sub-Saharan Africa, cervical cancer is the leading cause of cancer-related death among women (Bosch and others 2013; Lozano and others 2012).

In a meta-analysis involving nearly 200 studies and more than 1 million women who had a normal cervical cytologic examination, HPV DNA was detected in nearly 12 percent of women globally, although with marked geographic variation. Regions of frequent HPV detection include the Caribbean (35 percent) and Eastern Africa (34 percent), yet frequency is only 10 percent or less in Northern Europe (10 percent), Northern Africa (9 percent), Western Europe (9 percent), Southern Europe (9 percent), Southern Asia (7 percent), North America (5 percent), and Western Asia (2 percent) (Bruni and others 2010).

More than 100 types of HPV exist, but HPV 16 and 18 cause 70 percent of cancers. HIV may increase cervical cancer risk by increasing the rates of persistent HPV infection, in contrast to HPV in women without HIV whose immune systems often clear the infection (Ahdieh and others 2000).

The risk of cervical cancer in women with HIV increases with age and has no direct association with CD4 T-cell count (Yanik and others 2013); the risk, however, is reduced in women receiving ART (Blitz and others 2013). For all women, comprehensive screening and treatment programs dramatically reduce deaths from this disease.

Kaposi Sarcoma

KS, the most common HIV-associated malignancy worldwide, is caused by infection with human herpes virus 8 (HHV-8). In the United States and Europe, KS is 10 times more common among men than women; in Sub-Saharan Africa, the rates are nearly equal. In part, KS incidence mirrors HHV-8 prevalence, which is high among MSM in HICs and endemic in many parts of Sub-Saharan Africa (Nguyen and Casper 2010).

KS incidence declined nearly tenfold by 1996, the year after potent ART became available in the United States (Eltom and others 2002); it has declined more slowly in Sub-Saharan Africa since ART was rolled out (Mutyaba and others 2015). Mortality from KS is unusual in HICs, although the disease persists in up to 50 percent of patients treated with ART and chemotherapy (Achenbach and others 2011; Nguyen and others 2008). In LMICs, KS mortality is high and response to treatment is poor (Gondos and others 2005; Mosam and others 2012). Taken together, these factors mean that prevention of KS is paramount, calling for new therapies.

Lymphoma

The pathogenesis of AIDS-related lymphomas is often attributable to tumor-causing viruses, including Epstein-Barr virus, HHV-8, and hepatitis C virus. Although the incidence of such NHLs has significantly decreased since the widespread implementation of ART, incidence among people with HIV remains approximately 10 times greater than in the general population (Robbins and others 2014; van Leeuwen and others 2009). Patients with more severe immunodeficiency, as measured by CD4 T-cell count, are at an even greater risk (Guiguet and others 2009).

The incidence of Hodgkin lymphoma is significantly increased among people with HIV, and its incidence has not declined in parallel with the falling incidence of NHL. Data suggest, however, that prolonged ART use does reduce the risk of Hodgkin's lymphoma (Kowalkowski and others 2014).

People with HIV who also have lymphoma are more likely to present with symptomatic extranodal and central nervous system involvement (Carbone and Gloghini 2005). Independent of these factors, cancer-specific mortality among these patients is higher compared with patients without HIV (Coghill and others 2015).

Hepatocellular Carcinoma

HCC is the seventh most common cause of all cancers globally and the third leading cause of cancer-related death; nearly 85 percent of cases of HCC and of death secondary to HCC occur in LMICs (Ferlay and others 2013). Although the pathogenesis is not entirely clear, most cases of HCC worldwide are secondary to hepatitis B, a double-stranded DNA virus that can be transmitted sexually and can lead to chronic infection. A significant proportion of the remaining burden is secondary to hepatitis C (Arzumanyan, Reis, and Feitelson 2013; McGlynn, Petrick, and London 2015).

HIV routes of transmission are similar to those of hepatitis B virus and hepatitis C virus, so co-infection is high. In a cohort study of more than 3,000 patients, approximately one-third of people with HIV were co-infected with hepatitis C virus (Fultz and others 2003). The prevalence of hepatitis C virus infection tends to be higher, and the aggressiveness of hepatitis C virus disease is greater, among people with HIV (Puoti and others 2004). A separate analysis documented that nearly 10 percent of HIV patients were chronic carriers of hepatitis B virus. Accordingly, cancer prevention efforts need to target the treatment of hepatitis B and hepatitis C before the development of HCC.

Persons with HIV and chronic viral hepatitis do not progress more rapidly to HCC than do HIV negative persons, in marked contrast to other viral-associated malignancies. However, the use of antiviral medications in the treatment of HIV or associated diseases, including interferon and nucleoside or nucleotide analogs, markedly reduces the risk of developing HCC in both HIV positive and HIV negative persons (Sung and others 2008). Although current treatment options for hepatitis C virus are effective, the high cost of treatment is limiting widespread global implementation (Jacobson and others 2011; Poordad and others 2011). Chapter 16 of this volume (Wiktor 2017) provides additional information on viral hepatitis.

Anal Cancer

Anal cancer, like other urogenital cancers, is caused primarily by HPV infection. Anal cancer is nearly 30 times more common among people with HIV (Grulich and others 2007). Despite long-term use of ART, however, the incidence of anal cancer among people with HIV has not declined (Piketty and others 2012). One large cohort study in the United States revealed that rates of anal cancer had increased fivefold over those before 1996, that is, before ART became potent (Crum-Cianflone and others 2010).

Although anal-cancer-specific mortality among patients with HIV does not appear elevated (Coghill and others 2015), prevention strategies to reduce morbidity, including anal cytology and high resolution anoscopy, merit further consideration (Chiao and others 2006) and are being evaluated.

Lung Cancer

HIV infection is associated with approximately a three-fold increased risk of lung cancer, which is the most common NADC and third most common cancer overall (Engels and others 2006; Kirk and others 2007; Robbins and others 2015). Although the higher incidence of lung cancer among HIV patients appears to be in part independent of tobacco use, the prevalence of tobacco use is several-fold higher among patients with HIV in the United States compared with the general population (Mdodo and others 2015). Smoking is associated with lung-cancer-specific mortality, which has increased in the era of ART (Kirk and others 2007). Mortality from lung cancer has not been associated with either immunosuppression or HIV viral load (Clifford and others 2012).

Strategies for Prevention of HIV-Associated Malignancies

Vaccines

Vaccines against HPV and hepatitis B virus offer outstanding opportunities to reduce the burden of cancer in people with HIV. The most current HPV vaccine targets nine HPV types and is capable of eliminating more than 90 percent of cervical cancer cases. The effect of the vaccine on other HPV-related cancers and the efficacy among people with HIV are yet to be determined.

The World Health Organization (WHO) recommends universal vaccination of girls ages 9–13 years.

Uptake has been limited globally by gaps in funding and, in the United States, by sensitivities around vaccines for sexually transmitted diseases. Furthermore, this age group is not covered by the routine Expanded Program on Immunization, and alternative delivery strategies such as school-based vaccination need to be further explored (Watson-Jones and others 2015). Although HPV vaccines are approved for three doses administered over a six-month period, a two-dose HPV vaccine schedule in HIV-negative populations has been shown to be non-inferior (Dobson and others 2013; Kreimer and others 2015).

The use of the HPV vaccine among people with existing HIV infection has been the subject of several studies; preliminary data show good rates of seroconversion and lower peak antibody levels, but efficacy data are pending (Money and others 2016). A highly effective vaccine against hepatitis B has been seen to reduce the incidence of HCC in hepatitis B–endemic regions (Chang and others 1997; Chang and others 2009; Hsu and others 1988).

The WHO recommends universal vaccination against hepatitis B with the primary infant vaccination series; this vaccine is now included in national infant immunization programs in more than 90 percent of countries (Kane 1995, 2012).

Although vaccination against hepatitis B virus in susceptible people with HIV is part of national and international guidelines (CDC 2006; WHO 2013a), the hepatitis B virus vaccine has reduced immunogenicity in people with HIV (Landrum and others 2009). Programs for catch-up vaccinations among groups at high risk of HIV infection are also absent in low-resource settings.

Screening

Women in the general population in the United States, ages 21–65 years, are recommended to have cervical cancer screening with cytology every three years (Moyer 2012); the recommendation for women with HIV, in contrast, is screening twice in the first year after initial diagnosis and then annually for the rest of their lives (Panel on Opportunistic Infections in HIV-Infected Adults and Adolescents 2016). The WHO, however, recommends that if a woman with HIV has an initial negative screening test (that is, normal cytology, negative visual inspection with acetic acid, or negative cervical HPV screening test), then she should undergo subsequent screening within three years (WHO 2013b).

Such screening recommendations, independent of the screening modality, may not be feasible in low-income countries (LICs) with stressed health care systems. Additionally, the economic costs and the human resources required for standard cervical screening through either cytology or HPV testing are limited in LICs. Low-cost screening techniques (for example, visual inspection with acetic acid) are being widely adopted, although the accuracy of these tests in high-risk populations needs to be more completely defined (Campos and others 2015; Chung and others 2013; Moses and others 2015). Novel approaches, including self-swabbing testing for oncogenic HPV, are being evaluated for use in LMICs. High-risk lesions detected during screening can be locally ablated to prevent the development of invasive cervical cancer (WHO 2013b).

Few other HIV-associated cancers have been shown to be preventable with screening efforts. Because of the biological similarities between cervical and anal cancer, screening for preinvasive anal cancer has been evaluated. When performed by highly trained and experienced clinicians and laboratories, screening techniques such as high-resolution anoscopy can detect high-grade dysplasia (Dalla Pria and others 2014). However, evidence is still lacking from prospective randomized trials that ablation of these high-grade lesions reduces the risk of invasive anal cancer.

Screening for lung cancer with computed tomography has been evaluated among patients with HIV and may be effective. However, the incidence of the disease is low, and strategies for targeting screening efforts are needed (Hulbert and others 2014).

Chemoprevention of Cancer

Increasing evidence suggests that the risk of cancer in people with HIV can be reduced through the use of ART. In a randomized trial of early or delayed initiation of ART in people recently diagnosed with HIV, the risk of cancer overall was reduced by nearly two-thirds among people who initiated therapy at a CD4 T-cell count of more than 500 cells/mm^3, compared with those who initiated at CD4 T-cell of less than 350 cells/mm^3 (Klingman and others 2015). The findings included a 50 percent reduction in NADCs, a 91 percent reduction in KS, and a 70 percent reduction in lymphoma. The use of ART is also active in preventing the acquisition of some viral oncogens, such as hepatitis B, which in turn reduces the risk of cancer (Heuft and others 2014).

Finally, treatment with antiviral therapy of chronic infections that cause cancer, such as hepatitis B or hepatitis C, has been shown to reduce the risk of HCC (Shen and others 2012), although the efficacy of this strategy in people with HIV has not been further evaluated.

Other Approaches to Prevention of HIV-Associated Malignancies

Behavioral interventions to reduce smoking among people with HIV have been moderately effective and may reduce a broad spectrum of HIV comorbidities (Keith and others 2016).

HIV and Cancer Conclusions

Cancer is an increasingly common complication and is a leading cause of death in people with HIV. Strategies for cancer prevention—including vaccination, screening, and early ART initiation—can reduce the cancer burden, but additional strategies for reducing the burden of HIVAMs are needed.

IMPACT OF HIV AND OTHER SEXUALLY TRANSMITTED INFECTIONS ON FEMALE REPRODUCTIVE HEALTH

The ongoing burden of HIV in women is substantial, with 1,000 new infections per day (UNAIDS 2014). This concentration of the HIV epidemic has therefore had substantial impact on women's reproductive health, and intersects with the ongoing and long-standing burden of other sexually transmitted infections (STIs) in women.

Impact of HIV Infection on Family Planning Methods and Conception

Family Planning

Girls and women at risk of HIV or who are already infected are particularly vulnerable to the global problems of access to adequate reproductive choice and contraceptive options (WHO 2006). HIV often magnifies the lack of personal control over reproductive decisions. Beyond the importance of reproductive health for women themselves, transmission of HIV from mother to infant at a population level can most effectively be prevented by providing improved protection from HIV to women of reproductive age and preventing unplanned and unwanted pregnancies (WHO 2006).

Among contraceptive methods, barrier methods such as male condoms, female condoms, and cervical caps are suboptimal in preventing pregnancy, but they do protect against HIV acquisition and transmission (Weller and Davis 2002). Dual methods of protection and contraception, such as condoms and oral contraceptives, are not acceptable to many couples, resulting in inferior methods of contraception being used in partnerships in which one partner is HIV positive and the other partner is HIV negative (serodiscordant couples) (Heffron and others 2010; Nieves and others 2015).

Concerns about the potential interactions between antiretroviral drugs and the estrogen component in combination oral contraceptives notwithstanding (Robinson, Jamshidi, and Burke 2012; Thurman, Anderson, and Doncel 2014), recent data suggest that contraception efficacy for women with HIV is not inferior to that for other women (Pyra and others 2015).

Long-acting, injectable progestin or progestin-based implants offer effective contraception. However, concerns have arisen about declining bone mineral density with long-term progesterone use in women with HIV, who are already more susceptible to bone loss (Lopez and others 2014).

Furthermore, a prospective trial of preexposure prophylaxis (PrEP) with ART for serodiscordant couples found that women using injectable hormonal contraception were more likely than other women to acquire or transmit HIV infection (Heffron and others 2012). Formal studies of this association are underway.

Other relevant factors include the regional differences in cost, acceptability, and access to contraception. More recently, data suggest that intrauterine devices are safe in women with HIV and are highly effective, yet affordability limits their uptake (Wanyenze and others 2013).

Infertility

HIV affects fertility in women in a variety of ways. Women with HIV may wish to prevent transmission by avoiding sexual contact with partners; additionally, the biology of HIV itself may have an impact on fertility. Some studies have found higher infertility in women with HIV (Yaro and others 2001), although most such studies involved cohorts with inadequately managed HIV disease; no data support the notion that infertility is higher among women with HIV and who are in good health on ART.

For women with HIV whose partners do not have HIV, timed self-insemination with partner sperm is a simple and effective way to prevent risk of transmission to the male partner. However, many serodiscordant couples will choose to have unprotected sex if the female partner is on adequate suppressive ART (Loutfy and others 2012). Suppressive ART has been shown to eliminate the risk of HIV transmission between serodiscordant couples, at least in one study (Rodger and others 2016).

For women without HIV whose male partners have HIV, prevention of acquisition from the male partner ideally includes ensuring that the male partner is on fully suppressive ART. However, with individuals not engaged in care or in regions where access to ART is limited, alternative approaches are important (Loutfy and others 2012). One option is for the woman to use PrEP. Among women given oral tenofovir and emtricitabine PrEP who became pregnant, the PrEP was discontinued when the pregnancy became known. Of note, in this study, pregnancy outcomes and infant growth did not differ in women taking PrEP compared with those taking a placebo (Mugo and others 2014).

Overall, most HIV serodiscordant couples cannot afford the expensive assisted reproductive treatments for reduction of HIV transmission. In vitro fertilization and intracytoplasmic sperm injection have been used to decrease male-to-female HIV transmission; more recently, sperm washing and intrauterine insemination provides a less complex, less costly alternative and appears to be safe, with no reported cases of HIV transmission (Barnes and others 2014; Ohl and others 2005).

Although no data suggest that couples in which both partners have HIV have higher rates of infertility than other couples, they may face infertility treatment issues if they coincidentally have other fertility issues. In addition to issues of access and affordability, women with HIV may also face discrimination in infertility treatment. A cross-sectional study in the United States found that public attitudes toward people with HIV who seek infertility treatment are typically negative; only 38 percent of respondents favor offering it (Mok-Lin and others 2011). However, health care providers have generally been supportive of women with HIV who want children; in a facility in Ghana, 94.3 percent of health care workers providing care to women with HIV were supportive of their rights to reproduction (Laar 2013).

Regarding pregnancy outcomes after infertility treatment, a case-control study of women who received in vitro fertilization treatment showed that well-controlled HIV had no impact on fertility outcomes for women with HIV compared with those without HIV (Nurudeen and others 2013). Beyond fertility, greater risks of stillbirth, premature birth, and low birth weight have been observed in pregnancies of women with HIV (Turner and others 2013).

HIV prevention strategies aimed at men have included voluntary male circumcision, most widely offered in high-endemic areas in Sub-Saharan Africa. A review of published literature in this area suggests that opportunities for more extensive engagement of adolescents in sexual and reproductive health care have been missed (Kaufman and others 2016).

Other Sexually Transmitted Infections

Human Papillomavirus
HPV infection is associated with the great majority of squamous cell cancers of the cervix, vulva, vagina, penis, anus, and oropharynx. Women with HIV are at greater risk of contracting a persistent HPV infection and are often infected by a broader range of HPV genotypes (Salters and others 2016).

Infection with HPV may also serve as a marker of increased risk for HIV infection because both infections may be sexually transmitted. Massad and others (2004) found that women with HIV were four times as likely to have vulvar intraepithelial neoplasia and almost five

times more likely to have genital warts. This risk can be reduced in individuals with suppressed HIV (Blitz and others 2013).

Among women undergoing in vitro fertilization, detection of HPV in the cervix was associated with substantial reduction in pregnancy (Depuydt and others 2016). Detection of HPV in semen was associated with substantially lower rates of pregnancy after intrauterine insemination, and also associated with more miscarriages (Garolla and others 2016).

Herpes Simplex Virus
Global distribution, incidence, and prevalence of infection with HSV—HSV-1 and HSV-2—vary widely by country, region, and population subgroup. Women are more susceptible than men to HSV-2 infection. Primary HSV infection contracted in the third trimester of pregnancy may result in neurocognitive problems in the fetus, developmental delays, or death if the infant becomes infected (Watts and others 2003). For women with recurrent HSV or primary HSV infection occurring before 34 weeks gestation, prevention of transmission to the infant can be achieved with acyclovir or valacyclovir suppression therapy during pregnancy (Workowski and Bolan 2015).

In the United States, the prevalence of HSV-2 among adult men and women with HIV is three times higher than in the general population (Patel and others 2012). HSV-2 may also accelerate HIV disease progression in co-infected individuals. However, in a randomized clinical trial involving couples in which the HIV-1–infected partner was co-infected with HSV-2, acyclovir did not reduce the risk of HIV-1 transmission, despite a reduction in plasma HIV-1 RNA and a 73 percent reduction in the occurrence of genital ulcers due to the HSV-2 virus (Celum and others 2010).

Pelvic Inflammatory Disease
Pelvic inflammatory disease is classically associated with the ascension of microorganisms, including *Neisseria gonorrhoeae, Chlamydia trachomatis, Mycoplasma genitalium,* from the lower genital tract to the upper genital tract and of bacterial vaginosis-associated organisms from the vagina or cervix into the endometrium and fallopian tubes (Cohen and others 1998). Long-term consequences of pelvic inflammatory disease can include ectopic pregnancy, chronic pelvic pain, tubal infertility, adnexal tenderness, tubo-ovarian abscesses, fallopian tube dysfunction, difficult or painful sexual intercourse (dyspareunia), pelvic adhesions, and recurrent pelvic inflammatory disease.

Among women with pelvic inflammatory disease, those with HIV present with tubo-ovarian abscess more often than women without HIV. Among Kenyan women with lower abdominal pain and suspected pelvic inflammatory disease, histologically confirmed endometritis was three times more common in those with HIV than among those without (Cohen and others 1998). Nevertheless, treatment of pelvic inflammatory disease has been found to be equally successful in all women, regardless of HIV status (Bukusi and others 1999).

Bacterial Vaginosis

A meta-analysis of 23 studies found a significantly increased risk of HIV incidence among women with bacterial vaginosis (relative risk 1.6, 95 percent confidence interval 1.2, 2.1) (Atashili and others 2008). In a case-control analysis of 5,110 women in South Africa, bacterial vaginosis at baseline enrollment was associated with double the risk of acquiring HIV infection during 36 months' follow-up, after adjusting for demographic characteristics, other STIs, and sexual behavior (Myer and others 2005). Bacterial vaginosis is also associated with higher risk of transmission of HIV to a male partner (Cohen and others 2012).

In addition, bacterial vaginosis has been associated with increased risk of acquiring other STIs, with developing pelvic inflammatory disease, with several adverse outcomes of pregnancy (for example, fetal loss, spontaneous abortion, stillbirth, preterm delivery, low birth weight, and disease in the offspring), and with infertility. A large and growing number of possible mechanisms by which any vaginal dysbiosis may contribute to these complications have been identified (Brotman 2011; Hillier and others 1995).

Sexually Transmitted Intestinal and Enteric Infections

A study early in the HIV epidemic identified diverse pathogens, often of a polymicrobial nature, associated with proctitis, proctocolitis, and enteritis (Quinn and others 1983). Sexually associated proctitis, proctocolitis, or enteritis, which occur more commonly in MSM, but also in heterosexual women and men through unprotected anal intercourse, may increase susceptibility to HIV (Fleming and Wasserheit 1999). Such infections are occurring with greater frequency (Cone and Whitlow 2013).

HIV and Women's Reproductive Health Conclusions

HIV and other STIs have been associated with major direct and indirect harm to the reproductive health of women in many settings and populations.

IMPACT OF NONCOMMUNICABLE CHRONIC COMORBIDITIES IN PEOPLE WITH HIV

Expanded access to ART and accompanying increases in longevity of people with HIV have led to an increase in NCCs, including cardiovascular disease (CVD), diabetes and other metabolic conditions, renal disease, liver disease, cancers, and mental illness. Data demonstrating the importance of these conditions among people with HIV are often predominantly from HICs. Unfortunately, much less of the data and research advances for these conditions are from LMICs, where most people with HIV live (Narayan and others 2014). In many regions, such as Sub-Saharan Africa, HIV care, including with ART, is more widely available, but is not accompanied by care for NCCs, resulting in preventable morbidity and death (Narayan and others 2014).

Cardiovascular Disease

Burden and Epidemiology of CVD in People with HIV
CVD is one of the most important causes of NCC among people with HIV for several reasons. First, CVD, specifically ischemic heart disease, was the number one cause of death, years of life lost, and disability-adjusted life years in 2010 in the United States, and the number one cause of disability-adjusted life years globally (Murray and Lopez 2013). CVD and its risk factors are increasing in many LMICs as an emerging epidemic, even among those without HIV (Mensah 2008).

Second, rates of CVD, particularly myocardial infarction, are much higher among people with HIV than among those without, most likely due in part to chronic inflammation and immune activation (Freiberg and others 2013; Silverberg and others 2014; Triant 2014). The clinical classification of myocardial infarction was divided into five types in 2007 as part of the universal myocardial infarction definition (Thygesen and others 2007); type 1 and type 2 constitute almost the entirety. Type 1 or primary myocardial infarction events result spontaneously from atherosclerotic plaque instability. Type 2 myocardial infarction events are secondary events due to other illnesses or causes resulting in myocardial ischemia from increased oxygen demand or decreased supply, as can occur in the setting of hypotension or hypoxia. Little is known about myocardial infarction types in people with HIV in either HICs or LMICs. However, in the United States, type 2 myocardial infarction events make up close to half of all myocardial infarction events among people with HIV, a much higher proportion than in the general population. Understanding myocardial infarction types among people with HIV may help clarify unanswered questions regarding risk factors and higher prevalence among people with HIV (Crane and others 2014).

Third, the effect of CVD among people with HIV may be even more profound in LMICs than in HICs, given that most people with HIV live in LMICs and may have additional CVD risk factors unique to these areas (Bloomfield and others 2014). In a comparison of NCCs among two cohort studies of people with HIV on ART, one from Botswana and one from Tennessee, event rates were higher in Botswana in comparisons standardized to the U.S. population; the largest discrepancies were for CVD disease (Wester and others 2011). As a result, the major public health impact of CVD among people with HIV has been increasingly recognized in HICs and LMICs (Bloomfield and others 2014; Currier and others 2003).

Factors Associated with CVD among People with HIV

Causes of CVD among people with HIV are multifactorial and include long-term HIV exposure, consequences of ongoing inflammation, progressive immune dysfunction, and possible adverse effects associated with ART (Aberg 2009). These factors are compounded by the aging of the population of people with HIV in many regions and by higher rates of traditional CVD risk factors such as smoking, diabetes, and dyslipidemia (Silverberg and others 2014; Triant 2014).

While modifying traditional CVD risk factors may be important in preventing CVD, these factors have not been shown to explain the entire CVD risk increase among people with HIV, highlighting the importance of novel and HIV-specific factors influencing CVD risk (Triant 2014). HIV may also accelerate CVD through chronic inflammation. The increase in myocardial infarction risk in people with HIV is similar to that in inflammatory diseases like rheumatoid arthritis (Solomon and others 2003). Inflammatory and coagulation markers have been shown to predict CVD (Ford and others 2010; Triant, Meigs, and Grinspoon 2009), but the most appropriate intervention targets remain unclear.

Impact of ART on CVD Risk

ART has greatly reduced morbidity and mortality (Palella and others 1998); paradoxically, however, ART may theoretically increase CVD risk (Friis-Moller and others 2007) because of altered metabolism or atherogenic effects (Behrens and others 1999; Holmberg, Moorman, and Greenberg 2004; Holmberg and others 2002). CVD risk may be higher with longer ART or protease inhibitor duration (Currier and others 2003; DAD Study Investigators 2004; Friis-Moller and others 2007; Holmberg and others 2002), or with recent abacavir or

didanosine use (Sabin and others 2008), although both are controversial (Cutrell and others 2008).

The Strategies for Management of Antiretroviral Therapy (SMART) study found a trend toward increased CVD with delayed ART or ART interruptions (El-Sadr and others 2006), suggesting that despite potential metabolic impacts of ART, the overall effect is protective. This finding is several years old; in most regions, current regimens now have even lower negative metabolic impacts.

Several studies have found that low recent and nadir CD4 T-cell counts are associated with CVD (Drozd and others 2014; Lang and others 2012; Silverberg and others 2014). Elevated or detectable HIV RNA levels (viremia) have also been associated with CVD (Drozd and others 2014; Freiberg and others 2013; Lang and others 2012; Silverberg and others 2014). These studies, as well as findings from the SMART trial, support the hypothesis that CVD risk is reduced by control of HIV itself, and they provide additional support for recommendations for earlier ART initiation (Silverberg and others 2014; Triant 2014). However, overall risk and relative contributions of specific risk factors require more study in HICs and LMICs, including assessment of the effects of interventions that address these risk factors.

Other CVD Outcomes

Although much of the CVD and HIV literature has focused on myocardial infarction, this is not the only CVD outcome of relevance to people with HIV. In the United States, people with HIV have 1.8 times the risk of heart failure (Butt and others 2011); a meta-analysis suggested a prevalence of 8 percent for systolic dysfunction and 43 percent for diastolic dysfunction (Cerrato and others 2013).

Data on cardiac dysfunction are more limited in other parts of the world; several studies present such data, but they precede the widespread availability of ART. In Zimbabwe, 50 percent of people with HIV had cardiac dysfunction, including 22 percent with left-ventricular dysfunction, 6 percent with isolated right-ventricular dilation, and 9 percent with dilated cardiomyopathy (Hakim, Matenga, and Siziya 1996). A Rwanda study showed dilated cardiomyopathy in 18 percent of people with HIV who were not receiving ART (Twagirumukiza and others 2007).

More recently, in South Africa, cardiomyopathy was the most common cardiac disease manifestation (38 percent) among people with HIV with newly diagnosed heart disease (Sliwa and others 2012). These findings suggest that heart failure and cardiomyopathy are important complications among people with HIV. However, the data are insufficient to address whether these outcomes are more common among people with HIV in LMICs than in

HICs (Bloomfield and others 2014), how accurate these estimates might be in the current treatment era, and how these outcomes may have improved in LMICs with more widely available ART or in HICs with earlier initiation of ART.

Factors associated with CVD outcomes, such as heart failure, among people with HIV also include traditional risk factors such as smoking, prior myocardial infarction, hypertension, and higher age (Cerrato and others 2013). Other factors possibly associated with cardiomyopathy among patients in Sub-Saharan Africa not receiving ART include nutritional factors, low CD4 T-cell counts, higher viral load, and advanced HIV stage (Nzuobontane, Blackett, and Kuaban 2002; Twagirumukiza and others 2007).

Type 2 Diabetes Mellitus

Burden and Epidemiology of Diabetes Mellitus in People with HIV

In North America and Europe, people with HIV more often have glucose abnormalities and type 2 diabetes mellitus than do people without HIV (Brown and others 2005; Guaraldi and others 2011). In analyses adjusted for age and body mass index, men with HIV who were not receiving ART had 2.2 times the prevalence of diabetes mellitus than men without HIV (Brown and others 2005). The prevalence was more than four times higher among men with HIV who were receiving ART than among uninfected men (Brown and others 2005). Estimated prevalence rates among people with HIV have varied based on the patient population, from 3 percent to 21 percent (Hadigan and others 2001; Salehian and others 2005; Visnegarwala and others 2005). Diabetes mellitus prevalence and impaired glucose tolerance rates are higher among those older than age 60 years (Guaraldi and others 2011), ranging from 21 percent to 66 percent (Arama and others 2013; Araujo and others 2014; Hadigan and others 2001).

More is known about rates of diabetes mellitus and impaired glucose tolerance in HICs than in LICs. The estimated prevalence of diabetes mellitus among people with HIV is higher in HICs than in LMICs; however, the estimated absolute number of people with HIV with diabetes mellitus is greater in LMICs (Ali and others 2014). A study of countries in South America estimated diabetes mellitus prevalence rates to be from 0.8 percent in Columbia to 6.5 percent in Brazil (Cahn and others 2010).

Although the data on people with HIV in Asia are particularly limited, a study in Thailand found that among 580 people with HIV, 4.7 percent had hyperglycemia; this rate was higher among ART-experienced than among ART-naive individuals (Jantarapakde and others 2014).

In Uganda, people with HIV had slightly higher mean glucose levels over time, as evidenced by elevations in HbA1c measurements, compared with those without HIV (Dillon and others 2013).

The incidence of diabetes mellitus in people with HIV was higher in the earlier years of the ART era than in recent years (Capeau and others 2012). The decline in diabetes mellitus incidence during the ART era is likely because ART medications, such as didanosine, were more often used earlier and had greater negative metabolic impacts. These more toxic agents are used less often today, suggesting the global incidence of diabetes mellitus among people with HIV may continue to decline. However, other factors may serve to increase the risk of diabetes mellitus in the contemporary ART era, especially the increasing burden of diabetes in countries moving from low- to middle-income status.

Factors Associated with Diabetes Mellitus among People with HIV

Factors that may predispose people with HIV to diabetes mellitus are often similar to those of the general population, including older age (Butt and others 2004; Capeau and others 2012; Hughes and others 2005), obesity (Hughes and others 2005), and racial or ethnic minority group (Butt and others 2004; Hughes and others 2005). In many parts of the world, including the United States, increasing obesity and sedentary lifestyles will contribute to increasing diabetes mellitus incidence among people with and without HIV (Samaras 2009).

Hepatitis C virus is another established risk factor for diabetes mellitus in the general population (Fallahi and others 2013). Hepatitis C virus has a higher prevalence in many populations of people with HIV; as such, it may be a more important risk factor in individuals co-infected with HIV and hepatitis C virus (Butt and others 2004; Visnegarwala and others 2005).

HIV-specific risk factors for diabetes mellitus include the use of protease inhibitors, particularly indinavir (Capeau and others 2012) or ritonavir (Brown and others 2005), and longer duration of exposure to NRTIs (Tien and others 2007), particularly didanosine and stavudine (Capeau and others 2012). However, a meta-analysis of Sub-Saharan African studies found that among people with HIV, ART use was associated with a lower HbA1c value (Dillon and others 2013). People with HIV with a lower CD4 T-cell nadir (< 300 cells/mm^3) have a higher incidence of abnormal glucose metabolism than those with a higher CD4 T-cell nadir (Brown and others 2005). This finding suggests that current treatment recommendations that include starting people with

HIV on ART at higher CD4 T-cell counts may contribute to a decrease in diabetes mellitus incidence among people with HIV.

Dyslipidemia

Burden and Epidemiology of Dyslipidemia in HIV

Dyslipidemia is an important NCC, given both the high prevalence among people with HIV and impact of dyslipidemia on CVD risk (Giannarelli, Klein, and Badimon 2011). The condition is common among people with HIV who are untreated and is the most common metabolic abnormality associated with ART (Friis-Moller and others 2003).

HIV infection itself, before initiating effective ART, has been associated with changes in lipids, including reductions in total cholesterol, low-density lipoprotein cholesterol (LDL), and high-density lipoprotein cholesterol (HDL), as well as increases in triglyceride values, particularly among those with more advanced HIV disease (Riddler and others 2003).

Among people with HIV on ART, HIV-associated dyslipidemia may include decreased HDL, increased LDL, increased non-HDL cholesterol, and hypertriglyceridemia. Some of the lipid changes after ART initiation are due to a return to health with HIV treatment (Liu and others 2013). One large cross-sectional study found elevated total cholesterol levels in 27 percent of people with HIV receiving protease inhibitors and 23 percent receiving non-nucleoside reverse transcriptase inhibitors (NNRTI), compared with 8 percent of ART-naive people with HIV (Friis-Moller and others 2003). Cohort studies have suggested that the effect of ART on lipids may be greatest in the first six months after ART initiation (Papadopoulos and others 2012).

A large cross-sectional study of people with HIV in New York City, most of whom were receiving ART, found that the prevalence of elevated LDL was 37 percent in men and 31 percent in women (Myerson and others 2014). Furthermore, 30 percent of black people with HIV, 40 percent of Hispanic people with HIV, and 37 percent of white people with HIV had elevated LDL levels (Myerson and others 2014). Women with HIV have lower HDL and higher triglyceride values compared with women without HIV (Schwartz and others 2014).

Although less is known about dyslipidemia in people with HIV in LMICs than in HICs, it remains one of the better investigated NCCs in LMICs. Cross-sectional studies from Cameroon and Tanzania of people with HIV not receiving ART found low HDL levels and elevated triglyceride levels; high triglyceride levels were particularly associated with advanced stages of immunodeficiency (Armstrong and others 2011; Nguemaim and others 2010).

South Africa has one of the highest prevalence rates of HIV, but the prevalence and effect of dyslipidemia is less clear. Black Africans often exhibit lower fasting triglyceride, total cholesterol, and LDL levels, and higher HDL levels, than white Africans (Seedat 1999); however, in 300 black individuals in South Africa newly diagnosed with HIV, HDL levels were found to be lower than levels normally associated with increased CVD risk (Fourie and others 2010). A cross-sectional study of 580 people with HIV in Thailand found that 41 percent had triglyceride levels greater than 150 milligrams per deciliter (mg/dL), 40 percent had total cholesterol values greater than 200 mg/dL, and 12 percent had LDL values greater than 160 mg/dL (Jantarapakde and others 2014). A study of 129 people with HIV from Thailand who had survived with HIV more than 10 years found that more than 50 percent had lipid abnormalities (Kiertiburanakul, Luengroongroj, and Sungkanuparph 2012).

Factors Associated with Dyslipidemia among People with HIV

Dyslipidemia among people with HIV is associated with a number of factors, such as gender, older age, race, and CD4 T-cell count (Crane and others 2011). However, ART is likely to be one of the most important factors in dyslipidemia risk among people with HIV. Dyslipidemia is associated with most protease inhibitors; among the protease inhibitors, darunavir and atazanavir have been found to have better lipid profiles than older protease inhibitors (Carey and others 2010; Mills and others 2009) (table 3.1).

The NNRTIs tend to have a smaller impact on lipid levels than the protease inhibitors, except for atazanavir and darunavir (Daar and others 2011). Etravirine and rilpivirine, in particular, are NNRTIs with less impact

Table 3.1 Antiretroviral Medications Associated with Little or Less Negative Impact on Lipid Levels

Class	Agents
Protease inhibitors	Atazanavir
	Darunavir
NNRTI	Etravirine
	Rilpivirine
Integrase inhibitors	Raltegravir
	Dolutegravir
	Elvitegravir
NRTI	Tenofovir

Note: NNRTI = non-nucleoside reverse transcriptase inhibitors; NRTI = nucleoside reverse transcriptase inhibitors.

on lipid levels than other NNRTIs (Cohen and others 2013; Fatkenheuer and others 2012) (see table 3.1). Integrase inhibitors are increasingly important components of both follow-up or salvage regimens (Capetti and others 2014) and naive regimens (Gunthard and others 2014). Their use will likely continue to increase, particularly in regions with access to the once-daily integrase inhibitor dolutegravir and the single daily pill coformulation of dolutegravir with the NRTIs abacavir and lamivudine.

An important advantage of the integrase inhibitors is their minimal impact on lipid levels. In ART-naive people with HIV initiating a regimen with raltegravir or efavirenz, those on raltegravir had smaller increases in total cholesterol, HDL, LDL, and triglycerides with up to five years of follow-up (Gotuzzo and others 2012; Rockstroh and others 2013). The impact of dolutegravir is likely similar to raltegravir (Raffi and others 2013).

The impact of the NRTI class of agents on lipids is variable. Among the NRTIs, tenofovir has the least negative impact on lipid levels (see table 3.1). A study of treatment-naive people with HIV who initiated atazanavir/ritonavir or efavirenz with abacavir/lamivudine or tenofovir/emtricitabine found that those on abacavir/lamivudine generally had greater increases in lipid levels, including total cholesterol, LDL, and HDL levels, than those on tenofovir/emtricitabine at 48 and 96 weeks (Sax and others 2011). A United States–based cohort study found that people whose ART regimen contained tenofovir (in combination with lamivudine or emtricitabine) had lower concentrations of total cholesterol, LDL, non-HDL cholesterol, HDL, and triglyceride levels, compared with other pairs of NRTIs (Crane and others 2011). Those who received didanosine and stavudine—a combination that is no longer recommended—had the highest levels of LDL (Crane and others 2011). While stavudine leads to elevated total cholesterol and triglyceride values, it is rarely used in the United States any longer; however, it has been more widely used in LMICs (Ali and others 2014). Unfortunately, many of the newer agents with little or no impact on lipid levels are not as widely available in LMICs (Ali and others 2014).

Several studies in LMICs have examined the influence of ART in general on lipid levels; fewer studies in LMICs have focused on individual ART regimens or agents. Dyslipidemia, such as low HDL levels, was more common among patients with longer exposure to ART in several studies from South America (Albuquerque and others 2005; Cahn and others 2010). However, a Brazilian study found that low HDL was common before ART initiation; with initiation of ART, increased triglyceride levels were much more notable, with half of the patients having elevated triglyceride levels after ART (Pinto Neto and others 2013).

In Cameroon and Ethiopia, lipid levels were higher among people with HIV on NNRTI-based ART compared with those not on therapy (Abebe and others 2014; Pefura Yone and others 2011). Similarly, Nigerian people with HIV on ART had higher total cholesterol levels and lower HDL levels than those who were ART naive (Muhammad, Sani, and Okeahialam 2013).

Among Sub-Saharan African women randomized to regimens containing nelfinavir versus lopinavir/ritonavir, larger increases in lipid levels except HDL were found over time among those on lopinavir/ritonavir (Shaffer and others 2014). Variable increases in triglyceride, LDL, and HDL values have been reported after ART initiation (Ceccato and others 2011). Among Ugandan people with HIV with CD4 T-cell $< 200/mm^3$ or symptomatic HIV who initiated predominantly stavudine/lamivudine/nevirapine, substantial increases in HDL occurred during the initial 24 months of ART, with less frequent elevations in total cholesterol, LDL, and triglyceride values (Buchacz and others 2008). Among patients in Tanzania, one of the largest longitudinal studies found low HDL and high triglyceride levels were common before ART initiation; after ART was initiated, unfavorable changes were more common among those on stavudine and efavirenz compared with zidovudine- and nevirapine-based regimens (Liu and others 2013).

Summary of HIV and Dyslipidemia

To summarize, HIV itself is associated with changes in lipid levels, particularly elevated triglyceride levels, most notably among those with more pronounced immune deficiency. Initiating ART is also associated with dyslipidemia, but the effect is variable, depending on the regimen. Protease inhibitors as a class are associated with increased lipid levels, particularly triglycerides, but darunavir and atazanavir have less effect.

Other classes of ART are more variable. NNRTIs raise lipid levels, but etravirine and rilpivirine have less impact, as do integrase inhibitors such as raltegravir and dolutegravir. Among the NRTIs, tenofovir has little effect, while agents such as stavudine have a substantial negative impact on lipids. Data from LMICs on class- and agent-specific impacts, particularly of newer regimens, are sparse.

Recommendations for initial ART regimens have varied over time but more recently have included regimens less likely to cause dyslipidemia than those used a few years ago (Gunthard and others 2014), suggesting that in HICs the rate of newly developed dyslipidemia may drop. However, these benefits may not apply to other regions of the world where these regimen choices are less widely available.

HIV and NCCs Conclusions

NCCs among people with HIV present an increasing global health challenge in the era of increasing access to ART, which is leading to older populations of people with HIV.

Even though this chapter briefly summarizes several NCCs, many serious NCCs are not addressed here because of space considerations. These include strokes, bone disease, cognitive impairment, renal disease, and frailty. A very important NCC is liver disease, which is an area in flux, with increasing treatment options for hepatitis C virus (chapter 16 in this volume, Wiktor 2017).

Those covered here can be considered the tip of the iceberg. As access to ART continues to expand, particularly in LMICs, access to care for NCCs will also be needed to avoid widespread preventable morbidity and death. Notably, a theme common to many NCCs is the benefit of early ART. Many NCCs are worsened by the lack of treatment or late treatment initiation, leading to increased burden of illness. Focused efforts on engagement in care, expanded access to ART, and earlier initiation of ART are likely to reduce the rates of these NCCs, particularly in areas with access to newer ART agents with less metabolic and other associated toxicities.

However, as the population of people with HIV ages, the burden of many NCCs will continue to increase. The importance of NCCs among people with HIV as a global health challenge cannot be underestimated.

Data demonstrating the importance of these conditions among people with HIV are predominantly from HICs; unfortunately, much less of the data and research advances for these conditions are from LMICs, where most people with HIV live (Narayan and others 2014).

In many areas, such as Sub-Saharan Africa, HIV care, including ART, is more widely available than it has previously been, but this care is not accompanied by care for NCCs, resulting in preventable morbidity and death (Narayan and others 2014).

CONCLUSIONS

This chapter reviews the complex association of HIV with a host of other diseases and conditions; not least is the rise in those that have occurred because people with HIV have been living longer thanks to the widespread availability of ART. In the era of effective therapy for HIV, health professionals will need to deploy more complex strategies and treatments that recognize the rising impact of comorbidities complicating long-term HIV infection.

Cancer Prevention

Strategies for cancer prevention, including vaccination, screening, and early ART initiation, can reduce the cancer burden, but additional strategies for reducing the burden of HIVAMs are needed.

Reproductive Health

In the areas of reproductive health beyond fertility issues, evidence has also suggested a greater risk of stillbirth, premature birth, or low birth weight in pregnancies of women with HIV. Providing women with access to appropriate fertility and contraception to ensure safe and planned pregnancies will be paramount in strategies to reduce these risks associated with HIV and reproduction.

Noncommunicable Chronic Comorbidities

Among NCCs, ART has changed the nature of the global health challenge. This chapter only brushes the surface of a major issue, leaving out other diseases associated with HIV. Notably, and as with cancers, a theme common to many NCCs is the benefit of early ART. Many of the diseases are worsened by lack of treatment or late treatment. Better care, expanded access, and earlier initiation of ART are likely to help lower disease rates. Because populations of people with HIV will continue to rise, however, these comorbidities cannot be underestimated as a looming public health challenge.

The burden of NCCs will be concentrated in areas of the world, such as Sub-Saharan Africa, where the number of HIV infections continue to rise and access to life-prolonging ART is expanding.

Taken together, the great success in treating HIV has been met by a set of considerable challenges for persons with the infection and for the public health community in the form of chronic noncommunicable diseases. However, improvements in the treatment of HIV infection, attention to preventive measures for chronic disease in persons at high risk for their complications, and increased research and awareness offer hope that the same successes enjoyed in the fight against HIV infection can be brought to bear to reduce the complications of long-term infection.

NOTE

World Bank Income Classifications as of July 2014 are as follows, based on estimates of gross national income (GNI) per capita for 2013:

- Low-income countries (LICs) = US$1,045 or less
- Middle-income countries (MICs) are subdivided:
  (a) lower-middle-income = US$1,046 to US$4,125
  (b) upper-middle-income (UMICs) = US$4,126 to US$12,745
- High-income countries (HICs) = US$12,746 or more.

REFERENCES

Abebe, M., S. Kinde, G. Belay, A. Gebreegziabxier, F. Challa, and others. 2014. "Antiretroviral Treatment Associated Hyperglycemia and Dyslipidemia among HIV Infected Patients at Burayu Health Center, Addis Ababa, Ethiopia: A Cross-Sectional Comparative Study." *BMC Research Notes* 7: 380. doi:10.1186/1756-0500-7-380.

Aberg, J. A. 2009. "Cardiovascular Complications in HIV Management: Past, Present and Future." *Journal of Acquired Immune Deficiency Syndromes* 50 (1): 54–64.

Achenbach, C. J., S. R. Cole, M. M. Kitahata, C. Casper, J. H. Willig, and others. 2011. "Mortality after Cancer Diagnosis in HIV-Infected Individuals Treated with Antiretroviral Therapy." *AIDS* 25 (5): 691–700. doi:10.1097/QAD.0b013e3283437f77.

Ahdieh, L., A. Munoz, D. Vlahov, C. L. Trimble, L. A. Timpson, and K. Shah. 2000. "Cervical Neoplasia and Repeated Positivity of Human Papillomavirus Infection in Human Immunodeficiency Virus-Seropositive and -Seronegative Women." *American Journal of Epidemiology* 151 (12): 1148–57.

Akarolo-Anthony, S. N., L. D. Maso, F. Igbinoba, S. M. Mbulaiteye, and C. A. Adebamowo. 2014. "Cancer Burden among HIV-Positive Persons in Nigeria: Preliminary Findings from the Nigerian AIDS-Cancer Match Study." *Infectious Agents and Cancer* 9 (1): 1. doi:10.1186/1750-9378-9-1.

Albuquerque, E. M., E. C. de Faria, H. C. Oliveira, D. O. Magro, and L. N. Castilho. 2005. "High Frequency of Fredrickson's Phenotypes IV and IIb in Brazilians Infected by Human Immunodeficiency Virus." *BMC Infectious Diseases* 5: 47. doi:10.1186/1471-2334-5-47.

Ali, M. K., M. J. Magee, J. A. Dave, I. Ofotokun, M. Tungsiripat, and others. 2014. "HIV and Metabolic, Body, and Bone Disorders: What We Know from Low- and Middle-Income Countries." *Journal of Acquired Immune Deficiency Syndromes* 67 (Suppl 1): S27–39. doi:10.1097/QAI.0000000000000256.

Arama, V., C. Tiliscan, A. Streinu-Cercel, D. Ion, R. Mihailescu, and others. 2013. "Insulin Resistance and Adipokines Serum Levels in a Caucasian Cohort of HIV-Positive Patients Undergoing Antiretroviral Therapy: A Cross Sectional Study." *BMC Endocrine Disorders* 13: 4. doi:10.1186/1472-6823-13-4.

Araujo, S., S. Banon, I. Machuca, A. Moreno, M. J. Perez-Elias, and J. L. Casado. 2014. "Prevalence of Insulin Resistance and Risk of Diabetes Mellitus in HIV-Infected Patients Receiving Current Antiretroviral Drugs." *European Journal of Endocrinology* 171 (5): 545–54. doi:10.1530/EJE-14–0337.

Armstrong, C., E. Liu, J. Okuma, D. Spiegelman, C. Guerino, and others. 2011. "Dyslipidemia in an HIV-Positive Antiretroviral Treatment-Naive Population in Dar es Salaam, Tanzania." *Journal of Acquired Immune Deficiency Syndromes* 57 (2): 141–45. doi:10.1097/QAI.0b013e318219a3d1.

Arzumanyan, A., H. M. Reis, and M. A. Feitelson. 2013. "Pathogenic Mechanisms in HBV- and Hepatitis C Virus-Associated Hepatocellular Carcinoma." *Nature Reviews Cancer* 13 (2): 123–35. doi:10.1038/nrc3449.

Atashili, J., C. Poole, P. M. Ndumbe, A. A. Adimora, and J. S. Smith. 2008. "Bacterial Vaginosis and HIV Acquisition: A Meta-Analysis of Published Studies." *AIDS* 22 (12): 1493–501. doi:10.1097/QAD.0b013e3283021a37.

Barnes, A., D. Riche, L. Mena, T. Sison, L. Barry, and others. 2014. "Efficacy and Safety of Intrauterine Insemination and Assisted Reproductive Technology in Populations Serodiscordant for Human Immunodeficiency Virus: A Systematic Review and Meta-Analysis." *Fertility and Sterility* 102 (2): 424–34. doi:10.1016/j.fertnstert.2014.05.001.

Behrens, G., A. Dejam, H. Schmidt, H. J. Balks, G. Brabant, and others. 1999. "Impaired Glucose Tolerance, Beta Cell Function and Lipid Metabolism in HIV Patients under Treatment with Protease Inhibitors." *AIDS* 13 (10): F63–70.

Biggar, R. J., A. K. Chaturvedi, J. J. Goedert, E. A. Engels, and HIV AIDS Cancer Match Study. 2007. "AIDS-Related Cancer and Severity of Immunosuppression in Persons with AIDS." *Journal of the National Cancer Institute* 99 (12): 962–72. doi:10.1093/jnci/djm010.

Blitz, S., J. Baxter, J. Raboud, S. Walmsley, A. Rachlis, and others. 2013. "Evaluation of HIV and Highly Active Antiretroviral Therapy on the Natural History of Human Papillomavirus Infection and Cervical Cytopathologic Findings in HIV-Positive and High-Risk HIV-Negative Women." *Journal of Infectious Diseases* 208 (3): 454–62. doi:10.1093/infdis/jit181.

Bloomfield, G. S., P. Khazanie, A. Morris, C. Rabadan-Diehl, L. A. Benjamin, and others. 2014. "HIV and Noncommunicable Cardiovascular and Pulmonary Diseases in Low- and Middle-Income Countries in the ART Era: What We Know and Best Directions for Future Research." *Journal of Acquired Immune Deficiency Syndromes* 67 (Suppl 1): S40–53.

Bonnet, F., C. Lewden, T. May, L. Heripret, E. Jougla, and others. 2004. "Malignancy-Related Causes of Death in Human Immunodeficiency Virus-Infected Patients in the Era of Highly Active Antiretroviral Therapy." *Cancer* 101 (2): 317–24.

Bosch, F. X., T. R. Broker, D. Forman, A. B. Moscicki, M. L. Gillison, and others. 2013. "Comprehensive Control of Human Papillomavirus Infections and Related Diseases." *Vaccine* 31 (Suppl 7): H1–31. doi:10.1016/j.vaccine.2013.10.003.

Brotman, R. M. 2011. "Vaginal Microbiome and Sexually Transmitted Infections: An Epidemiologic Perspective." *Journal of Clinical Investigation* 121 (12): 4610–17. doi:10.1172/JCI57172.

Brown, T. T., S. R. Cole, X. Li, L. A. Kingsley, F. J. Palella, and others. 2005. "Antiretroviral Therapy and the Prevalence and Incidence of Diabetes Mellitus in the Multicenter AIDS Cohort Study." *Archives of Internal Medicine* 165 (10): 1179–84.

Bruni, L., M. Diaz, X. Castellsague, E. Ferrer, F. X. Bosch, and S. de Sanjose. 2010. "Cervical Human Papillomavirus Prevalence in 5 Continents: Meta-Analysis of 1 Million Women with Normal Cytological Findings." *Journal of Infectious Diseases* 202 (12): 1789–99. doi:10.1086/657321.

Bruyand, M., R. Thiebaut, S. Lawson-Ayayi, P. Joly, A. J. Sasco, and others. 2009. "Role of Uncontrolled HIV RNA Level and Immunodeficiency in the Occurrence of Malignancy in HIV-Infected Patients during the Combination Antiretroviral Therapy Era: Agence Nationale de Recherche sur le Sida (ANRS) CO3 Aquitaine Cohort." *Clinical Infectious Diseases* 49 (7): 1109–16. doi:10.1086/605594.

Buchacz, K., P. J. Weidle, D. Moore, W. Were, J. Mermin, and others. 2008. "Changes in Lipid Profile over 24 Months among Adults on First-Line Highly Active Antiretroviral Therapy in the Home-Based AIDS Care Program in Rural Uganda." *Journal of Acquired Immune Deficiency Syndromes* 47 (3): 304–11.

Bukusi, E. A., C. R. Cohen, C. E. Stevens, S. Sinei, M. Reilly, and others. 1999. "Effects of Human Immunodeficiency Virus 1 Infection on Microbial Origins of Pelvic Inflammatory Disease and on Efficacy of Ambulatory Oral Therapy." *American Journal of Obstetrics and Gynecology* 181 (6): 1374–81.

Butt, A. A., C. C. Chang, L. Kuller, M. B. Goetz, D. Leaf, and others. 2011. "Risk of Heart Failure with Human Immunodeficiency Virus without Prior Diagnosis of Coronary Heart Disease." *Archives of Internal Medicine* 171 (8): 737–43. doi:10.1001/archinternmed.2011.151.

Butt, A. A., S. L. Fultz, C. K. Kwoh, D. Kelley, M. Skanderson, and others. 2004. "Risk of Diabetes in HIV Infected Veterans Pre- and Post-HAART and the Role of Hepatitis C Virus Coinfection." *Hepatology* 40 (1): 115–19.

Cahn, P., O. Leite, A. Rosales, R. Cabello, C. A. Alvarez, and others. 2010. "Metabolic Profile and Cardiovascular Risk Factors among Latin American HIV-Infected Patients Receiving HAART." *Brazilian Journal of Infectious Diseases* 14 (2): 158–66. doi:S1413–86702010000200008 [pii].

Campos, N. G., P. E. Castle, T. C. Wright Jr., and J. J. Kim. 2015. "Cervical Cancer Screening in Low-Resource Settings: A Cost-Effectiveness Framework for Valuing Tradeoffs between Test Performance and Program Coverage." *International Journal of Cancer* 137 (9): 2208–19. doi:10.1002/ijc.29594.

Capeau, J., V. Bouteloup, C. Katlama, J. P. Bastard, V. Guiyedi, and others. 2012. "Ten-Year Diabetes Incidence in 1046 HIV-Infected Patients Started on a Combination Antiretroviral Treatment." *AIDS* 26 (3): 303–14. doi:10.1097/QAD.0b013e32834e8776.

Capetti, A., P. Meraviglia, S. Landonio, G. Sterrantino, A. Di Biagio, and others. 2014. "Four Years Data of Raltegravir-Based Salvage Therapy in HIV-1-Infected, Treatment-Experienced Patients: The SALIR-E Study." *International*

Journal of Antimicrobial Agents 43 (2): 189–94. doi:10.1016/j.ijantimicag.2013.10.013.

Carbone, A., and A. Gloghini. 2005. "AIDS-Related Lymphomas: From Pathogenesis to Pathology." *British Journal of Haematology* 130 (5): 662–70. doi:10.1111/j.1365–2141.2005.05613.x.

Carey, D., J. Amin, M. Boyd, K. Petoumenos, and S. Emery. 2010. "Lipid Profiles in HIV-Infected Adults Receiving Atazanavir and Atazanavir/Ritonavir: Systematic Review and Meta-Analysis of Randomized Controlled Trials." *Journal of Antimicrobial Chemotherapy* 65 (9): 1878–88. doi:10.1093/jac/dkq231.

CDC (Centers for Disease Control and Prevention). 1992. "1993 Revised Classification System for HIV Infection and Expanded Surveillance Case Definition for AIDS among Adolescents and Adults." *MMWR Recommendations and Reports* 41 (RR-17): 1–19.

———. 2006. "A Comprehensive Immunization Strategy to Eliminate Transmission of Hepatitis B Virus Infection in the United States." *Morbidity and Mortality Weekly Reports* 55.

Ceccato, M. G., P. F. Bonolo, A. I. Souza Neto, F. S. Araujo, and M. I. Freitas. 2011. "Antiretroviral Therapy–Associated Dyslipidemia in Patients from a Reference Center in Brazil." *Brazilian Journal of Medical and Biological Research* 44 (11): 1177–83.

Celum, C., A. Wald, J. R. Lingappa, A. S. Magaret, R. S. Wang, and others. 2010. "Acyclovir and Transmission of HIV-1 from Persons Infected with HIV-1 and HSV-2." *New England Journal of Medicine* 62 (5): 427–39. doi:10.1056/NEJMoa0904849.

Cerrato, E., F. D'Ascenzo, G. Biondi-Zoccai, A. Calcagno, S. Frea, and others. 2013. "Cardiac Dysfunction in Pauci Symptomatic Human Immunodeficiency Virus Patients: A Meta-Analysis in the Highly Active Antiretroviral Therapy Era." *European Heart Journal* 34 (19): 1432–36. doi:10.1093/eurheartj/ehs471.

Chang, M. H., C. J. Chen, M. S. Lai, H. M. Hsu, T. C. Wu, and others. 1997. "Universal Hepatitis B Vaccination in Taiwan and the Incidence of Hepatocellular Carcinoma in Children. Taiwan Childhood Hepatoma Study Group." *New England Journal of Medicine* 336 (26): 1855–59. doi:10.1056/nejm199706263362602.

Chang, M. H., S. L. You, C. J. Chen, C. J. Liu, C. M. Lee, and others. 2009. "Decreased Incidence of Hepatocellular Carcinoma in Hepatitis B Vaccinees: A 20-Year Follow-Up Study." *Journal of the National Cancer Institute* 101 (19): 1348–55. doi:10.1093/jnci/djp288.

Chiao, E. Y., T. P. Giordano, J. M. Palefsky, S. Tyring, and H. El Serag. 2006. "Screening HIV-Infected Individuals for Anal Cancer Precursor Lesions: A Systematic Review." *Clinical Infectious Diseases* 43 (2): 223–33. doi:10.1086/505219.

Chung, M. H., K. P. McKenzie, H. De Vuyst, B. A. Richardson, F. Rana, and others. 2013. "Comparing Papanicolau Smear, Visual Inspection with Acetic Acid and Human Papillomavirus Cervical Cancer Screening Methods among HIV-Positive Women by Immune Status and Antiretroviral Therapy." *AIDS* 27 (18): 2909–19. doi:10.1097/01.aids.0000432472.92120.1b.

Clifford, G. M., M. Lise, S. Francesshi, M. Egger, C. Bouchardy, and others. 2012. "Lung Cancer in the Swiss HIV Cohort Study: Role of Smoking, Immunodeficiency, and Pulmonary Infection." *British Journal of Cancer* 106 (3): 447–52.

Coghill, A. E., P. A. Newcomb, M. M. Madeleine, B. A. Richardson, I. Mutyaba, and others. 2013. "Contribution of HIV Infection to Mortality among Cancer Patients in Uganda." *AIDS* 27 (18): 2933–42. doi:10.1097/01.aids.0000433236.55937.cb.

Coghill, A. E., M. S. Shiels, G. Suneja, and E. A. Engels. 2015. "Elevated Cancer-Specific Mortality among HIV-Infected Patients in the United States." *Journal of Clinical Oncology* 3 (21): 2376–83. doi:10.1200/JCO.2014.59.5967.

Cohen, C. J., J. M. Molina, I. Cassetti, P. Chetchotisakd, A. Lazzarin, and others. 2013. "Week 96 Efficacy and Safety of Rilpivirine in Treatment-Naive, HIV-1 Patients in Two Phase III Randomized Trials." *AIDS* 27 (6): 939–50. doi:10.1097/QAD.0b013e32835cee6e.

Cohen, C. R., J. R. Lingappa, J. M. Baeten, M. O. Ngayo, C. A. Spiegel, and others. 2012. "Bacterial Vaginosis Associated with Increased Risk of Female-to-Male HIV-1 Transmission: A Prospective Cohort Analysis among African Couples." *PLoS Medicine* 9 (6): e1001251. doi:10.1371/journal.pmed.1001251.

Cohen, C. R., S. Sinei, M. Reilly, E. Bukusi, D. Eschenbach, and others. 1998. "Effect of Human Immunodeficiency Virus Type 1 Infection upon Acute Salpingitis: A Laparoscopic Study." *Journal of Infectious Diseases* 178 (5): 1352–58.

Cone, M. M., and C. B. Whitlow. 2013. "Sexually Transmitted and Anorectal Infectious Diseases." *Gastroenterology Clinics of North America* 42 (4): 877–92. doi:10.1016/j.gtc.2013.09.003.

Crane, H. M., C. Grunfeld, J. H. Willig, M. J. Mugavero, S. Van Rompaey, and others. 2011. "Impact of NRTIs on Lipid Levels among a Large HIV-Infected Cohort Initiating Antiretroviral Therapy in Clinical Care." *AIDS* 25 (2): 185–95. doi:10.1097/QAD.0b013e328341f925.

Crane, H. M., S. R. Heckbert, D. R. Drozd, M. J. Budoff, J. A. C. Delaney, and others. 2014. "Lessons Learned from the Design and Implementation of Myocardial Infarction Adjudication Tailored for HIV Clinical Cohorts." *American Journal of Epidemiology* 179 (8): 996–1005.

Crum-Cianflone, N. F., K. H. Hullsiek, V. C. Marconi, A. Ganesan, A. Weintrob, and others. 2010. "Anal Cancers among HIV-Infected Persons: HAART Is Not Slowing Rising Incidence." *AIDS* 24 (4): 535–43.

Currier, J. S., A. Taylor, F. Boyd, C. M. Dezii, H. Kawabata, and others. 2003. "Coronary Heart Disease in HIV-Infected Individuals." *Journal of Acquired Immune Deficiency Syndromes* 33 (4): 506–12.

Cutrell, A., C. Brothers, J. Yeo, J. Hernandez, and D. Lapierre. 2008. "Abacavir and the Potential Risk of Myocardial Infarction." *The Lancet* 371 (9622): 1413.

Daar, E. S., C. Tierney, M. A. Fischl, P. E. Sax, K. Mollan, and others. 2011. "Atazanavir Plus Ritonavir or Efavirenz as Part of a 3-Drug Regimen for Initial Treatment of HIV-1." *Annals of Internal Medicine* 154 (7): 445–56. doi:10.7326/0003-4819-154-7-201104050-00316.

DAD (Diabetes and Depression) Study Investigators. 2004. "Cardio- and Cerebrovascular Events in HIV-Infected Persons." *AIDS* 18 (13): 1811–17.

Dalla Pria, A., M. Alfa-Wali, P. Fox, P. Holmes, J. Weir, and others. 2014. "High-Resolution Anoscopy Screening of HIV-Positive MSM: Longitudinal Results from a Pilot Study." *AIDS* 28 (6): 861–67. doi:10.1097/QAD.0000000000000160.

Depuydt, C. E., L. Verstraete, M. Berth, J. Beert, J. P. Bogers, and others. 2016. "Human Papillomavirus Positivity in Women Undergoing Intrauterine Insemination Has a Negative Effect on Pregnancy Rates." *Gynecology and Obstetric Investigation* 81 (1): 41–46. doi:10.1159/000434749.

De Vuyst, H., L. Alemany, C. Lacey, C. J. Chibwesha, V. Sahasrabuddhe, and others. 2013. "The Burden of Human Papillomavirus Infections and Related Diseases in Sub-Saharan Africa." *Vaccine* 31 (Suppl 5): F32–46. doi:10.1016/j.vaccine.2012.07.092.

Dillon, D. G., D. Gurdasani, J. Riha, K. Ekoru, G. Asiki, and others. 2013. "Association of HIV and ART with Cardiometabolic Traits in Sub-Saharan Africa: A Systematic Review and Meta-Analysis." *International Journal of Epidemiology* 42 (6): 1754–71. doi:10.1093/ije/dyt198.

Dobson, S. R., S. McNeil, M. Dionne, M. Dawar, G. Ogilvie, and others. 2013. "Immunogenicity of 2 Doses of HPV Vaccine in Younger Adolescents vs. 3 Doses in Young Women: A Randomized Clinical Trial." *Journal of the American Medical Association* 309 (17): 1793–802. doi:10.1001/jama.2013.1625.

Drozd, D. R., R. M. Nance, J. A. C. Delaney, G. A. Burkholder, W. C. Mathews, and others. 2014. "Lower CD4 T-Cell Count and Higher Viral Load Are Associated with Increased Risk of Myocardial Infarction." Conference on Retroviruses and Opportunistic Infections (CROI), Boston, MA, March 3–6.

El-Sadr, W. M., J. D. Lundgren, J. D. Neaton, F. Gordin, D. Abrams, and others. 2006. "CD4 T-cell+ Count-Guided Interruption of Antiretroviral Treatment." *New England Journal of Medicine* 355 (22): 2283–96.

Eltom, M. A., A. Jemal, S. M. Mbulaiteye, S. S. Devesa, and R. J. Biggar. 2002. "Trends in Kaposi's Sarcoma and Non-Hodgkin's Lymphoma Incidence in the United States from 1973 through 1998." *Journal of the National Cancer Institute* 94 (16): 1204–10.

Engels, E. A., M. V. Brock, J. Chen, C. M. Hooker, M. Gillison, and others. 2006. "Elevated Incidence of Lung Cancer among HIV-Infected Individuals." *Journal of Clinical Oncology* 24 (9): 1383–88. doi:10.1200/JCO.2005.03.4413.

Fallahi, P., S. M. Ferrari, M. Colaci, I. Ruffilli, R. Vita, and others. 2013. "Hepatitis C Virus Infection and Type 2 Diabetes." *Clinical Therapeutics* 164 (5): e393–404. doi:10.7417/CT.2013.1620.

Fatkenheuer, G., C. Duvivier, A. Rieger, J. Durant, D. Rey, and others. 2012. "Lipid Profiles for Etravirine versus Efavirenz in Treatment-Naive Patients in the Randomized, Double-Blind SENSE Trial." *Journal of Antimicrobial Chemotherapy* 67 (3): 685–90. doi:10.1093/jac/dkr533.

Ferlay, J., I. Soerjomataram, M. Ervik, R. Dikshit, S. Eser, and others. 2013. "GLOBOCAN 2012 v1.0; Cancer Incidence and Mortality Worldwide." IARC CancerBase 11.

Fleming, D. T., and J. N. Wasserheit. 1999. "From Epidemiological Synergy to Public Health Policy and Practice: The Contribution of Other Sexually Transmitted Diseases to Sexual Transmission of HIV Infection." *Sexually Transmitted Infections* 75 (1): 3–17.

Ford, E. S., J. H. Greenwald, A. G. Richterman, A. Rupert, and others. 2010. "Traditional Risk Factors and D-Dimer Predict Incident Cardiovascular Disease Events in Chronic HIV Infection." *AIDS* 24 (10): 1509–17. doi:10.1097/QAD.0b013e32833ad914.

Forman, D., C. de Martel, C. J. Lacey, I. Soerjomataram, J. Lortet-Tieulent, and others. 2012. "Global Burden of Human Papillomavirus and Related Diseases." *Vaccine* 30 (Suppl 5): F12–23. doi:10.1016/j.vaccine.2012.07.055.

Fourie, C. M., J. M. Van Rooyen, A. Kruger, and A. E. Schutte. 2010. "Lipid Abnormalities in a Never-Treated HIV-1 Subtype C-Infected African Population." *Lipids* 45 (1): 73–80. doi:10.1007/s11745–009–3369–4.

Freiberg, M. S., C. C. Chang, L. H. Kuller, M. Skanderson, E. Lowy, and others. 2013. "HIV Infection and the Risk of Acute Myocardial Infarction." *JAMA Internal Medicine* 173 (8): 614–22. doi:1659742[pii]10.1001/jamainternmed.2013.3728.

Friis-Moller, N., P. Reiss, C. A. Sabin, R. Weber, A. Monforte, and others. 2007. "Class of Antiretroviral Drugs and the Risk of Myocardial Infarction." *New England Journal of Medicine* 356 (17): 1723–35.

Friis-Moller, N., R. Weber, P. Reiss, R. Thiebaut, O. Kirk, and others. 2003. "Cardiovascular Disease Risk Factors in HIV Patients—Association with Antiretroviral Therapy: Results from the DAD Study." *AIDS* 17 (8): 1179–93.

Fultz, S. L., A. C. Justice, A. A. Butt, L. Rabeneck, S. Weissman, and others. 2003. "Testing, Referral, and Treatment Patterns for Hepatitis C Virus Coinfection in a Cohort of Veterans with Human Immunodeficiency Virus Infection." *Clinical Infectious Diseases* 36 (8): 1039–46. doi:10.1086/374049.

Gantt, S., C. Casper, and R. F. Ambinder. 2013. "Insights into the Broad Cellular Effects of Nelfinavir and the HIV Protease Inhibitors Supporting Their Role in Cancer Treatment and Prevention." *Current Opinions in Oncology* 25 (5): 495–502. doi:10.1097/CCO.0b013e328363dfee.

Garolla, A., B. Engl, D. Pizzol, M. Ghezzi, A. Bertoldo, and others. 2016. "Spontaneous Fertility and In Vitro Fertilization Outcome: New Evidence of Human Papillomavirus Sperm Infection." *Fertility and Sterility* 105 (1): 65–72 e1. doi:10.1016/j.fertnstert.2015.09.018.

Giannarelli, C., R. S. Klein, and J. J. Badimon. 2011. "Cardiovascular Implications of HIV-Induced Dyslipidemia." *Atherosclerosis* 219 (2): 384–89. doi:10.1016/j.atherosclerosis.2011.06.003.

Gondos, A., H. Brenner, H. Wabinga, and D. M. Parkin. 2005. "Cancer Survival in Kampala, Uganda." *British Journal of Cancer* 92 (9): 1808–12.

Gotuzzo, E., M. Markowitz, W. Ratanasuwan, G. Smith, G. Prada, and others. 2012. "Sustained Efficacy and Safety of Raltegravir after 5 Years of Combination Antiretroviral Therapy as Initial Treatment of HIV-1 Infection: Final Results of a Randomized, Controlled, Phase II Study (Protocol 004)." *Journal of Acquired Immune Deficiency Syndromes* 61 (1): 73–77. doi:10.1097/QAI.0b013e318263277e.

Grulich, A. E., M. T. van Leeuwen, M. O. Falster, and C. M. Vajdic. 2007. "Incidence of Cancers in People with HIV/AIDS Compared with Immunosuppressed Transplant Recipients: A Meta-Analysis." *The Lancet* 370 (9581): 59–67. doi:10.1016/s0140–6736(07)61050–2.

Guaraldi, G., G. Orlando, S. Zona, M. Menozzi, F. Carli, and others. 2011. "Premature Age-Related Comorbidities among HIV-Infected Persons Compared with the General Population." *Clinical Infectious Diseases* 53 (11): 1120–6. doi:10.1093/cid/cir627.

Guiguet, M., F. Boue, J. Cadranel, J. M. Lang, E. Rosenthal, and others. 2009. "Effect of Immunodeficiency, HIV Viral Load, and Antiretroviral Therapy on the Risk of Individual Malignancies (FHDH-ANRS CO4): A Prospective Cohort Study." *The Lancet Oncology* 10 (12): 1152–59. doi:10.1016/s1470–2045(09)70282–7.

Gunthard, H. F., J. A. Aberg, J. J. Eron, J. F. Hoy, A. Telenti, and others. 2014. "Antiretroviral Treatment of Adult HIV Infection: 2014 Recommendations of the International Antiviral Society-USA Panel." *Journal of the American Medical Association* 312 (4): 410–25. doi:10.1001/jama.2014.8722.

Hadigan, C., J. B. Meigs, C. Corcoran, P. Rietschel, S. Piecuch, and others 2001. "Metabolic Abnormalities and Cardiovascular Disease Risk Factors in Adults with Human Immunodeficiency Virus Infection and Lipodystrophy." *Clinical Infectious Diseases* 32 (1): 130–39. doi:CID000838 [pii]10.1086/317541.

Hakim, J. G., J. A. Matenga, and S. Siziya. 1996. "Myocardial Dysfunction in Human Immunodeficiency Virus Infection: An Echocardiographic Study of 157 Patients in Hospital in Zimbabwe." *Heart* 76 (2): 161–65.

Heffron, R., D. Donnell, H. Rees, C. Celum, N. Mugo, and others. 2012. "Use of Hormonal Contraceptives and Risk of HIV-1 Transmission: A Prospective Cohort Study." *The Lancet Infectious Diseases* 12 (1): 19–26. doi:10.1016/S1473–3099(11)70247-X.

Heffron, R., E. Were, C. Celum, N. Mugo, K. Ngure, and others. 2010. "A Prospective Study of Contraceptive Use among African Women in HIV-1 Serodiscordant Partnerships." *Sexually Transmitted Diseases* 37 (10): 621–28. doi:10.1097/OLQ.0b013e3181e1a162.

Heuft, M. M., S. M. Houba, G. E. van den Berk, T. Smissaert van de Haere, and others. 2014. "Protective Effect of Hepatitis B Virus–Active Antiretroviral Therapy against Primary Hepatitis B Virus Infection." *AIDS* 28 (7): 999–1005. doi:10.1097/QAD.0000000000000180.

Hillier, S. L., R. P. Nugent, D. A. Eschenbach, M. A. Krohn, R. S. Gibbs, and others. 1995. "Association between Bacterial Vaginosis and Preterm Delivery of a Low-Birth-Weight Infant. The Vaginal Infections and Prematurity Study Group." *New England Journal of Medicine* 333 (26): 1737–42. doi:10.1056/NEJM199512283332604.

Holmberg, S. D., A. C. Moorman, and A. E. Greenberg. 2004. "Trends in Rates of Myocardial Infarction among Patients with HIV." *New England Journal of Medicine* 350 (7): 730–32.

Holmberg, S. D., A. C. Moorman, J. M. Williamson, T. C. Tong, D. J. Ward, and others. 2002. "Protease Inhibitors and Cardiovascular Outcomes in Patients with HIV-1." *The Lancet* 360 (9347): 1747–48.

Hsu, H. M., D. S. Chen, C. H. Chuang, J. C. Lu, D. M. Jwo, and others. 1988. "Efficacy of a Mass Hepatitis B Vaccination Program in Taiwan. Studies on 3464 Infants of Hepatitis B Surface Antigen-Carrier Mothers." *Journal of the American Medical Association* 260 (15): 2231–35.

Hughes, C. A., R. P. Cashin, D. T. Eurich, and S. Houston. 2005. "Risk Factors for New-Onset Diabetes Mellitus in Patients Receiving Protease Inhibitor Therapy." *Cancer Journal of Infectious Diseases Medical Microbiology* 16 (4): 230–22.

Hulbert, A., C. M. Hooker, J. C. Keruly, T. Brown, K. Horton, and others. 2014. "Prospective CT Screening for Lung Cancer in a High-Risk Population: HIV-Positive Smokers." *Journal of Thoracic Oncology* 9 (6): 752–59.

Hymes, K. B., T. Cheung, J. B. Greene, N. S. Prose, A. Marcus, and others. 1981. "Kaposi's Sarcoma in Homosexual Men—A Report of Eight Cases." *The Lancet* 2 (8247): 598–600.

Jacobson, I. M., J. G. McHutchison, G. Dusheiko, A. M. Di Bisceglie, K. R. Reddy, and others. 2011. "Telaprevir for Previously Untreated Chronic Hepatitis C Virus Infection." *New England Journal of Medicine* 364 (25): 2405–16. doi:10.1056/NEJMoa1012912.

Jantarapakde, J., N. Phanuphak, C. Chaturawit, S. Pengnonyang, P. Mathajittiphan, and others. 2014. "Prevalence of Metabolic Syndrome among Antiretroviral-Naive and Antiretroviral-Experienced HIV-1 Infected Thai Adults." *AIDS Patient Care and STDs* 28 (7): 331–40. doi:10.1089/apc.2013.0294.

Kane, M. A. 1995. "Global Programme for Control of Hepatitis B Infection." *Vaccine* 13 (Suppl 1): S47–49.

———. 2012. "Preventing Cancer with Vaccines: Progress in the Global Control of Cancer." *Cancer Prevention Research* 5 (1): 24–29. doi:10.1158/1940–6207.capr-11–0533.

Kaufman, M. R., M. Smelyanskaya, L. M. Van Lith, E. C. Mallalieu and others. 2016. "Adolescent Sexual and Reproductive Health Services and Implications for the Provision of Voluntary Medical Male Circumcision: Results of a Systematic Literature Review." *PLoS One* 11 (3): e0149892. doi:10.1371/journal.pone.0149892.

Keith, A., Y. Dong, J. Shuter, and S. Himelhoch. 2016. "Behavioral Interventions for Tobacco Use in HIV-Infected Smokers: A Meta-Analysis." *Journal of Acquired Immune Deficiency Syndromes* 72 (5): 527–33.

Kiertiburanakul, S., P. Luengroongroj, and S. Sungkanuparph. 2012. "Clinical Characteristics of HIV-Infected Patients Who Survive after the Diagnosis of HIV Infection for More than 10 Years in a Resource-Limited Setting." *Journal of the International Association of Physicians in AIDS Care* 11 (6): 361–65. doi:10.1177/1545109712449191.

Kirk, G. D., C. Merlo, P. O' Driscoll, S. H. Mehta, N. Galai, and others. 2007. "HIV Infection Is Associated with an Increased Risk for Lung Cancer, Independent of Smoking." *Clinical Infectious Diseases* 45 (1): 103–10. doi:10.1086/518606.

Klingman, K., J. D. Lundgren, A. Babiker, F. Gordin, S. Emery, and others. 2015. "Risk of Both AIDS-Related and Non-AIDS-Related Cancers Decreased by Early Initiation of Antiretroviral Therapy: Results from the START Trial (INSIGHT 001)." 15th International Conference on Malignancies in AIDS and Other Acquired Immunodeficiencies, Bethesda, MD, October 26.

Kowalkowski, M., M. Mims, R. Day, X. Du, W. Chan, and E Chiao. 2014. "Longer Duration of Combination Antiretroviral Therapy Reduces the Risk of Hodgkin Lymphoma: A Cohort Study of HIV-Infected Male Veterans." *Cancer Epidemiology* 38 (4): 386–92.

Kowalska, J. D., J. Reekie, A. Mocroft, P. Reiss, B. Ledergerber, and others. 2012. "Long-Term Exposure to Combination Antiretroviral Therapy and Risk of Death from Specific Causes: No Evidence for Any Previously Unidentified Increased Risk Due to Antiretroviral Therapy." *AIDS* 26 (3): 315–323. doi:10.1097/QAD.0b013e32834e8805.

Kreimer, A. R., M. E. Sherman, V. V. Sahasrabuddhe, and M. Safaeian. 2015. "The Case for Conducting a Randomized Clinical Trial to Assess the Efficacy of a Single Dose of Prophylactic HPV Vaccines among Adolescents." *Journal of the National Cancer Institute* 107 (3). doi:10.1093/jnci/dju436.

Laar, A. K. 2013. "Reproductive Rights and Options Available to Women Infected with HIV in Ghana: Perspectives of Service Providers from Three Ghanaian Health Facilities." *BMC Womens Health* 13: 13. doi:10.1186/1472–6874–13–13.

Landrum, M. L., K. Huppler Hullsiek, A. Ganesan, A. C. Weintrob, N. F. Crum-Cianflone, and others. 2009. "Hepatitis B Vaccine Responses in a Large U.S. Military Cohort of HIV-Infected Individuals: Another Benefit of HAART in those with Preserved CD4 T-Cell Count." *Vaccine* 27 (34): 4731–38. doi:10.1016/j.vaccine.2009.04.016.

Lang, S., M. Mary-Krause, A. Simon, M. Partisani, J. Gilquin, and others. 2012. "HIV Replication and Immune Status Are Independent Predictors of the Risk of Myocardial Infarction in HIV-Infected Individuals." *Clinical Infectious Diseases* 55 (4): 600–07. doi:10.1093/cid/cis489.

Liu, E., C. Armstrong, D. Spiegelman, G. Chalamilla, M. Njelekela, and others. 2013. "First-Line Antiretroviral Therapy and Changes in Lipid Levels over 3 Years among HIV-Infected Adults in Tanzania." *Clinical Infectious Diseases* 56 (12): 1820–28. doi:10.1093/cid/cit120.

Lopez, L. M., D. A. Grimes, K. F. Schulz, K. M. Curtis, and M. Chen. 2014. "Steroidal Contraceptives: Effect on Bone Fractures in Women." *Cochrane Database of Systematic Reviews* 6: CD006033.

Loutfy, M. R., S. Margolese, D. M. Money, M. Gysler, S. Hamilton, and others. 2012. "Canadian HIV Pregnancy Planning Guidelines." *Journal of Obstetrics and Gynaecology* 34 (6): 575–90.

Lozano, R., M. Naghavi, K. Foreman, S. Lim, K. Shibuya, and others. 2012. "Global and Regional Mortality from 235 Causes of Death for 20 Age Groups in 1990 and 2010: A Systematic Analysis for the Global Burden of Disease Study 2010." *The Lancet* 380 (9859): 2095–128. doi:10.1016/s0140–6736(12)61728–0.

Massad, L. S., M. J. Silverberg, G. Springer, H. Minkoff, N. Hessol, and others. 2004. "Effect of Antiretroviral Therapy on the Incidence of Genital Warts and Vulvar Neoplasia among Women with the Human Immunodeficiency Virus." *American Journal of Obstetrics and Gynecology* 190 (5): 1241–48.

Mbulaiteye, S. M., E. T. Katabira, H. Wabinga, D. M. Parkin, P. Virgo, and others. 2006. "Spectrum of Cancers among HIV-Infected Persons in Africa: The Uganda AIDS-Cancer Registry Match Study." *International Journal of Cancer* 118 (4): 985–90.

McGlynn, K. A., J. L. Petrick, and W. T. London. 2015. "Global Epidemiology of Hepatocellular Carcinoma: An Emphasis on Demographic and Regional Variability." *Clinical Liver Disease* 19 (2): 223–38. doi:10.1016/j.cld .2015.01.001.

Mdodo, R., E. L Frazier, S. R. Dube, C. L Mattson, M. Y. Sutton, and others. 2015. "Cigarette Smoking Prevalence among Adults with HIV Compared with the General Adult Population in the United States: Cross-Sectional Surveys." *Annals of Internal Medicine* 162 (5): 335–44.

Mensah, G. A. 2008. "Ischaemic Heart Disease in Africa." *Heart* 94 (7): 836–43. doi:10.1136/hrt.2007.136523.

Mills, A. M., M. Nelson, D. Jayaweera, K. Ruxrungtham, I. Cassetti, and others. 2009. "Once-Daily Darunavir/Ritonavir vs. Lopinavir/Ritonavir in Treatment-Naive, HIV-1-Infected Patients: 96-Week Analysis." *AIDS* 23 (13): 1679–88. doi:10.1097/QAD.0b013e32832d7350.

Mok-Lin, E., S. Missmer, K. Berry, L. S. Lehmann, and E. S. Ginsburg. 2011. "Public Perceptions of Providing IVF Services to Cancer and HIV Patients." *Fertility and Sterility* 96 (3): 722–27. doi:10.1016/j.fertnstert.2011.06.051.

Money, D. M., E. Moses, S. Blitz, S. M. Vandriel, N. Lipsky, and others. 2016. "HIV Viral Suppression Results in Higher Antibody Responses in HIV-Positive Women Vaccinated with the Quadrivalent Human Papillomavirus Vaccine." *Vaccine* 34 (40): 4799–806.

Mosam, A., F. Shaik, T. S. Uldrick, T. Esterhuizen, G. H. Friedland, and others. 2012. "A Randomized Controlled Trial of Highly Active Antiretroviral Therapy versus Highly Active Antiretroviral Therapy and Chemotherapy in Therapy-Naive Patients with HIV-Associated Kaposi Sarcoma in South Africa." *Journal of Acquired Immune Deficiency Syndromes* 60 (2): 150–57. doi:10.1097/QAI.0b013e318251aedd.

Moses, E., H. N. Pedersen, S. M. Mitchell, M. Sekikubo, D. Mwesigwa, and others. 2015. "Uptake of Community-Based, Self-Collected HPV Testing vs. Visual Inspection with Acetic Acid for Cervical Cancer Screening in Kampala, Uganda: Preliminary Results of a Randomised Controlled Trial." *Tropical Medicine and International Health* 10 (20): 1355–67. doi:10.1111/tmi.12549.

Moyer, V. A. 2012. "Screening for Cervical Cancer: U.S. Preventive Services Task Force Recommendation Statement." *Annals of Internal Medicine* 156 (12): 880–91, W312. doi:10.7326/0003-4819-156-12-201206190-00424.

Mugo, N. R., T. Hong, C. Celum, D. Donnell, E. A. Bukusi, and others. 2014. "Pregnancy Incidence and Outcomes among Women Receiving Preexposure Prophylaxis for HIV Prevention: A Randomized Clinical Trial." *Journal of the American Medical Association* 312 (4): 362–71. doi:10.1001 /jama.2014.8735.

Muhammad, S., M. U. Sani, and B. N. Okeahialam. 2013. "Prevalence of Dyslipidemia among Human Immunodeficiency Virus Infected Nigerians." *Annals of*

African Medicine 12 (1): 24–28. doi:10.4103/1596–3519 .108246.

Murray, C. J., and A. D. Lopez. 2013. "Measuring the Global Burden of Disease." *New England Journal of Medicine* 369 (5): 448–57. doi:10.1056/NEJMra1201534.

Mutyaba, I., W. Phipps, E. M. Krantz, J. D. Goldman, S. Nambooze, and others. 2015. "A Population-Level Evaluation of the Effect of Antiretroviral Therapy on Cancer Incidence in Kyadondo County, Uganda, 1999–2008." *Journal of Acquired Immune Deficiency Syndromes* 69 (4): 481–86.

Myer, L., L. Denny, R. Telerant, M. de Souza, T. C. Wright Jr., and L. Kuhn. 2005. "Bacterial Vaginosis and Susceptibility to HIV Infection in South African Women: A Nested Case-Control Study." *Journal of Infectious Diseases* 192 (8): 1372–80. doi:10.1086/462427.

Myerson, M., E. Poltavskiy, E. J. Armstrong, S. Kim, V. Sharp, and H. Bang. 2014. "Prevalence, Treatment, and Control of Dyslipidemia and Hypertension in 4278 HIV Outpatients." *Journal of Acquired Immune Deficiency Syndromes* 66 (4): 370–77. doi:10.1097/QAI.0000000000000168.

Narayan, K. M., P. G. Miotti, N. P. Anand, L. M. Kline, C. Harmston, and others. 2014. "HIV and Noncommunicable Disease Comorbidities in the Era of Antiretroviral Therapy: A Vital Agenda for Research in Low- and Middle-Income Country Settings." *Journal of Acquired Immune Deficiency Syndromes* 67 (Suppl 1): S2–7. doi:10.1097/QAI .0000000000000267.

Nguemaim, N. F., J. Mbuagbaw, T. Nkoa, G. Alemnji, G. Teto, and others. 2010. "Serum Lipid Profile in Highly Active Antiretroviral Therapy–Naive HIV-Infected Patients in Cameroon: A Case-Control Study." *HIV Medicine* 11 (6): 353–59. doi:10.1111/j.1468–1293.2009.00784.x.

Nguyen, H. Q., and C. Casper. 2010. "The Epidemiology of Kaposi Sarcoma." In *Kaposi Sarcoma: A Model of Oncogenesis*, edited by L. Pantanowitz, J. Stebbing, and B. J. Dezube, 197–232. Kerala, India: Research Signpost.

Nguyen, H. Q., A. S. Magaret, S. E. Van Rompaey, M. M. Kitahata, A. Wald, and others. 2008. "Persistent Kaposi Sarcoma in the Era of HAART: Characterizing the Predictors of Clinical Response." *AIDS* 22 (8): 937–45.

Nieves, C. I., A. Kaida, G. R. Seage, J. Kabakyenga, W. Muyindike, and others. 2015. "The Influence of Partnership on Contraceptive Use among HIV-Infected Women Accessing Antiretroviral Therapy in Rural Uganda." *Contraception* 92 (2): 152–59. doi:10.1016/j.contraception.2015.04.011.

Nurudeen, S. K., L. C. Grossman, L. Bourne, M. M. Guarnaccia, M. V. Sauer, and others. 2013. "Reproductive Outcomes of HIV Seropositive Women Treated by Assisted Reproduction." *Journal of Women's Health* 22 (3): 243–49. doi:10.1089/jwh .2012.3855.

Nzuobontane, D., K. N. Blackett, and C. Kuaban. 2002. "Cardiac Involvement in HIV Infected People in Yaounde, Cameroon." *Postgraduate Medical Journal* 78 (925): 678–81.

Ohl, J., M. Partisani, C. Wittemer, J. M. Lang, S. Viville, and R. Favre. 2005. "Encouraging Results Despite Complexity of Multidisciplinary Care of HIV-Infected Women Using Assisted Reproduction Techniques." *Human Reproduction* 20 (11): 3136–40. doi:10.1093/humrep/dei185.

Palella, F. J., Jr., K. M. Delaney, A. C. Moorman, M. O. Loveless, J. Fuhrer, and others. 1998. "Declining Morbidity and Mortality among Patients with Advanced Human Immunodeficiency Virus Infection. HIV Outpatient Study Investigators." *New England Journal of Medicine* 338 (13): 853–60.

Panel on Opportunistic Infections in HIV-Infected Adults and Adolescents. 2016. "Guidelines for the Prevention and Treatment of Opportunistic Infections in HIV-infected Adults and Adolescents: Recommendations from the Centers for Disease Control and Prevention, the National Institutes of Health, and the HIV Medicine Association of the Infectious Diseases Society of America." http://aidsinfo .nih.gov/contentfiles/lvguidelines/adult_oi.pdf.

Papadopoulos, A., N. Pantazis, P. Panagopoulos, S. Kourkounti, G. Xylomenos, and others. 2012. "Effects of First Antiretroviral Regimen on Lipid Levels in HIV (+) Individuals." *Journal of Chemotherapy* 24 (1): 38–47. doi:10.1179/1120009X12Z .0000000008.

Patel, P., T. Bush, K. H. Mayer, S. Desai, K. Henry, and others. 2012. "Prevalence and Risk Factors Associated with Herpes Simplex Virus-2 Infection in a Contemporary Cohort of HIV-Infected Persons in the United States." *Sexually Transmitted Diseases* 39 (2): 154–60.

Patel, P., D. L. Hanson, P. S. Sullivan, R. M. Novak, A. C. Moorman, and others. 2008. "Incidence of Types of Cancer among HIV-Infected Persons Compared with the General Population in the United States, 1992–2003." *Annals of Internal Medicine* 148 (10): 728–U29.

Pefura Yone, E. W., A. F. Betyoumin, A. P. Kengne, F. J. Kaze Folefack, and J. Ngogang. 2011. "First-Line Antiretroviral Therapy and Dyslipidemia in People Living with HIV-1 in Cameroon: A Cross-Sectional Study." *AIDS Research and Therapy* 8: 33. doi:10.1186/1742–6405-8-33.

Petoumenos, K., E. Hui, N. Kumarasamy, S. J. Kerr, J. Y. Choi, and others. 2010. "Cancers in the TREAT Asia HIV Observational Database (TAHOD): A Retrospective Analysis of Risk Factors." *Journal of the International AIDS Society* 13 (51).

Piketty, C., H. Selinger-Leneman, A. M. Bouvier, A. Belot, M. Mary-Krause, and others. 2012. "Incidence of HIV-Related Anal Cancer Remains Increased Despite Long-Term Combined Antiretroviral Treatment: Results from the French Hospital Database on HIV." *Journal of Clinical Oncology* 30 (35): 4360–66. doi:10.1200/JCO.2012.44.5486.

Pinto Neto, L. F., M. B. das Neves, R. Ribeiro-Rodrigues, K. Page, and A. E. Miranda. 2013. "Dyslipidemia and Fasting Glucose Impairment among HIV Patients Three Years after the First Antiretroviral Regimen in a Brazilian AIDS Outpatient Clinic." *Brazilian Journal of Infectious Diseases* 17 (4): 438–43. doi:10.1016/j.bjid.2012.12.006.

Poordad, F., J. McCone Jr., B. R. Bacon, S. Bruno, M. P. Manns, and others. 2011. "Boceprevir for Untreated Chronic Hepatitis C Virus Genotype 1 Infection." *New England Journal of Medicine* 364 (13): 1195–206. doi:10.1056/NEJMoa1010494.

Puoti, M., R. Bruno, V. Soriano, F. Donato, G. B. Gaeta, and others. 2004. "Hepatocellular Carcinoma in HIV-Infected Patients: Epidemiological Features, Clinical Presentation and Outcome." *AIDS* 18 (17): 2285–93.

Pyra, M., R. Heffron, N. R. Mugo, K. Nanda, K. K. Thomas, and others. 2015. "Effectiveness of Hormonal Contraception in HIV-Infected Women Using Antiretroviral Therapy." *AIDS* 29 (17): 2353–59.

Quinn, T. C., W. E. Stamm, S. E. Goodell, E. Mkrtichian, J. Benedetti, and others. 1983. "The Polymicrobial Origin of Intestinal Infections in Homosexual Men." *New England Journal of Medicine* 309 (10): 576–82.

Raffi, F., A. Rachlis, H. J. Stellbrink, W. D. Hardy, C. Torti, and others. 2013. "Once-Daily Dolutegravir versus Raltegravir in Antiretroviral-Naive Adults with HIV-1 Infection: 48 Week Results from the Randomised, Double-Blind, Non-Inferiority SPRING-2 Study." *The Lancet* 381 (9868): 735–43. doi:10.1016/S0140–6736(12)61853–4.

Riddler, S. A., E. Smit, S. R. Cole, R. Li, J. S. Chmiel, and others. 2003. "Impact of HIV Infection and HAART on Serum Lipids in Men." *Journal of the American Medical Association* 289 (22): 2978–82.

Riedel, D. J., E. I. Mwangi, L. E. Fantry, C. Alexander, M. B. Hossain, and others. 2013. "High Cancer-Related Mortality in an Urban, Predominantly African-American, HIV-Infected Population." *AIDS* 27 (7): 1109–17. doi:10.1097 /QAD.0b013e32835dc068.

Robbins, H. A., R. M. Pfeiffer, M. S. Shiels, J. Li, H. I. Hall, and E. A. Engels. 2015. "Excess Cancers among HIV-Infected People in the United States." *Journal of the National Cancer Institute* 107 (4). doi:10.1093/jnci/dju503.

Robbins, H. A., M. S. Shiels, R. M. Pfeiffer, and E. A. Engels. 2014. "Epidemiologic Contributions to Recent Cancer Trends among HIV-Infected People in the United States." *AIDS* 28 (6): 881–90. doi:10.1097/qad.0000000000000163.

Robinson, J. A., R. Jamshidi, and A. E. Burke. 2012. "Contraception for the HIV-Positive Woman: A Review of Interactions between Hormonal Contraception and Antiretroviral Therapy." *Infectious Diseases in Obstetrics and Gynecology* 2012 (890160).

Rockstroh, J. K., E. DeJesus, J. L. Lennox, Y. Yazdanpanah, M. S. Saag, and others. 2013. "Durable Efficacy and Safety of Raltegravir versus Efavirenz When Combined with Tenofovir/Emtricitabine in Treatment-Naive HIV-1-Infected Patients: Final 5-Year Results from STARTMRK." *Journal of Acquired Immune Deficiency Syndromes* 63 (1): 77–85. doi:10.1097/QAI.0b013e31828ace69.

Rodger, A. J., V. Cambiano, T. Bruun, P. Vernazza, S. Collins, and others. 2016. "Sexual Activity without Condoms and Risk of HIV Transmission in Serodifferent Couples When the HIV Positive Partner Is Using Suppressive Antiretroviral Therapy." *Journal of the American Medical Association* 316 (2): 171–81.

Sabin, C. A., S. W. Worm, R. Weber, P. Reiss, W. El-Sadr, and others. 2008. "Use of Nucleoside Reverse Transcriptase Inhibitors and Risk of Myocardial Infarction in HIV-Infected Patients Enrolled in the DAD Study: A Multicohort Collaboration." *The Lancet* 371 (9622): 1417–26.

Salehian, B., J. Bilas, M. Bazargan, and M. Abbasian. 2005. "Prevalence and Incidence of Diabetes in HIV-Infected Minority Patients on Protease Inhibitors." *Journal of the National Medical Association* 97 (8): 1088–92.

Salters, K. A., A. Cescon, W. Zhang, G. Ogilvie, M. Murray, and others. 2016. "Cancer Incidence among HIV-Positive Women in British Columbia, Canada: Heightened Risk of Virus-Related Malignancies." *HIV Medicine* 17 (3): 188–95. doi:10.1111/hiv.12290.

Samaras, K. 2009. "Prevalence and Pathogenesis of Diabetes Mellitus in HIV-1 Infection Treated with Combined Antiretroviral Therapy." *Journal of Acquired Immune Deficiency Syndromes* 50 (5): 499–505. doi:10.1097/QAI.0b013e31819c291b.

Sax, P. E., C. Tierney, A. C. Collier, E. S. Daar, K. Mollan, and others. 2011. "Abacavir/Lamivudine versus Tenofovir Df/Emtricitabine as Part of Combination Regimens for Initial Treatment of HIV: Final Results." *Journal of Infectious Diseases* 204 (8): 1191–201. doi:10.1093/infdis/jir505.

Schwartz, J. B., K. L. Moore, M. Yin, A. Sharma, D. Merenstein, and others. 2014. "Relationship of Vitamin D, HIV, HIV Treatment, and Lipid Levels in the Women's Interagency HIV Study of HIV-Infected and Uninfected Women in the United States." *Journal of the International Association of Providers of AIDS Care* 13 (3): 250–59. doi:10.1177/2325957413506748.

Seedat, Y. K. 1999. "Hypertension in Black South Africans." *Journal of Human Hypertension* 13 (2): 96–10.

Sengayi, M., A. Spoerri, M. Egger, D. Kielkowski, T. Crankshaw, and others. 2016. "Record Linkage to Correct Under-Ascertainment of Cancers in HIV Cohorts: The Sinikithemba HIV Clinic Linkage Project." *International Journal of Cancer* 139 (6): 1209–16.

Shaffer, D., M. D. Hughes, F. Sawe, Y. Bao, A. Moses, and others. 2014. "Cardiovascular Disease Risk Factors in HIV-Infected Women after Initiation of Lopinavir/Ritonavir– and Nevirapine–Based Antiretroviral Therapy in Sub-Saharan Africa: A5208 (OCTANE)." *Journal of Acquired Immune Deficiency Syndromes* 66 (2): 155–63. doi:10.1097/QAI.0000000000000131.

Shen, Y. C., C. Hsu, C. C. Cheng, F. C. Hu, and A. L. Cheng. 2012. "A Critical Evaluation of the Preventive Effect of Antiviral Therapy on the Development of Hepatocellular Carcinoma in Patients with Chronic Hepatitis C or B: A Novel Approach by Using Meta-Regression." *Oncology* 82 (5): 275–89. doi:10.1159/000337293.

Shiels, M. S., R. M. Pfeiffer, M. H. Gail, H. I. Hall, J. Li, and others. 2011. "Cancer Burden in the HIV-Infected Population in the United States." *Journal of the National Cancer Institute* 103 (9): 753–62. doi:10.1093/jnci/djr076.

Silverberg, M. J., B. Lau, C. J. Achenbach, Y. Jing, K.N. Althoff, and others. 2015. "Cumulative Incidence of Cancer among Persons with HIV in North America: A Cohort Study." *Annals of Internal Medicine* 163 (7): 507–18.

Silverberg, M. J., W. A. Leyden, L. Xu, M. A. Horberg, C. R. Chao, and others. 2014. "Immunodeficiency and Risk of Myocardial Infarction among HIV-Positive Individuals with Access to Care." *Journal of Acquired Immune Deficiency Syndromes* 65 (2): 160–66. doi:10.1097/QAI.0000000000000009.

Sliwa, K., M. J. Carrington, A. Becker, F. Thienemann, M. Ntsekhe, and others. 2012. "Contribution of the Human Immunodeficiency Virus/Acquired Immunodeficiency Syndrome Epidemic to De Novo Presentations of Heart Disease in the Heart of Soweto Study Cohort." *European Heart Journal* 33 (7): 866–74. doi:10.1093/eurheartj/ehr398.

Smith, C. J., L. Ryom, R. Weber, P. Morlat, C. Pradier, and others. 2014. "Trends in Underlying Causes of Death in People with HIV from 1999 to 2011 (DAD): A Multicohort Collaboration." *The Lancet* 384 (9939): 241–48. doi:10.1016/s0140–6736(14)60604–8.

Solomon, D. H., E. W. Karlson, E. B. Rimm, C. C. Cannuscio, L. A. Mandl, and others. 2003. "Cardiovascular Morbidity and Mortality in Women Diagnosed with Rheumatoid Arthritis." *Circulation* 107 (9): 1303–07.

Sung, J. J., K. K. Tsoi, V. W. Wong, K. C. Li, and H. L. Chan. 2008. "Meta-Analysis: Treatment of Hepatitis B Infection Reduces Risk of Hepatocellular Carcinoma." *Alimentary Pharmacology and Therapeutics* 28 (9): 1067–77. doi:10.1111/j.1365–2036.2008.03816.x.

Thurman, A. R., S. Anderson, and G. F. Doncel. 2014. "Effects of Hormonal Contraception on Antiretroviral Drug Metabolism, Pharmacokinetics and Pharmacodynamics." *American Journal of Reproductive Immunology* 71 (6): 523–30. doi:10.1111/aji.12210.

Thygesen, K., J. S. Alpert, H. D. White, A. S. Jaffe, F. S. Apple, and others. 2007. "Universal Definition of Myocardial Infarction." *Circulation* 116 (22): 2634–53.

Tien, P. C., M. F. Schneider, S. R. Cole, A. M. Levine, M. Cohen, and others. 2007. "Antiretroviral Therapy Exposure and Incidence of Diabetes Mellitus in the Women's Interagency HIV Study." *AIDS* 21 (13): 1739–1745.

Triant, V. A. 2014. "Epidemiology of Coronary Heart Disease in Patients with Human Immunodeficiency Virus." *Reviews of Cardiovascular Medicine* 15 (Suppl 1): S1–8.

Triant, V. A., J. B. Meigs, and S. K. Grinspoon. 2009. "Association of C-Reactive Protein and HIV Infection with Acute Myocardial Infarction." *Journal of Acquired Immune Deficiency Syndromes* 51 (3): 268–73. doi:10.1097/QAI.0b013e3181a9992c.

Turner, A. N., S. Tabbah, V. Mwapasa, S. J. Rogerson, S. R. Meshnick, and others. 2013. "Severity of Maternal HIV-1 Disease Is Associated with Adverse Birth Outcomes in Malawian Women: A Cohort Study." *Journal of Acquired Immune Deficiency Syndromes* 64 (4): 392–99.

Twagirumukiza, M., E. Nkeramihigo, B. Seminega, E. Gasakure, F. Boccara, and others. 2007. "Prevalence of Dilated Cardiomyopathy in HIV-Infected African Patients Not Receiving HAART: A Multicenter, Observational, Prospective, Cohort Study in Rwanda." *Current HIV Research* 5 (1): 129–37.

UNAIDS (Joint United Nations Programme on HIV/AIDS). 2014. *The Gap Report*. UNAIDS, Geneva.

van Leeuwen, M. T., C. M. Vajdic, M. G. Middleton, A. M. McDonald, M. Law, and others. 2009. "Continuing Declines in Some but Not All HIV-Associated Cancers in Australia after Widespread Use of Antiretroviral Therapy." *AIDS* 23 (16): 2183–90. doi:10.1097/QAD.0b013e328331d384.

Venkatesh, K. K., S. Saghayam, B. Devaleenal, S. Poongulali, T. P. Flanigan, and others. 2012. "Spectrum of Malignancies among HIV-Infected Patients in South India." *Indian Journal of Cancer* 49 (1): 176–80. doi:10.4103/0019–509X.98947.

Visnegarwala, F., L. Chen, S. Raghavan, and E. Tedaldi. 2005. "Prevalence of Diabetes Mellitus and Dyslipidemia among Antiretroviral Naive Patients Co-Infected with Hepatitis C Virus (HCV) and HIV-1 Compared to Patients without Co-Infection." *Journal of Infection* 50 (4): 331–37.

Wanyenze, R. K., G. J. Wagner, N. M. Tumwesigye, M. Nannyonga, F. Wabwire-Mangen, and others. 2013. "Fertility and Contraceptive Decision-Making and Support for HIV Infected Individuals: Client and Provider Experiences and Perceptions at Two HIV Clinics in Uganda." *BMC Public Health* 13: 98. doi:10.1186/1471–2458–13–98.

Watson-Jones, D., N. Mugo, S. Lees, M. Mathai, S. Vusha, and others. 2015. "Access and Attitudes to HPV Vaccination amongst Hard-to-Reach Populations in Kenya." *PLoS One* 10 (6): e0123701. doi:10.1371/journal.pone.0123701.

Watts, D. H., Z. A. Brown, D. Money, S. Selke, M. L. Huang, and others. 2003. "A Double-Blind, Randomized, Placebo-Controlled Trial of Acyclovir in Late Pregnancy for the Reduction of Herpes Simplex Virus Shedding and Cesarean Delivery." *American Journal of Obstetrics and Gynecology* 188 (3): 836–43.

Weller, S., and K. Davis. 2002. "Condom Effectiveness in Reducing Heterosexual HIV Transmission." *Cochrane Database of Systematic Reviews* (1): CD003255. doi:10.1002/14651858.CD003255.

Wester, C. W., J. R. Koethe, B. E. Shepherd, S. E. Stinnette, P. F. Rebeiro, and others. 2011. "Non-AIDS-Defining Events among HIV-1-Infected Adults Receiving Combination Antiretroviral Therapy in Resource-Replete versus Resource-Limited Urban Setting." *AIDS* 25 (12): 1471–79. doi:10.1097/QAD.0b013e328347f9d4.

WHO (World Health Organization). 2006. *Sexual and Reproductive Health of Women Living with HIV/AIDS.* Geneva: WHO.

———. 2013a. *Global Policy Report on the Prevention and Control of Viral Hepatitis in WHO Member States.* Geneva: WHO.

———. 2013b. *WHO Guidelines for Screening and Treatment of Precancerous Lesions for Cervical Cancer Prevention.* Geneva: WHO.

Wiktor, S. Z. 2017. "Viral Hepatitis." In *Disease Control Priorities* (third edition): Volume 6, *Major Infectious Diseases*, edited by K. K. Holmes, S. Bertozzi, B. R. Bloom, and P. Jha. Washington, DC: World Bank.

Workowski, K. A., and G. A. Bolan. 2015. "Sexually Transmitted Diseases Treatment Guidelines, 2015." *MMWR Recommendations and Reports* 64 (RR-03): 1–137.

Yanik, E. L., S. Napravnik, S. R. Cole, C. J. Achenbach, S. Gopal, and others. 2013. "Incidence and Timing of Cancer in HIV-Infected Individuals Following Initiation of Combination Antiretroviral Therapy." *Clinical Infectious Diseases* 57 (5): 756–64. doi:10.1093/cid/cit369.

Yaro, S., N. Meda, A. Desgrees Du Lou, I. Sombie, M. Cartoux, and others. 2001. "[Impaired Fertility in Women Infected with HIV-1. Implications for Sentinel Serosurveillance]." *Rev Epidemiol Sante Publique* 49 (3): 221–28.

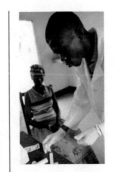

Chapter 4

HIV Care Continuum in Adults and Children: Cost-Effectiveness Considerations

Katherine Harripersaud, Margaret McNairy, Saeed Ahmed,
Elaine J. Abrams, Harsha Thirumurthy, and Wafaa M. El-Sadr

INTRODUCTION

The management of human immunodeficiency virus (HIV) infection has evolved substantially since the advent of the HIV/acquired immune deficiency syndrome (HIV/AIDS) epidemic in the 1980s. The discovery of effective antiretroviral therapy (ART) transformed the lives of persons living with HIV (Deeks, Lewin, and Havlir 2013) by achieving a substantial drop in morbidity and mortality (Danel and others 2015; START Study Group 2015). Additionally, evidence supports the efficacy of ART in preventing the transmission of HIV infection (Cohen and others 2011).

Progress in controlling the HIV epidemic, however, requires the achievement of virologic suppression among all HIV-infected individuals, which, in turn, requires the identification of such individuals and their retention across the care continuum—from conducting HIV testing, linking HIV-positive individuals to care, retaining them in care, and achieving viral suppression (figure 4.1) (Gardner and others 2011). For each step of the continuum, this chapter discusses the rationale, relevant guidelines, measurements of each parameter, barriers to achieving successful outcomes, interventions demonstrated to be effective, and available data on the costs and cost-effectiveness of interventions.

The chapter includes information from peer-reviewed manuscripts identified through a targeted literature review focused on publications pertinent to low- and middle-income countries (LMICs), with a focus on Sub-Saharan Africa. Studies conducted in other LMIC regions and high-income countries are referenced when they address a key relevant issue. A table summarizing approaches to improving HIV testing, linkage to and engagement with HIV care, retention in HIV care, and adherence to HIV treatment is included in annex 4A.

HIV TESTING SERVICES

Rationale and Coverage

HIV testing services (HTS) are essential for identifying HIV-positive persons in need of care and ART, as well as for identifying at-risk HIV-negative persons for referral and engagement in HIV prevention programs (Celum and others 2013). Despite the importance of HIV testing, the Joint United Nations Programme on HIV/AIDS (UNAIDS) estimates that nearly half of the 36.9 million people living with HIV globally in 2014 were unaware of their infection (UNAIDS 2015a). Similarly, only 44 percent of pregnant women in LMICs access HIV testing (WHO 2014c). Recent findings from

Corresponding author: Wafaa M. El-Sadr, ICAP, Mailman School of Public Health, Columbia University, New York, New York, United States; wme1@cumc.columbia.edu.

Figure 4.1 HIV Care Continuum

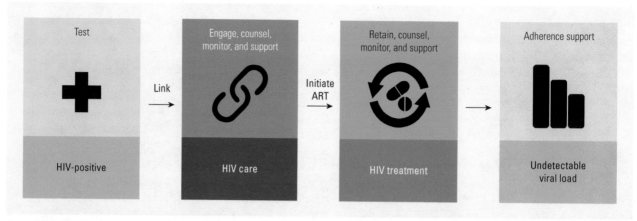

Source: McNairy and El-Sadr 2012. Adapted with permission from Wolters Kluwer.
Note: ART = antiretroviral treatment; HIV = human immunodeficiency virus.

the Population HIV Impact Assessment (PHIA) surveys completed in Malawi, Zambia, and Zimbabwe suggest the need to enhance HIV testing coverage; in these surveys of random samples of households, 70.4 percent of individuals found to be HIV-positive were aware of HIV infection (ICAP 2016).

HIV testing is especially critical for pregnant women and children. HIV-infected pregnant women must be identified early during pregnancy to benefit from ART for their own health and for the prevention of vertical transmission; HIV-negative pregnant and postpartum women require repeat testing during pregnancy and the postpartum period (Drake and others 2014).

HIV testing and ART initiation for HIV-infected infants in the first months of life has been demonstrated to markedly reduce mortality (Violari and others 2008). However, only 46 percent of HIV-exposed infants in LMICs received an early infant diagnostic (EID) test for HIV in 2014 (UNICEF 2015).

Adolescents are another high-risk group in need of increased access to and uptake of HIV testing. In 2015, there were 1.8 million adolescents ages 10–19 years living with HIV (UNAIDS 2015b). Since 2004, mortality has decreased 30 percent among adults but increased 50 percent among adolescents (Porth and others 2014). In the PHIA surveys cited above, only 46.4 percent of young individuals (15–24 years old) found to be HIV-positive in the population surveys were aware of their HIV infection (ICAP 2016).

Guidelines

The World Health Organization (WHO) recommends universal testing in countries with generalized HIV epidemics (WHO 2013b). Provider-initiated testing and counseling (PITC) is recommended for women as a routine component of antenatal care, with retesting before delivery for persons with a first negative test (WHO 2015a).

All infants of HIV-infected pregnant women should be tested for infection at age four to six weeks using a virologic test that directly detects the virus, including deoxyribonucleic acid (DNA), ribonucleic acid (RNA), or DNA polymerase chain reaction (PCR) assays (WHO 2015a). Infants testing positive should be initiated on ART, while those testing negative should be tested again with virologic or serologic assays (depending on their age) after the risk period for mother-to-child transmission ends with cessation of breastfeeding.

For children ages 18 months or older, the WHO recommends serological testing when HIV infection is suspected or exposure has occurred; and in high-prevalence settings, HIV testing should be routinely available to children attending immunization, under-five, malnutrition, and tuberculosis clinics; all hospitalized children; and those receiving services for orphans and vulnerable children (WHO 2015a). In generalized HIV epidemic settings, HTS, with links to prevention, treatment, and care, are recommended for all adolescents (WHO 2015a).

For populations at substantial risk for HIV, including persons who inject drugs (PWID), sex workers (SWs), and men who have sex with men (MSM), frequent, voluntary, community-based HTS, linked to prevention, treatment, and care, are recommended.

Measurement

Common measures of HIV testing include the number of tests conducted and the number of individuals who are tested, counseled, and receive their results (PEPFAR 2013). However, these measures do not assess the effectiveness of HIV testing in identifying all persons with HIV infection in a community. Others have highlighted the importance of measuring the proportion of individuals who test positive for HIV who then link to care (El-Sadr, Gamble, and Cohen 2013).

Barriers

Individual-level barriers to testing include perceived low risk of infection, anticipated psychological burden of living with HIV, fear of HIV-related stigma, direct and indirect financial costs of accessing HIV testing, and gender inequality (Musheke and others 2013). Testing of children and adolescents is complicated by the need to obtain consent from a parent or legal guardian (WHO 2013b, 2014b). System-level barriers include high patient load, test kit shortages, inadequate counseling space, and poor counseling skills (Larsson and others 2011; Nuti, Kabengula, and Msuya 2011). For pregnant women, low uptake of antenatal services in some settings remains an impediment to achieving universal HIV testing.

Approaches to Improve HTS Uptake

Voluntary counseling and testing (VCT) is dependent on individuals' actively seeking HIV testing at a clinic, hospital, mobile health unit, or free-standing site (Matovu and Makumbi 2007). However, VCT is of limited value among individuals who do not perceive themselves to be at risk. Moreover, children rarely access VCT services, because caregivers fear stigma and disclosure of their own serostatus (Ahmed and others 2013).

In 2007, the WHO and UNAIDS released guidance recommending PITC for all patients in high-prevalence settings and for all patients, irrespective of epidemic setting, whose clinical presentation suggests HIV infection (Kennedy and others 2013; Roura and others 2013; WHO 2007). A systematic review of PITC in Sub-Saharan Africa reported increased uptake of HIV testing after PITC was implemented in antenatal and family planning, tuberculosis, sexually transmitted infection, and outpatient clinics (Kennedy and others 2013). PITC uptake is lower among men and among women who are not pregnant, however (Baggaley and others 2012; Hensen and others 2012; MacPherson and others 2012). PITC has been effective in identifying HIV-infected and -exposed infants in inpatient settings, but it is not widely implemented for children (Kankasa and others 2009).

Community-based testing (CBT) strategies, including testing in homes, schools, the workplace, or other community venues (Bateganya, Abdulwadud, and Kiene 2010; Coates and others 2014), have demonstrated promise for expanding knowledge of HIV status. Compared with facility-based testing, CBT has been associated with increased testing, higher proportions of first-time testers, higher proportions of HIV-infected individuals identified with CD4 cell count greater than 350 cells per microliter, and an overall lower seropositivity rate (Suthar, Ford, and others 2013). Home-based testing has been highly acceptable, with 83 percent accepting testing in a meta-analysis (Sabapathy and others 2012). It was also found to be cost-effective for reaching youth, men, and rural populations (Sweat and others 2011; van Rooyen, McGrath, and others 2013; Wachira and others 2014). Home-based testing has also been more effective than facility-based testing at diagnosing people with less advanced disease and has increased linking of HIV-positive persons to care (Wachira, Kimaiyo, and others 2012).

CBT has also shown promise for pediatric case finding (Ahmed and others 2015). Among members of households with HIV-infected individuals in Uganda, home-based testing increased identification of HIV-infected persons, including children, compared with clinic-based care (Lugada and others 2010).

Mass campaigns that provide HTS in conjunction with other health services have also been used. In Kenya and Uganda, HTS were provided along with free bed nets, water purification kits, condoms, and cotrimoxazole to those who tested HIV-positive (Lugada and others 2010; Tumwesigye and others 2010). In Kenya, 80 percent of the population in a catchment area was tested for HIV in a period of one week; in Uganda, 63 percent of households were tested through such a campaign. In Tanzania, a CBT campaign for children identified 108 new pediatric cases (3.6 percent) (Shea and others 2013). Mass campaigns that include HIV testing have been less successful in reaching young adults and adult males (Chamie and others 2014; Ostermann and others 2011).

Couples' testing is another approach to identifying concordant HIV-positive couples in need of ART and serodiscordant couples in need of ART for positive partner or preexposure prophylaxis (PrEP) or voluntary medical male circumcision for negative partner (Baeten and others 2012; Gray and others 2007).

Self-testing for HIV holds promise (Choko and others 2011; Pant Pai and others 2013; Thirumurthy and others 2016). In Malawi, self-testing with oral test kits was acceptable among 92 percent of persons, and 99 percent of results were accurate (Choko and others 2011).

More research is needed to evaluate linking of HIV-positive patients to care, as well as disclosure of results to partners among persons who self-test positive.

Limited access to the specialized tests (nucleic acid tests including DNA and RNA PCR) for diagnosis of HIV infection in infants resulted in high mortality among HIV-infected babies (Creek and others 2008). The introduction of new laboratory technology at centralized laboratories in many Sub-Saharan African countries, coupled with the use of dried blood spots for specimen collection, improved access and uptake of early infant diagnosis (Essajee and others 2015; Ghadrshenas and others 2013). The use of text message printers and computerized tracking systems has increased the rate of return of EID results to clinics and families (Essajee and others 2015; Finocchario-Kessler and others 2014).

In South Africa, couples-based HIV testing in MSM appears to be effective (Stephenson and others 2013). In China, peer-driven counseling sessions significantly increased testing rates among MSM (Menzies and others 2009). Text reminders also increased testing rates (Bourne and others 2011). For PWID, venue-based testing at methadone clinics and drop-in sites was successful in increasing knowledge of HIV status (Xia and others 2013). Additionally, a qualitative study noted that female sex workers (FSWs) in Benin would more likely access HIV-testing services if paired with outreach strategies (Dugas and others 2015).

A systematic review of seven partner notification studies in LMICs to achieve testing of partners described the use of email, text messaging, and social networking, with most clients choosing to send notifications via text rather than email to enhance testing of partners of HIV-positive individuals (Hochberg, Berringer, and Schneider 2015). In a study from Malawi, only 25 percent of partners in the passive referral arm returned for HIV testing, compared with 51 percent in both the contract and the provider referral arms ($p < 0.001$) (Brown and others 2011). Similarly, a cohort study in Cameroon reported that 46 percent of partners in the passive referral group returned for testing as compared with 60 percent in the provider group and 61 percent in the contract referral arm (Henley and others 2013).

Cost-Effectiveness Considerations

Table 4.1 describes cost and cost-effectiveness studies regarding HTS.

Voluntary Counseling and Testing

Evidence suggests that while VCT and CBT have low costs per person tested, the cost per HIV-infected person tested is lower for PITC.

In East Africa, VCT can be delivered for US$10–US$30 per person tested, and the overall cost-effectiveness of VCT has been favorable in the few available studies (Grabbe and others 2010; Menzies and others 2009). In Tanzania, the cost per disability-adjusted life year (DALY) averted was estimated to be US$13–US$18 and the cost per HIV infection averted to be US$249–US$346 (Sweat and others 2000). Offering VCT for free was highly cost-effective (Thielman and others 2006). Because utilization levels for VCT services are an important driver of the costs per client, demand creation for VCT is essential for reducing costs. In addition, many studies underestimate the cost-effectiveness of HIV testing by neglecting the prevention benefits of knowing HIV-positive status, which leads to a decrease in risk behaviors, and the cost-effectiveness of ART provision to individuals identified as HIV-infected.

The costs of VCT approaches to HIV testing are higher when calculated per HIV-infected person identified rather than per individual tested. Costs per HIV-infected person identified are often lower for alternative testing approaches such as PITC (including hospital-based testing) than for VCT. In Uganda, hospital-based testing costs US$12 per client tested and US$43 per HIV-infected person identified (Menzies and others 2009). In contrast, VCT costs US$19 per person tested and US$101 per HIV-infected person identified.

Community-Based Testing

Evidence is emerging on the costs of approaches to CBT. Studies have found the costs of such approaches to be lower than or comparable to the costs of VCT, at approximately US$8–US$15 per person tested (Grabbe and others 2010; Menzies and others 2009). In Kenya and Uganda, mobile HTS had a lower cost per person tested than VCT. The cost per HIV-infected person identified was lower for mobile HTS than VCT in Kenya, but higher in Uganda. A modeling analysis for South Africa that estimated the incremental cost-effectiveness ratios (ICERs) per DALY averted of home-based HIV testing and counseling along with enhanced links to care found a high level of cost-effectiveness (Smith and others 2015). The cost per DALY averted was US$1,340 at an ART threshold of CD4 count less than 200 cells per microliter and US$1,360 at universal access to ART.

Although not high-prevalence settings, studies conducted in China and India have provided additional evidence on the cost-effectiveness of targeted use of VCT among key populations and high-risk groups. In China, among populations at higher risk of HIV acquisition, such as MSM, VCT was cost saving (Wang, Moss, and Hiller 2011). In Indonesia, costs per HIV-infected person identified were lower in prisons than in

Table 4.1 Cost-Effectiveness of Approaches to the HIV Care Continuum

Intervention	Study	Region or country	Cost per outcome	Cost (C) or cost-effectiveness (CE)	Unit of outcome	Currency as presented (year)	Cost in 2012 US$
HIV testing and counseling							
	Grabbe and others 2010	Sub-Saharan Africa, Kenya	$26.75	CE	per HTC client	2007 US$	$41.81
			$43.69	CE	per new HTC client	2007 US$	$68.28
			$189.14	CE	per HIV-positive client	2007 US$	$295.59
			$237.60	CE	per new HIV-positive client identified	2007 US$	$371.32
All mobile compared with stand-alone			$14.91	CE	per HTC client	2007 US$	$23.30
			$16.58	CE	per new HTC client	2007 US$	$25.91
			$157.21	CE	per HIV-positive client	2007 US$	$245.69
			$178.10	CE	per new HIV-positive client identified	2007 US$	$278.34
Community-site mobile compared with stand-alone			$8.82	CE	per HTC client	2007 US$	$13.78
			$9.73	CE	per new HTC client	2007 US$	$15.21
Semimobile container compared with stand-alone			$17.23	CE	per HTC client	2007 US$	$26.93
			$20.06	CE	per new HTC client	2007 US$	$31.35
Fully mobile truck compared with stand-alone			$20.38	CE	per HTC client	2007 US$	$31.85
			$23.39	CE	per new HTC client	2007 US$	$36.55
VCT	Sweat and others 2000	Sub-Saharan Africa, Kenya	$12.77	CE	per DALY averted	1998 US$	$17.47
VCT, enrolled as couples			$2.75–$3.48	CE	per DALY averted; HIV-1-positive males and females	1998 US$	$3.47–$4.73
			$19.48–$21.86	CE	per DALY averted; HIV-1-negative females and males	1998 US$	$26.38–$29.60
Free VCT campaign	Thielman and others 2006	Sub-Saharan Africa, Tanzania	$5.40	CE	per DALY averted	2003 US$	$8.09
Sustained free VCT			$4.72	CE	per DALY averted	2003 US$	$7.07
Scaled-up, community-based VCT	Tromp and others 2013	East Asia and Pacific, Indonesia	$9.17	CE	per DALY averted	2008 US$	$12.59

table continues next page

Table 4.1 Cost-Effectiveness of Approaches to the HIV Care Continuum (continued)

Intervention	Study	Region or country	Cost per outcome	Cost (C) or cost-effectiveness (CE)	Unit of outcome	Currency as presented (year)	Cost in 2012 US$
VCT	Wang, Moss, and Hiller 2011	East Asia and Pacific, China	1,087,669 yuan	CE	Incremental cost per HIV infection averted (including averted cost) in general population	2002 yuan	$228,514.82
			53,317 yuan	CE	Incremental cost per DALY averted (including averted cost) in general population	2002 yuan	$11,201.68
Stand-alone HTC	Menzies and others 2009	Sub-Saharan Africa, Uganda	$19.26	C	Cost per client tested	2007 US$	$25.07
Hospital-based HTC			$11.68	C	Cost per client tested	2007 US$	$15.20
Household-member HTC			$13.85	C	Cost per client tested	2007 US$	$18.03
Door-to-door HTC			$8.29	C	Cost per client tested	2007 US$	$10.79
Stand-alone HTC			$100.59	C	Cost per HIV-positive individual identified	2007 US$	$130.92
Hospital-based HTC			$43.10	C	Cost per HIV-positive individual identified	2007 US$	$56.09
Household-member HTC			$231.65	C	Cost per HIV-positive individual identified	2007 US$	$301.49
Door-to-door HTC			$163.93	C	Cost per HIV-positive individual identified	2007 US$	$213.35
HTC in prisons, HIV community clinics, and hospitals	Siregar and others 2011	East Asia and Pacific, Indonesia	$23.00	C	per VCT in prison	2008 US$	$31.58
			$39.00	C	per VCT in HIV community clinics	2008 US$	$53.56
			$65.00	C	per VCT in STI community clinics	2008 US$	$89.26
			$74.00	C	per VCT in hospitals	2008 US$	$101.62
VCT	Sweat and others 2000	Sub-Saharan Africa, Kenya and Tanzania	$249.00–$346.00	CE	per infection averted	1998 US$	$473.46–$722.66
Free VCT	Thielman and others 2006	Sub-Saharan Africa, Tanzania	$92.00	CE	per infection averted	2003 US$	$137.78

table continues next page

Table 4.1 Cost-Effectiveness of Approaches to the HIV Care Continuum (continued)

Intervention	Study	Region or country	Cost per outcome	Cost (C) or cost-effectiveness (CE)	Unit of outcome	Currency as presented (year)	Cost in 2012 US$
VCT at community health centers	Tromp and others 2013	East Asia and Pacific, Indonesia	$248.00	CE	per HIV infection averted	2008 US$	$340.56
VCT	Wang, Moss, and Hiller 2011	East Asia and Pacific, China	165,067 yuan	C	Lifetime cost of HIV care and treatment per person in MSM population and in general population	2002 yuan	$34,679.90
VCT	Venkatesh and others 2013	India	$800.00–$1,900.00	CE	per YLS	2010 US$	$912.27–$2,166.65
Home-based HTC with enhanced link to care	Smith and others 2015	Sub-Saharan Africa, South Africa	$1,090.00–$1,360.00	CE	per DALY averted	2013 US$	—
DNA-PCR for EID compared with use of rapid HIV tests to screen out HIV-uninfected infants	Menzies and others 2009	Sub-Saharan Africa, Uganda	$1,489.00	C	per infant correctly diagnosed and informed of result for DNA-PCR versus modified algorithm	2007 US$	$1,937.90
Improvement of retention and adherence							
HBC, FBC, and MCC for provision of ART	Babigumira and others 2009	Sub-Saharan Africa, Uganda	$2,615.00	CE	per QALY, ICER for MCC versus FBC	2008 US$	$3,200.86
			$2,814.00	CE	per QALY, ICER for HBC versus FBC	2008 US$	$3,444.44
			$2,241.00	CE	per life year, ICER for MCC versus FBC	2008 US$	$2,743.07
			$2,251.00	CE	per life year, ICER for HBC versus FBC	2008 US$	$2,755.31
Interventions to prevent LTFU: $22/intervention/person/year	Losina and others 2009	Sub-Saharan Africa, Côte d'Ivoire	$1,200–$3,100 depending on efficacy in reducing LTFU (10%–75%)	CE	per YLS	2006 US$	$1,489.27–$3,847.28
Interventions to prevent LTFU: $41/intervention/person/year			$1,500–$4,900 depending on efficacy in reducing LTFU (10%–75%)	CE	per YLS	2006 US$	$1,861.59–$6,081.18

table continues next page

Table 4.1 Cost-Effectiveness of Approaches to the HIV Care Continuum (continued)

Intervention	Study	Region or country	Cost per outcome	Cost (C) or cost-effectiveness (CE)	Unit of outcome	Currency as presented (year)	Cost in 2012 US$
Interventions to prevent LTFU: $77/intervention/person/year			$2,000–$8,400 depending on efficacy in reducing LTFU (10%–75%)	CE	per YLS	2006 US$	$2,482.12–$10,424.88
Patient tracer to follow up lost patients	Rosen and Ketlhapile 2010	Sub-Saharan Africa, South Africa	$432.00	C	per patient returned to care	2009 US$	$552.10
Patient tracer to follow up lost patients			$18.00	C	per patient attempted to be traced in the intervention, including those who could not be found through tracing	2009 US$	$23.00
Peer health workers for adherence monitoring and social support	Chang and others 2013	Sub-Saharan Africa, Uganda	$189.00	C	per virologic failure averted	2012 US$	$231.34
			$1,025.00	C	per LTFU averted	2012 US$	$1,254.64
Case management to improve adherence	Marseille 2011	Sub-Saharan Africa, Ethiopia	$33.00	C	per patient served	2009 US$	$42.11
Case management to improve adherence			$84.00	C	per "successful exit" from the case management program	2009 US$	$107.20

Note: — = not available; ART = antiretroviral therapy; DALY = disability-adjusted life year; DNA = deoxyribonucleic acid; EID = early infant diagnostic; FBC = facility-based care; HBC = home-based care; HIV = human immunodeficiency virus; HTC = HIV testing and counseling; ICER = incremental cost-effectiveness ratio; LTFU = loss to follow-up; MCC = mobile clinic care; MSM = men who have sex with men; PCR = polymerase chain reaction; QALY = quality-adjusted life year; STI = sexually transmitted infection; VCT = voluntary counseling and testing; YLS = year of life saved.

hospitals, underscoring the importance of identifying high-risk locations for HIV testing (Siregar and others 2011). In India, one-time voluntary HIV testing in the population was found to be very cost-effective (ICER of US$1,100 per life year saved). The cost-effectiveness of such screening was even greater in high-prevalence areas (ICER of US$1,100 per life year saved) and high-risk groups (US$800 per life year saved) (Venkatesh and others 2013). A strategy of annual screening in high-prevalence districts and high-risk groups was also found to be cost-effective, as was screening every five years in the national population.

Early Infant Diagnosis

In Uganda, one study assessed the cost-effectiveness of incorporating initial screening with rapid HIV tests into the conventional testing algorithm of DNA-PCR to screen out HIV-uninfected infants (Suthar, Ford, and others 2013). Costs per infant were US$23.47 for DNA-PCR screening, compared with US$7.58 and US$22.75 for the modified algorithm that used rapid HIV tests. The modified algorithm was significantly less costly for infants older than age three months. Cost-effectiveness was assessed by calculating the incremental cost per infected infant correctly diagnosed, with parents informed of results. The conventional algorithm had cost-effectiveness ranging from US$539 to US$7,139 per infant correctly diagnosed and with family informed of result, suggesting that screening infants with rapid HIV tests before DNA-PCR is potentially cost-effective in infants older than age three months.

LINKING TO AND ENGAGEMENT WITH HIV CARE

Rationale and Coverage

Linking to HIV care and treatment services after a positive HIV test is a critical, but poorly documented, step in the HIV care continuum. The verbal or written referral process is often insufficient, with significant loss to follow-up (El-Sadr, Gamble, and Cohen 2013; Mugglin and others 2012). In a systematic review of 28 studies from Sub-Saharan Africa, a median of 59 percent of patients testing HIV-positive linked to care (Rosen and Fox 2011). It is important to note that based on the PHIA surveys completed and reported, of all HIV-positive individuals identified through the populations surveys in Malawi, Zambia, and Zimbabwe, a substantial proportion (87%) indicated that they were receiving ART, suggesting excellent ART initiation (ICAP 2016). However, these data do not inform the time from an HIV-positive test to linkage to care and treatment.

A systematic review of linkage of HIV-infected pregnant women revealed a failure to initiate ART among 38 percent to 88 percent of women known to be eligible (Ferguson and others 2012; Psaros and others 2015). Although infants born to a known HIV-infected mother should be engaged in care, linking HIV-exposed infants to appropriate follow-up services has been inadequate (Ahmed and others 2013; Chatterjee and others 2011; Ghadrshenas and others 2013). For children found to be HIV-infected, linking with and entry into care is similarly difficult (Phelps and others 2013).

Guidelines

The WHO identifies linking to HIV care as necessary to realize the full health and prevention benefits of ART (WHO 2013a). However, no consistent guidance exists on the optimal timing from receipt of a positive HIV test to linking to HIV care. The International Association of Physicians in AIDS Care and the Centers for Disease Control and Prevention recommend that individuals testing HIV-positive be linked to care within three months of diagnosis (CDC 2013b; Thompson and others 2012).

Measurements of Linkage to Care

Measuring successful linkage from HIV testing to care is often not feasible because HTS typically record aggregate data on number of tests without individual identifiers (McNairy and El-Sadr 2012). In addition, some studies report links within 30–90 days of an HIV-positive test, while others do not specify the time interval (Medley and others 2013; van Rooyen, Barnabas, and others 2013).

Some HIV programs require HIV-positive individuals to register in the HIV clinic and receive a medical record number and an appointment date for a clinic visit, but not necessarily documentation of an encounter with a clinician (Elul and others 2014). Other programs prefer evidence of receipt of clinical evaluation or a CD4 cell count test (Rosen and Fox 2011).

Barriers

One review of 24 studies (21 of which were from Sub-Saharan Africa) cited the multiple steps needed to enroll HIV-positive individuals into care (Bogart and others 2013; Govindasamy and others 2014). Reasons reported for not linking include fear that HIV-positive status will be purposefully or inadvertently disclosed (Hatcher and others 2012), fear of discrimination and spousal violence or separation (Bogart and others 2013;

Gari and others 2013), and distance to the health facility and transportation costs (Bogart and others 2013; Hensen and others 2012; Posse and Baltussen 2009).

System-level barriers include inconvenient clinic hours; long waiting times; shortages of skilled health care workers; and delays in CD4 cell count, viral load, and EID results. Furthermore, improperly trained or overworked health care workers and clinics where space limits privacy discourage patients from engaging in care (Fayorsey and others 2013; Hensen and others 2012; Posse and Baltussen 2009; Tran and others 2012).

Approaches to Improving Linkage to Care

Individual-Level Approaches
A study from Uganda demonstrated that patients who received extended posttest counseling and monthly visits by peer support workers were 80 percent more likely than other patients to access HIV care (Muhamadi and others 2011). Such programs are encouraged among populations less likely to access and sustain HIV care (Wouters and others 2012). Training for counseling that emphasizes linkage could be a simple and feasible approach to more effectively engage HIV-infected individuals in care.

Use of community health workers (CHWs) and peer educators, who are often themselves HIV-positive, to provide support, guidance, and help with navigation to HIV-positive individuals has shown considerable promise for improving linkage to care (Ackerman Gulaid and Kiragu 2012; Hatcher and others 2012; Kim and others 2012). A study from the United States found that newly diagnosed HIV-positive persons were more successfully linked to care when supported by a case manager (Craw and others 2008). In Kenya, 63.2 percent of patients who received home visits by peers were enrolled in ART within three months (Kohler and others 2011). Similarly, when CHWs were assigned to HIV-infected pregnant women in Malawi at the time of diagnosis, more than 70 percent of eligible women and eligible children received ART (Ahmed and others 2015; Kim and others 2012).

Incentives, including food, conditional cash transfers, and vouchers, have been used to encourage linkage to care (Kundu and others 2012; Solomon and others 2014). In India among PWID, modest voucher incentives significantly improved linkage to HIV care (Solomon and others 2014).

Text messages can help remind patients of appointments, testing, and medication adherence (van Velthoven and others 2013). The HIV Infant Tracking System in Kenya improved linkage to HIV services for HIV-exposed infants, with increased uptake of EID testing and linkage to care for those found HIV-positive, as well as prompt ART initiation (Finocchario-Kessler and others 2014).

Structural-Level Approaches
Point-of-care (POC) CD4 testing has been shown to increase likelihood of timely access to care (Wynberg and others 2014); for those eligible for ART, it has been shown to increase likelihood of initiating ART (Faal and others 2011; Larson and others 2012; Larson and others 2013; Patten and others 2013; Wynberg and others 2014). In South Africa, initiating POC CD4 testing at the time of HIV diagnosis more than doubled the likelihood that patients would initiate ART (Faal and others 2011).

Many countries, particularly in Sub-Saharan Africa, have successfully decentralized HIV care to the primary care level, reducing transport time and costs for patients (Govindasamy, Ford, and Kranzer 2012; Suthar, Hoos, and others 2013). Task-shifting and task-sharing—allowing trained peer health workers, nurses, and other nonphysician cadres to administer HIV services—has enabled decentralization and the scale-up of HIV services. These approaches were implemented in Malawi and Uganda with improved linkage to care and minimal increases to costs (Arem and others 2011; McCollum and others 2010).

Colocating HIV testing and care services may also enhance linkage to care (Torian and others 2008). The effectiveness of this approach has perhaps been best demonstrated with the integration of prevention of mother-to-child transmission into antenatal care services, with dramatic increases in enrollment into care for HIV-infected pregnant and breastfeeding women (Ferguson and others 2012).

Home-based services, including HIV testing, POC CD4 testing, and immediate initiation of ART, may increase linkage to care, especially in rural areas and in settings with high stigma (Helleringer and others 2009; Lahuerta and others 2013; Myer and others 2013). In South Africa, home-based HIV testing, followed by POC CD4 testing, counseling, and referral, was associated with 86 percent of patients' initiating ART within three months (van Rooyen, Barnabas, and others 2013). In Malawi, a program that offered self-testing and immediate ART initiation for those testing HIV-positive showed a significant increase in ART initiation (MacPherson and others 2014).

Cost-Effectiveness Considerations

Individual-Level Approaches
Few of the studies assessing individual-level approaches to promoting linkage to care have evaluated their

cost-effectiveness. In a study of nonmonetary incentives to promote linkage to care in India, an incentive worth US$4 was effective in increasing ART initiation, suggesting that relatively low-cost interventions are capable of making a difference in this step of the care cascade (Solomon and others 2014).

Given that HIV-infected patients gain individual health benefits and generate positive health externalities once they initiate ART, allocating resources to approaches that promote linkage to care has the potential to be more cost-effective than allocating resources to approaches that promote HIV testing in the general population.

Structural-Level Approaches

A study of home-based HIV testing and counseling accompanied by POC CD4 testing and lay counselor follow-up visits in South Africa reported ICERs of US$1,090–US$1,360 per DALY averted depending on the ART initiation criteria used (Smith and others 2015).

RETENTION IN HIV CARE

Rationale and Coverage

Based on evidence of the benefits of ART when initiated at early stages of HIV disease, it is anticipated that the period from diagnosis to ART initiation will be shortened with adoption of the WHO's 2016 guidelines for universal ART (START Study Group 2015; WHO 2015b). A systematic review of 28 studies from Sub-Saharan Africa found that mean retention of adult patients before ART initiation was only 46 percent, and mean retention from determination of ART eligibility to ART initiation was 68 percent (Rosen and Fox 2011). A systematic review indicated that retention on ART among adult patients was 80 percent, 70 percent, and 65 percent at 12, 24, and 36 months, respectively (Fox and Rosen 2010). Loss to follow-up and death were more frequent among men, adolescents and young adults, and pregnant women (DeSilva and others 2009; Lamb and others 2014; Lawn and others 2008; Phillips and others 2014).

Retention in care remains a major challenge for prevention of mother-to-child transmission programs, including those implementing the Option B+ approach— universal treatment for all pregnant and breastfeeding women. Studies demonstrate significant loss to follow-up for pregnant women on ART, especially those newly diagnosed during antenatal care, those who are diagnosed late in pregnancy, younger women, and those at earlier HIV disease stages (Haas and others 2016; Tenthani and others 2014).

A systematic review of eight studies from Sub-Saharan Africa, with a total of 10,741 children, reported that 78 percent to 97 percent of HIV-infected children had a CD4+ cell count measured; 63.2 percent to 90.7 percent of children were assessed for ART initiation; and 39.5 percent to 99.4 percent of eligible children started ART (Mugglin and others 2013). Loss to follow-up and death are significantly higher among children younger than age one year and among those with advanced disease (McNairy and others 2013).

Globally, approximately 1.7 million PWID are living with HIV, only 38 percent of whom are estimated to be receiving ART (WHO 2014c). A systematic review found that loss to follow up among FSWs was only 6 percent, albeit from few available studies (Mountain and others 2014). In a study from Zimbabwe, an estimated 50 percent to 70 percent of HIV-infected FSWs reported being enrolled in HIV care, and only 25 percent to 35 percent accessed ART (Cowan and others 2013). Among MSM in LMICs, data on access to HIV treatment remains limited (Arreola and others 2012; UNAIDS 2014).

Guidelines

The WHO guidelines highlight the importance of retention in care to enable achievement of viral suppression (WHO 2016), including for adults, children, adolescents, and pregnant women. Strategies to increase retention in care include community-level interventions for adults and interventions to enhance retention among pregnant women during the postpartum period, highlighting the importance of follow-up among caregivers for children and development of adolescent-friendly services.

Measurement of Retention in Care

Retention in care is defined as the proportion of patients who remain in care as evidenced by a clinical visit or pharmacy visit within a defined period. For example, for an HIV program that recommends a clinical visit every 3 months, a patient is retained at 12 months if the patient has completed a visit within 3 months of the scheduled 12-month visit.

Barriers

Barriers to retention in care are multifactorial (Bogart and others 2013; Geng and others 2010; Ware and others 2013). Structural barriers include financial constraints such as transport costs and lost work wages, long wait times and inconvenient clinic hours, mobility to seek employment, health care worker attitudes, and perceived low-quality care (Geng and others 2010; Maskew and others 2007). Psychosocial and behavioral barriers include anxiety and hopelessness, stigma, lack of perceived severity of HIV disease, lack of social support, and reluctance to return after a hiatus from clinic attendance (Wringe and others 2009). Biomedical barriers include inadequate opportunistic infection prevention and management that may hinder clinic attendance and contribute to deteriorating health (Brinkhof, Pujades-Rodriguez, and Egger 2009). In a meta-analysis of 17 studies evaluating loss to follow-up in patients on ART, the most common reasons reported were lack of money, improving or deteriorating health, and transfer to another HIV care site (Brinkhof, Pujades-Rodriguez, and Egger 2009).

Women are often lost to care when they return to their home villages or towns for delivery and postpartum care, and postdelivery when they make the transition to routine ART services (Colvin and others 2014; Phillips and others 2015; Schnippel and others 2015). Retention is particularly challenging for children, who depend on caregivers to bring them for clinic visits. Caregiver fear of disclosing HIV status to the child, unstable family structure, and unsympathetic school environments may lead to loss to follow-up for children (Busza and others 2014; Wachira, Middlestadt, and others 2012).

Engagement and retention in care are particularly difficult for key populations because of systematic exclusion, social and institutionalized stigma, harassment, and other psychosocial barriers that discourage engagement in care after an HIV-positive diagnosis (Baral and others 2012; Mtetwa and others 2013; WHO 2014c).

Approaches to Improving Retention

Several interventions have been noted to enhance retention in care.

Provision of free cotrimoxazole improved 12-month retention by 20 percent among pre-ART patients in Kenya (Kohler and others 2011), and food assistance was associated with increased clinic attendance in Haiti (Ivers and others 2010). Weekly mobile phone communication via text messages to encourage retention is being evaluated in an ongoing study in Kenya (van der Kop and others 2013). HIV treatment programs that include staff or peer workers who conduct outreach for patients who fail to attend clinic visits had higher retention, higher estimated mortality (resulting from more accurate ascertainment of outcomes among those lost to follow-up), and lower loss to follow-up (McMahon and others 2013).

Task-shifting from physician- to nurse-led HIV management has been associated with improved patient retention in several studies from Sub-Saharan Africa (Assefa and others 2012; Brennan and others 2011; Emdin, Chong, and Millson 2013; Fairall and others 2012; Iwu and Holzemer 2014; Sherr and others 2010; Shumbusho and others 2009; Thurman and others 2010). Evidence suggests improved retention for patients who initiate and maintain ART at primary health facilities (full decentralization) versus patients who initiate at secondary health facilities and are maintained at primary health facilities (partial decentralization) (Auld and others 2015; Reidy and others 2014).

In a study from rural Uganda, provision of US$2.50–US$7.00 to patients on ART to cover transportation costs was associated with increased retention at 12 months of between 87 percent and 92 percent (Emenyonu, Thirumurthy, and Muyindike 2010). Several programmatic and research studies are now examining how best to optimize retention of HIV-infected pregnant women (Sturke and others 2014).

Patient ART groups in Mozambique and South Africa, in which one individual is designated to pick up medications for the group, showed more than 95 percent retention in care of patients over 12 months, as well as favorable longer-term outcomes (Luque-Fernandez and others 2013; Rasschaert and others 2014).

For key populations, intensified posttest counseling combined with follow-up counseling by CHWs significantly increased the proportion that were enrolled and retained in HIV care (WHO 2014b; Wouters and others 2012).

Cost-Effectiveness Considerations

Few studies have assessed the cost-effectiveness of approaches to improve retention in HIV care (table 4.1).

Using Treatment Supporters

The cost-effectiveness of approaches that rely on treatment supporters has been assessed in South Africa, where the costs of using patient tracers to determine the status of patients lost to follow-up and to assist patients in returning to care were determined (Rosen and Ketlhapile 2010). Although the average cost per patient attempted to be traced in the intervention (including those not found through tracing) was reasonably low at US$18, because information systems to track deaths and monitor patients who transferred to other sites were not available, the cost of the intervention per patient returned to care was high at US$432.

Eliminating Patient Costs and Providing Incentives

A modeling study estimated the long-term clinical benefits and cost-effectiveness of retention interventions in Côte d'Ivoire (Losina and others 2009), including eliminating ART copayments, eliminating charges to patients for opportunistic-infection-related drugs, improving personnel training, and providing meals and transportation reimbursements for patients. The intervention costs varied from US$22 per person per year to US$77 per person per year. The results suggest that for a US$22 per person per year intervention that reduces loss to follow-up by 10 percent, the cost-effectiveness ratio of the intervention (compared to no intervention) would be US$3,100 per year of life saved. Using the WHO threshold for cost-effectiveness of 3 × per capita GDP, such an intervention would be cost-effective if it had an efficacy of at least 12 percent (WHO 2014a). Similarly, the more costly US$77 per person per year intervention is also cost-effective, with an efficacy of at least 41 percent.

ADHERENCE TO HIV TREATMENT

Rationale and Coverage

The clinical effectiveness of ART for individuals and to reduce transmission depends on adherence to treatment (Cohen and others 2011; START Study Group 2015). A meta-analysis published in 2006 found that adherence among patients on ART in Sub-Saharan Africa and North America was 77 percent and 55 percent, respectively (Mills, Nachega, Buchan, and others 2006). However, a systematic review of findings from 53 countries indicated that 62 percent of adolescents and young adults (ages 12–24 years) receiving treatment were at least 85 percent adherent to ART (Kim and others 2014). Among children, adherence varies considerably by age and medication formulation but has been estimated to be 75 percent in Sub-Saharan Africa (Vreeman and others 2008). A systematic review of 51 studies reporting on adherence during and after pregnancy found that 77 percent of pregnant women had adequate adherence, but adherence decreased during the postpartum period to 53 percent (Nachega and others 2012).

Lastly, a systematic review of HIV-infected PWID found that ART adherence ranged from 33 percent to 97 percent in LMICs (Feelemyer and others 2015); another systematic review determined that 76 percent of FSWs globally adhered to ART (Mountain and others 2014). ART adherence rates among MSM populations in LMICs have not been reliably estimated.

The lack of broad availability of viral load measurement in LMICs has limited the ability to assess adherence through the effect on viral suppression (Lecher and others 2015). The recently conducted PHIA surveys provide encouraging findings. Overall, the first three surveys completed in Zimbabwe, Malawi and Zambia showed that 88.6 percent of HIV-positive patients who indicated that they were on ART had viral suppression.

Guidelines

Guidelines from both the WHO and the International Association of Providers of AIDS Care recommend a once-daily, fixed-dose regimen, with the goal of facilitating adherence (Thompson and others 2012; WHO 2016). The guidelines also recognize the centrality of excellent adherence to the success of ART for individual as well as population health and the complexity of maintaining adherence to lifetime treatment. To support patient adherence, the WHO recommends implementation of evidence-based interventions, including peer counselors, mobile phone text messages, reminder devices, cognitive behavioral therapy, and behavioral skills training.

Measurement

Adherence measures include self-reporting, pill counts, and pharmacy claims, or more reliably, directly observed therapy (Chaiyachati and others 2011; Kabore and others 2015; Simoni and others 2006). In research contexts, measures include determination of drug concentration in blood samples and use of Medication Event Monitoring System caps on prescription containers (Bulgiba and others 2013; Liu, Ma, and Zhang 2010; Thompson and others 2012).

Barriers

A systematic review of patient-related barriers found that fear of disclosure, stigma, concomitant substance abuse, forgetfulness, suspicions of treatment, regimens that are too complicated, high pill burden, decreased quality of life, work and family responsibilities, food insecurity, and limited access to medication are commonly reported barriers (Mills, Nachega, Bangsberg, and others 2006; Young and others 2014). System-level barriers include lack of awareness about ART, stigma, perceived high costs for antiretrovirals and related services, lack of financial means, distance and duration of travel to health providers, lack of consistency and coordination across services, limited involvement of the community in the program planning process, poor clinical practices and health care worker attitudes toward patients, and stock outs of antiretroviral drugs (Bezabhe and others 2014; Coetzee, Kagee, and Vermeulen 2011; Kagee and others 2011).

For pregnant women, additional barriers to adherence include medication side effects, disparate locations for delivery of ART (antenatal care versus ART clinic), and health worker attitudes (Gourlay and others 2013; Hodgson and others 2014; Thompson and others 2012). For children and adolescents, barriers include high pill burden, poorly tolerated formulations, ART side effects, concerns about stigma and discrimination, and a lack of youth-friendly clinical services (Denison and others 2015; Hudelson and Cluver 2015; Lall and others 2015).

Among MSM (Beyrer and others 2010), PWID (Feelemyer and others 2015), and SWs (Mountain and others 2014), mental illness, stigma and discrimination, lack of confidentiality, health worker discrimination, violence, and lack of tailored services, as well as structural barriers such as social and legal critical enablers, frequently discourage HIV-infected patients from adhering to ART care (Grubb and others 2014; WHO 2014b).

Approaches to Enhancing Adherence

A systematic review of adherence interventions in Sub-Saharan Africa identified six interventions that demonstrate efficacy: text messages and other reminder devices, treatment supporters, directly observed therapy, education and counseling, food supplements, and different care-delivery models (Bärnighausen and others 2011).

Data on patient-reported barriers to adherence suggest that efforts to reduce pill burden (with fixed dose combinations) and drug-specific side effects may result in higher adherence (Nachega and others 2014). While data on other strategies targeting HIV-infected pregnant women are limited, adoption of Option B+ may improve adherence when it consists of a once-daily, fixed-dose combination regimen (Ahmed, Kim, and Abrams 2013; Vitalis 2013).

In Sub-Saharan Africa, two randomized trials have shown that text message reminders to patients to take their medication can significantly increase adherence. The overall effect of text messaging was influenced by level of education, gender, and timing and interactivity of the message (Lester and others 2010; Mbuagbaw and others 2013). A recent review of studies evaluating the effect of text messaging on ART adherence noted one study that found that weekly one-way text messages to patients increased the proportion of patients with greater than 90 percent adherence, while another study found that weekly two-way messages (that is, messages sent to the patient with provider follow-up based on the patient's response) increased the proportion of patients with

greater than 95 percent adherence and viral suppression (Horvath and others 2012). Another meta-analysis of eight studies reported higher adherence among text message recipients than among controls (Finitsis, Pellowski, and Johnson 2014).

Community adherence support delivered by peers—peer educators or patient advocates—improved retention among both adults and children on ART in South Africa and was associated with decreased mortality (Bemelmans and others 2014; Grimwood and others 2012; Root and Whiteside 2013).

Studies also report significantly improved viral load suppression among patients in HIV programs with peer workers (Chang and others 2010; Pearson and others 2007; Taiwo and others 2010). A randomized controlled study in Rakai, Uganda, observed decreased virologic failure rates among patients at clinics with peer workers compared with those without peer workers (Chang and others 2010).

Decentralizing HIV services from secondary and tertiary health facilities to primary care facilities or community-based adherence clubs has improved virologic suppression (Chishinga and others 2014; Grimsrud and others 2015). Adherence clubs implemented in Cape Town, South Africa, that decentralize care to CHWs and include peer support and self-management features demonstrated only 6 percent loss to follow-up, and fewer than 2 percent of patients experienced viral rebound (Grimsrud and others 2015).

Interventions have been explored to enhance ART adherence among children and adolescents, including counseling, peer support group therapy, medication diaries, directly observed therapy, and improved antiretroviral formulations (Denison and others 2015). A qualitative study of HIV-infected adolescents in Zimbabwe suggested benefit from support group interventions (Mupambireyi and others 2014). A study in Zambia highlighted the importance of family support and life-skills training to enhance adherence to ART for adolescents living with HIV (Denison and others 2015). The introduction of Option B+ with a simplified once-daily, fixed-dose combination regimen is expected to improve adherence among pregnant and breastfeeding women (CDC 2013a).

Among PWID, those who receive care in supportive environments have ART outcomes similar to outcomes of non-PWID HIV-infected individuals (Wolfe, Carrieri, and Shepard 2010). Creating an enabling environment is also critical, including supporting legislation, making policy and financial commitments, decriminalizing behaviors of key populations, addressing stigma and discrimination, empowering specific communities, and addressing violence against people from key populations

(WHO 2014b). Among PWID, opioid substitution therapy was associated with greater ART adherence, supporting the need for integration of drug treatment and HIV treatment services (Malta and others 2008; Milloy, Montaner, and Wood 2012). Among SWs, interventions similar to those mentioned above but tailored to the specific needs of this population have been noted to be effective in improving ART adherence, including adherence counseling and monthly support groups (Graham and others 2013; Huet and others 2011; Konate and others 2011).

Food incentives provided at scheduled appointments have increased ART adherence and have modestly enhanced nutritional status (Cantrell and others 2008).

Cost-Effectiveness Considerations

Only a few approaches to promoting adherence have been assessed for cost-effectiveness (table 4.1). A number of studies that evaluated the efficacy of adherence interventions did not include cost-effectiveness analyses (Bärnighausen and others 2011). In South Africa, it has been estimated that higher ART adherence can reduce health care costs, particularly hospitalization costs (Nachega and others 2010), suggesting that effective adherence approaches could be highly cost-effective and possibly cost saving as well.

Peer Counseling

While the cost-effectiveness of using peer health workers has not been determined in studies, one study has reported on the costs of this approach. In Uganda, an approach that used peer health workers to provide clinical and adherence monitoring and psychosocial support to patients at clinics and during monthly home visits cost US$189 per virologic failure averted and US$1,025 per patient loss to follow-up averted (Chang and others 2013).

Decentralized Care

A study in Uganda that assessed the cost-effectiveness of facility-based care (FBC), home-based care (HBC), and mobile clinics indicated that facility-based ART provision was the least costly, and the ICER for mobile clinic care relative to FBC was US$2,615 per quality-adjusted life year (Babigumira and others 2009). The ICER for HBC relative to FBC was US$2,814 per quality-adjusted life year. Thus, though patient outcomes are often better with mobile care and HBC, their costs result in cost-effectiveness ratios that in some countries exceed the threshold of three times per capita GDP. Nevertheless, these approaches may be warranted in cases in which patient populations reside far from facilities or if the costs of these approaches can be reduced.

CONCLUSIONS

The global HIV response is at a critical crossroads. Although declines in the number of new infections and in HIV-related mortality have been noteworthy, more remains to be done, both to sustain these gains and to accelerate epidemic control (Piot and others 2015).

Achievement of optimal outcomes for HIV-infected individuals and for the prevention of transmission to others is dependent on optimizing every step of the HIV care continuum. As described in this chapter, many promising and efficacious approaches exist to address specific gaps. The findings from the PHIA surveys are encouraging and demonstrate, at least for the first three countries surveyed, good progress toward the UNAIDS 90/90/90 targets, with certain gaps identified particularly in terms of reaching the first 90 target, engaging men and adolescents and young adults. However, for key populations, large gaps remain in achieving the 90/90/90 targets and in addressing the gaps in the HIV care continuum (ICAP 2016).

It is important to note that enhancing one step in the continuum will be insufficient to achieve the overall desired outcome of HIV programs. Thus, research efforts should focus on identifying effective combinations of interventions that target multiple steps along the continuum. Similarly, research studies need to assess the cost-effectiveness of such interventions and packages of interventions across the care continuum. Having information on cost-effectiveness is critical to motivating policy change and resource mobilization.

Now more than ever, identifying cost-effective methods that enable the achievement of high service coverage and quality is essential to controlling the HIV epidemic.

ANNEX

The annex to this chapter is as follows. It is available at http://www.dcp-3.org/infectiousdiseases.

- Annex 4A. Effectiveness of HIV Interventions

ACKNOWLEDGMENTS

Partial funding support was provided to Wafaa M. El-Sadr and Katherine Harripersaud through the National Institutes of Health, National Institute of Allergy and Infectious Diseases Cooperative Agreement under cooperative agreement #UM1 AI068619; to Elaine J. Abrams from the Eunice Kennedy Shriver National Institute for Child Health and Human Development under award 1RO1HD074558; and to Harsha Thirumurthy from the

Eunice Kennedy Shriver National Institute for Child Health and Human Development under award K01HD061605.

NOTE

World Bank Income Classifications as of July 2014 are as follows, based on estimates of gross national income (GNI) per capita for 2013:

- Low-income countries (LICs) = US$1,045 or less
- Middle-income countries (MICs) are subdivided:
    (a) lower-middle-income = US$1,046 to US$4,125
    (b) upper-middle-income (UMICs) = US$4,126 to US$12,745
- High-income countries (HICs) = US$12,746 or more.

REFERENCES

Ackerman Gulaid, L., and K. Kiragu. 2012. "Lessons Learnt from Promising Practices in Community Engagement for the Elimination of New HIV Infections in Children by 2015 and Keeping Their Mothers Alive: Summary of a Desk Review." *Journal of the International AIDS Society* 15 (Suppl 2): 17390.

Ahmed, S., M. H. Kim, and E. J. Abrams. 2013. "Risks and Benefits of Lifelong Antiretroviral Treatment for Pregnant and Breastfeeding Women: A Review of the Evidence for the Option B+ Approach." *Current Opinion in HIV and AIDS* 8 (5): 474–89.

Ahmed, S., M. H. Kim, A. C. Dave, R. Sabelli, K. Kanjelo, and others. 2015. "Improved Identification and Enrolment into Care of HIV-Exposed and -Infected Infants and Children Following a Community Health Worker Intervention in Lilongwe, Malawi." *Journal of the International AIDS Society* 18 (1): 19305.

Ahmed, S., M. H. Kim, N. Sugandhi, B. R. Phelps, R. Sabelli, and others. 2013. "Beyond Early Infant Diagnosis: Case Finding Strategies for Identification of HIV-Infected Infants and Children." *AIDS* 27 (Suppl 2): S235–45.

Arem, H., N. Nakyanjo, J. Kagaayi, J. Mulamba, G. Nakigozi, and others. 2011. "Peer Health Workers and AIDS Care in Rakai, Uganda: A Mixed Methods Operations Research Evaluation of a Cluster-Randomized Trial." *AIDS Patient Care and STDs* 25 (12): 719–24.

Arreola, S., P. Hebert, K. Makofane, J. Beck, and G. Ayala. 2012. *Access to HIV Prevention and Treatment for Men Who Have Sex with Men: Findings from the 2012 Global Men's Health and Rights Study (GMHR)*. Oakland, CA: Global Forum on MSM and HIV (MSMGF).

Assefa, Y., A. Kiflie, B. Tekle, D. H. Mariam, M. Laga, and others. 2012. "Effectiveness and Acceptability of Delivery of Antiretroviral Treatment in Health Centres by Health Officers and Nurses in Ethiopia." *Journal of Health Services Research and Policy* 17 (1): 24–29.

Auld, A. F., H. Kamiru, C. Azih, A. L. Baughman, H. Nuwagaba-Biribonwoha, and others. 2015. "Implementation and Operational Research: Evaluation of Swaziland's Hub-and-Spoke Model for Decentralizing Access to Antiretroviral Therapy Services." *Journal of Acquired Immune Deficiency Syndromes* 69 (1): e1–12.

Babigumira, J. B., A. K. Sethi, K. A. Smyth, and M. E. Singer. 2009. "Cost Effectiveness of Facility-Based Care, Home-Based Care, and Mobile Clinics for Provision of Antiretroviral Therapy in Uganda." *Pharmacoeconomics* 27 (11): 963–73.

Baeten, J. M., D. Donnell, P. Ndase, N. R. Mugo, J. D. Campbell, and others. 2012. "Antiretroviral Prophylaxis for HIV Prevention in Heterosexual Men and Women." *New England Journal of Medicine* 367 (5): 399–410.

Baggaley, R., B. Hensen, O. Ajose, K. L. Grabbe, V. J. Wong, and others. 2012. "From Caution to Urgency: The Evolution of HIV Testing and Counselling in Africa." *Bulletin of the World Health Organization* 90 (9): 652–58B.

Baral, S., C. Beyrer, K. Muessig, T. Poteat, A. L. Wirtz, and others. 2012. "Burden of HIV among Female Sex Workers in Low-Income and Middle-Income Countries: A Systematic Review and Meta-Analysis." *The Lancet Infectious Diseases* 12 (7): 538–49.

Bärnighausen, T., K. Chaiyachati, N. Chimbindi, A. Peoples, J. Haberer, and others. 2011. "Interventions to Increase Antiretroviral Adherence in Sub-Saharan Africa: A Systematic Review of Evaluation Studies." *The Lancet Infectious Diseases* 11 (12): 942–51.

Bateganya, M., O. A. Abdulwadud, and S. M. Kiene. 2010. "Home-Based HIV Voluntary Counselling and Testing (VCT) for Improving Uptake of HIV Testing." *Cochrane Database of Systematic Reviews* 7 (July): CD006493.

Bemelmans, M., S. Baert, E. Goemaere, L. Wilkinson, M. Vandendyck, and others. 2014. "Community-Supported Models of Care for People on HIV Treatment in Sub-Saharan Africa." *Tropical Medicine and International Health* 19 (8): 968–77.

Beyrer, C., S. D. Baral, D. Walker, A. L. Wirtz, B. Johns, and others. 2010. "The Expanding Epidemics of HIV Type 1 among Men Who Have Sex with Men in Low- and Middle-Income Countries: Diversity and Consistency." *Epidemiologic Reviews* 32 (June): 137–51.

Bezabhe, W. M., L. Chalmers, L. R. Bereznicki, G. M. Peterson, M. A. Bimirew, and others. 2014. "Barriers and Facilitators of Adherence to Antiretroviral Drug Therapy and Retention in Care among Adult HIV-Positive Patients: A Qualitative Study from Ethiopia." *PLoS One* 9 (5): e97353.

Bogart, L. M., S. Chetty, J. Giddy, A. Sypek, L. Sticklor, and others. 2013. "Barriers to Care among People Living with HIV in South Africa: Contrasts between Patient and Healthcare Provider Perspectives." *AIDS Care* 25 (7): 843–53.

Bourne, C., V. Knight, R. Guy, H. Wand, H. Lu, and others. 2011. "Short Message Service Reminder Intervention Doubles Sexually Transmitted Infection/HIV Re-Testing Rates among Men Who Have Sex with Men." *Sexually Transmitted Infections* 87 (3): 229–231.

Brennan, A. T., L. Long, M. Maskew, I. Sanne, I. Jaffray, and others. 2011. "Outcomes of Stable HIV-Positive Patients Down-Referred from a Doctor-Managed Antiretroviral

Therapy Clinic to a Nurse-Managed Primary Health Clinic for Monitoring and Treatment." *AIDS* 25 (16): 2027–36.

Brinkhof, M. W., M. Pujades-Rodriguez, and M. Egger. 2009. "Mortality of Patients Lost to Follow-Up in Antiretroviral Treatment Programmes in Resource-Limited Settings: Systematic Review and Meta-Analysis." *PLoS One* 4 (6): e5790.

Brown, L. B., W. C. Miller, G. Kamanga, N. Nyirenda, P. Mmodzi, and others. 2011. "HIV Partner Notification Is Effective and Feasible in Sub-Saharan Africa: Opportunities for HIV Treatment and Prevention." *Journal of Acquired Immune Deficiency Syndromes* 56 (5): 437–42.

Bulgiba, A., U. Y. Mohammed, Z. Chik, C. Lee, and D. Peramalah. 2013. "How Well Does Self-Reported Adherence Fare Compared to Therapeutic Drug Monitoring in HAART?" *Preventive Medicine* 57 (Suppl): S34–36.

Busza, J., E. Dauya, T. Bandason, H. Mujuru, and R. A. Ferrand. 2014. "'I Don't Want Financial Support but Verbal Support.' How Do Caregivers Manage Children's Access to and Retention in HIV Care in Urban Zimbabwe?" *Journal of the International AIDS Society* 17 (1): 18839.

Cantrell, R. A., M. Sinkala, K. Megazzini, S. Lawson-Marriott, S. Washington, and others. 2008. "A Pilot Study of Food Supplementation to Improve Adherence to Antiretroviral Therapy among Food-Insecure Adults in Lusaka, Zambia." *Journal of Acquired Immune Deficiency Syndromes* 49 (2): 190–95.

CDC (Centers for Disease Control and Prevention). 2013a. "Impact of an Innovative Approach to Prevent Mother-to-Child Transmission of HIV—Malawi, July 2011–September 2012." *Morbidity and Mortality Weekly Report* 62 (8): 148–51.

———. 2013b. *Recommended Prevention Services: Linkage to and Retention in HIV Medical Care*. Atlanta, GA: CDC. http://www.cdc.gov/hiv/prevention/programs/pwp/linkage.html.

Celum, C., J. M. Baeten, J. P. Hughes, R. Barnabas, A. Liu, and others. 2013. "Integrated Strategies for Combination HIV Prevention: Principles and Examples for Men Who Have Sex with Men in the Americas and Heterosexual African Populations." *Journal of Acquired Immune Deficiency Syndromes* 63 (Suppl 2): S213–20.

Chaiyachati, K., L. R. Hirschhorn, F. Tanser, M. L. Newell, and T. Bärnighausen. 2011. "Validating Five Questions of Antiretroviral Nonadherence in a Public-Sector Treatment Program in Rural South Africa." *AIDS Patient Care and STDs* 25 (3): 163–70.

Chamie, G., D. Kwarisiima, T. D. Clark, J. Kabami, V. Jain, and others. 2014. "Uptake of Community-Based HIV Testing during a Multi-Disease Health Campaign in Rural Uganda." *PLoS One* 9 (1): e84317.

Chang, L. W., J. Kagaayi, G. Nakigozi, D. Serwada, T. C. Quinn, and others. 2013. "Cost Analyses of Peer Health Worker and mHealth Support Interventions for Improving AIDS Care in Rakai, Uganda." *AIDS Care* 25 (5): 652–56.

Chang, L. W., J. Kagaayi, G. Nakigozi, V. Ssempijja, A. H. Packer, and others. 2010. "Effect of Peer Health Workers on AIDS Care in Rakai, Uganda: A Cluster-Randomized Trial." *PLoS One* 5 (6): e10923.

Chatterjee, A., S. Tripathi, R. Gass, N. Hamunime, S. Panha, and others. 2011. "Implementing Services for Early Infant Diagnosis (EID) of HIV: A Comparative Descriptive Analysis of National Programs in Four Countries." *BMC Public Health* 11 (July): 553.

Chishinga, N., P. Godfrey-Faussett, K. Fielding, and H. Ayles. 2014. "Effect of Home-Based Interventions on Virologic Outcomes in Adults Receiving Antiretroviral Therapy in Africa: A Meta-Analysis." *BMC Public Health* 14 (1): 239.

Choko, A. T., N. Desmond, E. L. Webb, K. Chavula, S. Napierala-Mavedzenge, and others. 2011. "The Uptake and Accuracy of Oral Kits for HIV Self-Testing in High HIV Prevalence Setting: A Cross-Sectional Feasibility Study in Blantyre, Malawi." *PLoS Medicine* 8 (10): e1001102.

Coates, T. J., M. Kulich, D. D. Celentano, C. E. Zelaya, S. Chariyalertsak, and others. 2014. "Effect of Community-Based Voluntary Counselling and Testing on HIV Incidence and Social and Behavioural Outcomes (NIMH Project Accept; HPTN 043): A Cluster-Randomised Trial." *The Lancet Global Health* 2 (5): e267–77.

Coetzee, B., A. Kagee, and N. Vermeulen. 2011. "Structural Barriers to Adherence to Antiretroviral Therapy in a Resource-Constrained Setting: The Perspectives of Health Care Providers." *AIDS Care* 23 (2): 146–51.

Cohen, M. S., Y. Q. Chen, M. McCauley, T. Gamble, M. C. Hosseinipour, and others. 2011. "Prevention of HIV-1 Infection with Early Antiretroviral Therapy." *New England Journal of Medicine* 365 (6): 493–505.

Colvin, C. J., S. Konopka, J. C. Chalker, E. Jonas, J. Albertini, and others. 2014. "A Systematic Review of Health System Barriers and Enablers for Antiretroviral Therapy (ART) for HIV-Infected Pregnant and Postpartum Women." *PLoS One* 9 (10): e108150.

Cowan, F. M., S. Mtetwa, C. Davey, E. Fearon, J. Dirawo, and others. 2013. "Engagement with HIV Prevention Treatment and Care among Female Sex Workers in Zimbabwe: A Respondent-Driven Sampling Survey." *PLoS One* 8 (10): e77080.

Craw, J. A., L. I. Gardner, G. Marks, R. C. Rapp, J. Bosshart, and others. 2008. "Brief Strengths-Based Case Management Promotes Entry into HIV Medical Care: Results of the Antiretroviral Treatment Access Study-II." *Journal of Acquired Immune Deficiency Syndromes* 47 (5): 597–606.

Creek, T., A. Tanuri, M. Smith, K. Seipone, M. Smit, and others. 2008. "Early Diagnosis of Human Immunodeficiency Virus in Infants Using Polymerase Chain Reaction on Dried Blood Spots in Botswana's National Program for Prevention of Mother-to-Child Transmission." *Pediatric Infectious Disease Journal* 27 (1): 22–26.

Danel, C., R. Moh, D. Gabillard, A. Badje, J. Le Carrou, and others. 2015. "A Trial of Early Antiretrovirals and Isoniazid Preventive Therapy in Africa." *New England Journal of Medicine* 373 (9): 808–22.

Deeks, S. G., S. R. Lewin, and D. V. Havlir. 2013. "The End of AIDS: HIV Infection as a Chronic Disease." *The Lancet* 382 (9903): 1525–33.

Denison, J. A., H. Banda, A. C. Dennis, C. Packer, N. Nyambe, and others. 2015. "'The Sky Is the Limit': Adhering to Antiretroviral Therapy and HIV Self-Management from the Perspectives of Adolescents Living with HIV and Their Adult Caregivers." *Journal of the International AIDS Society* 18 (1): 19358.

DeSilva, M. B., S. P. Merry, P. R. Fischer, J. E. Rohrer, C. O. Isichei, and others. 2009. "Youth, Unemployment, and Male Gender Predict Mortality in AIDS Patients Started on HAART in Nigeria." *AIDS Care* 21 (1): 70–77.

Drake, A. L., A. Wagner, B. Richardson, and G. John-Stewart. 2014. "Incident HIV during Pregnancy and Postpartum and Risk of Mother-to-Child HIV Transmission: A Systematic Review and Meta-Analysis." *PLoS Medicine* 11 (2): e1001608.

Dugas, M., E. Bedard, G. Batona, A. C. Kpatchavi, F. A. Guedou, and others. 2015. "Outreach Strategies for the Promotion of HIV Testing and Care: Closing the Gap between Health Services and Female Sex Workers in Benin." *Journal of Acquired Immune Deficiency Syndromes* 68 (Suppl 2): S198–205.

El-Sadr, W. M., T. R. Gamble, and M. S. Cohen. 2013. "Linkage from HIV Testing to Care: A Positive Test Often Leads Nowhere." *Sexually Transmitted Diseases* 40 (1): 26–27.

Elul, B., M. Lahuerta, F. Abacassamo, M. R. Lamb, L. Ahoua, and others. 2014. "A Combination Strategy for Enhancing Linkage to and Retention in HIV Care among Adults Newly Diagnosed with HIV in Mozambique: Study Protocol for a Site-Randomized Implementation Science Study." *BMC Infectious Diseases* 14 (1): 549.

Emdin, C. A., N. J. Chong, and P. E. Millson. 2013. "Non-Physician Clinician Provided HIV Treatment Results in Equivalent Outcomes as Physician-Provided Care: A Meta-Analysis." *Journal of the International AIDS Society* 16 (July): 18445.

Emenyonu, N., H. Thirumurthy, and W. Muyindike. 2010. "Cash Transfers to Cover Clinic Transportation Costs Improve Adherence and Retention in Care in a HIV Treatment Program in Rural Uganda." Prepared for the Seventeenth Conference on Retroviruses and Opportunistic Infections, San Francisco, CA, February 16–19.

Essajee, S., L. Vojnov, M. Penazzato, I. Jani, G. K. Siberry, and others. 2015. "Reducing Mortality in HIV-Infected Infants and Achieving the 90-90-90 Target through Innovative Diagnosis Approaches." *Journal of the International AIDS Society* 18 (Suppl 6): 20299.

Faal, M., N. Naidoo, D. K. Glencross, W. D. Venter, and R. Osih. 2011. "Providing Immediate CD4 Count Results at HIV Testing Improves ART Initiation." *Journal of Acquired Immune Deficiency Syndromes* 58 (3): e54–59.

Fairall, L., M. O. Bachmann, C. Lombard, V. Timmerman, K. Uebel, and others. 2012. "Task Shifting of Antiretroviral Treatment from Doctors to Primary-Care Nurses in South Africa (STRETCH): A Pragmatic, Parallel, Cluster-Randomised Trial." *The Lancet* 380 (9845): 889–98.

Fayorsey, R. N., S. Saito, R. J. Carter, E. Gusmao, K. Frederix, and others. 2013. "Decentralization of Pediatric HIV Care and Treatment in Five Sub-Saharan African Countries." *Journal of Acquired Immune Deficiency Syndromes* 62 (5): e124–30.

Feelemyer, J., D. Des Jarlais, K. Arasteh, and A. Uuskula. 2015. "Adherence to Antiretroviral Medications among Persons Who Inject Drugs in Transitional, Low, and Middle Income Countries: An International Systematic Review." *AIDS and Behavior* 19 (4): 575–83.

Ferguson, L., A. D. Grant, D. Watson-Jones, T. Kahawita, J. O. Ong'ech, and others. 2012. "Linking Women Who Test HIV-Positive in Pregnancy-Related Services to Long-Term HIV Care and Treatment Services: A Systematic Review." *Tropical Medicine and International Health* 17 (5): 564–80.

Finitsis, D. J., J. A. Pellowski, and B. T. Johnson. 2014. "Text Message Intervention Designs to Promote Adherence to Antiretroviral Therapy (ART): A Meta-Analysis of Randomized Controlled Trials." *PLoS One* 9 (2): e88166.

Finocchario-Kessler, S., B. J. Gautney, S. Khamadi, V. Okoth, K. Goggin, and others. 2014. "If You Text Them, They Will Come: Using the HIV Infant Tracking System to Improve Early Infant Diagnosis Quality and Retention in Kenya." *AIDS* 28 (Suppl 3): S313–21.

Fox, M. P., and S. Rosen. 2010. "Patient Retention in Antiretroviral Therapy Programs up to Three Years on Treatment in Sub-Saharan Africa, 2007–2009: Systematic Review." *Tropical Medicine and International Health* 15 (Suppl 1): 1–15.

Gardner, E. M., M. P. McLees, J. F. Steiner, C. Del Rio, and W. J. Burman. 2011. "The Spectrum of Engagement in HIV Care and Its Relevance to Test-and-Treat Strategies for Prevention of HIV Infection." *Clinical Infectious Diseases* 52 (6): 793–800.

Gari, S., C. Doig-Acuna, T. Smail, J. R. Malungo, A. Martin-Hilber, and others. 2013. "Access to HIV/AIDS Care: A Systematic Review of Socio-Cultural Determinants in Low- and High-Income Countries." *BMC Health Services Research* 13 (May): 198.

Geng, E. H., D. Nash, A. Kambugu, Y. Zhang, P. Braitstein, and others. 2010. "Retention in Care among HIV-Infected Patients in Resource-Limited Settings: Emerging Insights and New Directions." *Current HIV/AIDS Reports* 7 (4): 234–44.

Ghadrshenas, A., Y. Ben Amor, J. Chang, H. Dale, G. Sherman, and others. 2013. "Improved Access to Early Infant Diagnosis Is a Critical Part of a Child-Centric Prevention of Mother-to-Child Transmission Agenda." *AIDS* 27 (Suppl 2): S197–205.

Gourlay, A., I. Birdthistle, G. Mburu, K. Iorpenda, and A. Wringe. 2013. "Barriers and Facilitating Factors to the Uptake of Antiretroviral Drugs for Prevention of Mother-to-Child Transmission of HIV in Sub-Saharan Africa: A Systematic Review." *Journal of the International AIDS Society* 16 (1): 18588.

Govindasamy, D., N. Ford, and K. Kranzer. 2012. "Risk Factors, Barriers, and Facilitators for Linkage to Antiretroviral Therapy Care: A Systematic Review." *AIDS* 26 (16): 2059–67.

Govindasamy, D., J. Meghij, E. Kebede Negussi, R. Clare Baggaley, N. Ford, and others. 2014. "Interventions to Improve or Facilitate Linkage to or Retention in Pre-ART (HIV) Care and Initiation of ART in Low- and Middle-Income Settings: A Systematic Review." *Journal of the International AIDS Society* 17 (August): 19032.

Grabbe, K. L., N. Menzies, M. Taegtmeyer, G. Emukule, P. Angala, and others. 2010. "Increasing Access to HIV Counseling and Testing through Mobile Services in Kenya: Strategies, Utilization, and Cost-Effectiveness." *Journal of Acquired Immune Deficiency Syndromes* 54 (3): 317.

Graham, S. M., P. Mugo, E. Gichuru, A. Thiong'o, M. Macharia, and others. 2013. "Adherence to Antiretroviral Therapy and Clinical Outcomes among Young Adults Reporting High-Risk Sexual Behavior, Including Men Who Have Sex with Men, in Coastal Kenya." *AIDS and Behavior* 17 (4): 1255–65.

Gray, R. H., G. Kigozi, D. Serwadda, F. Makumbi, S. Watya, and others. 2007. "Male Circumcision for HIV Prevention in Men in Rakai, Uganda: A Randomised Trial." *The Lancet* 369 (9562): 657–66.

Grimsrud, A., J. Sharp, C. Kalombo, L. G. Bekker, and L. Myer. 2015. "Implementation of Community-Based Adherence Clubs for Stable Antiretroviral Therapy Patients in Cape Town, South Africa." *Journal of the International AIDS Society* 18 (May): 19984.

Grimwood, A., G. Fatti, E. Mothibi, M. Malahlela, J. Shea, and others. 2012. "Community Adherence Support Improves Programme Retention in Children on Antiretroviral Treatment: A Multicentre Cohort Study in South Africa." *Journal of the International AIDS Society* 15 (2): 17381.

Grubb, I. R., S. W. Beckham, M. Kazatchkine, R. M. Thomas, E. R. Albers, and others. 2014. "Maximizing the Benefits of Antiretroviral Therapy for Key Affected Populations." *Journal of the International AIDS Society* 17 (July): 19320.

Haas, A. D., L. Tenthani, M. T. Msukwa, K. Tal, A. Jahn, and others. 2016. "Retention in Care during the First 3 Years of Antiretroviral Therapy for Women in Malawi's Option B+ Programme: An Observational Cohort Study." *The Lancet HIV* 3 (4): e175–82.

Hatcher, A. M., J. M. Turan, H. H. Leslie, L. W. Kanya, Z. Kwena, and others. 2012. "Predictors of Linkage to Care Following Community-Based HIV Counseling and Testing in Rural Kenya." *AIDS and Behavior* 16 (5): 1295–307.

Helleringer, S., H. P. Kohler, J. A. Frimpong, and J. Mkandawire. 2009. "Increasing Uptake of HIV Testing and Counseling among the Poorest in Sub-Saharan Countries through Home-Based Service Provision." *Journal of Acquired Immune Deficiency Syndromes* 51 (2): 185–93.

Henley, C., G. Forgwei, T. Welty, M. Golden, A. Adimora, and others. 2013. "Scale-Up and Case-Finding Effectiveness of an HIV Partner Services Program in Cameroon: An Innovative HIV Prevention Intervention for Developing Countries." *Sexually Transmitted Diseases* 40 (12): 909–14.

Hensen, B., R. Baggaley, V. J. Wong, K. L. Grabbe, N. Shaffer, and others. 2012. "Universal Voluntary HIV Testing in Antenatal Care Settings: A Review of the Contribution of Provider-Initiated Testing and Counselling." *Tropical Medicine and International Health* 17 (1): 59–70.

Hochberg, C. H., K. Berringer, and J. A. Schneider. 2015. "Next-Generation Methods for HIV Partner Services: A Systematic Review." *Sexually Transmitted Diseases* 42 (9): 533–39.

Hodgson, I., M. L. Plummer, S. N. Konopka, C. J. Colvin, E. Jonas, and others. 2014. "A Systematic Review of Individual and Contextual Factors Affecting ART Initiation, Adherence, and Retention for HIV-Infected Pregnant and Postpartum Women." *PLoS One* 9 (11): e111421.

Horvath, T., H. Azman, G. E. Kennedy, and G. W. Rutherford. 2012. "Mobile Phone Text Messaging for Promoting Adherence to Antiretroviral Therapy in Patients with HIV Infection." *Cochrane Database of Systematic Reviews* 3: CD009756.

Hudelson, C., and L. Cluver. 2015. "Factors Associated with Adherence to Antiretroviral Therapy among Adolescents Living with HIV/AIDS in Low- and Middle-Income Countries: A Systematic Review." *AIDS Care* 27 (7): 805–16.

Huet, C., A. Ouedraogo, I. Konate, I. Traore, F. Rouet, and others. 2011. "Long-Term Virological, Immunological, and Mortality Outcomes in a Cohort of HIV-Infected Female Sex Workers Treated with Highly Active Antiretroviral Therapy in Africa." *BMC Public Health* 11 (December): 700.

ICAP (International Center for AIDS Care and Treatment Programs). 2016. "The PHIA [Population HIV Impact Assessment] Project." ICAP, Mailman School of Public Health, Columbia University, New York. http://phia.icap.columbia.edu/.

Ivers, L. C., Y. Chang, J. Gregory Jerome, and K. A. Freedberg. 2010. "Food Assistance Is Associated with Improved Body Mass Index, Food Security, and Attendance at Clinic in an HIV Program in Central Haiti: A Prospective Observational Cohort Study." *AIDS Research and Therapy* 7 (August): 33.

Iwu, E. N., and W. L. Holzemer. 2014. "Task Shifting of HIV Management from Doctors to Nurses in Africa: Clinical Outcomes and Evidence on Nurse Self-Efficacy and Job Satisfaction." *AIDS Care* 26 (1): 42–52.

Kabore, L., P. Muntner, E. Chamot, A. Zinski, G. Burkholder, and others. 2015. "Self-Report Measures in the Assessment of Antiretroviral Medication Adherence: Comparison with Medication Possession Ratio and HIV Viral Load." *Journal of the International Association of Providers of AIDS Care* 14 (2): 156–62.

Kagee, A., R. H. Remien, A. Berkman, S. Hoffman, L. Campos, and others. 2011. "Structural Barriers to ART Adherence in Southern Africa: Challenges and Potential Ways Forward." *Global Public Health* 6 (1): 83–97.

Kankasa, C., R. J. Carter, N. Briggs, M. Bulterys, E. Chama, and others. 2009. "Routine Offering of HIV Testing to Hospitalized Pediatric Patients at University Teaching Hospital, Lusaka, Zambia: Acceptability and Feasibility." *Journal of Acquired Immune Deficiency Syndromes* 51 (2): 202–8.

Kennedy, C. E., V. A. Fonner, M. D. Sweat, F. Amolo Okero, R. Baggaley, and others. 2013. "Provider-Initiated HIV

Testing and Counseling in Low- and Middle-Income Countries: A Systematic Review." *AIDS and Behavior* 17 (5): 1571–90.

Kim, M. H., S. Ahmed, W. C. Buck, G. A. Preidis, M. C. Hosseinipour, and others. 2012. "The Tingathe Programme: A Pilot Intervention Using Community Health Workers to Create a Continuum of Care in the Prevention of Mother to Child Transmission of HIV (PMTCT) Cascade of Services in Malawi." *Journal of the International AIDS Society* 15 (Suppl 2): 17389.

Kim, S. H., S. M. Gerver, S. Fidler, and H. Ward. 2014. "Adherence to Antiretroviral Therapy in Adolescents Living with HIV: Systematic Review and Meta-Analysis." *AIDS* 28 (13): 1945–56.

Kohler, P. K., M. H. Chung, C. J. McGrath, S. F. Benki-Nugent, J. W. Thiga, and others. 2011. "Implementation of Free Cotrimoxazole Prophylaxis Improves Clinic Retention among Antiretroviral Therapy–Ineligible Clients in Kenya." *AIDS* 25 (13): 1657–61.

Konate, I., L. Traore, A. Ouedraogo, A. Sanon, R. Diallo, and others. 2011. "Linking HIV Prevention and Care for Community Interventions among High-Risk Women in Burkina Faso: The ARNS 1222 'Yerelon' Cohort." *Journal of Acquired Immune Deficiency Syndromes* 57 (Suppl 1): S50–54.

Kundu, C. K., M. Samanta, M. Sarkar, S. Bhattacharyya, and S. Chatterjee. 2012. "Food Supplementation as an Incentive to Improve Pre-Antiretroviral Therapy Clinic Adherence in HIV-Positive Children: Experience from Eastern India." *Journal of Tropical Pediatrics* 58 (1): 31–37.

Lahuerta, M., F. Ue, S. Hoffman, B. Elul, S. G. Kulkarni, and others. 2013. "The Problem of Late ART Initiation in Sub-Saharan Africa: A Transient Aspect of Scale-Up or a Long-Term Phenomenon?" *Journal of Health Care for the Poor and Underserved* 24 (1): 359–83.

Lall, P., S. H. Lim, N. Khairuddin, and A. Kamarulzaman. 2015. "Review: An Urgent Need for Research on Factors Impacting Adherence to and Retention in Care among HIV-Positive Youth and Adolescents from Key Populations." *Journal of the International AIDS Society* 18 (2, Suppl 1): 19393.

Lamb, M. R., R. Fayorsey, H. Nuwagaba-Biribonwoha, V. Viola, V. Mutabazi, and others. 2014. "High Attrition before and after ART Initiation among Youth (15–24 Years of Age) Enrolled in HIV Care." *AIDS* 28 (4): 559–68.

Larson, B. A., K. Schnippel, A. Brennan, L. Long, T. Xulu, and others. 2013. "Same-Day CD4 Testing to Improve Uptake of HIV Care and Treatment in South Africa: Point-of-Care Is Not Enough." *AIDS Research and Treatment* 2013: 941493.

Larson, B. A., K. Schnippel, B. Ndibongo, T. Xulu, A. Brennan, and others. 2012. "Rapid Point-of-Care CD4 Testing at Mobile HIV Testing Sites to Increase Linkage to Care: An Evaluation of a Pilot Program in South Africa." *Journal of Acquired Immune Deficiency Syndromes* 61 (2): e13–17.

Larsson, E. C., A. Thorson, G. Pariyo, P. Conrad, M. Arinaitwe, and others. 2011. "Opt-Out HIV Testing during Antenatal

Care: Experiences of Pregnant Women in Rural Uganda." *Health Policy and Planning* 27 (1): 69–75.

Lawn, S. D., A. D. Harries, X. Anglaret, L. Myer, and R. Wood. 2008. "Early Mortality among Adults Accessing Antiretroviral Treatment Programmes in Sub-Saharan Africa." *AIDS* 22 (15): 1897–908.

Lecher, S, D. Ellenberger, A. A. Kim, P. N. Fonjungo, S. Agolory, M. Y. Borget, and others. 2015. "Scale-up of HIV Viral Load Monitoring—Seven Sub-Saharan African Countries." *Morbidity and Mortality Weekly Report* 64 (46): 1287–90.

Lester, R. T., P. Ritvo, E. J. Mills, A. Kariri, S. Karanja, and others. 2010. "Effects of a Mobile Phone Short Message Service on Antiretroviral Treatment Adherence in Kenya (WelTel Kenya1): A Randomised Trial." *The Lancet* 376 (9755): 1838–45.

Liu, X., Q. Ma, and F. Zhang. 2010. "Therapeutic Drug Monitoring in Highly Active Antiretroviral Therapy." *Expert Opinion on Drug Safety* 9 (5): 743–58.

Losina, E., H. Toure, L. M. Uhler, X. Anglaret, A. D. Paltiel, and others. 2009. "Cost-Effectiveness of Preventing Loss to Follow-Up in HIV Treatment Programs: A Côte d'Ivoire Appraisal." *PLoS Medicine* 6 (10): e1000173.

Lugada, E., J. Levin, B. Abang, J. Mermin, E. Mugalanzi, and others. 2010. "Comparison of Home- and Clinic-Based HIV Testing among Household Members of Persons Taking Antiretroviral Therapy in Uganda: Results from a Randomized Trial." *Journal of Acquired Immune Deficiency Syndromes* 55 (2): 245–52.

Luque-Fernandez, M. A., G. Van Cutsem, E. Goemaere, K. Hilderbrand, M. Schomaker, and others. 2013. "Effectiveness of Patient Adherence Groups as a Model of Care for Stable Patients on Antiretroviral Therapy in Khayelitsha, Cape Town, South Africa." *PLoS One* 8 (2): e56088.

MacPherson, P., D. G. Lalloo, A. T. Choko, G. H. Mann, S. B. Squire, and others. 2012. "Suboptimal Patterns of Provider-Initiated HIV Testing and Counselling, Antiretroviral Therapy Eligibility Assessment and Referral in Primary Health Clinic Attendees in Blantyre, Malawi." *Tropical Medicine and International Health* 17 (4): 507–17.

MacPherson, P., D. G. Lalloo, E. L. Webb, H. Maheswaran, A. T. Choko, and others. 2014. "Effect of Optional Home Initiation of HIV Care Following HIV Self-Testing on Antiretroviral Therapy Initiation among Adults in Malawi: A Randomized Clinical Trial." *Journal of the American Medical Association* 312 (4): 372–79.

Malta, M., S. A. Strathdee, M. M. Magnanini, and F. I. Bastos. 2008. "Adherence to Antiretroviral Therapy for Human Immunodeficiency Virus/Acquired Immune Deficiency Syndrome among Drug Users: A Systematic Review." *Addiction* 103 (8): 1242–57.

Marseille, E. A. 2011. "Case Management to Improve Adherence for HIV-Infected Patients Receiving Antiretroviral Therapy in Ethiopia: A Micro-Costing Study." *Cost Effectiveness and Resource Allocation* 20 (9): 18.

Maskew, M., P. MacPhail, C. Menezes, and D. Rubel. 2007. "Lost to Follow-Up: Contributing Factors and Challenges in South African Patients on Antiretroviral Therapy." *South African Medical Journal* 97 (9): 853–57.

Matovu, J. K., and F. E. Makumbi. 2007. "Expanding Access to Voluntary HIV Counselling and Testing in Sub-Saharan Africa: Alternative Approaches for Improving Uptake, 2001–2007." *Tropical Medicine and International Health* 12 (11): 1315–22.

Mbuagbaw, L., M. L. van der Kop, R. T. Lester, H. Thirumurthy, C. Pop-Eleches, and others. 2013. "Mobile Phone Text Messages for Improving Adherence to Antiretroviral Therapy (ART): An Individual Patient Data Meta-Analysis of Randomised Trials." *BMJ Open* 3 (12): e003950.

McCollum, E. D., G. A. Preidis, M. M. Kabue, E. B. Singogo, C. Mwansambo, and others. 2010. "Task Shifting Routine Inpatient Pediatric HIV Testing Improves Program Outcomes in Urban Malawi: A Retrospective Observational Study." *PLoS One* 5 (3): e9626.

McMahon, J. H., J. H. Elliott, S. Y. Hong, S. Bertagnolio, and M. R. Jordan. 2013. "Effects of Physical Tracing on Estimates of Loss to Follow-Up, Mortality, and Retention in Low- and Middle-Income Country Antiretroviral Therapy Programs: A Systematic Review." *PLoS One* 8 (2): e56047.

McNairy, M. L., and W. M. El-Sadr. 2012. "The HIV Care Continuum: No Partial Credit Given." *AIDS* 26 (14): 1735–38.

McNairy, M. L., M. R. Lamb, R. J. Carter, R. Fayorsey, G. Tene, and others. 2013. "Retention of HIV-Infected Children on Antiretroviral Treatment in HIV Care and Treatment Programs in Kenya, Mozambique, Rwanda, and Tanzania." *Journal of Acquired Immune Deficiency Syndromes* 62 (3): e70–81.

Medley, A., M. Ackers, M. Amolloh, P. Owuor, H. Muttai, and others. 2013. "Early Uptake of HIV Clinical Care after Testing HIV-Positive during Home-Based Testing and Counseling in Western Kenya." *AIDS and Behavior* 17 (1): 224–34.

Menzies, N., B. Abang, R. Wanyenze, F. Nuwaha, B. Mugisha, and others. 2009. "The Costs and Effectiveness of Four HIV Counseling and Testing Strategies in Uganda." *AIDS* 23 (3): 395–401.

Milloy, M. J., J. Montaner, and E. Wood. 2012. "Barriers to HIV Treatment among People Who Use Injection Drugs: Implications for 'Treatment as Prevention.'" *Current Opinion in HIV/AIDS* 7 (4): 332–38.

Mills, E. J., J. B. Nachega, D. R. Bangsberg, S. Singh, B. Rachlis, and others. 2006. "Adherence to HAART: A Systematic Review of Developed and Developing Nation Patient-Reported Barriers and Facilitators." *PLoS Medicine* 3 (11): e438.

Mills, E. J., J. B. Nachega, I. Buchan, J. Orbinski, A. Attaran, and others. 2006. "Adherence to Antiretroviral Therapy in Sub-Saharan Africa and North America: A Meta-Analysis." *Journal of the American Medical Association* 296 (6): 679–90.

Mountain, E., S. Mishra, P. Vickerman, M. Pickles, C. Gilks, and others. 2014. "Antiretroviral Therapy Uptake, Attrition, Adherence, and Outcomes among HIV-Infected Female Sex Workers: A Systematic Review and Meta-Analysis." *PLoS One* 9 (9): e105645.

Mtetwa, S., J. Busza, S. Chidiya, S. Mungofa, and F. Cowan. 2013. "'You Are Wasting Our Drugs': Health Service Barriers to HIV Treatment for Sex Workers in Zimbabwe." *BMC Public Health* 13 (July): 698.

Mugglin, C., J. Estill, G. Wandeler, N. Bender, M. Egger, and others. 2012. "Loss to Programme between HIV Diagnosis and Initiation of Antiretroviral Therapy in Sub-Saharan Africa: Systematic Review and Meta-Analysis." *Tropical Medicine and International Health* 17 (12): 1509–20.

Mugglin, C., G. Wandeler, J. Estill, M. Egger, N. Bender, and others. 2013. "Retention in Care of HIV-Infected Children from HIV Test to Start of Antiretroviral Therapy: Systematic Review." *PLoS One* 8 (2): e56446.

Muhamadi, L., N. M. Tumwesigye, D. Kadobera, G. Marrone, F. Wabwire-Mangen, and others. 2011. "A Single-Blind Randomized Controlled Trial to Evaluate the Effect of Extended Counseling on Uptake of Pre-Antiretroviral Care in Eastern Uganda." *Trials* 12 (July): 184.

Mupambireyi, Z., S. Bernays, M. Bwakura-Dangarembizi, and F. M. Cowan. 2014. "'I Don't Feel Shy Because I Will Be among Others Who Are Just Like Me…': The Role of Support Groups for Children Perinatally Infected with HIV in Zimbabwe." *Children and Youth Services Review* 45 (October): 106–13.

Musheke, M., H. Ntalasha, S. Gari, O. McKenzie, V. Bond, and others. 2013. "A Systematic Review of Qualitative Findings on Factors Enabling and Deterring Uptake of HIV Testing in Sub-Saharan Africa." *BMC Public Health* 13 (March): 220.

Myer, L., K. Daskilewicz, J. McIntyre, and L. G. Bekker. 2013. "Comparison of Point-of-Care versus Laboratory-Based CD4 Cell Enumeration in HIV-Positive Pregnant Women." *Journal of the International AIDS Society* 16 (1): 18649.

Nachega, J. B., R. Leisegang, D. Bishai, H. Nguyen, M. Hislop, and others. 2010. "Association of Antiretroviral Therapy Adherence and Health Care Costs." *Annals of Internal Medicine* 152 (1): 18–25.

Nachega, J. B., J. J. Parienti, O. A. Uthman, R. Gross, D. W. Dowdy, and others. 2014. "Lower Pill Burden and Once-Daily Antiretroviral Treatment Regimens for HIV Infection: A Meta-Analysis of Randomized Controlled Trials." *Clinical Infectious Diseases* 58 (9): 1297–307.

Nachega, J. B., O. A. Uthman, J. Anderson, K. Peltzer, S. Wampold, and others. 2012. "Adherence to Antiretroviral Therapy during and after Pregnancy in Low-Income, Middle-Income, and High-Income Countries: A Systematic Review and Meta-Analysis." *AIDS* 26 (16): 2039–52.

Nuti, K. A., J. S. Kabengula, and S. E. Msuya. 2011. "Perceived Barriers and Attitudes of Health Care Providers towards Provider-Initiated HIV Testing and Counseling in Mbeya Region, Southern Highland Zone of Tanzania." *Pan African Medical Journal* 8 (March): 17.

Ostermann, J., E. A. Reddy, M. M. Shorter, C. Muiruri, A. Mtalo, and others. 2011. "Who Tests, Who Doesn't, and Why? Uptake of Mobile HIV Counseling and Testing in the Kilimanjaro Region of Tanzania." *PLoS One* 6 (1): e16488.

Pant Pai, N., J. Sharma, S. Shivkumar, S. Pillay, C. Vadnais, and others. 2013. "Supervised and Unsupervised Self-Testing for HIV in High- and Low-Risk Populations: A Systematic Review." *PLoS Medicine* 10 (4): e1001414.

Patten, G. E., L. Wilkinson, K. Conradie, P. Isaakidis, A. D. Harries, and others. 2013. "Impact on ART Initiation of Point-of-Care CD4 Testing at HIV Diagnosis among HIV-Positive Youth in Khayelitsha, South Africa." *Journal of the International AIDS Society* 16 (July): 18518.

Pearson, C. R., M. A. Micek, J. M. Simoni, P. D. Hoff, E. Matediana, and others. 2007. "Randomized Control Trial of Peer-Delivered, Modified Directly Observed Therapy for HAART in Mozambique." *Journal of Acquired Immune Deficiency Syndromes* 46 (2): 238–44.

PEPFAR (President's Emergency Plan for AIDS Relief). 2013. *PEPFAR Next Generation Indicators Reference Guide.* Washington, DC: PEPFAR.

Phelps, B. R., S. Ahmed, A. Amzel, M. O. Diallo, T. Jacobs, and others. 2013. "Linkage, Initiation and Retention of Children in the Antiretroviral Therapy Cascade: An Overview." *AIDS* 27 (Suppl 2): S207–13.

Phillips, T., M. L. McNairy, A. Zerbe, L. Myer, and E. J. Abrams. 2015. "Implementation and Operational Research: Postpartum Transfer of Care among HIV-Infected Women Initiating Antiretroviral Therapy during Pregnancy." *Journal of Acquired Immune Deficiency Syndromes* 70 (3): e102–9.

Phillips, T., E. Thebus, L.-G. Bekker, J. Mcintyre, E. J. Abrams, and others. 2014. "Disengagement of HIV-Positive Pregnant and Postpartum Women from Antiretroviral Therapy Services: A Cohort Study." *Journal of the International AIDS Society* 17 (1): 19242.

Piot, P., S. S. Abdool Karim, R. Hecht, H. Legido-Quigley, K. Buse, and others. 2015. "Defeating AIDS: Advancing Global Health." *The Lancet* 386 (9989): 171–218.

Porth, T., C. Suzuki, A. Gillespie, S. Kasedde, and I. Idele. 2014. "Disparities and Trends in AIDS Mortality among Adolescents Living with HIV in Low- and Middle-Income Countries." Paper prepared for the Twentieth International AIDS Conference, Melbourne, Australia, July 20–25.

Posse, M., and R. Baltussen. 2009. "Barriers to Access to Antiretroviral Treatment in Mozambique, as Perceived by Patients and Health Workers in Urban and Rural Settings." *AIDS Patient Care and STDs* 23 (10): 867–75.

Psaros, C., J. E. Remmert, D. R. Bangsberg, S. A. Safren, and J. A. Smit. 2015. "Adherence to HIV Care after Pregnancy among Women in Sub-Saharan Africa: Falling off the Cliff of the Treatment Cascade." *Current HIV/AIDS Reports* 12 (1): 1–5.

Rasschaert, F., T. Decroo, D. Remartinez, B. Telfer, F. Lessitala, and others. 2014. "Sustainability of a Community-Based Anti-Retroviral Care Delivery Model: A Qualitative Research Study in Tete, Mozambique." *Journal of the International AIDS Society* 17 (October): 18910.

Reidy, W. J., M. Sheriff, C. Wang, M. Hawken, E. Koech, and others. 2014. "Decentralization of HIV Care and Treatment

Services in Central Province, Kenya." *Journal of Acquired Immune Deficiency Syndromes* 67 (1): e34–40.

Root, R., and A. Whiteside. 2013. "A Qualitative Study of Community Home-Based Care and Antiretroviral Adherence in Swaziland." *Journal of the International AIDS Society* 16 (October): 17978.

Rosen, S., and M. P. Fox. 2011. "Retention in HIV Care between Testing and Treatment in Sub-Saharan Africa: A Systematic Review." *PLoS Medicine* 8 (7): e1001056.

Rosen, S., and M. Ketlhapile. 2010. "Cost of Using a Patient Tracer to Reduce Loss to Follow-Up and Ascertain Patient Status in a Large Antiretroviral Therapy Program in Johannesburg, South Africa." *Tropical Medicine and International Health* 15 (Suppl 1): 98–104.

Roura, M., D. Watson-Jones, T. M. Kahawita, L. Ferguson, and D. A. Ross. 2013. "Provider-Initiated Testing and Counselling Programmes in Sub-Saharan Africa: A Systematic Review of Their Operational Implementation." *AIDS* 27 (4): 617–26.

Sabapathy, K., R. Van den Bergh, S. Fidler, R. Hayes, and N. Ford. 2012. "Uptake of Home-Based Voluntary HIV Testing in Sub-Saharan Africa: A Systematic Review and Meta-Analysis." *PLoS Medicine* 9 (12): e1001351.

Schnippel, K., C. Mongwenyana, L. C. Long, and B. A. Larson. 2015. "Delays, Interruptions, and Losses from Prevention of Mother-to-Child Transmission of HIV Services during Antenatal Care in Johannesburg, South Africa: A Cohort Analysis." *BMC Infectious Diseases* 15 (1): 46.

Shea, S. R. M., S. Makungu, I. Sultan, M. Minde, B. Anosike, and others. 2013. "Know Your Child's Status Testing Events: A Targeted Strategy for Paediatric HIV Case Identification in the Lake Zone of Tanzania." Prepared for the Seventh International AIDS Conference, Kuala Lumpur, June 30–July 3.

Sherr, K. H., M. A. Micek, S. O. Gimbel, S. S. Gloyd, J. P. Hughes, and others. 2010. "Quality of HIV Care Provided by Non-Physician Clinicians and Physicians in Mozambique: A Retrospective Cohort Study." *AIDS* 24 (Suppl 1): S59–66.

Shumbusho, F., J. van Griensven, D. Lowrance, I. Turate, M. A. Weaver, and others. 2009. "Task Shifting for Scale-Up of HIV Care: Evaluation of Nurse-Centered Antiretroviral Treatment at Rural Health Centers in Rwanda." *PLoS Medicine* 6 (10): e1000163.

Simoni, J. M., C. R. Pearson, D. W. Pantalone, G. Marks, and N. Crepaz. 2006. "Efficacy of Interventions in Improving Highly Active Antiretroviral Therapy Adherence and HIV-1 RNA Viral Load: A Meta-Analytic Review of Randomized Controlled Trials." *Journal of Acquired Immune Deficiency Syndromes* 43 (Suppl 1): S23–35.

Siregar, A. Y., D. Komarudin, R. Wisaksana, R. van Crevel, and R. Baltussen. 2011. "Costs and Outcomes of VCT Delivery Models in the Context of Scaling up Services in Indonesia." *Tropical Medicine and International Health* 16 (2): 193–99.

Smith, J. A., M. Sharma, C. Levin, J. M. Baeten, H. van Rooyen, and others. 2015. "Cost-Effectiveness of Community-Based Strategies to Strengthen the Continuum of HIV Care in Rural South Africa: A Health Economic Modelling Analysis." *The Lancet HIV* 2 (4): e159–68.

Solomon, S. S., A. K. Srikrishnan, C. K. Vasudevan, S. Anand, M. S. Kumar, and others. 2014. "Voucher Incentives Improve Linkage to and Retention in Care among HIV-Infected Drug Users in Chennai, India." *Clinical Infectious Diseases* 59 (4): 589–95.

START Study Group. 2015. "Initiation of Antiretroviral Therapy in Early Asymptomatic HIV Infection." *New England Journal of Medicine* 373 (August): 795–807.

Stephenson, R., C. Rentsch, P. Sullivan, A. McAdams-Mahmoud, G. Jobson, and others. 2013. "Attitudes toward Couples-Based HIV Counseling and Testing among MSM in Cape Town, South Africa." *AIDS and Behavior* 17 (Suppl 1): S43–50.

Sturke, R., C. Harmston, R. J. Simonds, L. M. Mofenson, G. K. Siberry, and others. 2014. "A Multi-Disciplinary Approach to Implementation Science: The NIH-PEPFAR PMTCT Implementation Science Alliance." *Journal of Acquired Immune Deficiency Syndromes* 67 (Suppl 2): S163–67.

Suthar, A. B., N. Ford, P. J. Bachanas, V. J. Wong, J. S. Rajan, and others. 2013. "Towards Universal Voluntary HIV Testing and Counselling: A Systematic Review and Meta-Analysis of Community-Based Approaches." *PLoS Medicine* 10 (8): e1001496.

Suthar, A. B., D. Hoos, A. Beqiri, K. Lorenz-Dehne, C. McClure, and others. 2013. "Integrating Antiretroviral Therapy into Antenatal Care and Maternal and Child Health Settings: A Systematic Review and Meta-Analysis." *Bulletin of the World Health Organization* 91 (1): 46–56.

Sweat, M., S. Gregorich, G. Sangiwa, C. Furlonge, D. Balmer, and others. 2000. "Cost-Effectiveness of Voluntary HIV-1 Counselling and Testing in Reducing Sexual Transmission of HIV-1 in Kenya and Tanzania." *The Lancet* 356 (9224): 113–21.

Sweat, M., S. Morin, D. Celentano, M. Mulawa, B. Singh, and others. 2011. "Community-Based Intervention to Increase HIV Testing and Case Detection in People Aged 16–32 Years in Tanzania, Zimbabwe, and Thailand (NIMH Project Accept, HPTN 043): A Randomised Study." *The Lancet Infectious Diseases* 11 (7): 525–32.

Taiwo, B. O., J. A. Idoko, L. J. Welty, I. Otoh, G. Job, and others. 2010. "Assessing the Viorologic and Adherence Benefits of Patient-Selected HIV Treatment Partners in a Resource-Limited Setting." *Journal of Acquired Immune Deficiency Syndromes* 54 (1): 85–92.

Tenthani, L., A. D. Haas, H. Tweya, A. Jahn, J. J. van Oosterhout, and others. 2014. "Retention in Care under Universal Antiretroviral Therapy for HIV-Infected Pregnant and Breastfeeding Women ('Option B+') in Malawi." *AIDS* 28 (4): 589–98.

Thielman, N. M., H. Y. Chu, J. Ostermann, D. K. Itemba, A. Mgonja, and others. 2006. "Cost-Effectiveness of Free HIV Voluntary Counseling and Testing through a Community-Based AIDS Service Organization in Northern Tanzania." *American Journal of Public Health* 96 (1): 114–19.

Thirumurthy, H., S. H. Masters, S. N. Mavedzenge, S. Maman, E. Omanga, and others. 2016. "Promoting Male Partner HIV Testing and Safer Sexual Decision Making through Secondary Distribution of Self-Tests by HIV-Negative Female Sex Workers and Women Receiving Antenatal and Post-Partum Care in Kenya: A Cohort Study." *The Lancet HIV* 3 (6): e266–74.

Thompson, M. A., M. J. Mugavero, K. R. Amico, V. A. Cargill, L. W. Chang, and others. 2012. "Guidelines for Improving Entry into and Retention in Care and Antiretroviral Adherence for Persons with HIV: Evidence-Based Recommendations from an International Association of Physicians in AIDS Care Panel." *Annals of Internal Medicine* 156 (11): 817–33, w-284–94.

Thurman, T. R., L. J. Haas, A. Dushimimana, B. Lavin, and N. Mock. 2010. "Evaluation of a Case Management Program for HIV Clients in Rwanda." *AIDS Care* 22 (6): 759–65.

Torian, L. V., E. W. Wiewel, K. L. Liu, J. E. Sackoff, and T. R. Frieden. 2008. "Risk Factors for Delayed Initiation of Medical Care after Diagnosis of Human Immunodeficiency Virus." *Archives of Internal Medicine* 168 (11): 1181–87.

Tran, D. A., A. Shakeshaft, A. D. Ngo, J. Rule, D. P. Wilson, and others. 2012. "Structural Barriers to Timely Initiation of Antiretroviral Treatment in Vietnam: Findings from Six Outpatient Clinics." *PLoS One* 7 (12): e51289.

Tromp, N., A. Siregar, B. Leuwol, D. Komarudin, A. van der Ven, and others. 2013. "Cost-Effectiveness of Scaling up Voluntary Counselling and Testing in West-Java, Indonesia." *Acta Medica Indonesiana* 45 (1): 17–25. .

Tumwesigye, E., G. Wana, S. Kasasa, E. Muganzi, and F. Nuwaha. 2010. "High Uptake of Home-Based, District-Wide, HIV Counseling and Testing in Uganda." *AIDS Patient Care and STDs* 24 (11): 735–41.

UNAIDS (Joint United Nations Programme on HIV/AIDS). 2014. *UNAIDS: The Gap Report.* Geneva: UNAIDS.

———. 2015a. *How AIDS Changed Everything—MDG6: 15 Years, 15 Lessons of Hope from the AIDS Response.* Geneva: UNAIDS.

———.2015b. "AIDSinfo." Geneva: UNAIDS. http://aidsinfo.unaids.org/.

UNICEF (United Nations Children's Fund). 2015. "Situation—Global Statistics Tables: Children and AIDS 2015 Statistical Update." UNICEF. http://www.childrenandaids.org/situation.

van der Kop, M. L., D. I. Ojakaa, A. Patel, L. Thabane, K. Kinagwi, and others. 2013. "The Effect of Weekly Short Message Service Communication on Patient Retention in Care in the First Year after HIV Diagnosis: Study Protocol for a Randomised Controlled Trial (WelTel Retain)." *BMJ Open* 3 (6): e003155.

van Rooyen, H., R. V. Barnabas, J. M. Baeten, Z. Phakathi, P. Joseph, and others. 2013. "High HIV Testing Uptake and Linkage to Care in a Novel Program of Home-Based HIV Counseling and Testing with Facilitated Referral in KwaZulu-Natal, South Africa." *Journal of Acquired Immune Deficiency Syndromes* 64 (1): e1–8.

van Rooyen, H., N. McGrath, A. Chirowodza, P. Joseph, A. Fiamma, and others. 2013. "Mobile VCT: Reaching Men and Young People in Urban and Rural South African Pilot Studies (NIMH Project Accept, HPTN 043)." *AIDS and Behavior* 17 (9): 2946–53.

van Velthoven, M. H., S. Brusamento, A. Majeed, and J. Car. 2013. "Scope and Effectiveness of Mobile Phone Messaging for HIV/AIDS Care: A Systematic Review." *Psychology, Health, and Medicine* 18 (2): 182–202.

Venkatesh, K. K., J. E. Becker, N. Kumarasamy, Y. M. Nakamura, K. H. Mayer, and others. 2013. "Clinical Impact and Cost-Effectiveness of Expanded Voluntary HIV Testing in India." *PLoS One* 8 (5): e64604.

Violari, A., M. F. Cotton, D. M. Gibb, A. G. Babiker, J. Steyn, and others. 2008. "Early Antiretroviral Therapy and Mortality among HIV-Infected Infants." *New England Journal of Medicine* 359 (21): 2233–44.

Vitalis, D. 2013. "Factors Affecting Antiretroviral Therapy Adherence among HIV-Positive Pregnant and Postpartum Women: An Adapted Systematic Review." *International Journal of STD and AIDS* 24 (6): 427–32.

Vreeman, R. C., S. E. Wiehe, E. C. Pearce, and W. M. Nyandiko. 2008. "A Systematic Review of Pediatric Adherence to Antiretroviral Therapy in Low- and Middle-Income Countries." *Pediatric Infectious Disease Journal* 27 (8): 686–91.

Wachira, J., S. Kimaiyo, S. Ndege, J. Mamlin, and P. Braitstein. 2012. "What Is the Impact of Home-Based HIV Counseling and Testing on the Clinical Status of Newly Enrolled Adults in a Large HIV Care Program in Western Kenya?" *Clinical Infectious Diseases* 54 (2): 275–81.

Wachira, J., S. E. Middlestadt, R. Vreeman, and P. Braitstein. 2012. "Factors Underlying Taking a Child to HIV Care: Implications for Reducing Loss to Follow-Up among HIV-Infected and -Exposed Children." *Sahara Journal* 9 (1): 20–29.

Wachira, J., S. Ndege, J. Koech, R. C. Vreeman, P. Ayuo, and others. 2014. "HIV Testing Uptake and Prevalence among Adolescents and Adults in a Large Home-Based HIV Testing Program in Western Kenya." *Journal of Acquired Immune Deficiency Syndromes* 65 (2): e58–66.

Wang, S., J. R. Moss, and J. E. Hiller. 2011. "The Cost-Effectiveness of HIV Voluntary Counseling and Testing in China." *Asia-Pacific Journal of Public Health* 23 (4): 620–33.

Ware, N. C., M. A. Wyatt, E. H. Geng, S. F. Kaaya, O. O. Agbaji, and others. 2013. "Toward an Understanding of Disengagement from HIV Treatment and Care in Sub-Saharan Africa: A Qualitative Study." *PLoS Medicine* 10 (1): e1001369.

WHO (World Health Organization). 2007. *Guidance on Provider-Initiated HIV Testing and Counselling in Health Facilities*. Geneva: WHO.

———. 2013a. *Consolidated Guidelines on the Use of Antiretroviral Drugs for Treating and Preventing HIV Infection: Recommendations for a Public Health Approach*. Geneva: WHO.

———. 2013b. "WHO Guidelines Approved by the Guidelines Review Committee." In *HIV and Adolescents: Guidance for HIV Testing and Counselling and Care for Adolescents Living with HIV; Recommendations for a Public Health Approach and Considerations for Policy-Makers and Managers*. Geneva: WHO.

———. 2014a. *Choosing Interventions that Are Cost-Effective (WHO-CHOICE)*. Geneva: WHO. http://www.who.int /choice/en/.

———. 2014b. *Consolidated Guidelines on HIV Prevention, Diagnosis, Treatment, and Care for Key Populations*. Geneva: WHO.

———. 2014c. *Global Update on the Health Sector Response to HIV, 2014*. Geneva: WHO.

———. 2015a. *Consolidated Guidelines on HIV Testing Services*. Geneva: WHO.

———. 2015b. *Guideline on When to Start Antiretroviral Therapy and on Pre-Exposure Prophylaxis for HIV*. Geneva: WHO.

———. 2016. *Consolidated Guidelines on the Use of Antiretroviral Drugs for Treating and Preventing HIV Infection: Recommendations for a Public Health Approach*. Geneva: WHO.

Wolfe, D., M. P. Carrieri, and D. Shepard. 2010. "Treatment and Care for Injecting Drug Users with HIV Infection: A Review of Barriers and Ways Forward." *The Lancet* 376 (9738): 355–66.

Wouters, E., W. Van Damme, D. van Rensburg, C. Masquillier, and H. Meulemans. 2012. "Impact of Community-Based Support Services on Antiretroviral Treatment Programme Delivery and Outcomes in Resource-Limited Countries: A Synthetic Review." *BMC Health Services Research* 12 (July): 194.

Wringe, A., M. Roura, M. Urassa, J. Busza, V. Athanas, and others. 2009. "Doubts, Denial, and Divine Intervention: Understanding Delayed Attendance and Poor Retention Rates at a HIV Treatment Programme in Rural Tanzania." *AIDS Care* 21 (5): 632–37.

Wynberg, E., G. Cooke, A. Shroufi, S. D. Reid, and N. Ford. 2014. "Impact of Point-of-Care CD4 Testing on Linkage to HIV Care: A Systematic Review." *Journal of the International AIDS Society* 17 (January): 18809.

Xia, Y. H., W. Chen, J. D. Tucker, C. Wang, and L. Ling. 2013. "HIV and Hepatitis C Virus Test Uptake at Methadone Clinics in Southern China: Opportunities for Expanding Detection of Bloodborne Infections." *BMC Public Health* 13 (September): 899.

Young, S., A. C. Wheeler, S. I. McCoy, and S. D. Weiser. 2014. "A Review of the Role of Food Insecurity in Adherence to Care and Treatment among Adult and Pediatric Populations Living with HIV and AIDS." *AIDS and Behavior* 18 (Suppl 5): S505–15.

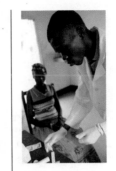

Chapter 5

Effectiveness and Cost-Effectiveness of Treatment as Prevention for HIV

Charles B. Holmes, Timothy B. Hallett, Rochelle P. Walensky,
Till Bärnighausen, Yogan Pillay, and Myron S. Cohen

INTRODUCTION

The beneficial effects of antiretroviral therapy (ART) on individual health are well established, and ART is widely used to reduce the morbidity and mortality due to the human immunodeficiency virus (HIV) (WHO 2016). Recent evidence has strengthened the case for initiating ART as early in the disease stage as possible (Danel and others 2015; INSIGHT START Study Group 2015). Similarly, using ART to prevent mother-to-child transmission of HIV is supported with conclusive evidence and has been adopted into clinical policies worldwide, as discussed in chapter 6 of this volume (John-Stewart and others 2017). Years of accumulating biological and observational evidence also suggest that ART may reduce sexual transmission of HIV, although the field lacked conclusive evidence until recently (Donnell and others 2010; Nachega and others 2013).

The evidence base and attention to "treatment as/for prevention" strengthened substantially in 2011 with the interim results from HIV Prevention Trials Network (HPTN) 052, a randomized controlled trial of early versus delayed use of ART among serodiscordant couples (Cohen and others 2011). The trial demonstrated a 96 percent reduction in new infections with earlier initiation of ART and provided strong evidence that ART reduces the sexual transmission of HIV. Final results of this trial with nearly 10,000 person-years of follow-up with similar conclusions were published in 2016 (Cohen and others 2016).

This emerging evidence stimulated a range of questions regarding the biological mechanisms of HIV treatment as prevention (TasP), variations in efficacy across subgroups, differences in at-risk populations, optimal implementation strategies, and potential implications for public health (Cohen, Holmes, and others 2012; Delva and others 2012). Recognition of the dual benefits of treatment has resulted in the reevaluation of the cost-effectiveness of ART, as well as of the paradigms of HIV prevention (Garnett and others 2017) and has led to policy discussions about how best to value the risks and benefits of treatment for personal and public health.

Even as substantial research and evaluation have improved the understanding of these trade-offs, clinical and public health policy and funding decisions are being made at the program, national, and global levels. This chapter examines the concept of HIV TasP, focusing on the underlying biological mechanisms, effectiveness, and cost-effectiveness of various strategies and settings and assessing how these factors may influence resource allocation, policy decisions, and research agendas at the national and global levels.

Corresponding author: Charles B. Holmes, Johns Hopkins University, Baltimore, Maryland, United States, and Centre for Infectious Disease Research in Zambia (CIDRZ); Charles.Holmes@cidrz.org.

THE BIOLOGY OF TRANSMISSION

HIV is transmitted in three ways: from parenteral exposure to contaminated blood and blood products; from exposure of many mucosal sites to infected genital secretions; and from mother to baby before, during, or after delivery (Royce and others 1997). These routes of transmission have been studied extensively and found to have different probabilities of transmission, given exposure. In each case, the biology of transmission is believed to be defined by the infectiousness of the host and the susceptibility of the person exposed (Cohen and others 2010; Cope and others 2014; Pilcher and others 2004).

HIV-infected fluids contain cells infected and not infected with HIV. The replication of HIV generates a very large number of viral variants—viruses that have different nucleic acid sequences—that constitute an infectious swarm. Within the swarm, some viruses are capable of producing infection; others are defective or less fit for transmission (Ho and others 2013). The likelihood that HIV will cause infection is governed by the number of viruses—the inoculum (Baeten and others 2011; Donnell and others 2010; Laeyendecker and others 2012; Quinn and others 2000)—and the genotypic and phenotypic characteristics of HIV in the swarm (Martin and others 2014). The probability of HIV transmission in heterosexual couples directly reflects the concentration of HIV in the fluid studied (Baeten and others 2011; Quinn and others 2000). In a landmark study of heterosexual transmission, Quinn and others (2000) observed no transmission when the blood plasma viral load was less than 1,500 copies per milliliter, and the most transmission when the viral load was more than 37,500 copies per milliliter. Unprotected anal intercourse appears to have high risk of transmission per contact (Baggaley, Dimitrov, and others 2013), explaining the high incidence of HIV in men who have sex with men (MSM), but the viral load required for transmission by this route has not been determined.

The phenotype of the founder viruses that initiate infection helps determine the probability of HIV transmission above and beyond the inoculum effects (Carlson and others 2014; Parrish and others 2013; Ping and others 2013). HIV variants that cause infection are dual tropic—that is, they use both CD4 and CCR5 receptors (Joseph and others 2014; Ping and others 2013; Shaw and Hunter 2012). Only one to three founder viruses are generally transmitted, and the number of variants may reflect the route of exposure (Keele and others 2008). Transmission from penile-vaginal exposure has the fewest variants, followed by anal exposure, followed by parenteral exposure (Li and others 2010).

Susceptibility to infection varies greatly. The only proven relative immunity to HIV results from deletion in the CCR5 receptor, which has been observed in about 1 of 100 Caucasians and less commonly in non-Caucasians (O'Brien and others 2000). Many studies have tried to define factors that allow some people to remain exposed and uninfected (McLaren and others 2013). By definition, all HIV-discordant couples include a partner who is exposed and uninfected (Muessig and Cohen 2014). Yet, many people in this group will become infected.

There is little evidence to suggest that innate immunity, antibodies, or T-cell responses provide durable or reliable resistance to HIV. More likely, "apparent resistance" reflects the absence of factors that amplify transmission (Pilcher and others 2007). Inflammation from any source will cause defects in the mucosa, evoke a large number of receptive cells, increase the number of receptors expressed, and activate cells that favor HIV replication. For example, bacterial vaginosis characterized by a change in vaginal flora and watery discharge is strongly associated with HIV acquisition in women (Taha and others 1998). Unique cytokine profiles may also favor these conditions (Olivier and others 2014).

TasP uses ART to reduce the replication of HIV in the blood and mucosal secretions profoundly, quickly, and reliably. The hypothesis that treatment could serve as prevention began as soon as the first ART was developed (Henry 1988). Numerous groups have since demonstrated the ability of ART to penetrate and suppress viral replication in the male and female genital tract (Thompson, Cohen, and Kashuba 2013). Many antiretroviral agents achieve similar or higher concentrations in the genital tract as in blood (Kwara and others 2008). However, the body's ability to metabolize and eliminate the medications may compromise the prevention benefits of treatment, and viruses isolated from areas of low or variable drug levels have demonstrated site-specific resistance.

To date, few cases of HIV transmission have been documented when a person with HIV has been treated sufficiently to prevent viral replication (Cohen and others 2016; Rodger and others 2016). However, HIV can be found in the male and female genital tract secretions even when HIV is suppressed in the blood (Anderson and Cu-Uvin 2011; Reichelderfer and others 2000). The implication is that the HIV detected in the genital tract under these conditions may be defective and incapable of causing infection (Zhang and others 1998).

An additional concern is the pharmacology of ART in the genital tract, which is considered a special compartment. Studies of the female genital tract and colorectum have noted that the concentrations of tenofovir and emtricitabine and their active metabolites vary according to the type of mucosal tissue (Patterson and others 2011). Differential penetration or metabolism of ART offers further insight into the highly variable level of protection conferred by these agents (Hendrix and others 2008). The results from preexposure prophylaxis (PrEP) clinical trials suggest that the use of ART for prevention can be optimized by choosing agents that (1) preferentially penetrate sites of HIV acquisition or transmission or (2) have a long tissue half-life that might provide a pharmacologic buffer for imperfect drug adherence. In summary, extensive studies of HIV transmission have been completed, and the results help illuminate the understanding of the ways to use ART to maximize the prevention of transmission.

EVIDENCE OF THE EFFECTIVENESS OF TREATMENT AS PREVENTION

Four lines of complementary evidence support the idea that treatment in HIV-infected individuals reduces their transmission of HIV to others:

- Observational studies of serodiscordant couples
- A randomized controlled trial
- Ecologic studies
- Population-based studies.

Observational Studies of Serodiscordant Couples

As shown in annex 5A, 14 observational studies of serodiscordant couples have been reported (Muessig and Cohen 2014). In 11 of these, ART was associated with the prevention of HIV transmission. The two studies from China failed to note a prevention benefit from ART (Lu and others 2010; Wang and others 2010). A larger retrospective analysis of 38,862 serodiscordant heterosexual couples across China noted a 26 percent relative reduction in transmission when the index case received ART (Jia and others 2012). In most of these studies (including studies in China), it is not known either whether the HIV-infected person receiving ART was actually using the agents prescribed or what degree of viral suppression was achieved.

Several systematic reviews of TasP studies have been conducted. Attia and others (2009) reviewed 11 cohorts reporting on 5,021 heterosexual couples and 461 transmission events. The transmission rate overall from patients on ART was 0.46 per 100 person-years, based on five events. The transmission rate from a seropositive partner with a viral load less than 400 copies per milliliter was zero for persons on ART and 0.16 per 100 person-years for persons not on ART, based on five studies and one event. A meta-analysis of studies of serodiscordant heterosexual couples where the HIV-positive partner was on ART and virally suppressed found zero transmissions per 100 person-years (Loutfy and others 2013); a similar review of partners on combination ART for at least six months found a transmission risk of between 1 and 13 per 100,000 sex acts. Another meta-analysis of 50 publications found a 91 percent (79 percent to 96 percent) reduction in incidence of HIV-1 per partner among couples when the index case used ART (Baggaley, White, and others 2013). Supervie and others (2014) reported at most one HIV transmission over an estimated 113,480 sex acts—of which 17 percent were not condom protected—among 1,672 serodiscordant couples where the index partner had been treated for more than six months.

The PARTNER Study is assessing the occurrence of linked transmission among serodiscordant heterosexual and MSM couples who have condomless sex, are not taking PrEP, and have a recent viral load of less than 200 cells per cubic millimeter (cells/mm^3). No linked transmissions among MSM couples were observed among 1,238 couple-years of follow-up (Rodger and others 2016), implying that ART treatment prevented transmission of HIV during unprotected anal intercourse.

The HPTN 052 Randomized Controlled Trial

HPTN 052 was a randomized controlled trial designed to provide an understanding of the magnitude and durability of ART for prevention. The study enrolled 1,562 serodiscordant couples at 13 sites in nine countries in Africa, Asia, and the Americas; it randomized infected men and women to start ART at CD4 T-cell counts of 200–250 cells/mm^3, compared with subjects who started ART at CD4 T-cell counts of 350–550 cells/mm^3 (median cell count of 446 cells/mm^3). All participants were offered couples counseling for prevention. In those receiving delayed ART, the counseling itself appeared to reduce HIV transmission to levels far lower than in earlier studies (less than 2 percent per year). However, the addition of early ART led to a 96 percent prevention of HIV transmission compared with delayed ART in an interim analysis. Infected subjects who were treated earlier not only had CD4 T-cell counts that rose quickly but also developed fewer infections (Grinsztejn and others 2014). After 8,494 person-years of follow-up, early ART maintained 93 percent effectiveness in the prevention of new linked infections compared with delayed ART (Cohen and others 2015; Cohen and others 2016).

Ecological and Population-Based Studies

As shown in annex 5B, a large number of ecological studies demonstrate the ability of ART to reduce the incidence of HIV (Smith and others 2012). Most of these are from North America (Castel and others 2012; Das and others 2010; Katz and others 2002; Montaner and others 2010; Porco and others 2004; Wood and others 2009); one is from Taiwan, China (Fang and others 2004); and one is from Australia (Law and others 2011). Each study used an ecological measure of exposure (access to ART), outcome (HIV incidence), or both. The reliability of the results lies in the strength of the measurements used for exposure and outcome.

The exposure of the entire HIV-infected population to ART can only be measured if every person infected with HIV can be identified and their treatment and virological suppression status assessed. Indeed, the hypothesis that use of ART by the entire population infected will decrease HIV incidence assumes that ongoing care will sustain viral suppression, thereby preventing transmission (Cohen and others 2011; Walensky and others 2010). However, in some settings, substantial numbers of HIV-infected persons are lost to follow-up along the path from testing to suppressive treatment (Gardner and others 2011). In the first population-based ART randomized controlled trial completed (AAAS 2016; Iwuji, Orne-Gliemann, Larmarange, and others 2016), individuals living in communities in KwaZulu-Natal, South Africa, receiving "immediate ART" irrespective of CD4 T-cell count did not have lower incidence of HIV than those in control (standard of care) communities; however, individuals in the immediate ART communities did not have the anticipated uptake and benefits of ART because of the difficulty of implementing this strategy. Several other community randomized TasP trials are underway (Boily and others 2012).

Challenges in the Measurement of Population-Level HIV Incidence

The ability to detect a benefit of TasP depends on the ability to detect changes in HIV incidence. Widely different methods have been developed to measure HIV incidence. Perhaps the most commonly used approach estimates population-based incidence using information on newly identified cases as a proxy for new infections (Castel and others 2012; Das and others 2010; Montaner and others 2010). Newly diagnosed patients acquired HIV at some unknown earlier time, and they are not "incident" in the traditional sense. Using new diagnoses as a proxy for incidence also misses people who do not seek testing; these people

may have less access to health care and a greater risk of acquiring HIV (Lopez-Quintero, Shtarkshall, and Neumark 2005; Spielberg and others 2003). Another approach is to use back-calculation from new diagnoses (Fang and others 2004), although this approach relies on assumptions related to disease progression markers such as the onset of symptoms and decline in CD4 T-cell count to estimate the time of infection (Holmes and others 2006; Novitsky and others 2010; Wand and others 2009; Wolbers and others 2010).

Longitudinal cohort follow-up data have also been used to define population incidence and are considered the gold standard of HIV incidence estimation, despite well-known sources of bias (Porco and others 2004; Wood and others 2009). In a striking example of the power of cohort studies, Tanser and others (2013) enrolled 16,000 HIV-negative people from 2005 to 2011 to receive HIV antibody testing every six months. An HIV-negative individual living in a community with 30 percent to 40 percent ART coverage was 38 percent less likely to acquire HIV than a person living in a community with less than 10 percent ART coverage. As noted above, no change in cohort incidence was observed in a cluster randomized controlled trial in the same area (Iwuji, Orne-Gliemann, Balestre, and others 2016). The likely reason for the failure of the trial to show effectiveness was that ART coverage was nearly the same in both the intervention and the control arms of the trial. Links to care were low, and the TasP intervention generally did not induce more people in the intervention arm to take up ART. In contrast, in the population-based cohort study by Tanser and others (2013), ART coverage across different geographic communities ranged from less than 10 percent to 30 percent to 40 percent.

Laboratory assays to identify persons with recent HIV infection can be applied to stored biospecimens collected in the course of routine surveillance or epidemiological research studies. The serologic testing algorithm for recent HIV seroconversion derives HIV incidence based on differences in antibodies generated in the weeks after infection (Janssen and others 1998), although logistical challenges in storing and tracking remnant blood can affect the completeness of data (Das and others 2010; Katz and others 2002). Even relatively new laboratory methods misclassify established and early infections (Le Vu and others 2008), but other methods are in development (Burns and others 2014). Currently, surveillance for recent infections in low- and middle-income countries (LMICs) is limited, which further constrains the ability to track the effect of intervention scale-up on the incidence of recent infections. However, successful development of serological detection of incidence infection would allow cross-sectional detection of incident HIV infection either in stored samples or in demographic surveys.

Modeling Population-Level Prevention Effectiveness

Mathematical modeling has been used extensively to gauge the potential of ART to reduce or eliminate the spread of HIV, and virtually all models report a benefit from ART; the magnitude of the benefit reflects the degree of coverage, model assumptions, and program quality issues such as retention and adherence (Cohen and others 2013; Maddali and others 2015). In a powerful and controversial analysis of the South African HIV epidemic, Granich and others (2009) projected that massive expansion of testing and treatment ("test and treat") along with best case program quality could substantially reduce and potentially eliminate the HIV epidemic in South Africa within 10 years. Wagner and Blower (2012) also demonstrated the theoretical possibility of HIV epidemic elimination in South Africa using a test-and-treat approach. However, they reported that it would take 40 years, and the cumulative costs would be much higher. The differences were partly attributable to differing model assumptions about survival time on ART and the costs of ART over time. A modeled analysis of expanded testing and treatment regardless of CD4 T-cell count in Washington, DC, found a more modest impact on HIV transmission (Walensky and others 2010). In a comparison of 12 independent mathematical models, Eaton and others (2012) reported broad agreement regarding the substantial potential to reduce HIV incidence in generalized epidemics in Sub-Saharan Africa, despite large differences in the structures of the models. For example, in South Africa and Zambia, expanding ART eligibility to all HIV-positive adults was projected to avert 9 percent to 40 percent of new infections over a 20-year time horizon, with greater reductions attributed to strategies involving increased testing and links to care.

Multiple investigators have also modeled the effects of various strategies incorporating TasP in concentrated epidemics in which the HIV epidemic has the largest burden among specific populations, such as persons who inject drugs (PWIDs), MSM, and female sex workers (FSWs) (Boily and Shubber 2014). In an analysis of the epidemic in Belgaum, India, the expansion of eligibility to all FSWs resulted in a 13 percent decline in projected HIV infections (Eaton and others 2012). Expanding eligibility to all HIV-positive adults, in conjunction with prioritized access for FSWs, resulted in 29 percent to 41 percent of new HIV infections being averted. In Vietnam, expanding eligibility to targeted groups produced small declines in HIV incidence: 2 percent in FSWs, 5 percent in MSM, and 5 percent in PWIDs; in contrast, expanding eligibility to all adults and prioritizing access for all three key populations resulted in a 30 percent cumulative decline in new infections (Eaton and others 2012).

A model assessing the impact of a test-and-treat strategy for urban MSM in New York City estimated a reduction in new cases of 39.3 percent over 20 years. The annual testing component of this approach provided the majority of the projected impact, whereas earlier treatment (at CD4 T-cell counts of less than 500 cells/mm^3) itself contributed to an 8.5 percent decline in new infections over 20 years (Sorensen and others 2012). A test-and-treat strategy for adults with HIV in British Columbia using a model specifically built to include the main drivers of the local epidemic demonstrated 37 percent to 62 percent reductions in new infections over 25 years (Lima and others 2008).

The effectiveness of TasP will be highly dependent on the elements of the HIV cascade, as outlined in detail in chapter 4 of this volume (Harrispersaud and others 2017), including testing frequency and coverage, links to care, adherence to treatment, virological suppression, and long-term retention in care (Delva and others 2012). Maddali and others (2015) projected that moving to early treatment in India resulted in a reduction from an estimated 1,285,000 new HIV infections to 1,050,000 infections under existing program conditions over a 20-year period. However, with enhanced testing, links to care, and retention in care, the projected number of new infections with early treatment was projected to fall further to 517,000. As pointed out by Wilson and Fraser (2014), country-level data on virological suppression are variable. For example, 26.1 percent of 266 individuals reporting ART use in the 2012 Kenya AIDS Indicator Survey were found to have a detectable viral load greater than 550 copies (Cherutich and others 2016; National AIDS and STI Control Programme 2013).

Efforts to project the impact of HIV TasP strategies have highlighted the importance of understanding the relative infectiousness of people with acute and early infection. HIV transmission is more efficient during acute infection, reflecting higher viral loads and phenotypic factors that favor transmission (Cohen, Dye, and others 2012). A study in Uganda reported that people with acute and early infection are 26 times more likely to transmit HIV than people with established infection (Hollingsworth, Anderson, and Fraser 2008). Viral phylogenetic results suggest that acute and early infections are responsible for one-third to one-half of new HIV cases in MSM (Brenner, Wainberg, and Roger 2013; Rieder and others 2010). A modeling study by Eaton and Hallett (2014) reported that a higher proportion of early infection lessened the impact of ART on estimated incidence in the first year in South Africa but did not have an important influence on the long-term effect on incidence (figure 5.1). Powers, Kretzschmar, and Miller (2014) have challenged the conclusions of this report, and the contribution of people with acute and early infection to the spread of HIV continues to be debated. The debate turns on numerous assumptions, including levels and distribution of risk behavior and epidemic patterns.

Regardless of acute infection's potential impact, diagnosing and linking people to care as early as possible are crucial. However, it is difficult to detect and diagnose people with acute and early infection. When acutely infected patients are identified, U.S. guidelines recommend immediate treatment to preserve CD4 T-cell count, shrink the viral reservoir, and reduce HIV transmission (DHHS 2014). The World Health Organization (WHO) has not yet issued specific guidelines related to acute infection, although it does recommend treatment for all HIV-infected individuals (WHO 2016).

Figure 5.1 Reduction in HIV Incidence Rate after 30 Years, by Relative Infectiousness during Early Infection

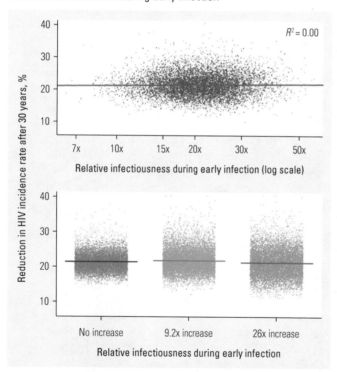

Source: Eaton and Hallet 2014.
Note: HIV = human immunodeficiency virus; x = times. This model showed no effect of relative infectiousness during early infection on the long-term (30-year) reduction in HIV incidence projected with scale-up of treatment as prevention. Relative infectiousness is increased 9.2 times and 26 times, neither of which had an effect on projected long-term incidence reduction.

In summary, the effectiveness of TasP has been well established through observational studies and clinical trials. Ecological studies and projection models further demonstrate the substantial potential for population-level HIV prevention from expanded treatment across a wide variety of geographies, epidemic types, and populations. Ongoing population-based studies will further evaluate the validity of these models and provide additional evidence on the impact of TasP strategies and the real-world effects of variable program quality along the HIV treatment cascade.

EVALUATING COST-EFFECTIVENESS

Metrics of Cost-Effectiveness

Given the effectiveness of treatment for reducing the sexual transmission of HIV, it is increasingly important for policy makers to consider the cost-effectiveness of TasP. Accordingly, analysts have begun to grapple with how best to represent the range of effects of ART.

In its simplest form, a narrow definition of cost-effectiveness has been represented as the incremental cost per infection averted by ART (Bärnighausen, Salomon, and Sangrujee 2012; Ying and others 2015). However, this outcome alone does not value ART's long-term health and health-related quality-of-life effects in the denominator of the cost-effectiveness ratio as recommended by consensus guidelines for cost-effectiveness (Gold and others 1996; Weinstein and others 1996). A trial-based cost-effectiveness analysis of HPTN 052 and other analyses used joint measures—for example, life-years saved, disability-adjusted life years (DALYs) averted—to value the impacts on both health and prevention (Eaton and others 2014; Walensky and others 2013). In this construct, life-years saved or DALYs averted by ART include both direct effects on health and downstream (discounted) effects on the prevention of new infections. Other analysts have reported the cost per death averted, which similarly values deaths directly averted by the therapeutic and preventive effects of ART, although this approach is less common and does not fully account for health-related quality of life (Bärnighausen, Bloom, and Humair 2012).

Cost-Effectiveness Estimates of Treatment

First-generation studies evaluated the cost-effectiveness of ART versus no ART and generally did not include the prevention effects of treatment. Second-generation cost-effectiveness studies of ART examine circumstances in which ART is widely used for its health benefits. Instead of comparisons with no ART, these studies look at expanding ART to various groups and include the effect of ART on sexual transmission (table 5.1). Most of these studies model the cost-effectiveness of earlier initiation of treatment compared with later initiation and typically include scenarios in which treatment is started at CD4 T-cell counts greater than 500 cells/mm³ or is started promptly regardless of CD4 T-cell count; in contrast, the 2010 WHO guidelines (WHO 2010) recommend beginning treatment at CD4 T-cell count of 350 cells/mm³. Some analyses also include related interventions, such as expanded testing and links to care, and compare ART with other prevention modalities, such as PrEP and voluntary medical male circumcision (VMMC).

These second-generation studies generally demonstrate more favorable cost-effectiveness than previous analyses. In a cost-effectiveness analysis that considered the sexual prevention–related effects of ART, Long, Brandeau, and Owens (2010) estimated that expanded treatment using prevailing eligibility criteria of CD4 T-cell levels < 200 cells/mm³ was very cost-effective in the United States and that increased frequency of HIV testing resulted in a substantial additional decrease in incidence and remained very cost-effective.

In generalized epidemics in Sub-Saharan Africa, all analyses demonstrated the cost-effectiveness of further ART expansion, including early ART. Five of the 10 published analyses focused exclusively on South Africa. In an extensive analysis, Eaton and others (2014) assessed the cost-effectiveness of earlier treatment using six independent models for South Africa and four for Zambia. The models incorporated a common costing framework and some common assumptions, although the models retained their individual structural features. The cost-effectiveness of starting treatment at CD4 T-cell counts of 500 cells/mm³ compared with CD4 T-cell counts of 350 cells/mm³ ranged from US$237 to US$1,691 per DALY averted in South Africa and from being cost saving to US$749 per DALY averted in Zambia over a 20-year time horizon (Eaton and others 2014). These estimates were considered likely to be very cost-effective in comparison with international benchmarks for each country and were similar to those in South Africa reported by Alistar, Grant, and Bendavid (2014). However, the threshold for determining whether an intervention is likely to be cost-effective is poorly known in many resource-limited settings. Granich and others (2012) reported lower costs per DALY averted over a shorter time frame of five years and found earlier treatment to be cost-saving over 40 years, using generally more optimistic measures of program quality.

More aggressive public health strategies included treatment at all CD4 T-cell counts and greater expansion of testing and links to the health system. Compared with existing conditions, these scenarios were very cost-effective over 20 years. However, they were less cost-effective over a shorter time horizon, in part because the effect of ART on HIV transmission is initially small but increases (Eaton and others 2014).

Walensky and others (2013) reported on the cost-effectiveness of earlier treatment in a trial-based analysis focused on earlier treatment of serodiscordant couples in South Africa. Treatment of all discordant couples was cost saving in South Africa over five years; over a lifetime, it cost US$590 per life-year saved in South Africa and US$530 per life-year saved in India, both considered very cost-effective. Another trial-based analysis of earlier treatment in serodiscordant couples in Uganda reported a cost per DALY averted of US$1,075 over 10 years (Ying and others 2015).

In the concentrated epidemic setting of India, Maddali and others (2015) and Eaton and others (2014) reported favorable cost-effectiveness ratios for broader strategies of earlier treatment, ranging from US$199 per DALY averted (Eaton and others 2014) to US$512 per quality-adjusted life year gained (Maddali and others 2015). Eaton and others (2014) noted that in the city of Belgaum in southern India, where the epidemic is driven largely by FSWs, the estimated incidence of new infections has fallen substantially since 2003 as a result of programs targeting this special population. They found that the incremental cost-effectiveness ratio for expanding ART to all, regardless of CD4 T-cell counts, was US$131 per DALY averted in the presence of these programs; it was slightly higher (US$241) in the theoretical case in which these programs did not exist. In Vietnam, where the epidemic is driven by FSWs, MSM, and IDUs, the incremental cost per DALY averted was US$289.

To guide resource allocation decisions for different interventions in the presence of budget constraints, Bärnighausen, Bloom, and Humair (2012) reported a favorable incremental cost per infection averted of ART initiated only in persons with CD4 T-cell counts of less than 350 cells/mm³ and VMMC scale-up (US$1,402), compared with early treatment and VMMC scale-up (US$7,325–US$10,083); however, this measure does not value the health- and quality-of-life-related effects of these interventions. This difference was less marked when using the measure of incremental cost-effectiveness of deaths averted (US$7,761–US$10,014 versus US$6,650). In a budgetary analysis, Bärnighausen, Bloom, and Humair (2012) found that VMMC combined with ART at CD4 T-cell counts of less than 350 cells/mm³ was cumulatively less expensive over 12 years and provided a similar incidence reduction as the expansion of treatment eligibility to those with

Table 5.1 Studies Estimating the Cost-Effectiveness of Treatment Direct and Indirect Benefits

Study	Study location	Study group	Intervention, comparison	Outcome	Conclusions
Alistar, Grant, and Bendavid 2014	South Africa	HIV-positive adults	ART scale-up at CD4 T-cell level < 350 cells/mm³ vs. test and treat at all CD4 T-cell levels; addition of focused (aimed at highest risk) or general PrEP	At 20 years, cost per QALY gained: US$362–US$370 (all CD4 T-cell levels); US$481–US$486 (< 350 cells/mm³); US$192–US$270 for ART at CD4 T-cell levels < 350 cells/mm³ and focused PrEP; US$1,078–US$1,125 for ART at CD4 T-cell levels < 350 cells/mm³ and general PrEP (2012 US$)	Scale-up of test-and-treat ART strategy is very cost-effective. Focused PrEP strategies, if feasible, would be highly cost-effective combined with ART.
Bärnighausen, Bloom, and Humair 2012	South Africa	HIV-positive persons; general population	ART at CD4 T-cell level < 350 cells/mm³ vs. at all CD4 T-cell levels; plus VMMC; varying levels of coverage of each intervention	At 12 years, US$1,402 per infection averted for ART (50% coverage) and VMMC (80% coverage); US$7,325–US$10,083 per infection averted for ART at all CD4 T-cell levels (20–80% coverage) and 80% VMMC; US$6,650 per death averted (50% ART at CD4 T-cell levels < 350 cells/mm³); US$7,761–US$10,014 per death averted (70–80% ART at CD4 T-cell levels < 350 cells/mm³, 20–80% ART at all CD4 T-cell levels; 80% VMMC). (2012 US$)	Using cost per infection averted as a measure, ART at CD4 T-cell levels < 350 cells/mm³ with VMMC scale-up has lowest cost-effectiveness ratios, whereas ART at all levels has higher ratios.[a]
Eaton and others 2014	South Africa; Zambia; Bangalore, Manipur, and Belgaum, India; Vietnam	HIV-positive adults, including key populations	ART at CD4 T-cell levels < 350 cells/mm³ vs. < 500 cells/mm³ and at all CD4 T-cell levels	At 20 years, costs per DALY averted at CD4 T-cell levels < 500 cells/mm³ vs. < 350 cells/mm³. South Africa: US$237–US$1,691; Zambia: dominating to US$749; Vietnam: US$290; at all levels vs. CD4 T-cell levels < 350 cells/mm³. South Africa: US$438–US$3,790; Zambia: dominating: US$790; India: US$131 (all) and US$199 (< 500 cells/mm³); Vietnam: US$289 (all) (2012 US$)	ART at CD4 T-cell levels < 500 cells/mm³ and ART at all levels is very cost-effective in South Africa, in Zambia, and for concentrated epidemic settings in India and Vietnam.
Granich and others 2012	South Africa	HIV-positive adults	Best-case testing and ART: CD4 T-cell levels < 200 cells/mm³, < 350 cells/mm³, and < 500 cells/mm³ vs. expanded testing and ART at all levels	At five years, ART at CD4 T-cell levels < 500 cells/mm³ vs. 350 cells/mm³: US$221 per DALY averted; ART at all CD4 T-cell levels: US$1,728 per DALY averted; with enhanced prevention (40% reduction in HIV incidence): US$233 for CD4 T-cell levels < 500 cells/mm³, and US$1,767 for all CD4 T-cell levels (2012 US$)	Early ART is very cost-effective when considering a short time frame of five years, with projected cost savings over a 40-year time horizon.
Hontelez and others 2011	Hlabisa, South Africa	HIV-positive adults	ART at CD4 T-cell levels ≤ 350 cells/mm³ or ≤ 200 cells/mm³	Costs of treating patients at CD4 T-cell levels ≤ 350 cells/mm³ or ≤ 200 cells/mm³ by 2017: breakeven of cumulative net costs in 2026 (2010 US$)	Front-loaded costs of treating at CD4 T-cell levels ≤ 350 cells/mm³ vs. ≤ 200 cells/mm³ may be offset by model-projected savings from health and prevention gains after 2026.

table continues next page

Table 5.1 Studies Estimating the Cost-Effectiveness of Treatment Direct and Indirect Benefits (continued)

Study	Study location	Study group	Intervention, comparison	Outcome	Conclusions
Hontelez and others 2016	10 countries in Sub-Saharan Africa[b]	HIV-positive adults	ART at all CD4 T-cell levels with continued scale-up vs. no further scale-up	Over 35 years, US$269 per life-year saved	Treatment scale-up at all CD4 T-cell levels was cost-effective.
Long, Brandeau, and Owens 2010	United States	HIV-positive adults; general population	Expanded ART (75% coverage) vs. status quo, testing and expanded ART	At 20 years, cost per QALY gained for expanded ART: US$21,647; testing (low risk once, high risk annually) and expanded ART: US$22,055; testing (low risk every three years, high risk annually) and expanded ART: US$31,274 (2012 US$)	Expansion of ART coverage in the United States is very cost-effective, and expanded testing increases QALYs gained. Expansion of ART alone decreases new infections by 10.3%; addition of testing (low risk once and high risk annually) decreases new infections by 17.3% over 20 years.
Maddali and others 2015	India	HIV-positive adults	Early (CD4 T-cell levels ≥ 350 cells/mm³) vs. delayed (CD4 T-cell levels < 350 cells/mm³) initiation of ART	At 20 years, cost per QALY gained: US$442 (ideal program conditions)—US$530 (realistic parameters for program performance) for ART at CD4 T-cell levels ≥ 350 cells/mm³ (2014 US$)	Early treatment is very cost-effective in India.
Nichols and others 2014	Macha, Zambia	HIV-positive adults; sexually active adults; general population	Early (CD4 T-cell levels < 500 cells/mm³) vs. delayed (CD4 T-cell levels < 350 cells/mm³) ART, with and without PrEP for most sexually active or general population	Cost per QALY gained: US$62 for ART at CD4 T-cell levels < 500 cells/mm³; ART at CD4 T-cell levels < 500 cells/mm³ and general population PrEP: $5,861 (2012 US$)	Early ART is very cost-effective in this rural setting. Adding PrEP was not cost-effective.
Walensky and others 2013	South Africa; India	HIV-positive partners in serodiscordant couples	Early (CD4 T-cell levels < 550 cells/mm³) vs. delayed (< 350 cells/mm³) initiation of ART	Five-year cost per life-life-year saved: South Africa: cost saving; India: US$1,800; lifetime horizon, incremental cost per life-year saved: South Africa: US$590; India: US$530 (2012 US$)	Early initiation was cost saving in South Africa over a five-year interval, cost-effective in India at five years, and very cost-effective in both countries over a lifetime.
Ying and others 2015	Kampala, Uganda	Partners in serodiscordant couples	Scale-up ART at CD4 T-cell levels < 500 cells/mm³ vs. current ART uptake; PrEP for serodiscordant couples	At 10 years: cost per DALY averted: US$1,075 for scale-up ART at CD4 T-cell levels < 500 cells/mm³ (2012 US$); cost per DALY averted: US$5,354 (2012 US$) for ART scale-up at CD4 T-cell levels < 500 cells/mm³ and PrEP	ART scale-up at CD4 T-cell levels < 500 cells/mm³ is very cost-effective compared with current ART uptake. The addition of PrEP to ART scale-up averted more DALYs, but was not cost-effective by per capita GDP standards.

Source: Commission on Macroeconomics and Health 2001.

Note: ART = antiretroviral therapy; DALY = disability-adjusted life year; HIV = human immunodeficiency virus; PrEP = preexposure prophylaxis; QALY = quality-adjusted life year; VMMC = voluntary medical male circumcision. This table follows the World Health Organization–endorsed convention, which classifies interventions in cost-effectiveness studies as (1) "cost-effective" when they avert a DALY (or gain a QALY) at a cost of three times per capita GDP or (2) "very cost-effective," when they avert a DALY (or gain a QALY) at a cost of one times per capita GDP. Dominating = one intervention dominates another intervention when it provides a greater health benefit at a lower cost (Eaton and others 2014, 26).

a. Cost per infection averted does not value ART's long-term health and health-related quality-of-life effects in the denominator of the cost-effectiveness ratio as recommended by consensus guidelines for cost-effectiveness.

b. Ethiopia, Kenya, Malawi, Mozambique, Nigeria, South Africa, Tanzania, Uganda, Zambia, and Zimbabwe.

CD4 T-cell counts of more than 350 cells/mm^3. Ying and others (2015) reported that scaling up ART to CD4 T-cell levels of less than 500 cells/mm^3 among serodiscordant couples in Uganda was very cost-effective compared with status quo uptake at CD4 T-cell levels less than or equal to 350 cells/mm^3, whereas the addition of PrEP raised the cost per DALY averted to more than three times the GDP per capita of Uganda. When using a denominator of infections averted that did not include health-related effects, they reported more favorable estimates of cost-effectiveness of the addition of PrEP to ART scale-up. The emerging issue of ART as a component of combination prevention strategies is further examined in chapter 7 of this volume (Garnett and others 2017).

In general, these myriad cost-effectiveness analyses present persuasive model-based projections of the incremental cost-effectiveness of expanding treatment access across a range of settings and populations in LMICs and high-income countries, especially where the costs of outreach are low and a long-term perspective is taken. The following sections consider further methodological issues in modeling the cost-effectiveness of TasP and the impact of TasP on global health recommendations and policy.

Key Considerations and Limitations of Models Projecting the Cost-Effectiveness of Treatment as Prevention

As with the modeling of nearly any intervention, many decisions must be made about model structure, and parameters need to be estimated. In general, model parameters can be easily explored in sensitivity analyses, whereas structural choices may have large impacts and their influence may be more difficult to ascertain. In the case of HIV cost-effectiveness, models have been calibrated, to the extent possible, with increasingly good inputs and outputs from real-life implementation of care and treatment programs. Even so, the HIV response in resource-limited settings has only been active for the past 11–12 years, and most modeling horizons are a lifetime; accordingly, certain parameter choices—especially as they relate to evolving drug costs and future lines of treatment—are likely to entail substantial uncertainty.

The best approach to calibrating effectiveness models to underlying HIV epidemic trends has been debated and managed differently by various groups (Hallett, Eaton, and Menzies 2014; Okano and Blower 2014). Modeling cost-effectiveness of TasP also requires examining initiation of treatment earlier in the course of disease than has been done in most LMICs.

The challenge of introducing earlier initiation, along with the valuation of the prevention effects of treatment, is the scarcity of programmatic data (outside of trials and well-studied cohorts) at this stage of the disease to guide parameter development. Many new parameters need to be considered and potentially included, which introduces greater uncertainty (Bärnighausen, Salomon, and Sangrujee 2012).

Substantial uncertainty exists about whether the unit costs of various elements of HIV care and treatment will remain constant as scale-up is accelerated, extended to persons with higher CD4 T-cell counts, or both. As Meyer-Rath and Over (2012) noted, many models rely either on fixed unit costs for a year of treatment or on cost accounting identities, in which each of the constituent costs of treatment is estimated and multiplied by health care utilization figures. These costs may need to be considered in a flexible cost-function manner, given the likely nonlinearities of inputs around scaling TasP, such as uneven need for new infrastructure (Meyer-Rath and Over 2012). Many models also assume constant antiretroviral prices into the future, but for any given drug, prices tend to decline over time (Holmes and others 2010). Conversely, when newer drugs replace existing drugs in guidelines, abrupt price increases may result (Waning and others 2009).

Most cost-effectiveness models further assume that ART retention and adherence do not vary by stage of the disease at initiation, the previous health experience of individuals, and other determinants of health-care-seeking behavior. However, earlier initiation may lead to reduced—or increased—overall retention and adherence, due to underlying differences in those facts. Finally, the preventive effects of TasP are likely to alter the composition of the HIV-infected population over time, changing its biological and behavioral characteristics and leading to different costs and outcomes (Bärnighausen, Salomon, and Sangrujee 2012; Smit and others 2015).

Risk compensation is another consideration that could have a positive or negative effect on projected benefits (Dukers and others 2001; Stolte and others 2004). Changes in HIV risk taking following ART scale-up have at times been considered risk compensation—that is, HIV-negative persons take more sexual risks as ART coverage lowers the average risk of HIV acquisition and ART availability reduces the potential health losses. However, persons could take fewer sexual risks, including changes in sexual behavior, substance use, and contraceptive use, in response to ART scale-up because of improved survival expectations and increased optimism for the future (Bor and others 2013; Raifman and others 2014). Future models of combination prevention modalities need to attempt to examine the presence of potential behavioral effects.

Select Policy Questions Addressed by Cost-Effectiveness Models

As with nearly all health policy decisions, there are trade-offs among benefits, costs, and risks as national and global decision makers consider possible strategies for their investments in treatment and prevention. Although most TasP scenarios are considered cost-effective or very cost-effective over reasonable horizons for decision making, they all have higher up-front costs. Therefore, optimal policy choices will vary greatly according to available funding, local HIV response, goals, and other elements of feasibility and local preference, such as the political environment. This section highlights several critical policy issues and illustrates the trade-offs involved in using select modeling and cost-effectiveness analyses.

What Trade-Offs Are Involved in Expanding Testing and Links to Care under Existing Treatment Guidelines, Compared with Expanding Earlier Treatment?

Eaton and others (2014) considered the comparative effects on new HIV infections and cost-effectiveness of a policy decision in South Africa, where estimated ART coverage under existing guidelines (CD4 T-cell counts of less than 350 cells/mm^3) was approximately 50 percent at the time of the analysis, and in Zambia, where reported ART coverage (CD4 T-cell counts of less than 350 cells/mm^3) was more than 90 percent. First, they found that expanding testing and linking patients to care under existing guidelines in South Africa had a substantial effect on lowering the incidence of new infections (6 percent to 28 percent, depending on the model). The approach averted more infections than changing eligibility to CD4 T-cell counts of less than 500 cells/mm^3 without expanding testing and links to care (5 percent to 12 percent of infections averted). In Zambia, where reported coverage was already high, simply expanding ART eligibility averted 21 percent to 40 percent of new infections, an impact greater than expanding both testing and links to care (8 percent to 17 percent). Given the high estimated coverage reported in Zambia, the model assumed that cases were being identified earlier and that expanding testing and links to care would have somewhat less of an impact than simply raising the threshold. Since the time of this analysis, Zambia has raised the treatment threshold to CD4 T-cell counts of less than 500 cells/mm^3.

From a cost-effectiveness perspective, Zambia's decision to expand eligibility was generally supported by assessments of costs per DALY averted. The picture for South Africa is less clear, and the conclusions from the models are conflicting. The up-front costs of expanding testing and links to care are high, and four of seven models favored simply expanding eligibility; three favored expanding testing and links to care at the current threshold of CD4 T-cell counts of less than 350 cells/mm^3 (Eaton and others 2014). In 2012–13, South Africa chose to expand coverage of persons with CD4 T-cell counts of less than 350 cells/mm^3 and to use less toxic antiretroviral medicines; in 2014–15, the country shifted to a policy of treating persons with CD4 T-cell counts of less than 500 cells/mm^3; in mid-2016, the government announced the intention to shift to a "treat all" policy consistent with updated WHO guidelines (WHO 2016).

How Might the Timing of the Costs and Benefits of TasP Affect Policy Makers' Decisions, and What Further Information Could Be Helpful?

Although numerous strategies are considered cost-effective, treating greater numbers of people brings greater up-front costs regardless of potential downstream (discounted) savings. Expanding access to persons with CD4 T-cell counts of less than 350 cells/mm^3 results in additional costs that tend to increase over time after a small initial spike (Eaton and others 2014). This increase occurs because increasing numbers of individuals live longer and incur costs to the health system.

In this analysis, increasing eligibility to persons with CD4 T-cell counts of less than 500 cells/mm^3, with or without expanded access, results in a greater initial spike in costs; however, as with the "treat all" strategy, the cost curve generally declines each subsequent year, in part because these strategies are expected to reduce the number of new HIV infections (Eaton and others 2014). Accordingly, later outlays could diminish with larger up-front investments, even when including the effects of discounting. Decision making will hinge on the assessment of potential impacts, relevance of model assumptions to the environment, validity of available model inputs, availability of funding and competing investments, and other local factors.

These types of models generally do not consider the financial costs to patients of starting treatment earlier. These costs are related largely to transport and opportunity costs; depending on the extent of decentralization of HIV services, they could be substantial (Rosen and others 2007). If treatment is more for prevention than for direct health benefits, these higher up-front costs may discourage patients from getting care, although this theoretical risk requires further empirical data. Several investigators have demonstrated greater productivity with HIV treatment in clinic- and population-based cohorts (Bor and others 2012), which is excluded in most model-based analyses. The extent to which productivity gains could offset transport and other costs among people starting treatment while healthier is unknown.

It is also difficult for models to reflect that, in the context of constrained budgets, additional spending on HIV treatment will lead to displaced resources for other interventions. If the treatment intervention generates health per cost at a rate greater than a certain threshold, then despite that displacement, there is a net gain in health. However, quantifying that threshold is difficult. International guidance has, until recently, suggested benchmarks related to the GDP per capita of a country; there are indications that a more realistic assessment of the opportunity costs of health expenditure would demand lower cost per health gain for an intervention to be likely to be cost-effective (Woods and others 2015).

Policy makers in many sectors, but particularly health, face a trade-off between higher up-front costs and longer-term gains. Unlike problems associated with non-communicable diseases, TasP could reduce the intensity and spread of a transmissible pandemic. In this time-dependent context, donors and policy makers have often leaned toward up-front investments.

What Approaches Could Improve the Cost-Effectiveness of Treatment as Prevention?

Innovations in care delivery, such as task-shifting elements of the delivery cascade to lower-level staff members, have been widely adopted and have facilitated reductions in the costs of delivering care. Innovators such as Médecins Sans Frontières and national governments have further pioneered methods of care delivery, now known as *differentiated care*, which target the intensity of care to the needs of patients (Duncombe and others 2015; Holmes and Sanne 2015). For example, the formation of community adherence groups among stable patients in Mozambique allowed for substantially less clinic contact and increased retention in care among those opting into these models (Decroo and others 2011). Greater attention to both the models of care and the costs of care delivery is another tool that can be used by in-country stakeholders to strive for greater efficiency and quality of care delivery. The President's Emergency Plan for AIDS Relief (PEPFAR) program's expenditure analysis approach entails the collection of detailed data that allow country-level decision makers to distinguish between low- and high-cost providers of quality care. A report of results from this methodology noted reductions in the heterogeneity of the costs of supporting not only ART, but also HIV testing and other key elements along the TasP cascade (PEPFAR 2012).

NATIONAL AND GLOBAL GUIDANCE, POLICIES, AND RESOURCE ALLOCATION

The release in May 2011 of the HPTN 052 data on the remarkable reduction of sexual transmission of HIV disease among serodiscordant couples sent ripples not only through the scientific community, but also through policy-making circles, including national governments, the WHO, and leading funders of HIV programs in low-resource settings (El Sadr and others 2011). After more than two decades of focusing on the health-related effects of ART, experts began to grapple with its role as a tool for the prevention of sexual transmission of HIV.

Members of the WHO Guidelines Group on Couples HIV Testing and Counseling incorporated the HPTN 052 findings in their review process (WHO 2012a), judging them to be directly and immediately applicable to couples counseling and testing. In addition to other potential interventions, the evidence for treatment in this setting was considered to be substantial. After stakeholder reviews, updated guidelines were released 11 months after the HPTN 052 results (box 5.1).

In April 2012, the WHO incorporated the findings of HPTN 052 and released the programmatic update on Option B+ (WHO 2012b). In addition to programmatic data from Malawi that supported full treatment for pregnant women, the potential effects of treatment on sexual prevention of HIV was considered as follows: "If Option B+ can be supported, funded, scaled up at the primary care level and sustained, it will also likely provide the best protection for the mother's health, and it offers a promising new approach to preventing sexual transmission and new HIV infections in the general population" (WHO 2012b, 4).

In 2013, the WHO combined all of its ART-related HIV guidance into a single guideline that considered the sexual prevention effects of treatment demonstrated in

---

Box 5.1

Recommendations from the WHO Couples HIV Testing and Counseling Guidelines

People with HIV whose partners do not have HIV and who are started on ART for their own health should be advised that ART is also recommended to reduce HIV transmission to uninfected partners. This is a strong recommendation based on high-quality evidence.

HPTN 052. The guidelines committee changed eligibility criteria to CD4 T-cell counts of 500 cells/mm³, persuaded by a combination of clinical benefits drawn mainly from LMIC settings (Kitahata and others 2009), along with evidence of reduced sexual transmission and tuberculosis among treated individuals. In addition, review of the evidence using the Grading of Recommendations Assessment, Development and Evaluation (GRADE) system led to recommendations for treatment regardless of CD4 T-cell count for pregnant women, serodiscordant couples, persons with tuberculosis, and persons with severe liver disease. The U.S. and European guidelines, which already counseled earlier initiation of treatment, also incorporated the benefits of TasP (DHHS 2014; European AIDS Clinical Society 2014). Updated WHO guidelines, reviewed in the setting of further evidence for the health benefits of earlier ART initiation, recommended offering treatment to all individuals with HIV, regardless of CD4 T-cell count (INSIGHT START Study Group 2015; TEMPRANO ANRS Study Group 2015; WHO 2016).

Since the release of the WHO documents recommending earlier treatment, national governments have weighed guidelines changes. As of 2015, the WHO reported that of the 58 WHO focus countries, 34 (59 percent) have adopted new guidelines for treatment of serodiscordant couples and 37 (64 percent) have raised their thresholds to CD4 T-cell counts of 500 cells/mm³. Rwanda's national guidelines support a TasP strategy (ART regardless of CD4 T-cell count) and universal testing. Other countries with limited health infrastructure and financial resources are struggling with high unmet needs at lower CD4 T-cell counts and have legitimate concerns about crowding out treatment slots for sicker patients (Linas and others 2006). The prevention effects of treatment have also substantially influenced policy and allocation decisions of major payers and funders of HIV programs in LMICs.

The results of HPTN 052 arrived during the latter stages of a global economic downturn and coincided with a leveling off of the rapid growth of HIV-related overseas development aid (Kaiser Family Foundation 2015). Despite these challenges, global leaders, advocates, and public health officials were energized by the potential impact of the addition of ART to the combination prevention armamentarium.

The PEPFAR program is the largest bilateral program supporting the HIV response in LMICs. Its federally chartered Scientific Advisory Board reviewed the HPTN 052 data, discussed its potential applications, and ultimately recommended that PEPFAR support the use of ART in specific populations with CD4 T-cell counts greater than 350 cells/mm³ to prevent transmission to others (El Sadr and others 2011). The board also recommended that "careful evaluations, including assessment of benefit/risk/impact/feasibility and modeling exercises are urgently needed to identify populations that should be prioritized for this intervention, given local conditions" (El Sadr and others 2011, 19). Following these and other recommendations, the U.S. government strongly endorsed accelerating combination prevention in 2011, including a 50 percent increase in persons on treatment over a two-year period. As overall allocations to HIV reached a plateau, PEPFAR weighted its financial allocations more heavily toward treatment and several other high-impact interventions (Cohen, Holmes, and others 2012; Goosby and others 2012; Holmes and others 2012; PEPFAR 2014). In 2014, PEPFAR took the further step of endorsing the UNAIDS (Joint United Nations Programme on HIV/AIDS) 90-90-90 targets, and in 2015 announced support for the ongoing expansion of treatment in the context of further studies on the effectiveness of earlier treatment on individual health (PEPFAR 2014, 2015).

ONGOING RESEARCH

Even as investigators have advanced the understanding of the preventive role of treatment, critical questions remain. Ongoing studies are evaluating the biological, pharmacologic, clinical, and public health elements of ART as a prevention modality, and priority areas for future research continue to emerge.

Biological and Pharmacological Studies

The quest to understand the biology of transmission revolves around the fitness requirements of the viral pathogen (Carlson and others 2014) and its susceptibility to innate host defenses (Borrow 2011). Successful viral suppression does not prevent intermittent viral shedding in the genital tracts of both men (Kalichman and others 2010) and women (Cu-Uvin and others 2010). However, observational studies suggest that the viruses being shed during viral suppression are likely compromised and not readily transmitted (Cohen and others 2013).

Perhaps the most important TasP consideration lies in the simplification of treatment itself. Successful suppression of viral replication virtually eliminates HIV transmission (Muessig and Cohen 2014). Accordingly, linked transmission events reflect failed treatment or resistance to the antiretroviral regimen being used. Failure to adhere to a treatment regimen is the greatest problem. Newer antiviral agents are very well tolerated but still require daily medication.

Glaxo-Smith-Kline and Janssen are exploring a combination of injectable agents, with one combination being tested in the Phase 2b LATTE (Long-Acting Antiretroviral Treatment Enabling) Trial (Margolis and others 2014). The trial includes a run-in of oral agents for safety testing, which has been completed, followed by maintenance injections every month or every two months. Injectable ART may be appropriate for several types of patients, but it is particularly attractive for people in serodiscordant sexual relationships.

Clinical, Public Health, and Population Effects Studies

Granich and others (2011) identified more than 50 ongoing studies covering the impact of treatment on prevention among serodiscordant couples and key populations and the secondary benefits of treatment for individuals infected with both tuberculosis and HIV. These studies examine HIV incidence and mortality in the general population and economic outcomes for patients receiving TasP.

Substantial funding has been allocated to research aimed at understanding the potential population-level impact of TasP. Four large studies underway are designed to demonstrate that TasP, as part of a package of prevention interventions, reduces population-level HIV incidence in generalized epidemics (box 5.2).

CONCLUSIONS

Treatment has well-known direct effects on the health outcomes of HIV-positive individuals; it has also been conclusively shown in observational studies and randomized clinical trials to prevent sexual transmission of HIV. These prevention effects are backed by years of basic science and clinical work that have established the effectiveness of ART in reducing HIV replication in blood and genital tissues and secretions. The projected effectiveness of early treatment on reductions in sexual transmission of HIV is dependent on the performance of the treatment cascade, including HIV testing and links to care, retention in care, and virological suppression. When the prevention effects of ART are included in analyses of the cost-effectiveness of earlier treatment, ART is generally found to be a highly cost-effective intervention in diverse settings of varied income levels, HIV

Box 5.2

Population-Level Effects of Treatment as Prevention: Select Studies

Population Effects of ART to Reduce HIV Transmission (PopART), also known as the HIV Prevention Trials Network 071, examines the effect of universal testing and treatment compared with treatment at CD4 T-cell counts of less than 350 cells/mm^3 or the standard of care. PopART includes 21 communities in two countries—South Africa and Zambia—with a total population of 1.2 million; results are expected in 2017–18 (Hayes and others 2014).

The Botswana Combination Prevention Project assesses the provision of treatment to all individuals with CD4 T-cell counts greater than 350 cells/mm^3 or with a viral load greater than or equal to 10,000 copies per milliliter, compared with individuals receiving the standard of care in the setting of scaled-up combination prevention (CDC 2013).

The Africa Centre and the Agence Nationale de Recherche sur le Sida 12249 TasP Trial was developed to establish the causal impact of TasP (treatment as prevention) on population-level HIV incidence and other health, economic, and social outcomes. The trial randomized 34 communities with a total adult population of 34,000 to receive home-based HIV testing and ART referral under either a TasP strategy (intervention) or the South African standard of care with home-based HIV testing (control) (Iwuji and others 2013). The only difference between the intervention and the control arm was whether HIV-positive people were offered immediate ART in early stages of the disease (intervention) vs. only in later disease stages (control).

The SEARCH (Sustainable East Africa Research on Community Health) Study, based in Kenya and Uganda, includes 32 communities of approximately 10,000 individuals each. The study compares early treatment to standard of care, with multiple health outcomes and a prevention outcome of community viral load (Chamie and others 2012; Jain and others 2013).

epidemic types, and risk populations. It is projected to be most effective and cost-effective when paired with efforts to identify infected individuals through expanded testing and links to care.

Ongoing population-based studies will provide further information on the wider prevention impact of earlier treatment as part of a package of combination prevention modalities.

ANNEXES

The annexes to this chapter are as follows. They are available at http://www.dcp-3.org/infectiousdiseases.

- Annex 5A. Studies of TasP in Serodiscordant Couples
- Annex 5B. Ecological Studies Examining the Effectiveness of ART on HIV Incidence

NOTES

The authors are indebted to Musonda Namuyemba and Megan Wolf, MPH, for their editorial assistance.

This chapter is linked closely with chapters on the HIV care continuum in adults and children (chapter 4, Harrispersaud and others 2017), prevention of mother-to-child transmission (chapter 6, John-Stewart and others 2017), and cost-effectiveness of interventions to prevent HIV acquisition (chapter 7, Garnett and others 2017).

World Bank Income Classifications as of July 2014 are as follows, based on estimates of gross national income (GNI) per capita for 2013:

- Low-income countries (LICs) = US$1,045 or less
- Middle-income countries (MICs) are subdivided:
  (a) lower-middle-income = US$1,046 to US$4,125
  (b) upper-middle-income (UMICs) = US$4,126 to US$12,745
- High-income countries (HICs) = US$12,746 or more.

REFERENCES

AAAS (American Association for the Advancement of Science). 2016. "Entering the Health-Care System: The Challenge of the Universal Test-and-Treat Strategy." Press release, Eurekalert, July 20. http://www.eurekalert.org /pub_releases/2016-07/a-eth071916.php#.V5TTdKRGkxo .email.

Alistar, S. S., P. M. Grant, and E. Bendavid. 2014. "Comparative Effectiveness and Cost-Effectiveness of Antiretroviral Therapy and Pre-Exposure Prophylaxis for HIV Prevention in South Africa." BMC Medicine 12 (46): 11.

Anderson, B. L., and S. C. Cu-Uvin. 2011. "Clinical Parameters Essential to Methodology and Interpretation of Mucosal Responses." American Journal of Reproductive Immunology 65 (3): 352–60.

Attia, S., M. Egger, M. Müller, M. Zwahlen, and N. Low. 2009. "Sexual Transmission of HIV According to Viral Load and Antiretroviral Therapy: Systematic Review and Meta-Analysis." AIDS 23 (11): 1397–404.

Baeten, J. M., E. Kahle, J. R. Lingappa, R. W. Coombs, S. Delany-Moretlwe, and others. 2011. "Genital HIV-1 RNA Quantity Predicts Risk of Heterosexual HIV-1 Transmission." Science Translational Medicine 3 (77): 77ra29.

Baggaley, R. F., D. Dimitrov, B. N. Owen, M. Pickles, A. R. Butler, and others. 2013. "Heterosexual Anal Intercourse: A Neglected Risk Factor for HIV?" American Journal of Reproductive Immunology 69 (1): 95–105.

Baggaley, R. F., R. G. White, T. D. Hollingsworth, and M. C. Boily. 2013. "Heterosexual HIV-1 Infectiousness and Antiretroviral Use: Systematic Review of Prospective Studies of Discordant Couples." Epidemiology 24 (1): 110–21.

Bärnighausen, T., D. E. Bloom, and S. Humair. 2012. "Economics of Antiretroviral Treatment vs. Circumcision for HIV Prevention." Proceedings of the National Academy of Sciences of the United States of America 109 (52): 21271–76.

Bärnighausen, T., J. A. Salomon, and N. Sangrujee. 2012. "HIV Treatment as Prevention: Issues in Economic Evaluation." PLoS Medicine 9 (7): e1001263.

Boily, M. C., B. Mâsse, R. Alsallaq, N. S. Padian, J. W. Eaton, and others. 2012. "HIV Treatment as Prevention: Considerations in the Design, Conduct, and Analysis of Cluster Randomized Controlled Trials of Combination HIV Prevention." PLoS Medicine 9 (7): e1001250.

Boily, M. C., and Z. Shubber. 2014. "Modelling in Concentrated Epidemics: Informing Epidemic Trajectories and Assessing Prevention Approaches." Current Opinion in HIV and AIDS 9 (2): 134–49.

Bor, J., A. J. Herbst, M.-L. Newell, and T. Bärnighausen. 2013. "Increases in Adult Life Expectancy in Rural South Africa: Valuing the Scale-Up of HIV Treatment." Science 339 (6122): 961–65.

Bor, J., F. Tanser, M.-L. Newell, and T. Bärnighausen. 2012. "Nearly Full Employment Recovery among South African HIV Patients on Antiretroviral Therapy: Evidence from a Large Population Cohort." Health Affairs 31 (7): 10.1377 /hlthaff.2012.0407.

Borrow, P. 2011. "Innate Immunity in Acute HIV-1 Infection." Current Opinion in HIV and AIDS 6 (5): 353–63.

Brenner, B., M. A. Wainberg, and M. Roger. 2013. "Phylogenetic Inferences on HIV-1 Transmission: Implications for the Design of Prevention and Treatment Interventions." AIDS 27 (7): 1045–57.

Burns, D. N., V. DeGruttola, C. D. Pilcher, M. Kretzschmar, C. M. Gordon, and others. 2014. "Toward an Endgame: Finding and Engaging People Unaware of Their HIV-1 Infection in Treatment and Prevention." AIDS Research and Human Retroviruses 30 (3): 217–24.

Carlson, J. M., M. Schaefer, D. C. Monaco, R. Batorsky, D. T. Claiborne, and others. 2014. "HIV Transmission: Selection Bias at the Heterosexual HIV-1 Transmission Bottleneck." Science 345 (6193): 1254031.

Castel, A. D., M. Befus, S. Willis, A. Griffin, S. Hader, and others. 2012. "Use of the Community Viral Load as a Population-Based Biomarker of HIV Burden." *AIDS* 26 (3): 345–53.

CDC (Centers for Disease Control and Prevention). 2013. "Botswana Combination Prevention Project (BCPP)." Atlanta, GA. https://clinicaltrials.gov/ct2/show/NCT01965470.

Chamie, G., D. Kwarisiima, T. D. Clark, J. Kabami, V. Jain, and others. 2012. "Leveraging Rapid Community-Based HIV Testing Campaigns for Non-Communicable Diseases in Rural Uganda." *PLoS One* 7 (8): e43400.

Cherutich, P., A. A. Kim, T. A. Kellogg, K. Sherr, A. Waruru, and others. 2016. "Detectable HIV Viral Load in Kenya: Data from a Population-Based Survey." *PLoS One* 11 (5): e0154318.

Cohen, M. S, Y. Chen, M. McCauley, T. Gamble, and M. Hosseinpour. 2015. "Final Results of the HPTN 052 Randomized Controlled Trial: Antiretroviral Therapy Prevents HIV Transmission." International AIDS Society 2015, 8th Conference on HIV Pathogenesis, Treatment, and Prevention, Vancouver, British Columbia, July 19–22.

Cohen, M. S., Y. Q. Chen, M. McCauley, T. Gamble, M. C. Hosseinipour, and others. 2011. "Prevention of HIV-1 Infection with Early Antiretroviral Therapy." *New England Journal of Medicine* 365 (6): 493–505.

Cohen, M. S., Y. Q. Chen, M. McCauley, T. Gamble, M. C. Hosseinipour, and others. 2016. "Antiretroviral Therapy for the Prevention of HIV-1 Transmission." *New England Journal of Medicine* 375: 830–39.

Cohen, M. S., C. Dye, C. Fraser, W. C. Miller, K. A. Power, and others. 2012. "HIV Treatment as Prevention: Debate and Commentary; Will Early Infection Compromise Treatment-as-Prevention Strategies?" *PLoS Medicine* 9 (7): e1001232.

Cohen, M. S., C. L. Gay, M. P. Busch, and F. M. Hecht. 2010. "The Detection of Acute HIV Infection." *Journal of Infectious Diseases* 202 (Suppl 2): S270–77.

Cohen, M. S., C. Holmes, N. Padian, M. Wolf, G. Himschall, and others. 2012. "HIV Treatment as Prevention: How Scientific Discovery Occurred and Translated Rapidly into Policy for the Global Response." *Health Affairs* 31 (7): 1439–49.

Cohen, M. S., M. K. Smith, K. E. Muessig, T. B. Hallett, K. A. Powers, and others. 2013. "Antiretroviral Treatment of HIV-1 Prevents Transmission of HIV-1: Where Do We Go from Here?" *The Lancet* 383 (9903): 1515–24.

Commission on Macroeconomics and Health. 2001. *Macroeconomics and Health: Investing in Health for Economic Development.* Geneva: World Health Organization.

Cope, A. B., A. M. Crooks, T. Chin, J. D. Kuruc, K. S. McGee, and others. 2014. "Incident Sexually Transmitted Infection as a Biomarker for High-Risk Sexual Behavior Following Diagnosis with Acute HIV." *Sexually Transmitted Diseases* 41 (7): 447–52.

Cu-Uvin, S., A. K. DeLong, K. K. Venkatesh, J. W. Hogan, J. Ingersoll, and others. 2010. "Genital Tract HIV-1 RNA Shedding among Women with Below Detectable Plasma Viral Load." *AIDS* 24 (16): 2489–97.

Danel, C., R. Moh, D. Gabillard, A. Badje, J. Le Carrou, and others. 2015. "A Trial of Early Antiretrovirals and Isoniazid Preventive Therapy in Africa." *New England Journal of Medicine* 373 (9): 808–22.

Das, M., P. L. Chu, G. M. Santos, S. Scheer, E. Vittinghoff, and others. 2010. "Decreases in Community Viral Load Are Accompanied by Reductions in New HIV Infections in San Francisco." *PLoS One* 5 (6): e11068. http://dx.doi.org/10.1371/journal.pone.0011068.

Decroo, T., B. Telfer, M. Biot, J. Maikere, S. Dezembro, and others. 2011. "Distribution of Antiretroviral Treatment through Self-Forming Groups of Patients in Tete Province, Mozambique." *Journal of Acquired Immune Deficiency Syndromes* 56 (2): e39–44.

Delva, W., D. P. Wilson, L. Abu-Raddad, M. Gorgens, D. Wilson, and others. 2012. "HIV Treatment as Prevention: Principles of Good HIV Epidemiology Modelling for Public Health Decision-Making in All Modes of Prevention and Evaluation." *PLoS Medicine* 9 (7): e1001239.

DHHS (Department of Health and Human Services). 2014. "Guidelines for the Use of Antiretroviral Agents in HIV-1-Infected Adults and Adolescents." Panel on Antiretroviral Guidelines for Adults and Adolescents, DHHS, Washington, DC.

Donnell, D., J. M. Baeten, J. Kiarie, K. Thomas, W. Stevens, and others. 2010. "Heterosexual HIV-1 Transmission after Initiation of Antiretroviral Therapy: A Prospective Cohort Analysis." *The Lancet* 375 (9731): 2092–98.

Dukers, N. H., J. Goudsmit, J. B. de Wit, M. Prins, G. J. Weverling, and others. 2001. "Sexual Risk Behaviour Relates to the Virological and Immunological Improvements during Highly Active Antiretroviral Therapy in HIV-1 Infection." *AIDS* 15 (3): 369–78.

Duncombe, C., S. Rosenblum, N. Hellman, C. Holmes, L. Wilkinson, and others. 2015. "Reframing HIV Care: Putting People at the Centre of Antiretroviral Delivery." *Tropical Medicine and International Health* 20 (4): 430–47.

Eaton, J. W., and T. B. Hallett. 2014. "Why the Proportion of Transmission during Early-Stage HIV Infection Does Not Predict the Long-Term Impact of Treatment on HIV Incidence." *Proceedings of the National Academy of Sciences of the United States of America* 111 (45): 16202–7.

Eaton, J. W., L. F. Johnson, J. A. Salomon, T. Bärnighausen, E. Bendavid, and others. 2012. "HIV Treatment as Prevention: Systematic Comparison of Mathematical Models of the Potential Impact of Antiretroviral Therapy on HIV Incidence in South Africa." *PLoS Medicine* 9 (7): e1001245.

Eaton, J. W., N. A. Menzies, J. Stover, V. Cambiano, L. Chindelevitch, and others. 2014. "Health Benefits, Costs, and Cost-Effectiveness of Earlier Eligibility for Adult Antiretroviral Therapy and Expanded Treatment Coverage: A Combined Analysis of 12 Mathematical Models." *The Lancet Global Health* 2 (1): e23–34. doi:10.1016/S2214-109X(13)70172-4.

El Sadr, W., M. S. Cohen, K. DeCock, L.-G. Bekker, S. Karim, and others. 2011. *PEPFAR Scientific Advisory Board Recommendations for the Office of the U.S. Global AIDS*

Coordinator: *Implications of HPTN 052 for PEPFAR's Treatment Programs.* Washington, DC: PEPFAR. https://www.pepfar.gov/documents/organization/177126.pdf.

European AIDS Clinical Society. 2014. *Guidelines, version 7.1.* Copenhagen: European AIDS Clinical Society. http://www.eacsociety.org/files/guidelines_english_71_141204.pdf.

Fang, C.-T., H.-M. Hsu, S.-J. Twu, M.-Y. Chen, Y. Y. Chang, and others. 2004. "Decreased HIV Transmission after a Policy of Providing Free Access to Highly Active Antiretroviral Therapy in Taiwan." *Journal of Infectious Diseases* 190 (5): 879–85.

Gardner, E. M., M. P. McLees, J. F. Steiner, C. Del Rio, and W. J. Burman. 2011. "The Spectrum of Engagement in HIV Care and Its Relevance to Test-and-Treat Strategies for Prevention of HIV Infection." *Clinical Infectious Diseases* 52 (6): 793–800.

Garnett, G., S. Krishnaratne, K. Harris, T. Hallet, M. Santos, and others. 2017. "Cost-Effectiveness of Interventions to Prevent HIV Acquisition." In *Disease Control Priorities* (third edition): Volume 6, *Major Infectious Diseases*, edited by K. K. Holmes, S. Bertozzi, B. R. Bloom, and P. Jha. Washington, DC: World Bank.

Gold, M. R., J. E. Siegel, L. B. Russell, and M. C. Weinstein. 1996. *Cost-Effectiveness in Health and Medicine: Report of the Panel on Cost-Effectiveness in Health and Medicine.* New York: Oxford University Press.

Goosby, E., D. Von Zinkernagel, C. B. Holmes, D. Haroz, and T. Walsh. 2012. "Raising the Bar: PEPFAR and New Paradigms for Global Health." *Journal of Acquired Immune Deficiency Syndromes* 60 (Suppl 3): S158–62.

Granich, R. M., C. F. Gilks, C. Dye, K. M. De Cock, and B. G. Williams. 2009. "Universal Voluntary HIV Testing with Immediate Antiretroviral Therapy as a Strategy for Elimination of HIV Transmission: A Mathematical Model." *The Lancet* 373 (9657): 48–57.

Granich, R. M., S. Gupta, A. B. Suthar, C. Smyth, D. Hoos, and others. 2011. "Antiretroviral Therapy in Prevention of HIV and TB: Update on Current Research Efforts." *Current HIV Research* 9 (6): 446–69.

Granich, R. M., J. G. Kahn, R. Bennett, C. B. Holmes, N. Garg, and others. 2012. "Expanding ART for Treatment and Prevention of HIV in South Africa: Estimated Cost and Cost-Effectiveness 2011–2050." *PLoS One* 7 (2): e30216.

Grinsztejn, B., M. C. Hosseinipour, H. J. Ribaudo, S. Swindells, J. Eron, and others. 2014. "Effects of Early Versus Delayed Initiation of Antiretroviral Treatment on Clinical Outcomes of HIV-1 Infection: Results from the Phase 3 HPTN 052 Randomised Controlled Trial." *The Lancet Infectious Diseases* 14 (4): 281–90.

Hallett, T. B., J. W. Eaton, and N. Menzies. 2014. "Beware of Using Invalid Transmission Models to Guide HIV Health Policy: Authors' Reply." *The Lancet Global Health* 2: e261.

Harrispersaud, K., M. McNairy, S. Ahmed, E. J. Abrams, H. Thirumurthy, and others. 2017. "HIV Care Continuum in Adults and Children: Cost-Effectiveness Considerations." In *Disease Control Priorities* (third edition): Volume 6, *Major Infectious Diseases*, edited by K.K. Holmes, S. Bertozzi, B. R. Bloom, and P. Jha. Washington, DC: World Bank.

Hayes, R., H. Ayles, N. Beyers, K. Sabapathy, S. Floyd, and others. 2014. "HPTN 071 (PopART): Rationale and Design of a Cluster-Randomised Trial of the Population Impact of an HIV Combination Prevention Intervention Including Universal Testing and Treatment: A Study Protocol for a Cluster Randomised Trial." *Trials* 15 (1): 57.

Hendrix, C. W., E. J. Fuchs, K. J. Macura, L. A. Lee, T. L. Parsons, and others. 2008. "Quantitative Imaging and Sigmoidoscopy to Assess Distribution of Rectal Microbicide Surrogates." *Clinical Pharmacology and Therapeutics* 83 (1): 97–105.

Henry, K. 1988. "Setting AIDS Priorities: The Need for a Closer Alliance of Public Health and Clinical Approaches toward the Control of AIDS." *American Journal of Public Health* 78 (9): 1210–12.

Ho, Y.-C., L. Shan, N. N. Hosmane, J. Wang, S. B. Laskey, and others. 2013. "Replication-Competent Non-Induced Proviruses in the Latent Reservoir Increase Barrier to HIV-1 Cure." *Cell* 155 (3): 540–51.

Hollingsworth, T. D., R. M. Anderson, and C. Fraser. 2008. "HIV-1 Transmission, by Stage of Infection." *Journal of Infectious Diseases* 198 (5): 687–93.

Holmes, C. B., J. M. Blandford, N. Sangrujee, S. R. Stewart, A. Dubois, and others. 2012. "PEPFAR's Past and Future Efforts to Cut Costs, Improve Efficiency, and Increase the Impact of Global HIV Programs." *Health Affairs* 31 (7): 1553–60.

Holmes, C. B., W. Coggin, D. Jamieson, H. Mihm, R. Granich, and others. 2010. "Use of Generic Antiretroviral Agents and Cost Savings in PEPFAR Treatment Programs." *Journal of the American Medical Association* 304 (3): 313–20.

Holmes, C. B., and I. Sanne. 2015. "Changing Models of Care to Improve Progression through the HIV Treatment Cascade in Different Populations." *Current Opinion in HIV and AIDS* 10 (6): 447–50.

Holmes, C. B., R. Wood, M. Badri, S. Zilber, B. Wang, and others. 2006. "CD4 Decline and Incidence of Opportunistic Infections in Cape Town, South Africa: Implications for Prophylaxis and Treatment." *Journal of Acquired Immune Deficiency Syndromes* 42 (4): 464–69.

Hontelez, J. A., A. Y. Chang, O. Ogbuoji, S. J. Vlas, T. Bärnighausen, and others. 2016. "Changing HIV Treatment Eligibility under Health System Constraints in Sub-Saharan Africa: Investment Needs, Population Health Gains, and Cost-Effectiveness." *AIDS* 30 (150): 2341–50.

Hontelez, J. A. C., S. J. de Vlas, F. Tanser, R. Bakker, T. Bärnighausen, and others. 2011. "The Impact of the New WHO Antiretroviral Treatment Guidelines on HIV Epidemic Dynamics and Cost in South Africa." *PLoS One* 6 (7): e21919.

INSIGHT START Study Group. 2015. "Initiation of Antiretroviral Therapy in Early Asymptomatic HIV Infection." *New England Journal of Medicine* 373 (9): 795–807.

Iwuji, C. C., J. Orne-Gliemann, E. Balestre, J. Larmarange, R. Thiebaut, and others. 2016. "The Impact of Universal

Test and Treat on HIV Incidence in a Rural South African Population: ANRS 12249 TasP Trial, 2012–2016." 21st International AIDS Conference (AIDS 2016), Durban, South Africa, July 18–22.

Iwuji, C., J. Orne-Gliemann, J. Larmarange, N. Okesola, F. Tanser, and others. 2016. "Uptake of Home-Based HIV Testing, Linkage to Care, and Community Attitudes about ART in Rural Kwazulu-Natal, South Africa: Descriptive Results from the First Phase of the ANRS 12249 TasP Cluster-Randomised Trial." *PLoS Medicine* 13 (8): e1002107.

Iwuji, C. C., J. Orne-Gliemann, F. Tanser, S. Boyer, R. J. Lessells, and others. 2013. "Evaluation of the Impact of Immediate Versus WHO Recommendations: Guided Antiretroviral Therapy Initiation on HIV Incidence; the ANRS 12249 TasP (Treatment as Prevention) Trial in Hlabisa Sub-district, KwaZulu-Natal, South Africa, Study Protocol for a Cluster Randomized Control Trial." *Trials* 14 (1): 230.

Jain, V., T. Liegler, J. Kabami, G. Chamie, T. D. Clark, and others. 2013. "Assessment of Community Viral Load in a Rural East African Setting Using a Fingerprick-Based Blood Collection Method." *Clinical Infectious Diseases* 56 (4): 598–605.

Janssen, R. S., G. A. Satten, S. L. Stramer, B. D. Rawal, T. R. O'Brien, and others. 1998. "New Testing Strategy to Detect Early HIV-1 Infection for Use in Incidence Estimates and for Clinical and Prevention Purposes." *Journal of the American Medical Association* 280 (1): 42–48.

Jia, Z., Y. Mao, F. Zhang, Y. Ruan, Y. Ma, and others. 2012. "Antiretroviral Therapy to Prevent HIV Transmission in Serodiscordant Couples in China (2003–11): A National Observational Cohort Study." *The Lancet* 382 (9899): 1195–203.

John-Stewart, G., R. Peeling, C. Levin, P. J. Garcia, D. Mabey, and others. 2017. "Elimination of Mother-to-Child Transmission of HIV and Syphilis." In *Disease Control Priorities* (third edition): Volume 6, *Major Infectious Diseases*, edited by K. K. Holmes, S. Bertozzi, B. R. Bloom, and P. Jha. Washington, DC: World Bank.

Joseph, S. B., K. T. Arrildt, A. E. Swanstrom, G. Schnell, B. Lee, and others. 2014. "Quantification of Entry Phenotypes of Macrophage-Tropic HIV-1 across a Wide Range of CD4 Densities." *Journal of Virology* 88 (4): 1858–69.

Kaiser Family Foundation. 2015. "Financing the Response to HIV in Low- and Middle-Income Countries: International Assistance from Donor Governments in 2015." Kaiser Family Foundation, Menlo Park, CA. http://files.kff.org/attachment/Financing-the-Response-to-HIV-in-Low-and-Middle-Income-Countries-International-Assistance-from-Donor-Governments-in-2015.

Kalichman, S. C., C. Cherry, C. M. Amaral, C. Swetzes, L. Eaton, and others. 2010. "Adherence to Antiretroviral Therapy and HIV Transmission Risks: Implications for Test-and-Treat Approaches to HIV Prevention." *AIDS Patient Care and STDs* 24 (5): 271–77.

Katz, M. H., S. K. Schwarcz, T. A. Kellogg, J. D. Klausner, J. W. Dilley, and others. 2002. "Impact of Highly Active Antiretroviral Treatment on HIV Seroincidence among Men Who Have Sex with Men: San Francisco." *American Journal of Public Health* 92 (3): 388–94.

Keele, B. F., E. E. Giorgi, J. F. Salazar-Gonzalez, J. M. Decker, K. T. Pham, and others. 2008. "Identification and Characterization of Transmitted and Early Founder Virus Envelopes in Primary HIV-1 Infection." *Proceedings of the National Academy of Sciences of the United States of America* 105 (21): 7552–57.

Kitahata, M. M., S. J. Gange, A. G. Abraham, B. Merriman, M. S. Saag, and others. 2009. "Effect of Early versus Deferred Antiretroviral Therapy for HIV on Survival." *New England Journal of Medicine* 360 (18): 1815–26.

Kwara, A., A. Delong, N. Rezk, J. Hogan, H. Burtwell, and others. 2008. "Antiretroviral Drug Concentrations and HIV RNA in the Genital Tract of HIV-Infected Women Receiving Long-Term Highly Active Antiretroviral Therapy." *Clinical Infectious Diseases* 46 (5): 719–25.

Laeyendecker, O., R. Brookmeyer, C. E. Mullis, D. Donnell, J. Lingappa, and others. 2012. "Specificity of Four Laboratory Approaches for Cross-Sectional HIV Incidence Determination: Analysis of Samples from Adults with Known Nonrecent HIV Infection from Five African Countries." *AIDS Research and Human Retroviruses* 28 (10): 1177–83.

Law, M. G., I. Woolley, D. J. Templeton, N. Roth, J. Chuah, and others. 2011. "Trends in Detectable Viral Load by Calendar Year in the Australian HIV Observational Database." *Journal of the International AIDS Society* 14 (1): 10.

Le Vu, S., J. Pillonel, C. Semaille, P. Bernillon, Y. Le Strat, and others. 2008. "Principles and Uses of HIV Incidence Estimation from Recent Infection Testing: A Review." *Eurosurveillance* 13 (36): 11–16.

Li, H., K. J. Bar, S. Wang, J. M. Decker, Y. Chen, and others. 2010. "High Multiplicity Infection by HIV-1 in Men Who Have Sex with Men." *PLoS Pathogens* 6 (5): e1000890.

Lima, V. D., K. Johnston, R. S. Hogg, A. R. Levy, P. R. Harrigan, and others. 2008. "Expanded Access to Highly Active Antiretroviral Therapy: A Potentially Powerful Strategy to Curb the Growth of the HIV Epidemic." *Journal of Infectious Diseases* 198 (1): 59–67.

Linas, B. P., H. Zheng, E. Losina, A. Rockwell, R. P. Walensky, and others. 2006. "Optimizing Resource Allocation in United States AIDS Drug Assistance Programs." *Clinical Infectious Diseases* 43 (10): 1357–64.

Long, E. F., M. L. Brandeau, and D. K. Owens. 2010. "The Cost-Effectiveness and Population Outcomes of Expanded HIV Screening and Antiretroviral Treatment in the United States." *Annals of Internal Medicine* 153 (12): 778–89.

Lopez-Quintero, C., R. Shtarkshall, and Y. D. Neumark. 2005. "Barriers to HIV-Testing among Hispanics in the United States: Analysis of the National Health Interview Survey." *AIDS Patient Care and STDs* 19 (10): 672–83.

Loutfy, M. R., W. Wu, M. Letchumanan, L. Bondy, T. Antoniou, and others. 2013. "Systematic Review of HIV Transmission between Heterosexual Serodiscordant Couples Where the HIV-Positive Partner Is Fully Suppressed on Antiretroviral Therapy." *PLoS One* 8 (2): e55747.

Lu, W., G. Zeng, J. Luo, S. Duo, G. Xing, and others. 2010. "HIV Transmission Risk among Serodiscordant Couples: A Retrospective Study of Former Plasma Donors in

Henan, China." *Journal of Acquired Immune Deficiency Syndromes* 55 (2): 2332–38

Maddali, M. V., D. W. Dowdy, A. Gupta, and M. Shah. 2015. "Economic and Epidemiological Impact of Early Antiretroviral Therapy Initiation in India." *Journal of the International AIDS Society* 18: 20217.

Margolis, D., C. Brinson, J. Eron, G. Richmond, R. LeBlanc, and others. 2014. "744 and Rilpivirine as Two-Drug Oral Maintenance Therapy: LAI116482 (LATTE) Week 48 Results." Special Issue: Abstracts from the 2014 Conference on Retroviruses and Opportunistic Infections. *Topics in Antiviral Medicine International* 22 (e-1): 34.

Martin, E., J. M. Carlson, A. Q. Le, D. R. Chopera, R. McGovern, and others. 2014. "Early Immune Adaptation in HIV-1 Revealed by Population-Level Approaches." *Retrovirology* 11 (64): 1–16.

McLaren, P. J., C. Coulonges, S. Ripke, L. van den Berg, S. Buchbinder, and others. 2013. "Association Study of Common Genetic Variants and HIV-1 Acquisition in 6,300 Infected Cases and 7,200 Controls." *PLoS Pathogens* 9 (7): e1003515.

Meyer-Rath, G., and M. Over. 2012. "HIV Treatment as Prevention: Modelling the Cost of Antiretroviral Treatment—State of the Art and Future Directions." *PLoS Medicine* 9 (7): e1001247.

Montaner, J. S., E. Wood, T. Kerr, V. Lima, R. Barrios, and others. 2010. "Expanded Highly Active Antiretroviral Therapy Coverage among HIV-Positive Drug Users to Improve Individual and Public Health Outcomes." *Journal of Acquired Immune Deficiency Syndromes* 55 (1): S5–S9.

Muessig, K. E., and M. S. Cohen. 2014. "Advances in HIV Prevention for Serodiscordant Couples." *Current HIV/AIDS Reports* 11 (4): 434–46.

Nachega, J. B., O. A. Uthman, E. J. Mills, and T. C. Quinn. 2013. "Adherence to Antiretroviral Therapy for the Success of Emerging Interventions to Prevent HIV Transmission: A Wake-Up Call." *Journal of AIDS and Clinical Research* (Suppl 4): 2039–52.

National AIDS and STI Control Programme. 2013. "Kenya AIDS Indicator Survey 2012." Ministry of Health, Nairobi, Kenya.

Nichols, B. E., R. Baltussen, J. H. van Dijk, P. Thuma, J. L. Nouwen, and others. 2014. "Cost-Effectiveness of PrEP in HIV/AIDS Control in Zambia: A Stochastic League Approach." *Journal of Acquired Immune Deficiency Syndromes* 66 (2): 221–28.

Novitsky, V., R. Wang, S. Lagakos, and M. Essex. 2010. "HIV-1 Subtype C Phylodynamics in the Global Epidemic." *Viruses* 2 (1): 33–54.

O'Brien, T. R., D. H. McDermott, J. P. Ioannidis, M. Carrington, P. M. Murphy, and others. 2000. "Effect of Chemokine Receptor Gene Polymorphisms on the Response to Potent Antiretroviral Therapy." *AIDS* 14 (7): 821–26.

Okano, J. T., and S. Blower. 2014. "Beware of Using Invalid Transmission Models to Guide HIV Health Policy." *The Lancet Global Health* 2 (5): e260.

Olivier, A. J., L. Masson, K. Ronacher, G. Walzl, D. Coetzee, and others. 2014. "Distinct Cytokine Patterns in Semen Influence Local HIV Shedding and HIV Target Cell Panel Activation." *Journal of Infectious Diseases* 209 (8): 1174–84.

Patterson, K. B., H. A. Prince, E. Kraft, A. J. Jenkins, N. J. Shaheen, and others. 2011. "Penetration of Tenofovir and Emtricitabine in Mucosal Tissues: Implications for Prevention of HIV-1 Transmission." *Science Translational Medicine* 3 (112): 112.

Parrish, N. F., F. Gao, H. Li, E. E. Giorgi, H. J. Barbian, and others. 2013. "Phenotypic Properties of Transmitted Founder HIV-1." *Proceedings of the National Academy of Sciences of the United States of America* 110 (17): 6626–33.

PEPFAR (President's Emergency Plan for AIDS Relief). 2012. "Report on Pilot Expenditure Analysis of PEPFAR Programs in Six Countries." Department of State, Washington, DC. http://www.pepfar.gov/documents/organization/195700.pdf.

———. 2014. *PEPFAR 3.0 Controlling the Epidemic: Delivering on the Promise of an AIDS-free Generation.* Washington, DC: The Office of the U.S. Global AIDS Coordinator. http://www.pepfar.gov/documents/organization/234744.pdf.

———. 2015. "2015 United Nations General Assembly Sustainable Development Summit." Fact Sheet, Department of State, Washington, DC. http://www.pepfar.gov/documents/organization/247548.pdf.

Pilcher, C. D., J. J. Eron Jr., S. Galvin, C. Gay, and M. S. Cohen. 2004. "Acute HIV Revisited: New Opportunities for Treatment and Prevention." *Journal of Clinical Investigation* 113 (7): 937–45.

Pilcher, C. D., G. Joak, I. F. Hoffman, F. E. A. Martinson, C. Mapanje, and others. 2007. "Amplified Transmission of HIV-1: Comparison of HIV-1 Concentrations in Semen and Blood during Acute and Chronic Infection." *AIDS* 21 (13): 1723–30.

Ping, L. H., S. B. Joseph, J. A. Anderson, M. R. Abrahams, J. F. Salazar-Gonzalez, and others. 2013. "Comparison of Viral Env Proteins from Acute and Chronic Infections with Subtype C Human Immunodeficiency Virus Type 1 Identifies Differences in Glycosylation and CCR5 Utilization and Suggests a New Strategy for Immunogen Design." *Journal of Virology* 87 (13): 7218–33.

Porco, T. C., J. N. Martin, K. A. Page-Shafer, A. Cheng, E. Charlebois, and others. 2004. "Decline in HIV Infectivity Following the Introduction of Highly Active Antiretroviral Therapy." *AIDS* 18 (1): 81–88.

Powers, K. A., M. E. Kretzschmar, and W. C. Miller. 2014. "Impact of Early-Stage HIV Transmission on Treatment as Prevention." *Proceedings of the National Academy of Sciences of the United States of America* 111 (45): 15867–68.

Quinn, T. C., M. J. Wawer, N. Sewankambo, D. Serwadda, C. Li, and others. 2000. "Viral Load and Heterosexual Transmission of Human Immunodeficiency Virus Type 1. Rakai Project Study Group." *New England Journal of Medicine* 342 (13): 921–29.

Raifman, J., T. Chetty, F. Tanser, T. Mutevedzi, P. Matthews, and others. 2014. "Preventing Unintended Pregnancy and HIV Transmission: Effects of the HIV Treatment Cascade on Contraceptive Use and Choice in Rural KwaZulu-Natal." *Journal of Acquired Immune Deficiency Syndromes* 67 (Suppl 4): S218–27.

Reichelderfer, P. S., R. W. Coombs, D. J. Wright, J. Cohn, D. N. Burns, and others. 2000. "Effect of Menstrual Cycle on HIV-1 Levels in the Peripheral Blood and Genital Tract: WHS 001 Study Team." *AIDS* 14 (14): 2101–7.

Rieder, P., B. Joos, V. von Wyl, H. Kuster, C. Grube, and others. 2010. "HIV-1 Transmission after Cessation of Early Antiretroviral Therapy among Men Having Sex with Men." *AIDS* 24 (8): 1177–83.

Rodger, A. J., V. Cambiano, T. Bruun, P. Vernazza, S. Collins, and others. 2016. "Sexual Activity without Condoms and Risk of HIV Transmission in Serodifferent Couples when the HIV-Positive Partner Is Using Suppressive Antiretroviral Therapy." *Journal of the American Medical Association* 316 (2): 171–81.

Rosen, S., M. Ketlhapile, I. Sanne, and M. B. De Silva. 2007. "Cost to Patients of Obtaining Treatment for HIV/AIDS in South Africa." *South African Medical Journal* 97 (7): 524–29.

Royce, R. A., A. Seña, W. Cates, and M. S. Cohen. 1997. "Sexual Transmission of HIV." *New England Journal of Medicine* 336: 1072–78.

Shaw, G. M., and E. Hunter. 2012. "HIV Transmission." *Cold Spring Harbor Perspectives in Medicine* 2 (11): a006965.

Smit, M., K. Brinkman, S. Geerlings, C. Smit, K. Thyagarajan, and others. 2015. "Future Challenges for Clinical Care of an Ageing Population Infected with HIV: A Modelling Study." *The Lancet Infectious Diseases* 15 (7): 810–18.

Smith, M. K., K. A. Powers, K. E. Muessig, W. C. Miller, and M. S. Cohen. 2012. "HIV Treatment as Prevention: The Utility and Limitations of Ecological Observation." *PLoS Medicine* 9 (7): e1001260.

Sorensen, S. W., S. L. Sansom, J. T. Brooks, G. Marks, E. M. Begier, and others. 2012. "A Mathematical Model of Comprehensive Test-and-Treat Services and HIV Incidence among Men Who Have Sex with Men in the United States." *PLoS One* 7 (2): e29098.

Spielberg, F., B. M. Branson, G. M. Goldbaum, D. Lockhart, A. Kurth, and others. 2003. "Overcoming Barriers to HIV Testing: Preferences for New Strategies among Clients of a Needle Exchange, a Sexually Transmitted Disease Clinic, and Sex Venues for Men Who Have Sex with Men." *Journal of Acquired Immune Deficiency Syndromes* 32 (3): 318–27.

Stolte, I. G., N. H. Dukers, R. B. Geskus, R. A. Coutinho, and J. B. de Wit. 2004. "Homosexual Men Change to Risky Sex When Perceiving Less Threat of HIV/AIDS since Availability of Highly Active Antiretroviral Therapy: A Longitudinal Study." *AIDS* 18 (2): 303–9.

Supervie, V., J. P. Viard, D. Costagliola, and R. Breban. 2014. "Heterosexual Risk of HIV Transmission per Sexual Act under Combined Antiretroviral Therapy: Systematic Review and Bayesian Modeling." *Clinical Infectious Diseases* 59 (1): 115–22.

Taha, T. E., D. R. Hoover, G. A. Dallabetta, N. I. Kumwenda, L. A. Mtimavalve, and others. 1998. "Bacterial Vaginosis and Disturbances of Vaginal Flora: Association with Increased Acquisition of HIV." *AIDS* 12 (13): 1699–706.

Tanser, F., T. Bärnighausen, E. Grapsa, J. Zaidi, and M. L Newell. 2013. "High Coverage of ART Associated with Decline in Risk of HIV Acquisition in Rural KwaZulu-Natal, South Africa." *Science* 339 (6122): 966–71.

TEMPRANO ANRS Study Group. 2015. "A Trial of Early Antiretrovirals and Isoniazid Preventive Therapy in Africa." *New England Journal of Medicine* 373: 808–22.

Thompson, C. G., M. S. Cohen, and A. D. M. Kashuba. 2013. "Antiretroviral Pharmacology in Mucosal Tissues." *Journal of Acquired Immune Deficiency Syndromes* 63 (2): S240–47.

Wagner, B. G., and S. Blower. 2012. "Universal Access to HIV Treatment versus Universal 'Test and Treat': Transmission, Drug Resistance, and Treatment Costs." *PLoS One* 7 (9): e41212.

Walensky, R. P., A. D. Paltiel, E. Losina, B. L. Morris, C. A. Schott, and others. 2010. "Test and Treat DC: Forecasting the Impact of a Comprehensive HIV Strategy in Washington, DC." *Clinical Infectious Diseases* 51 (4): 392–400.

Walensky, R. P., E. L. Ross, N. Kumarasmy, R. Wood, F. Noubary, and others. 2013. "Cost-Effectiveness of HIV Treatment as Prevention in Serodiscordant Couples." *New England Journal of Medicine* 369 (18): 1715–25.

Wand, H., D. Wilson, P. Yan, A. Gonnermann, A. McDonald, and others. 2009. "Characterizing Trends in HIV Infection among Men Who Have Sex with Men in Australia by Birth Cohorts: Results from a Modified Back-Projection Method." *Journal of the International AIDS Society* 12: 19.

Wang, L., G. E. Zeng, J. Luo, S. Duo, G. Xing, and others. 2010. "HIV Transmission Risk among Serodiscordant Couples: A Retrospective Study of Former Plasma Donors in Henan, China." *Journal of Acquired Immune Deficiency Syndromes* 55 (2): 232–38.

Waning, B., W. Kaplan, A. C. King, D. A. Lawrence, H. G. Leufkens, and others. 2009. "Global Strategies to Reduce the Price of Antiretroviral Medicines: Evidence from Transactional Databases." *Bulletin of the World Health Organization* 87 (7): 520–28.

Weinstein, M. C., J. E. Siegel, M. R. Gold, M. S. Kamlet, and L. B. Russell. 1996. "Recommendations of the Panel on Cost-Effectiveness in Health and Medicine." *Journal of the American Medical Association* 276 (15): 1253–58.

WHO (World Health Organization). 2010. *Antiretroviral Therapy for HIV Infection in Adults and Adolescents: Recommendations for a Public Health Approach.* Geneva: WHO.

———. 2012a. *Guidance on Couples HIV Testing and Counselling, Including Antiretroviral Therapy for Treatment and Prevention in Serodiscordant Couples.* Geneva: WHO.

———. 2012b. *Programmatic Update: Use of Antiretroviral Drugs for Treating Pregnant Women and Preventing HIV Infection in Infants.* Geneva: WHO.

———. 2016. *Consolidated Guidelines on the Use of Antiretroviral Drugs for Treating and Preventing HIV Infection: Recommendations for a Public Health Approach.* 2nd ed. Geneva: WHO.

Wilson, D., and N. Fraser. 2014. "Controlling the HIV Epidemic with Antiretrovirals: Who Pays and Why? Costs, Effectiveness, and Feasibility of HIV Treatment as Prevention." *Clinical Infectious Diseases* 59 (Suppl 1): S28–31.

Wolbers, M., A. Babiker, C. Sabin, J. Young, M. Dorrucci, and others. 2010. "Pretreatment CD4 Cell Slope and Progression to AIDS or Death in HIV-Infected Patients Initiating Antiretroviral Therapy: The CASCADE Collaboration; A Collaboration of 23 Cohort Studies." *PLoS Medicine* 7 (2): e1000239.

Wood, E., T. Kerr, B. D. L. Marshall, K. Li, R. Zhang, and others. 2009. "Longitudinal Community Plasma HIV-1 RNA Concentrations and Incidence of HIV-1 among Injecting Drug Users: Prospective Cohort Study." *BMJ* 338 (b1649).

Woods, B., P. Revill, M. Sculpher, and K. Claxton. 2015. "Country-Level Cost-Effectiveness Thresholds: Initial Estimates and the Need for Future Research." CHE Research Paper 109, Centre for Health Economics, University of York, United Kingdom.

Ying, R., M. Sharma, R. Heffron, C. L. Celum, J. M. Baeten, and others. 2015. "Cost-Effectiveness of Pre-Exposure Prophylaxis Targeted to High-Risk Serodiscordant Couples as a Bridge to Sustained ART Use in Kampala, Uganda." *Journal of the International AIDS Society* 18 (Suppl 3): 20013.

Zhang, H., G. Dornadula, M. Beumont, L. Livornese, B. Van Uitert, and others. 1998. "Human Immunodeficiency Virus Type 1 in the Semen of Men Receiving Highly Active Antiretroviral Therapy." *New England Journal of Medicine* 339 (25): 1803–9.

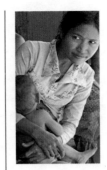

Prevention of Mother-to-Child Transmission of HIV and Syphilis

Grace John-Stewart, Rosanna W. Peeling, Carol Levin, Patricia J. Garcia, David Mabey, and John Kinuthia

INTRODUCTION

The past decade has yielded enormous progress in the prevention of mother-to-child transmission (PMTCT) of the human immunodeficiency virus (HIV) (UNAIDS 2015). Interventions that decrease mother-to-child transmission (MTCT) of HIV from more than 30 percent to 1 percent have been identified. Decentralized point-of-care (POC) approaches for detecting maternal HIV and immediate provision of comprehensive antiretroviral treatment (ART) have resulted in rapid decreases in the number of HIV-infected infants. Indeed, PMTCT has been credited with driving observed decreases in HIV incidence overall.

The guidelines for PMTCT of HIV have been dynamic: the World Health Organization (WHO) and Joint United Nations Programme on AIDS (UNAIDS) have revised their recommendations every two to five years, most recently to recommend combination lifelong ART for all pregnant HIV-infected women (WHO 2014a). The term *elimination of mother-to-child transmission* (EMTCT) was used to further spur global efforts to virtually eliminate pediatric HIV by 2015 (UNAIDS 2011; WHO 2014a).

PMTCT of syphilis *(Treponema pallidum)* has not received the same amount of attention as PMTCT of HIV, although syphilis is estimated to affect more children globally than HIV. PMTCT of syphilis requires less costly and less intensive interventions than HIV, making

its elimination potentially more feasible. The rollout of PMTCT of syphilis may be hampered by less political will to implement it than PMTCT of HIV, lack of accountability for monitoring PMTCT of syphilis, inconsistent availability of diagnostic tests, and use of tests that are not POC (WHO 2006). PMTCT of syphilis could readily leverage advances in PMTCT of HIV by using these programs to enhance the supply chain, lab testing, and accountability for prompt syphilis diagnosis and treatment.

The current momentum in PMTCT of HIV offers a unique opportunity to accelerate PMTCT of HIV and syphilis concurrently. Combining interventions for PMTCT of HIV and syphilis adds minimal cost while potentially benefiting twice as many mother-infant pairs as interventions focused solely on either HIV or syphilis. Health systems improvements for rapid diagnosis and treatment, partner engagement, and follow-up of mothers and infants can enhance both types of PMTCT programs. Combined PMTCT of HIV and syphilis will yield sustained and important benefits for women and children worldwide.

This chapter reviews the rates, burden, and consequences of mother-to-child transmission of HIV and syphilis; the effectiveness of interventions to decrease transmission; the estimated cost-effectiveness of these interventions; and several successful PMTCT programmatic approaches. The chapter also highlights

Corresponding author: Grace John-Stewart, Department of Global Health, University of Washington, Seattle, Washington, United States; gjohn@uw.edu.

opportunities for integrated programming to efficiently decrease the number of infants infected with these chronically debilitating pathogens. Because syphilis testing is already currently recommended by WHO for all pregnant women (WHO 2006) and is at least partially implemented in most antenatal clinics, new costs for improving the program may be minimal: adapting programs to incorporate dual POC tests to diagnose syphilis, providing training to improve adherence to guidelines, and increasing accountability for tracking outcomes in PMTCT of syphilis within clinics can be added to existing programs with limited additional investment.

In 2015, Cuba became the first country to eliminate perinatal HIV and syphilis (WHO 2015). This experience demonstrates that the goal of dual elimination is attainable and feasible with effective integration of PMTCT of HIV and syphilis. Children do not need to suffer from the consequences of either of these devastating infections when these PMTCT programs function synergistically.

GLOBAL BURDEN AND CONSEQUENCES OF MTCT OF HIV AND SYPHILIS

MTCT Rates and Cofactors

Comparisons of MTCT of syphilis and MTCT of HIV are difficult because of differences in the precision of infant diagnosis (and thus in the precision of MTCT risk estimates), and because of varied infant outcomes attributable to maternal infection, and differences in the timing and routes of transmission. Diagnosis of congenital syphilis is clinical and imprecise. In contrast, infant HIV diagnosis is based on a robust replicable measure—detection of HIV virus—that is highly sensitive and specific.

HIV Transmission

MTCT of HIV occurs either during pregnancy, at delivery, or through breastfeeding. Without intervention, HIV MTCT rates range from 20 percent to 35 percent in breastfed infants and from 15 percent to 20 percent in nonbreastfed infants (table 6.1) (De Cock and others 2000). Cofactors of MTCT of HIV include maternal viral burden (both systemically and in mucosal compartments to which the baby is exposed, such as genital secretions or breast milk), immunosuppression, and preterm birth (John and Kreiss 1996; John and others 2001).

Syphilis Transmission

MTCT of syphilis predominantly occurs during pregnancy, but few studies have been conducted on the estimated risk. The precision and accuracy of syphilis MTCT risk estimates are limited by the study design used (case control), varied diagnostic tests for maternal syphilis, and lack of a good diagnostic marker of infant infection. In a systematic review, Gomez and others (2013) screened 3,258 records and identified six studies

Table 6.1 Mother-to-Child Transmission of Syphilis and HIV, Selected Findings

Metric	Syphilis	HIV
Estimated annual number of pregnant women infected worldwide	1.36 million (summary from 2008 data [Newman and others 2013])	1.45 million (UNAIDS 2013)
Timing of transmission	In utero	In utero, intrapartum, postnatal (John and Kreiss 1996)
Method for detecting infant infection	Clinical manifestations, cerebrospinal fluid, and radiological	Detection of HIV virus by nucleic acid amplification tests
Transmission risk	15.5 percent of infants born to mothers with untreated syphilis have clinical signs of congenital syphilis (Gomez and others 2013)	20 to 35 percent infant HIV transmission depending on breastfeeding duration in the absence of maternal treatment or infant prophylaxis (De Cock and others 2000)
Adverse infant outcomes: fetal death, preterm birth, stillbirth, neonatal death, low birth weight	4.6-fold increased risk of combined adverse outcomes (66.5 percent among mothers with syphilis vs. 14.3 percent among mothers without syphilis) (Gomez and others 2013)	2-fold to 4-fold increased risk of combined adverse outcomes (Brocklehurst and French 1998)
Cofactors for MTCT	Maternal RPR level (Watson-Jones, Changalucha, and others 2002)	Maternal HIV viral load, other sexually transmitted infections, CD4 count, route of delivery, infant breastfeeding (John and others 2001)

Note: CD4 = cluster of differentiation 4 (blood count); HIV = human immunodeficiency virus; MTCT = mother-to-child transmission; RPR = rapid plasma reagin.

conducted between 1917 and 2000 (all case-control studies) to estimate the MTCT risk of syphilis. The estimated rates of congenital syphilis (diagnosed in infants showing signs of clinical infection) ranged from 2.2 percent to 40.9 percent, with a pooled MTCT rate of 15.5 percent (table 6.1). Cofactors of syphilis MTCT remain undefined (Gomez and others 2013); some evidence suggests that more recent maternal active syphilis (with high rapid plasma reagin [RPR] titer) is associated with increased adverse infant outcomes (Watson-Jones, Changalucha, and others 2002).

In contrast to studies of MTCT of HIV, outcomes of maternal syphilis often emphasize estimated attributable adverse infant outcomes in addition to infant infections, because of difficulties in infant diagnosis and strong evidence of numerous additional adverse outcomes. Accordingly, combined adverse infant outcomes prevented by treatment of maternal syphilis are used to estimate cost-effectiveness. Gomez and others' (2013) systematic review attributed multiple adverse infant outcomes—including spontaneous abortion, stillbirth, fetal death, preterm birth, low birth weight, neonatal death, and congenital syphilis—to untreated syphilis. The pooled frequency of these adverse infant outcomes was 66.5 percent in mothers with syphilis, compared with 14.3 percent in mothers without syphilis (Gomez and others 2013). The authors noted marked heterogeneity and potential for bias in the estimates. Newer syphilis molecular diagnostics (polymerase chain reaction [PCR] assays) have greater than 70 percent sensitivity. To date, however, these newer diagnostic tests for syphilis have not been used to estimate MTCT syphilis rates (Grimprel and others 1991; Palmer and others 2003; Sanchez and others 1993; Shields and others 2012).

Other Infant Impacts from MTCT of HIV

Estimates of the impact of maternal HIV infection on infants have focused predominantly on HIV transmission risk itself, without including multiple adverse infant outcomes. However, untreated maternal HIV may contribute to adverse infant outcomes in addition to infant HIV infection, including fetal death, preterm birth, infant mortality, stillbirth, and low birth weight. In a systematic review of 31 studies, HIV-infected mothers had increased risk of spontaneous abortion, perinatal mortality, infant mortality, intrauterine growth retardation, low birth weight, and preterm birth (Brocklehurst and French 1998).[1]

In addition, some of the new antiretroviral regimens for PMTCT may confer increased risk of adverse outcomes unrelated to HIV (Townsend and others 2007; Townsend and others 2010). The Promoting Maternal-Infant Survival Everywhere (PROMISE) study, which enrolled more than 3,500 mother-infant pairs, compared two types of antiretroviral regimens for pregnant women who did not meet cluster of differentiation 4 (CD4) or clinical criteria for triple ART. One regimen type, Option A, was a short-course antiretroviral regimen that included different single or double drug regimens in pregnancy, delivery, and postpartum.[2] Option B was a combined three-drug ART regimen administered to all women during pregnancy and postpartum.[3] Both regimens provided preventive antiretrovirals for breastfeeding MTCT; Option A relied on infant prophylaxis, while Option B relied on maternal ART with a six-week period of infant prophylaxis. Although Option A was inferior to Option B for PMTCT in this randomized controlled trial, Option B was associated with higher rates of prematurity, low birth weight, and neonatal death.[4] Among the two Option B alternatives, lamivudine-ART was safer for infants than tenofovir-ART. Thus, the PROMISE study showed that the antiretroviral regimens a woman receives can affect both MTCT rates and rates of adverse infant outcomes. The WHO guidelines recommend Option B+, both for enhanced PMTCT effectiveness and for programmatic feasibility. Future guidelines and programs may adapt specific Option B+ antiretroviral regimens to concurrently decrease HIV and other adverse child outcomes.

Maternal HIV and Syphilis Coinfection

Some evidence suggests that women coinfected with HIV and syphilis may have greater than twofold increased risk of HIV transmission than women with HIV infection alone; however, some studies have not found this association (Lee and others 1998; Mwapasa and others 2006; Schulte and others 2001; Yeganegh and others 2015). Children of coinfected mothers may have HIV-syphilis coinfection and poorer outcomes than those with either infection alone (Mwapasa and others 2006).

Maternal and Pediatric Burden of HIV and Syphilis

Maternal Burden of HIV and Syphilis

There are distinct regional and global patterns of maternal HIV and syphilis. In Sub-Saharan Africa, for example, both HIV and syphilis are highly prevalent; however, the distributions of HIV infection and syphilis vary distinctly by region. Consistently assessed national HIV and syphilis prevalence estimates are not produced; however, South Africa, which has a higher HIV prevalence, appears to have lower antenatal syphilis prevalence than do other southern and eastern African countries. China has higher syphilis but lower HIV prevalence than the Russian Federation. Although syphilis and HIV are both sexually transmitted infections (STIs), their distinct regional distribution may stem from differences in transmission epidemiology, sexual networks, treatment program effectiveness and coverage, notification and tracing guidelines, and measurement methods (WHO 2013).

Map 6.1 shows the global distribution of HIV prevalence in women ages 15–24 years, and map 6.2 shows the distribution of maternal antenatal syphilis seroprevalence.

Pediatric Burden of HIV

Annually, an estimated 1.5 million pregnant women worldwide are HIV infected, which, during the peak of the HIV epidemic in the mid-1990s, resulted in more than 500,000 infant HIV infections per year (UNAIDS 2013). However, with active PMTCT programs, infant HIV infections have steadily declined to about half that peak level; in 2015, an estimated 150,000 children younger than age 15 years were newly infected, as shown in map 6.3 (UNAIDS 2016a). This is a modeled estimate with confidence limits ranging from 110,000 to 190,000.

Although the annual number of HIV-infected infants has been decreasing, 1.8 million children younger than age 15 years are living with HIV, predominantly acquired through MTCT before the expansion of effective PMTCT programs, as shown in map 6.4 (UNAIDS 2016a). Many of these children remain undiagnosed and untreated until they become symptomatic. Although additional children older than age 15 years were infected with HIV in utero or at childbirth, it is difficult to estimate their numbers.

Pediatric Burden of Syphilis

Similar maps for congenital syphilis are not available, although map 6.5 approximates relative burdens by country. Children with syphilis are harder to diagnose, map, and count than those with HIV. Worldwide between 1997 and 2003, an estimated 2 million women with

Map 6.1 Global HIV Prevalence among Women Ages 15–24 Years, 2014

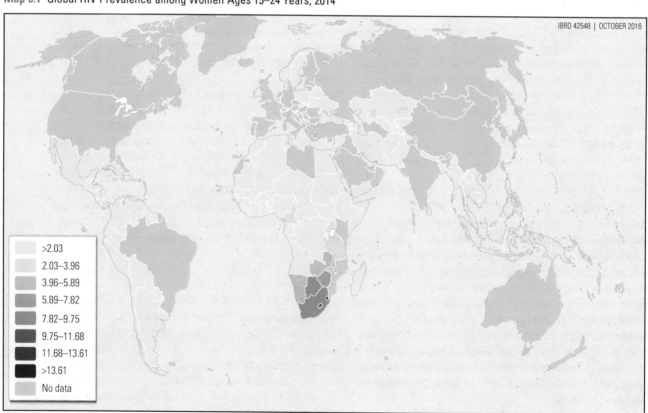

Source: World Bank (http://en.actualitix.com/country/wld/prevalence-of-hiv-women-15-24-years.php).
Note: HIV = human immunodeficiency virus.

Map 6.2 Global Syphilis Seroprevalence among Pregnant Women, 2012

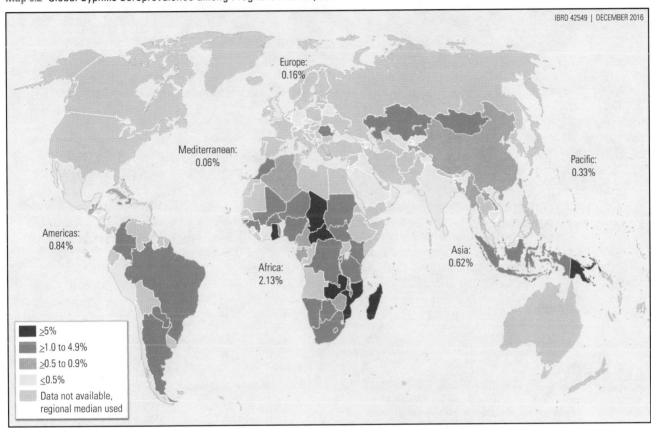

IBRD 42549 | DECEMBER 2016

Europe:
0.16%

Mediterranean:
0.06%

Pacific:
0.33%

Americas:
0.84%

Africa:
2.13%

Asia:
0.62%

≥5%
≥1.0 to 4.9%
≥0.5 to 0.9%
≤0.5%
Data not available,
regional median used

Source: Reprinted from "Global Health Estimates." 2013. Online Database. WHO, Geneva.

syphilis became pregnant, resulting in 728,000–1,527,000 new cases of congenital syphilis each year (Schmid and others 2007). This broad range in estimates of congenital syphilis is a result of poor ability to measure cases.

Other infant complications may also be partially extrapolated from maternal syphilis rates. The WHO estimated that, in 2008, 1.36 million pregnant women worldwide had active syphilis, of whom 80 percent had attended antenatal clinics (ANCs). Among those women, syphilis was responsible for more than 500,000 adverse pregnancy outcomes, including more than 200,000 stillbirths or early fetal deaths, 92,000 neonatal deaths, 65,000 preterm or low-birth-weight infants, and 152,000 infected newborns (Newman and others 2013). Two-thirds of these adverse outcomes occurred in women who had attended ANCs but were not screened or treated for syphilis (Newman and others 2013). The WHO estimates for 2012 illustrate a decline from 2008: 950,000 maternal syphilis infections

resulting in 360,000 adverse outcomes, including 150,000 early fetal deaths or stillbirths, 50,000 preterm or low-birth-weight infants, 60,000 neonatal deaths, and 110,000 infants with congenital infection (WHO 2013).

Consequences of Pediatric HIV and Syphilis

Consequences of Pediatric HIV

Infants who are infected with HIV through MTCT typically have a rapidly progressive course: about half die within two years (Newell and others 2004; Obimbo and others 2004). Infants with later MTCT of HIV through breastfeeding may have a more indolent course than infants with in utero or peripartum HIV acquisition (Becquet and others 2012; Obimbo and others 2009).

Children with untreated pediatric HIV infection have high risk of early mortality, severe malnutrition, and growth faltering, as well as recurrent infections,

Map 6.3 Estimated Number of Children Younger than Age 15 Years Newly Infected with HIV, by Region, 2015

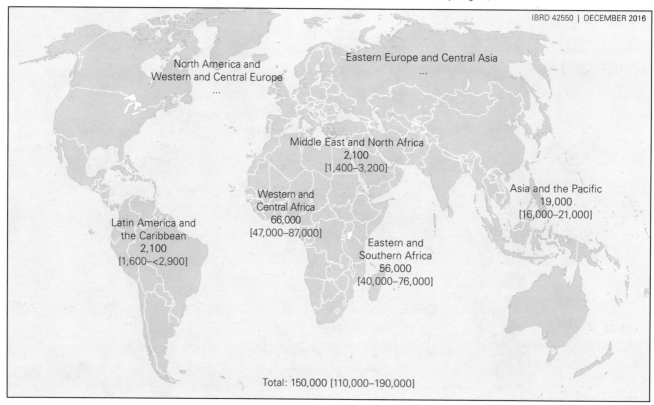

IBRD 42550 | DECEMBER 2016

North America and Western and Central Europe
...

Eastern Europe and Central Asia
...

Middle East and North Africa
2,100
[1,400–3,200]

Western and Central Africa
66,000
[47,000–87,000]

Latin America and the Caribbean
2,100
[1,600–<2,900]

Asia and the Pacific
19,000
[16,000–21,000]

Eastern and Southern Africa
56,000
[40,000–76,000]

Total: 150,000 [110,000–190,000]

Source: UNAIDS 2015. Reproduced, with permission, from UNAIDS; further permission required for reuse.
Note: HIV = human immunodeficiency virus. The estimated 150,000 new infections worldwide only include children younger than age 15 years.

including opportunistic infections such as tuberculosis (Obimbo and others 2004; Obimbo and others 2009), and neurocognitive delays. If given ART early, infants have significantly lower mortality but may have continued deficiencies in growth, persistent morbidity, and compromised neurocognitive ability (Wamalwa and others 2010).

Relative to uninfected mothers, HIV-infected mothers may have increases in other adverse outcomes of pregnancy, including stillbirth, prematurity, and low birth weight (Brocklehurst and French 1998). Their infants, if uninfected but HIV exposed, also have increased risk of morbidity and mortality compared with infants unexposed to HIV, perhaps because of increased immunologic susceptibility, sociodemographic factors, or increased exposure to other infectious diseases (Afran and others 2014; Mofenson and Watts 2014).

Consequences of Pediatric Syphilis

Children with congenital syphilis have a range of presentations, from asymptomatic to a variety of symptoms including rash; skeletal changes; hepatosplenomegaly; and neurologic, renal, pulmonary, or ocular involvement. Moreover, congenital syphilis may result in lifelong disability, particularly when undetected or detected late in infancy (Arnold and Ford-Jones 2000).

A study of women who had not been screened for syphilis in ANCs and delivered babies in a Tanzanian hospital found that, among those with serological evidence of active syphilis, 25 percent delivered a stillborn baby, 20 percent a premature baby, and 33 percent a low-birth-weight baby. Overall, adverse events were noted in 49 percent of infants born to those women, compared with 11 percent of women without syphilis (Watson-Jones, Changalucha, and others 2002). A systematic review of the impact of untreated syphilis on pregnancy outcomes found a consistently higher proportion of adverse pregnancy outcomes in women with untreated syphilis than in uninfected women (Gomez and others 2013). The pooled estimate of neonatal death was 12.3 percent in women with syphilis and 3 percent in women without syphilis.

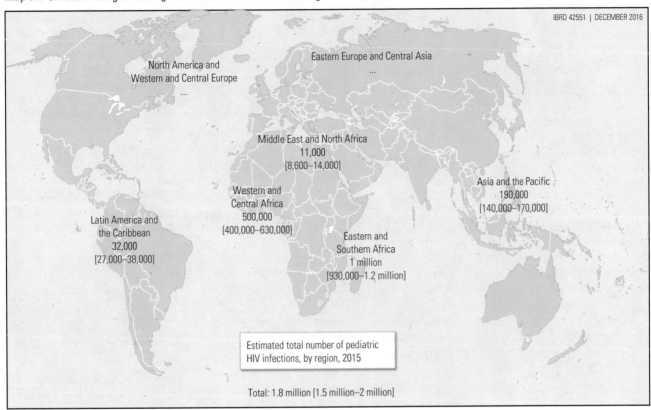

IBRD 42551 | DECEMBER 2016

North America and
Western and Central Europe
...

Eastern Europe and Central Asia
...

Middle East and North Africa
11,000
[8,600–14,000]

Western and
Central Africa
500,000
[400,000–630,000]

Asia and the Pacific
190,000
[140,000–170,000]

Latin America and
the Caribbean
32,000
[27,000–38,000]

Eastern and
Southern Africa
1 million
[930,000–1.2 million]

Estimated total number of pediatric
HIV infections, by region, 2015

Total: 1.8 million [1.5 million–2 million]

Source: UNAIDS 2015. Reproduced, with permission, from UNAIDS; further permission required for reuse.
Note: HIV = human immunodeficiency virus. The estimated 1.8 million infections worldwide only include children younger than age 15 years.

The pooled estimate for stillbirth or prematurity was 25.6 percent and for low birth weight was 12.1 percent among the infants of women with syphilis (Gomez and others 2013). Treatment of pregnant women is estimated to avert these outcomes as outlined in table 6.2.

EFFECTIVENESS AND COVERAGE OF PMTCT INTERVENTIONS

Effectiveness of Interventions for PMTCT of HIV

Identification of HIV during Pregnancy and in Infants
HIV testing during pregnancy initially used the enzyme-linked immunosorbent assay (ELISA) test with opt-in counseling, which resulted in attrition because women elected either not to have the test or not to return for results.[5] The introduction of opt-out HIV testing—in which routine HIV testing is offered to all women unless a woman opts out—has substantially increased the number of women who are tested for HIV (Creek and others 2007; Day and others 2004). In addition, rapid

HIV testing, which can provide results during the same visit, significantly increases the proportion of women who receive their test results (Malonza and others 2003).[6] Rapid HIV testing enables testing of women of unknown HIV status at any time they present to the health care system, including at delivery.

Testing for HIV needs to include not only diagnostic services but also careful counseling of women. Peer counselors and mother-to-mother models have been critically important for helping women cope with their diagnoses, make decisions about disclosure of their results to their partners, and adhere to their medication regimen (Futterman and others 2010; Shetty and others 2008; Shroufi and others 2013).

Women may become infected with HIV during pregnancy or postpartum, and repeat HIV testing is advised to detect and treat women with HIV seroconversion during this period. As PMTCT of HIV expands, women diagnosed with HIV at or before their first antenatal visit routinely receive HIV treatment. However, mothers who are initially seronegative but acquire HIV infection in pregnancy or postpartum are

Map 6.5 Relative Global Concentrations of Congenital Syphilis, by Country

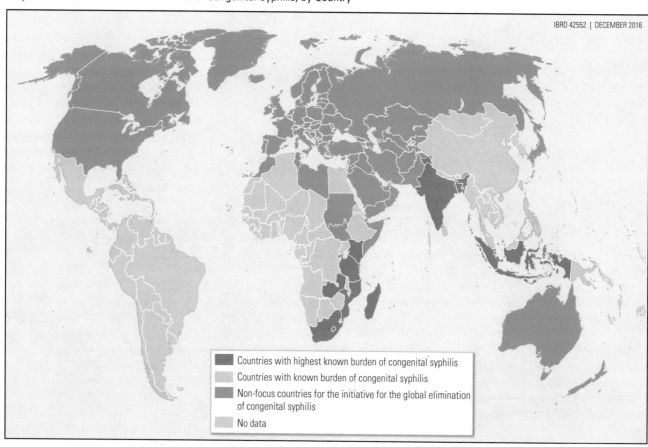

IBRD 42552 | DECEMBER 2016

■ Countries with highest known burden of congenital syphilis
□ Countries with known burden of congenital syphilis
■ Non-focus countries for the initiative for the global elimination of congenital syphilis
□ No data

Source: Reprinted from "Advancing MDGs 4, 5 and 6: Impact of Congenital Syphilis Elimination." Partner Brief, WHO, Geneva; http://apps.who.int/iris/bitstream/10665/70331/1/WHO_RHR _HRP_10.01_eng.pdf. 2010a.
Note: The Initiative for the Global Elimination of Congenital Syphilis was launched by the WHO in 2007 to support global efforts to achieve several of the Millennium Development Goals (MDGs): MDG 4 (reduce child mortality), MDG 5 (improve maternal health), and MDG 6 (combat HIV/AIDS, malaria, and other diseases) (WHO 2010a).

Table 6.2 Adverse Infant Outcomes Potentially Avertable by Treatment of Maternal Syphilis

Outcome	Outcomes averted by treatment (%)
Stillbirth	13.3
Miscarriage	8.1
Neonatal death (age 0–28 days)	9.3
Prematurity or low birth weight	5.8
Infant with clinical evidence of syphilis	19.4
Nonneonatal infant death (age 29–365 days)	3.4
Any adverse outcome	48.7*

Source: LSHTM 2011.
Note: "Treatment" refers to penicillin in pregnancy. * = "Any adverse outcome" is less than the sum of the individual outcomes because of differences in weighting and variance that occur when doing a meta-analysis, as well as the possibility of an infant's having more than one outcome.

often undiagnosed and contribute to an increasing proportion of infant HIV infections that may not be detected until the child presents with symptomatic disease (Drake and others 2014). Thus, repeat HIV testing during pregnancy and postpartum is recommended, although guidelines for frequency and timing of repeat HIV tests in follow-up vary by national setting.

Infants are born with maternal antibodies to HIV, making HIV serologic testing unhelpful for newborns. HIV DNA can be diagnosed from a dried blood spot (DBS) using PCR assays in a central laboratory. DBS HIV DNA virologic rather than serologic testing is recommended for infants (WHO 2010b). Early infant diagnosis (EID) is conducted using DBS HIV DNA tests at age six weeks, followed by testing at age nine months and again at six weeks following cessation of breastfeeding (Luzuriaga and Mofenson 2016). New POC assays for HIV DNA are becoming available that may be useful for decreasing turnaround time for EID results and expediting treatment of infants with HIV.

Antiretroviral Treatment for PMTCT of HIV
ART to decrease MTCT of HIV has been assessed in numerous randomized clinical trials (Siegfried and others 2011). Initial simple short-course regimens, such as single-dose maternal and infant nevirapine administered to the mother during labor and to infants, decreased transmission by 50 percent. Triple-ART and infant prophylaxis regimens increase intervention efficacy.[7] Evidence supporting the use of ART for PMTCT of HIV is Grading of Recommendations Assessment, Development and Evaluation (GRADE) A1 (with large decreases in HIV transmission risk—declining from more than 30 percent to less than 1 percent) (WHO 2012b and 2014b).

Effectiveness of Interventions for PMTCT of Syphilis

Identification of Syphilis during Pregnancy and in Infants
Because most pregnant women with syphilis do not have symptoms, a serological screening test is needed to identify those who are infected. A nontreponemal agglutination test such as the RPR test has traditionally been used. This test is cheap (less than US$0.10) and rapid, but the reagents need to be refrigerated, serum needs to be separated from whole blood, and a plate shaker is needed, meaning that a reliable electricity supply is required. Simple, lateral-flow POC tests have become available in recent years; these tests are sensitive, specific, can be stored at ambient temperature, and can be performed with a sample obtained by finger prick (Jafari and others 2013; Mabey and others 2006). These tests detect treponemal antibodies and cannot distinguish between active and past or treated infection. However, given the disease complications and the simplicity and effectiveness of treatment (penicillin), these tests can provide a net public health benefit (Kuznik and others 2013). A dual POC test for HIV and syphilis has become available that detects both treponemal and nontreponemal antibodies and is both sensitive and specific, with good test performance for the diagnosis of active syphilis (Yin and others 2013). The dual POC test is a pragmatic and attractive approach to promoting integration of PMTCT of HIV-syphilis programs (Kiarie and others 2015).

Women should be tested antenatally at their first visit in pregnancy, preferably before 16 weeks' gestation, and retested in the third trimester. Women who have not been tested before delivery should be tested at delivery.

Infants are born with maternal antibodies, limiting diagnostic utility of routine treponemal or nontreponemal tests. Clinical diagnosis may be made in symptomatic infants, with signs including mucocutaneous lesions, bone changes evident on radiographs, syphilitic rhinitis ("snuffles"), lymphadenopathy, and hematologic changes.

Penicillin Treatment for PMTCT of Syphilis
Women with evidence of syphilis from either a treponemal or nontreponemal test should receive treatment with penicillin (WHO 2006). In Tanzania, women with syphilis who received a single dose of benzathine penicillin before 28 weeks' gestation had the same incidence of adverse pregnancy outcomes as women without syphilis (Watson-Jones, Gumodoka, and others 2002). A systematic review of the impact of penicillin treatment on pregnancy outcomes in women with syphilis showed that treatment with at least 2.4 million units of penicillin reduced the incidence of clinical congenital syphilis by 97 percent (relative risk 0.03) (Blencowe and others 2011). The pooled estimate for reduction of stillbirths was 82 percent, 64 percent for reduction in preterm delivery, and 80 percent for reduction in neonatal death (Blencowe and others 2011). The effect estimates were large and consistent across studies, leading to a strong recommendation for screening and treatment according to the GRADE criteria (Blencowe and others 2011). Seropositive women should receive benzathine penicillin (2.4 million units), and partners should also receive penicillin treatment. Infants of these women should receive 50,000 units/kilogram of benzathine penicillin if asymptomatic or 10 days of crystalline or procaine penicillin if symptomatic. The combined cost of diagnosis and penicillin treatment of maternal syphilis is less than US$1.

PMTCT Implementation and Coverage

PMTCT of HIV
Concerns about stigma and loss of confidentiality motivated the initial intensive, opt-in voluntary counseling and HIV testing models. Routinizing HIV testing has led to much more efficient systems for PMTCT of HIV (Creek and others 2007). HIV stigma may continue to inhibit the likelihood of HIV testing or

ART adherence, but health-system bottlenecks appear to be a comparable or greater barrier to PMTCT implementation (Kinuthia and others 2011). On the positive side, male partner engagement may enhance maternal adherence to antenatal and postnatal care visits and ART, while also improving infant outcomes (Farquhar and others 2001; Taha and others 2007). Other implementation issues relevant to PMTCT effectiveness include the following:

ART Delays and Adherence Constraints. Previous PMTCT antiretroviral regimens, such as Option A, required waiting for CD4 count results to determine ART eligibility, which delayed ART initiation and compromised PMTCT programmatic effectiveness. Options B and B+ use an accelerated test-and-treat approach, with immediate ART following HIV diagnosis without waiting for a CD4 count (Taha and others 2007; WHO 2012b).[8] Long-term adherence to ART may decline for PMTCT regimens postpartum. In an early Option B+ program model in Malawi, initiation of Option B+ led to a rapid increase in the number of women receiving ART, but only 77 percent of women remained on ART at one year following delivery (CDC 2013). Option B or B+ also may decrease sexual transmission of HIV to male HIV-uninfected partners relative to Option A (Cohen and others 2011). The health costs and benefits of Option B versus Option B+ are not well defined (Watts and others 2009). However, between pregnancies, Option B+ with continued ART will encounter fewer health-system bottlenecks than Option B, in which episodic ART is administered only during pregnancy and breastfeeding. Specifically, the maternal and child health (MCH) system will not need to restart ART; however, there may be supply chain challenges in consistent drug procurement. It is also not clear whether young asymptomatic women will maintain long-term adherence to Option B+ between pregnancies, or which strategies may optimize long-term adherence to ART.

Lack of Tailored Counseling Approaches. Other issues facing PMTCT programs require improvement or innovation. As PMTCT programs and HIV care programs expand, an increasing number of women will have been previously diagnosed with HIV and will have begun receiving treatment before they become pregnant. Stratified counseling approaches to previously diagnosed and treated women versus newly diagnosed women do not exist. With Option B+, newly diagnosed women initiate ART for life in the context of pregnancy and need counseling and other interventions to motivate long-term ART adherence.

Lack of Diagnostic System Tracking and Coordination. Medical records of mothers are often not linked to infant medical records, which would facilitate tracking of maternal-to-infant outcomes (Chi, Bolton-Moore, and Holmes 2013). EID-of-HIV programs involve the collection of DBS from infants at age six weeks; the DBS are sent to a central laboratory for HIV PCR testing for detection of HIV DNA. Results from EID programs have unacceptably long turnaround times (Sutcliffe and others 2014; Woldesenbet and others 2014). Consequently, mothers often fail to receive infant results or remain unaware of infant HIV diagnosis, despite testing. Children may not get a diagnosis of HIV until they become ill, resulting in poor long-term outcomes. New POC EID assays may circumvent problems with existing infant HIV diagnostic systems (Jani and others 2014). EID detects perinatal infant HIV infections, but infants with negative early HIV tests remain at risk throughout the breastfeeding period, and repeat testing is important. In addition, in settings of high HIV prevalence, new maternal HIV infection acquired during the pregnancy and breastfeeding periods contributes appreciably to infant HIV infections despite good PMTCT programs (Drake and others 2014).

Late Postnatal Follow-Up during Breastfeeding. Following the six-week postnatal visit, retention decreases, and long-term follow-up to exclude or diagnose infant HIV is erratic. With the scale-up of Option B+, retention beyond the early infant period needs to be improved.

PMTCT of Syphilis

A 1996–97 survey of health ministries in 22 countries in Sub-Saharan Africa concluded that, although 73 percent of women attended ANCs overall, and although syphilis screening of ANC attendees was national policy in nearly all countries, only 38 percent of women were estimated to actually have been screened for syphilis (Gloyd, Chai, and Mercer 2001). Reported reasons for not performing screening in this survey included costs of testing, treatment, and transport; inadequate prioritization; sociocultural resistance; and lack of compliance or awareness by health care workers. In Tanzania, where screening and treatment of ANC attendees for syphilis is national policy, a survey in nine districts found that only 43 percent of 2,256 ANC attenders had been screened, and only 61 percent of seropositive women and 37 percent of their partners had been treated. Watson-Jones and others (2005) found that adequate training, continuity of supplies, supervision, and quality control are critical elements for effective antenatal services but were frequently overlooked. The WHO noted that in 2012, 95 percent coverage of syphilis testing was achieved in only 29 percent of 51 low- and middle-income countries (LMICs) surveyed.[9]

A review of syphilis screening in 13 ANCs in Nairobi, Kenya, where blood was sent to a central laboratory for syphilis serology, found that only 291 of 540 women (54 percent) had been tested. Of 11 who were seropositive, only 1 had been treated. However, after these clinics introduced same-day screening and treatment, 99.9 percent of ANC attendees were screened for syphilis, and 87.3 percent of seropositive women and 50 percent of their partners received treatment (Temmerman, Mohamedalf, and Fransen 1993). The new POC tests make it possible to offer same-day screening and treatment in any health facility, which increases the coverage of screening and treatment in many settings (Hawkes and others 2011; Jenniskens and others 1995).

Cross-Cutting Issues for PMTCT of HIV and Syphilis

MCH is addressed through public health systems and was prioritized in Millennium Development Goal (MDG) 4 (to reduce child mortality) and MDG 5 (to improve maternal health) (Chi, Bolton-Moore, and Holmes 2013); MCH is also part of Sustainable Development Goal 3 (health and well-being at all ages). PMTCT of HIV and PMTCT of syphilis are delivered through the same MCH system. Programs for PMTCT of HIV have used the cascade-of-care approach to identify bottlenecks in services.[10] In many settings, most pregnant women visit an ANC at least once during their pregnancy, at which time routine HIV and syphilis testing can occur. Downstream treatment of women with positive HIV results is measured systematically in countries targeted for PMTCT of HIV, specifically to assess whether mothers were started and maintained on ART, continued in follow-up care, and had their infants tested for HIV through EID programs (UNAIDS 2013). The MCH registers typically include information on syphilis testing. Registers could be enhanced to improve PMTCT of syphilis by leveraging current program evaluation of HIV PMTCT to include variables on syphilis indicators (table 6.3) (WHO 2014b). Enhancements should include monitoring infant receipt of antiretroviral prophylaxis and infant evaluation for clinical syphilis and treatment needs.

Other cross-cutting issue areas affecting PMTCT of both HIV and syphilis include the following:

Male Partner Involvement. Several studies have noted enhanced PMTCT and infant outcomes and treatment adherence among women whose male partners have participated in MCH programs, either through HIV testing or ANC attendance (Aluisio and others 2011; Kalembo and others 2013). A program offering home-based HIV testing to male partners noted high uptake of male HIV testing (Osoti and others 2014). It is difficult to discern whether these benefits are the result of male

Table 6.3 Cross-Cutting Health System Implementation Issues for PMTCT of HIV and Syphilis

Implementation need	PMTCT of syphilis	PMTCT of HIV
Community awareness	Community has not been mobilized	✓
Required ANC attendance	✓	✓
ANC attendance early in pregnancy (optimal for prevention)	✓	✓
MoH recommendation of maternal testing	✓	✓
Availability of POC diagnostic test	✓	✓
National use of POC diagnostic test	✓	✓
QA and QC of lab tests, good supply chain of lab tests	✓	✓
Use of opt-out approach	✓	✓
Availability of one-time treatment	✓	Needs lifelong treatment
Availability of low-cost treatment	✓	Not a one-time cost—ART currently provided by a combination of resources including from government, PEPFAR, or GAP
Usefulness of partner notification and engagement	✓	✓
Availability of standard infant diagnostic test	No laboratory test—clinical diagnosis	✓

Note: ANC = antenatal clinic; ART = antiretroviral treatment; HIV = human immunodeficiency virus; PMTCT = prevention of mother-to-child transmission; GAP = Global AIDS Program; MoH = Ministry of Health; PEPFAR = President's Emergency Plan for AIDS Relief; POC = point-of-care; QA = quality assurance; QC = quality control.

involvement or female self-efficacy, because few women involve male partners in ANC attendance. Efforts to increase this involvement include written invitations, weekend openings, initiatives to provide male partners with incentives to attend, male-friendly clinics, and home visits for male testing and education (Reece and others 2010). Rwanda made a concerted effort to mandate male attendance during antenatal care of women to improve maternal and infant outcomes (Irakoze and others 2012), and male HIV testing increased substantially in parallel with increased facility delivery. Conversely, this approach may stigmatize single mothers. In addition, since syphilis screening leads to male notification and treatment, such screening could be integrated into male partner programs for PMTCT of HIV.

Integration of Family Planning and Primary Maternal HIV and Syphilis Prevention. Postpartum visits are opportunities to increase uptake of contraception and to promote prevention of HIV and other STIs. However, family planning clinics and postpartum family planning clinics do not routinely incorporate HIV or STI prevention or testing.

Community Engagement to Reduce Stigma of Testing and Treatment. Both HIV and syphilis carry a community stigma as STIs. In the case of HIV infection, the combination of high community prevalence, mature epidemics, and increasing community knowledge and advocacy have led to vibrant activism and pragmatic peer mentoring and counseling (Namukwaya and others 2015). In contrast, syphilis awareness lacks community-level advocacy. Individuals are not familiar with the disease or its symptoms and typically do not know whether someone has been identified as having had syphilis. To our knowledge, peer mentoring is not used, and children and parents with syphilis do not have support groups comparable to HIV support groups.

Alignment of the Long-Term Health Benefits of Interventions with the MDGs and General MCH Goals. Comprehensive MCH requires detection and treatment of maternal HIV and syphilis to improve short-term and long-term outcomes for mothers and their children. Interventions may have impacts on multiple outcomes, including decreasing preterm birth, stillbirth, and other morbidity in addition to enhancement of growth, cognition, and survival.

Intersection of PMTCT Interventions with General Prevention and Treatment of HIV and Syphilis. Community-level HIV treatment and prevention

occur at voluntary counseling and testing centers, in comprehensive HIV care and treatment programs, and at PMTCT programs in MCH clinics. Women with HIV may shift between PMTCT and HIV care and treatment programs, and Options B and B+ approaches ensure comparable antiretroviral regimens during this process. Women's HIV care and treatment affect both sexual and mother-to-infant transmission and contribute to community HIV prevention. Because pregnancy is an identifiable trigger point for accessing HIV testing, it is often a sentinel event for family HIV diagnosis in young couples who do not perceive themselves at risk for HIV but who live in settings with high HIV prevalence.

Syphilis is similarly preferentially detected during pregnancy because of widespread access to care and testing. However, since no large syphilis care and treatment centers exist, prevention and detection of syphilis typically occur at primary health care visits or at sexually transmitted disease (STD) treatment programs. MCH clinics have limited experience with standard partner testing for STIs and often refer male partners to STD programs for syphilis testing. An alternative approach would be to include partner syphilis testing and follow-up in routine MCH care, analogous to HIV, without referral to STD services.

Methods for Assessing PMTCT Program Effectiveness

Program Evaluation Methodology for PMTCT of HIV

Standardized national surveys using routine infant DBS for HIV DNA testing at age six weeks can capture most mother-infant pairs, because uptake of routine six-week infant immunizations is high, regardless of HIV diagnosis or PMTCT intervention uptake (WHO 2012a). Thus, the evaluation of programs for PMTCT of HIV can be standardized because there is a hard outcome—infant HIV status. However, this outcome measure is not the final infant HIV outcome, because breastmilk transmission may occur until cessation of breastfeeding, particularly if women do not adhere to ART. Later time points—nine months and thereafter—for MCH visits are less well attended and do not include infants who become lost to follow-up or who die before assessment. Community household-based surveys may complement facility-based assessment, reach mother-infant pairs who do not attend facility services, and enable better estimation of HIV-free survival at later endpoints, but assessment of programmatic effectiveness may have shortcomings depending on participation and self-reporting (Conrad and others 2012; Kohler and others 2014; Larsson and others 2012).

UNAIDS has developed evaluation strategies for consistent assessment of national programs for PMTCT of HIV. In these surveys, several countries report higher than 90 percent PMTCT coverage, with a transmission risk of less than 5 percent (UNAIDS 2015). Remarkable progress has been made in Botswana, South Africa, and several eastern and southern African countries. Indeed, PMTCT interventions have been responsible for a substantial proportion of the declines in overall HIV incidence globally. However, although infant HIV infections have plummeted (figure 6.1), the world did not accomplish the UNAIDS PMTCT goal of no more than 15,000 infections by 2015 (UNAIDS 2016b).

Program Evaluation Methodology for PMTCT of Syphilis

The Rapid Syphilis Test Toolkit is a comprehensive guide for planning and management of syphilis prevention programs that includes guidelines on policy advocacy, supply chain, cost-effectiveness, clinical training, laboratory procedures, and monitoring and evaluation with clearly defined program indicators (LSHTM 2011). Specifically, it states that the number of women screened, who tested positive, and whose male partners were tested, as well as the number of syphilis-positive women who received same-day penicillin, should be summarized from clinic register data. In addition, the number of cases of congenital syphilis and other complications of syphilis should be summarized as a percentage of live

births. The guidelines also note the additional sequelae that are anticipated to decrease following implementation of an effective program for PMTCT of syphilis (figure 6.2 and table 6.4).

Combined Validation of PMTCT of HIV and Syphilis

In 2014, the WHO published a framework for validation of PMTCT of HIV and syphilis for program managers and policy makers (WHO 2014a). This framework was used to validate PMTCT of HIV and syphilis in Cuba in 2015. Measures assessed include MTCT of HIV and congenital syphilis rate, and coverage (greater than 95 percent) of antenatal syphilis and HIV testing and treatment (WHO 2015).

COST-EFFECTIVENESS OF PMTCT OF HIV AND SYPHILIS

Cost-effectiveness analyses allow policy makers to prioritize approaches for disease prevention. In this case, they help policy makers compare PMTCT of HIV with PMTCT of syphilis and potentially estimate the benefits of a dual approach to PMTCT. The cost-effectiveness studies presented are all from low- and middle-income settings. Tables 6.5 and 6.6 present cost-effectiveness estimates for PMTCT of HIV and PMTCT of syphilis, respectively, extracted from systematic reviews of the literature (Johri and Ako-Arrey 2011; Levin and Brouwer 2014) and using only those

Figure 6.1 Number of New HIV Infections among Children in 21 Global Plan Priority Countries, 2000–15

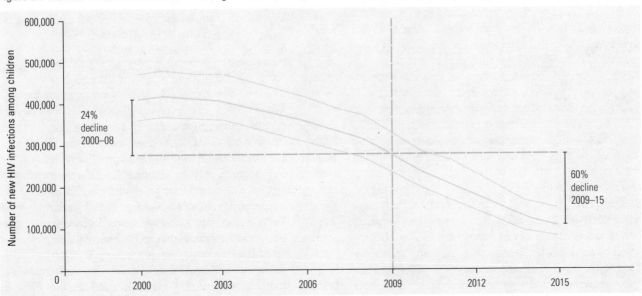

Source: UNAIDS 2016b.

Note: HIV = human immunodeficiency virus.

Figure 6.2 Syphilis Monitoring and Evaluation Results Pyramid

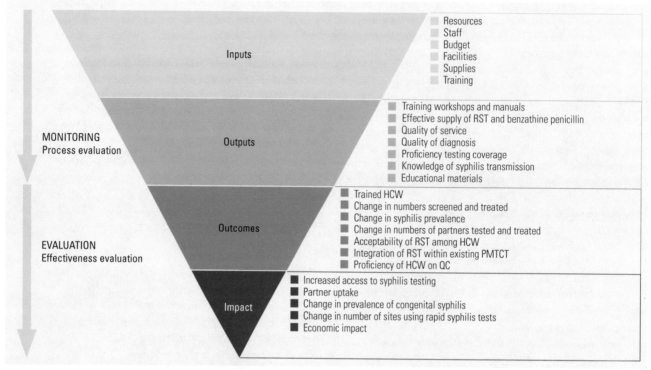

Source: Adapted from LSHTM 2011, figure 1; originally published in UNAIDS/World Bank, panel 1.
Note: HCW = health care workers; PMTCT = prevention of mother-to-child transmission; QC = quality control; RST = rapid syphilis test.

Table 6.4 Required Indicators for Global Validation of PMTCT of HIV and Syphilis

HIV

Impact indicators

Case rate of new pediatric HIV infections resulting from MTCT of HIV of ≤50 cases per 100,000 live births; AND

MTCT rate of HIV of <5 percent in breastfeeding populations OR MTCT rate of HIV of <2 percent in nonbreastfeeding populations

Process indicators

ANC coverage (at least one visit) of ≥95 percent

Coverage of pregnant women who know their HIV status of ≥95 percent

ARV coverage of HIV-positive pregnant women of ≥90 percent

Congenital syphilis

Impact indicator

Case rate of congenital syphilis ≤50 cases per 100,000 live births

Process indicators

ANC coverage (at least one visit) of ≥95 percent

Coverage of syphilis testing of pregnant women of ≥95 percent

Treatment of syphilis-seropositive pregnant women ≥95 percent

Source: WHO 2014a.
Note: ANC = antenatal care; ARV = antiretroviral; PMTCT = elimination of mother-to-child transmission; HIV = human immunodeficiency virus; MTCT = mother-to-child transmission.

articles published after 2000. In addition, a supplementary search yielded more recent studies published between 2010 and 2015. We extracted 24 cost-effectiveness metrics or ranges from 18 articles for PMTCT of HIV and 23 from 8 articles for PMTCT of syphilis and integrated approaches. All estimates have been converted into 2012 US dollars.

Cost-Effectiveness of PMTCT of HIV

The cost-effectiveness of extended combination prophylaxis for PMTCT of HIV is well established, especially in high-risk areas, compared with no intervention or the use of single-dose nevirapine or short-course prophylaxis (Johri and Ako-Arrey 2011). In high-risk regions such as Sub-Saharan Africa, regional models estimate that Option A is cost-effective, ranging from US$25 to US$730 per disability-adjusted life year (DALY) averted. Since 2010, country-specific studies have focused on comparing the incremental costs and benefits of new guidelines related to treatment Options A, B, or B+. For the LMICs shown in table 6.5, these options benefit infants and mothers, save money over time, and are cost-effective (Ciaranello and others 2013; Fasawe 2013). For resource-constrained countries with high risk of HIV, there are

Table 6.5 Cost-Effectiveness Analyses since 2000 of Interventions for PMTCT of HIV

Region	Intervention	Comparator	Country or region	Cost in 2012 US$	Unit of outcome	Study
Sub-Saharan Africa			Regional studies			
	Option A	No intervention	SSA	25.71–43.68	DALYs averted	Marseille and others 2000
	Option A	No intervention	SSA	184.48	Infection averted	Stringer and others 2000
	Option A	No intervention	SSA	136.67–730.49	DALYs averted	Sweat and others 2004
	Option A	No intervention	AFR-E	38.94	DALYs averted	Hogan and others 2005
			Country studies			
	Option A	No intervention	South Africa	47–99	DALYs averted	Wilkinson, Floyd, and Gilks 2000
	Option A and mass screening	No intervention	Chad	1,862	Infection averted	Hutton, Wyss, and N'Diekhor 2003
	Option B	Current practice	Malawi	40	DALYs averted	Orlando and others 2010
	Option B+	No intervention	Tanzania	251	DALYs averted	Robberstad and Evjen-Olsen 2010
	Option B	Option A	Nigeria	171	DALYs averted	Shah and others 2011
	Option B	Option A	Uganda	65–140	DALYs averted	Kuznik and others 2012
	Option B+	No intervention	Uganda	291–502	DALYs averted	Kuznik and others 2012
	Option B	Option A	South Africa	1,187	QALYs gained	Zulliger and others 2014
	Option B+	Option B	Zimbabwe	1370[a]	YLS	Ciaranello and others 2013
	Option A	Current practice[b]	Malawi	30	DALYs averted	Fasawe and others 2013
	Option B	Current practice[b]	Malawi	54	DALYs averted	Fasawe and others 2013
	Option B+	Current practice[b]	Malawi	50	DALYs averted	Fasawe and others 2013
	Option B	Option A	Zambia	82	QALYs gained	Ishikawa and others 2014
	Option B+	Option A	Zambia	145	QALYs gained	Ishikawa and others 2014
Latin America and the Caribbean						
	Option A and mass screening	No intervention	Peru	3,092–7,924	DALYs averted	Aldridge and others 2009
South Asia						
	Universal screening	No intervention	India	32	YLS	Kumar and others 2006
	Targeted screening	No intervention	India	68	YLS	Kumar and others 2006
East Asia and Pacific						
	Option A	No intervention	SEAR-D	355	DALYs averted	Hogan and others 2005
	Option B	Option A	Thailand	2,299–3,225	DALYs averted	Teerawattananon and others 2005
	Option B	Option A	Thailand	Cost saving	QALYs gained	Werayingyong and others 2013

Note: AFR-E = WHO member states Botswana, Burundi, the Central African Republic, the Republic of Congo, Côte d'Ivoire, the Democratic Republic of Congo, Eritrea, Ethiopia, Kenya, Lesotho, Malawi, Mozambique, Namibia, Rwanda, South Africa, Swaziland, Uganda, Tanzania, Zambia, and Zimbabwe; CEA = cost-effectiveness analysis; DALYs = disability-adjusted life years; PMTCT = prevention of mother-to-child transmission; HIV = human immunodeficiency virus; QALYs = quality-adjusted life years; SEAR-D = WHO member states Bangladesh, Bhutan, the Democratic People's Republic of Korea, India, Maldives, Myanmar, and Nepal; SSA = Sub-Saharan Africa; YLS = years of life saved.
a. This estimate is in 2013 US dollars, as in the publication, because a reliable consumer price index deflator was not available for Zimbabwe.
b. Mix of interventions including single-dose nevirapine, or dual-drug regimen containing zidovudine, or triple-drug antiretroviral prophylaxis until cessation of breastfeeding.

debates about the advantages and disadvantages of Option B+ (lifelong ART for all pregnant and HIV-infected women), in part because Option B+ is effective in saving lives but is associated with higher short-term costs compared with Options A and B (Saeed, Kim, and Abrams 2013). In low-prevalence settings, such as Thailand, PMTCT is cost-effective at US$2,299–US$3,225 per DALY averted; it may even be cost saving, depending on adherence to ART and relative costs of ARVs. HIV treatment guidelines and PMTCT intervention options are continuously evolving; country context (prevalence rates, drug costs, health utilization rates, health system capacity) will affect the relative cost-effectiveness of and the choice of best strategy from these and future options.

Table 6.6 Cost-Effectiveness Analyses since 2000 of Interventions for PMTCT of Syphilis

Region	Intervention	Comparator	Country or region	Cost in 2012 US$	Unit of outcome	Study
Sub-Saharan Africa			Global or regional			
	Rapid point-of-care ICS[a] screen and treat with penicillin	No screening	Sub-Saharan Africa	11	DALYs averted	Kuznik and others 2013
	Laboratory RPR[a] screen and treat with penicillin	No screening	Global low prevalence	24–111	DALYs averted	Kahn and others 2014
	Laboratory RPR[a] screen and treat with penicillin	No screening	Global high prevalence	Cost-saving	DALYs averted	Kahn and others 2014
			Country studies			
	Laboratory RPR[a] screen and treat with penicillin	No screening	Tanzania	23	DALYs averted	Terris-Prestholt and others 2015
			Tanzania	16	DALYs averted	Terris-Prestholt and others 2003
			Zambia	26	DALYs averted	Terris-Prestholt and others 2015
	Rapid point-of-care ICS[a] screen and treat with penicillin	No screening	Tanzania	17	DALYs averted	Terris-Prestholt and others 2015
			Zambia	16	DALYs averted	Terris-Prestholt and others 2015
	Dual screening with ICS[a] and RPR and treat with penicillin	No screening	Tanzania	18	DALYs averted	Terris-Prestholt and others 2015
			Zambia	70	DALYs averted	Terris-Prestholt and others 2015
	ICS screen and treat with penicillin	RPR screen and treat	Tanzania	16	DALYs averted	Terris-Prestholt and others 2015
			Zambia	11	DALYs averted	Terris-Prestholt and others 2015
	ICS screen and treat with penicillin	Current practice: 62 percent tested, 2.8 percent positive, 10.4 percent of positives treated	Zambia	453	DALYs averted	Larson and others 2014
		Improved treatment: 100 percent of positives treated	Zambia	48	DALYs averted	Larson and others 2014
		Improved screening and treatment: 100 percent tested and treated	Zambia	45	DALYs averted	Larson and others 2014
Latin America and the Caribbean						
	Laboratory RPR[a] screen and treat with penicillin	No screening	Peru	139	DALYs averted	Terris-Prestholt and others 2015
	Rapid point-of-care ICS[a] screen and treat with penicillin	No screening	Peru	54	DALYs averted	Terris-Prestholt and others 2015
	Dual screening with ICS and RPR and treat with penicillin	No screening	Peru	76	DALYs averted	Terris-Prestholt and others 2015
	ICS screen and treat with penicillin	RPR screen and treat	Peru	Cost-saving	DALYs averted	Terris-Prestholt and others 2015
	Rapid point-of-care ICS screen added to rapid HIV screen and treat	National HIV screening program with no syphilis screening	Haiti	21	DALYs averted	Schackman and others 2007

table continues next page

Table 6.6 Cost-Effectiveness Analyses since 2000 of Interventions for PMTCT of Syphilis (continued)

Region	Intervention	Comparator	Country or region	Cost in 2012 US$	Unit of outcome	Study
East Asia and Pacific						
	Laboratory TRUST[a] and TTPA[b] test and treat with penicillin	No screening	China	369	DALYs averted	Hong and others 2010
	Laboratory RPR screen and treat with penicillin	No screening	China	200	DALYs averted	Owusu-Edusei and others 2014
	Rapid ICS screen added to rapid HIV screen and treat		China	160	DALYs averted	Owusu-Edusei and others 2014

Note: DALYs = disability-adjusted life years; PMTCT = prevention of mother-to-child transmission; HIV = human immunodeficiency virus; ICS = point-of-care immunochromatographic strip; RPR = lab-based rapid plasma reagin test; TPPA = *T. pallidum* particle agglutination lab-based treponemal test; TRUST = lab-based Toluidine Red Unheated Serum Test.

a. Nontreponemal tests that cannot distinguish between recent and previous infection.

b. Treponemal test.

At this point, Option B+ is the recommended strategy and is aligned with the WHO 2015 recommendations to treat all individuals with lifelong ART.

Cost-Effectiveness of PMTCT of Syphilis

Several models have demonstrated the cost-effectiveness of PMTCT in Sub-Saharan Africa, demonstrating that antenatal syphilis screening is cost-effective, even at low prevalence rates; it may even be cost saving in high-prevalence settings (Blandford and others 2007; Kahn and others 2014; Kuznik and others 2013; Rydzak and Goldie 2008). In high-risk areas, PMTCT of syphilis is among one of the most cost-effective interventions available. For example, a study of the cost-effectiveness of prenatal syphilis screening in Tanzania found that the cost was US$1.44 per woman screened, US$20 per woman treated, US$16 per DALY averted, or US$10.56 per DALY averted if stillbirths averted were included in the calculation (Terris-Prestholt and others 2003). Operational costs of testing may influence cost-effectiveness (Levin 2007). Cost-effectiveness analysis using country-level evaluation data has been critical for informing the choice of screening strategy and for highlighting the importance of achieving higher screening rates and full adherence to guidelines (Larson and others 2014; Terris-Prestholt and others 2015). Of 10 screening and treatment approaches, Terris-Prestholt and others (2015) found that treponemal-based rapid POC syphilis test-and-treat strategies were the most cost-effective, at US$16–US$17 per DALY averted in Zambia and Tanzania and US$54 per DALY averted in Peru. In Peru, the incremental cost-effectiveness of switching from a lab-based test to a rapid POC test was cost saving.

Larson and others (2014) showed that the cost per DALY averted falls from US$628 to US$60 with full adherence to screening and treatment guidelines.

Cost-Effectiveness of Integrated PMTCT of Syphilis and HIV

Although information on the integration of PMTCT of syphilis and HIV is limited, two studies provide information on the potential benefit of adding syphilis diagnosis and treatment to existing PMTCT of HIV services. In Haiti, a high-prevalence country for both HIV and syphilis, adding an RPR test-and-treat model in rural areas cost US$6.83 per DALY averted, while the estimate for an urban program was US$9.95 per DALY averted (Schackman and others 2007). In a recent study in China—a low-prevalence country for both HIV and syphilis—syphilis screening or integrated HIV and syphilis screening were both more cost-effective than HIV screening alone (Owusu-Edusei and others 2014). This is a conservative finding, given the low prevalence of both HIV and syphilis. Based on the results from the Haiti and China studies, it is likely that in settings with higher prevalence rates for both HIV and syphilis, integrating HIV and syphilis services would be the most cost-effective option.

LESSONS FROM CASE STUDIES

PMTCT of HIV: Success in South Africa

As an upper-middle-income country, South Africa has been able to make enormous progress in implementing PMTCT. MTCT rates decreased from more than 30 percent to approximately 4 percent in a national programmatic evaluation of all six-week-old infants tested at 572 clinics throughout the country (Goga, Dinh, and

Jackson 2010). Maternal HIV seroprevalence had been 32 percent at the time of the study.[11] An astonishing 98 percent of pregnant women received testing, and almost 92 percent of HIV-positive women received ART. Gaps remained in CD4 testing and EID.

The study also illustrates that high maternal HIV seroprevalence contributes to the effectiveness of PMTCT programs. When large numbers of mothers in a given health center or community are HIV infected, large networks of peer counselors can lead to more effective peer counseling, dissemination of education and programs, and acceptability of HIV testing and ART.

PMTCT of Syphilis: Successful Rapid POC Models

A study conducted in six countries showed that the introduction of POC testing for syphilis in ANCs was well accepted in a wide variety of settings and delivery platforms, from the Amazon rain forest in Brazil to the cities of China, and from primary health posts to teaching hospitals. After the introduction of POC testing, more than 90 percent of those who attended ANCs were screened for syphilis in all six countries, and more than 90 percent of women testing positive received treatment on the same day (Mabey and others 2012).

Table 6.7 Estimated Costs and Benefits of Screening for HIV and Syphilis in Theoretical Sub-Saharan African Population of 20,000 Pregnant Women Yearly

	Syphilis	HIV*
Seroprevalence	8%	15%
Test positive	1,600	3,000
Result		
Stillbirth averted[a]	200 cases	—
LBW averted[a]	184 cases	—
HIV averted*	—	246 cases
Cost of counselling and testing per woman	$1.44	$18.50
Cost of treatment	$0.5–1.00	$4.00 for single-dose nevirapine
Cost per case averted	Stillbirth, $318; all adverse pregnancy outcomes, $44–187[b]	$506
Cost per DALY saved	$4.0–18.7[b]	$19.2

Source: Peeling and others 2004.
Note: DALY = disability-adjusted life year; HIV = human immunodeficiency virus; LBW = low birth weight; — = not available.
*Data from Sweat and others 2004; Marseille and others 2000.
a. Assuming 4 percent of women have rapid plasma reagin titer of 1:8 or more, of whom 25 percent will have stillbirth, and 33 percent will deliver live baby weighing below 2.5 kilograms, compared with 10 percent of seronegative women (Brocklehurst and French 1998; Grimprel and others 1991).
b. Range taken from studies summarized in UNAIDS 2013.

In Peru, 604 trained health providers implemented POC testing for syphilis using the two-for-one strategy: offering both syphilis and HIV testing with one finger prick. This approach resulted in testing and treatment on the first visit; before POC testing was introduced, a woman would typically not receive her syphilis result until her fifth clinic visit, 27 days later (Garcia and others 2013). In Uganda and Zambia, the integration of HIV and syphilis screening in ANCs, using two POC tests, was well accepted and led to increased coverage of syphilis screening (Strasser and others 2012).

PMTCT of HIV and Syphilis: An Integrated Model

Peeling and others (2004) described cases of infants born to HIV-infected mothers in Haiti who successfully escaped HIV transmission following ART and formula feeding but who acquired congenital syphilis. These cases highlight the lost opportunity to prevent syphilis among women attending ANCs; despite receiving interventions for PMTCT of HIV (testing and treatment), the women failed to access simple measures to detect and prevent congenital syphilis.

In the authors' assessment of a Sub-Saharan African population of pregnant women (table 6.7), the costs of testing and treatment per DALY averted were estimated to be lower for syphilis (US$4–US$18.70) than for HIV (US$19.20). They noted that more efficient POC diagnostic testing for syphilis and development of oral regimens could further enhance congenital syphilis prevention efforts.

CONCLUSIONS

During the next few years, the concerted efforts to prevent infant HIV infection will continue and perhaps accelerate (IATT 2014). This intensive focus on HIV provides an opportune time to leverage program improvements to similarly target elimination of congenital syphilis and other adverse outcomes of maternal syphilis. Programs that monitor HIV outcomes can also track syphilis testing, treatment, and transmission and motivate prompt, efficient management of newly diagnosed cases in pregnancy, as shown in China, Haiti, Peru, Uganda, and Zambia. In short, improving PMTCT of syphilis within PMTCT of HIV is a feasible, low-cost strategy that would yield enormous benefits to mothers and infants. The incremental cost is small and the gains—prevention of stillbirth, preterm birth, and long-term disability of children delivered by women with maternal syphilis—are substantial.

NOTES

World Bank Income Classifications as of July 2014 are as follows, based on estimates of gross national income (GNI) per capita for 2013:

- Low-income countries (LICs) = US$1,045 or less
- Middle-income countries (MICs) are subdivided:
  (a) lower-middle-income = US$1,046–US$4,125
  (b) upper-middle-income (UMICs) = US$4,126–US$12,745
- High-income countries (HICs) = US$12,746 or more.

1. Increased risk of spontaneous abortion: odds ratio (OR) 4.05, 95 percent confidence interval (CI) 2.75–5.96; perinatal mortality: OR 1.79, 95 percent CI 1.1–2.81; infant mortality: OR 3.69, 95 percent CI 3.03–4.49; intrauterine growth retardation: OR 1.7, 95 percent CI 1.43–2.02; low birth weight: OR 2.09, 95 percent CI 1.86–2.35; preterm birth: OR 1.83, 95 percent CI 1.63–2.06.

2. In Option A, women received zidovudine as early as 14 weeks into the pregnancy, a single dose of nevirapine during labor, and two weeks of tenofovir and emtricitabine after delivery.

3. In Option B, women received one of two triple anti-HIV drug regimens as early as 14 weeks into the pregnancy—either (1) lamivudine, zidovudine, and ritonavir-boosted lopinavir (called the "lamivudine combination"); or (2) tenofovir, emtricitabine, and ritonavir-boosted lopinavir (called the "tenofovir combination"). Option B+ is lifelong ART.

4. This study has not yet been published, but the press release noted increased adverse outcomes (NIH 2014).

5. The ELISA test detects antibodies to HIV, usually from either a blood sample (drawn from a vein) or saliva. A positive result is often confirmed with a follow-up test such as the Western blot, which is less likely than the ELISA test to yield a false positive result. Results from most ELISA tests and confirmatory Western blot tests are usually available within 2 to 14 days.

6. A rapid HIV test uses technology similar to the ELISA test (except blood is drawn from a finger prick instead of from a vein) but produces results in approximately 20 minutes. As with the ELISA test, however, a "preliminary positive" result must be confirmed with a second test, either a Western blot test or a second rapid test from another manufacturer.

7. The studied triple-ART in PROMISE was either lamivudine, zidovudine, and ritonavir-boosted lopinavir, or tenofovir, emtricitabine, and ritonavir-boosted lopinavir. All infants received six weeks of nevirapine prophylaxis.

8. Option B+ refers to lifelong ART initiated in pregnancy

9. WHO, Global Health Observatory Data Repository, Antenatal care (ANC) attendees tested for syphilis at first ANC visit, Data by country (http://apps.who.int/gho/data/node.main.A1358STI).

10. The cascade of care model refers to following interventions from diagnosis to receipt of interventions to continued retention in care.

11. Maternal HIV seroprevalence was 32.0 percent (95 percent CI 30.7–33.3).

REFERENCES

Afran, L., M. Garcia Knight, E. Nduati, B. C. Urban, R. S. Heyderman, and others. 2014. "HIV-Exposed Uninfected Children: A Growing Population with a Vulnerable Immune System?" *Clinical and Experimental Immunology* 176 (1): 11–22.

Aldridge R. W., D. Iglesias, C. F. Caceres, and J. J. Miranda. 2009. "Determining a Cost Effective Intervention Response to HIV/AIDS in Peru." *BMC Public Health* 9: 352. doi:10.1186/1471-2458-9-352.

Aluisio, A., B. A. Richardson, R. Bosire, G. John-Stewart, D. Mbori-Ngacha, and others. 2011. "Male Antenatal Attendance and HIV Testing Are Associated with Decreased Infant HIV Infection and Increased HIV-Free Survival." *Journal of Acquired Immune Deficiency Syndromes* 56 (1): 76–82.

Arnold, S. R., and E. L. Ford-Jones. 2000. "Congenital Syphilis: A Guide to Diagnosis and Management." *Paediatrics and Child Health* 5 (8): 463–69.

Becquet, R., M. Marston, F. Dabis, L. H. Moulton, G. Gray, and others. 2012. "Children Who Acquire HIV Infection Perinatally Are at Higher Risk of Early Death than Those Acquiring Infection through Breastmilk: A Meta-Analysis." *PLoS One* 7 (2): e28510.

Blandford, J. M., T. L. Gift, S. Vasaikar, D. Mwesigwa-Kayongo, P. Dlali, and others. 2007. "Cost-Effectiveness of On-Site Antenatal Screening to Prevent Congenital Syphilis in Rural Eastern Cape Province, Republic of South Africa." *Sexually Transmitted Diseases* 34 (Suppl 7): S61–66.

Blencowe, H., S. Cousens, M. Kamb, S. Berman, and J. E. Lawn. 2011. "Lives Saved Tool Supplement Detection and Treatment of Syphilis in Pregnancy to Reduce Syphilis Related Stillbirths and Neonatal Mortality." *BMC Public Health* 11 (Suppl 3): S9.

Brocklehurst, P., and R. French. 1998. "The Association between Maternal HIV Infection and Perinatal Outcome: A Systematic Review of the Literature and Meta-Analysis." *British Journal of Obstetrics and Gynaecology* 105 (8): 836–48.

CDC (Centers for Disease Control and Prevention). 2013. "Impact of an Innovative Approach to Prevent Mother-to-Child Transmission of HIV—Malawi, July 2011–September 2012." *Morbidity and Mortality Weekly Report* 62 (8): 148–51. http://www.cdc.gov/mmwr/preview/mmwrhtml/mm6208a3.htm.

Chi, B. H., C. Bolton-Moore, and C. B. Holmes. 2013. "Prevention of Mother-to-Child HIV Transmission within the Continuum of Maternal, Newborn, and Child Health Services." *Current Opinion in HIV and AIDS* 8 (5): 498–503.

Ciaranello, A. L., F. Perez, B. Engelsmann, R. P. Walensky, A. Mushavi, and others. 2013. "Cost-Effectiveness of World Health Organization 2010 Guidelines for Prevention of Mother-to-Child HIV Transmission in Zimbabwe." *Clinical Infectious Diseases* 56 (3): 430–46.

Cohen, M. S., Y. Q. Chen, M. McCauley, T. Gamble, M. C. Hosseinipour, and others. 2011. "Prevention of HIV-1

Infection with Early Antiretroviral Therapy." *New England Journal of Medicine* 365 (6): 493–505.

Conrad, P., M. De Allegri, A. Moses, E. C. Larsson, F. Neuhann, and others. 2012. "Antenatal Care Services in Rural Uganda: Missed Opportunities for Good-Quality Care." *Qualitative Health Research* 22 (5): 619–29.

Creek, T. L., R. Ntumy, K. Seipone, M. Smith, M. Mogodi, and others. 2007. "Successful Introduction of Routine Opt-Out HIV Testing in Antenatal Care in Botswana." *Journal of Acquired Immune Deficiency Syndromes* 45 (1): 102–7.

Day, S., D. Lakhani, M. Hankins, and C. A. Rodgers. 2004. "Improving Uptake of HIV Testing in Patients with a Confirmed STI." *International Journal of STD and AIDS* 15 (9): 626–28.

De Cock, K. M., M. G. Fowler, E. Mercier, I. de Vincenzi, J. Saba, and others. 2000. "Prevention of Mother-to-Child HIV Transmission in Resource-Poor Countries: Translating Research into Policy and Practice." *Journal of the American Medical Association* 283 (9): 1175–82.

Drake, A. L., A. Wagner, B. Richardson, and G. John-Stewart. 2014. "Incident HIV during Pregnancy and Postpartum and Risk of Mother-to-Child HIV Transmission: A Systematic Review and Meta-Analysis." *PLoS Medicine* 11 (2): e1001608.

Farquhar, C., D. A. Mbori-Ngacha, R. K. Bosire, R. W. Nduati, J. K. Kreiss, and others. 2001. "Partner Notification by HIV-1 Seropositive Pregnant Women: Association with Infant Feeding Decisions." *AIDS* 15 (6): 815–17.

Fasawe, O., C. Avila, N. Shaffer, E. Schouten, E. Chimbwandira, and others. 2013. "Cost-Effectiveness Analysis of Option B+ for HIV Prevention and Treatment of Mothers and Children in Malawi." *PLoS One* 8 (3): e57778. doi:10.1371/journal.pone.0057778.

Futterman, D., J. Shea, M. Besser, S. Stafford, K. Desmond, and others. 2010. "Mamekhaya: A Pilot Study Combining a Cognitive-Behavioral Intervention and Mentor Mothers with PMTCT Services in South Africa." *AIDS Care: Psychological and Socio-Medical Aspects of AIDS/HIV* 22 (9): 1093–100.

Garcia, P. J., C. P. Carcamo, M. Chiappe, M. Valderrama, S. La Rosa, and others. 2013. "Rapid Syphilis Tests as Catalysts for Health Systems Strengthening: A Case Study from Peru." *PLoS One* 8 (6): e66905.

Gloyd, S., S. Chai, and M. A. Mercer. 2001. "Antenatal Syphilis in Sub-Saharan Africa: Missed Opportunities for Mortality Reduction." *Health Policy and Planning* 16 (1): 29–34.

Goga, A., T.-H. Dinh, and D. Jackson. 2010. *Evaluation of the Effectiveness of the National Prevention of Mother-to-Child Transmission (PMTCT) Programme on Infant HIV Measured at Six Weeks Postpartum in South Africa*. Pretoria: Department of Health, Republic of South Africa.

Gomez, G. B., M. L. Kamb, L. M. Newman, J. Mark, N. Broutet, and others. 2013. "Untreated Maternal Syphilis and Adverse Outcomes of Pregnancy: A Systematic Review and Meta-Analysis." *Bulletin of the World Health Organization* 91 (3): 217–26.

Grimprel, E., P. J. Sanchez, G. D. Wendel, J. M. Burstain, G. H. McCracken Jr., and others. 1991. "Use of Polymerase Chain Reaction and Rabbit Infectivity Testing to Detect *Treponema pallidum* in Amniotic Fluid, Fetal and Neonatal Sera, and Cerebrospinal Fluid." *Journal of Clinical Microbiology* 29 (8): 1711–18.

Hawkes, S., N. Matin, N. Broutet, and N. Low. 2011. "Effectiveness of Interventions to Improve Screening for Syphilis in Pregnancy: A Systematic Review and Meta-Analysis." *The Lancet Infectious Diseases* 11 (9): 684–91.

Hogan, D. R., R. Baltussen, C. Hayashi, J. A. Lauer, and J. A. Salomon. 2005. "Cost Effectiveness Analysis of Strategies to Combat HIV/AIDS in Developing Countries." *British Medical Journal* 331 (7530): 1431–37.

Hong, F. C., J. B. Liu, T. J. Feng, X. L. Liu, P. Pan, and others. 2010. "Congenital Syphilis: An Economic Evaluation of a Prevention Program in China." *Sexually Transmitted Diseases* 37 (1): 26–31.

Hutton, G., K. Wyss, and Y. N'Diekhor. 2003. "Prioritization of Prevention Activities to Combat the Spread of HIV/AIDS in Resource Constrained Settings: A Cost-Effectiveness Analysis from Chad, Central Africa." *International Journal of Health Planning and Management* 18 (2): 117–36.

IATT (Inter-Agency Task Team). 2014. *HIV and Sexual and Reproductive Health Programming: Innovative Approaches to Integrated Service Delivery*. Compendium of Case Studies. New York, NY: IATT. https://sustainabledevelopment.un .org/content/documents/1779HIV_SRH_Programming _Integrated_Service_Delivery_Case_Studies_1.pdf.

Irakoze, A. A., S. Nsanzimana, M. Jennifer, E. Remera, C. Karangwa, and others. 2012. "Family Centered Approach in PMTCT Program, Rwanda 2005–2011." Presentation to the Coalition for Children Affected by AIDS Symposium, "Children and HIV: Closing the Gap," Washington, DC, July 20.

Ishikawa, N., T. Shimbo, S. Miyano, I. Sikazwe, A. Mwango, and others. 2014. "Health Outcomes and Cost Impact of the New WHO 2013 Guidelines on Prevention of Mother-to-Child Transmission of HIV in Zambia." *PLoS One* 9 (3): e90991.

Jafari, Y., R. W. Peeling, S. Shivkumar, C. Claessens, L. Joseph, and others. 2013. "Are *Treponema pallidum* Specific Rapid and Point-of-Care Tests for Syphilis Accurate Enough for Screening in Resource Limited Settings? Evidence from a Meta-Analysis." *PLoS One* 8 (2): e54695.

Jani, I. V., B. Meggi, N. Mabunda, A. Vubil, N. E. Sitoe, and others. 2014. "Accurate Early Infant HIV Diagnosis in Primary Health Clinics Using a Point-of-Care Nucleic Acid Test." *Journal of Acquired Immune Deficiency Syndromes* 67 (1): e1–4.

Jenniskens, F., E. Obwaka, S. Kirisuah, S. Moses, F. M. Yusufali, and others. 1995. "Syphilis Control in Pregnancy: Decentralization of Screening Facilities to Primary Care Level, a Demonstration Project in Nairobi, Kenya." *International Journal of Gynecology and Obstetrics* 48 (Suppl): S121–28.

John, G. C., and J. Kreiss. 1996. "Mother-to-Child Transmission of Human Immunodeficiency Virus Type 1." *Epidemiologic Reviews* 18 (2): 149–57.

John, G. C., R. W. Nduati, D. A. Mbori-Ngacha, B. A. Richardson, D. Panteleeff, and others. 2001. "Correlates of Mother-to-Child Human Immunodeficiency Virus Type 1 (HIV-1) Transmission: Association with Maternal Plasma HIV-1 RNA Load, Genital HIV-1 DNA Shedding, and Breast Infections." *Journal of Infectious Diseases* 183 (2): 206–12.

Johri, M., and D. Ako-Arrey. 2011. "The Cost-Effectiveness of Preventing Mother-to-Child Transmission of HIV in Low- and Middle-Income Countries: Systematic Review." *Cost Effectiveness and Resource Allocation* 9: 3.

Kahn, J. G., A. Jiwani, G. B. Gomez, S. J. Hawkes, H. W. Chesson, and others. 2014. "The Cost and Cost-Effectiveness of Scaling up Screening and Treatment of Syphilis in Pregnancy: A Model." *PLoS One* 9 (1): e87510.

Kalembo, F. W., M. Zgambo, A. N. Mulaga, D. Yukai, and N. I. Ahmed. 2013. "Association between Male Partner Involvement and the Uptake of Prevention of Mother-to-Child Transmission of HIV (PMTCT) Interventions in Mwanza District, Malawi: A Retrospective Cohort Study." *PLoS One* 8 (6): e66517.

Kiarie, J. N., C. K. Mishra, M. Temmerman, and L. Newman. 2015. "Accelerating the Dual Elimination of Mother-To-Child Transmission of Syphilis and HIV: Why Now?" *International Journal of Gynecology and Obstetrics* 130 (Suppl 1): S1–3.

Kinuthia, J., J. N. Kiarie, C. Farquhar, B. A. Richardson, R. Nduati, and others. 2011. "Uptake of Prevention of Mother to Child Transmission Interventions in Kenya: Health Systems Are More Influential than Stigma." *Journal of the International AIDS Society* 14: 61.

Kohler, P. K., J. Okanda, J. Kinuthia, L. A. Mills, G. Olilo, and others. 2014. "Community-Based Evaluation of PMTCT Uptake in Nyanza Province, Kenya." *PLoS One* 9 (10): e110110.

Kumar, M., S. Birch, A. Maturana, and A. Gafni. 2006. "Economic Evaluation of HIV Screening in Pregnant Women Attending Antenatal Clinics in India." *Health Policy* 77 (2): 233–43.

Kuznik, A., M. Lamorde, S. Hermans, B. Castelnuovo, B. Auerbach, and others. 2012. "Evaluating the Cost-Effectiveness of Combination Antiretroviral Therapy for the Prevention of Mother-to-Child Transmission of HIV in Uganda." *Bulletin of the World Health Organization* 90 (8): 595–603.

Kuznik, A., M. Lamorde, A. Nyabigambo, and Y. C. Manabe. 2013. "Antenatal Syphilis Screening Using Point-of-Care Testing in Sub-Saharan African Countries: A Cost-Effectiveness Analysis." *PLoS Medicine* 10 (11): e1001545.

Larson, B. A., D. Lembela-Bwalya, R. Bonawitz, E. E. Hammond, D. M. Thea, and others. 2014. "Finding a Needle in the Haystack: The Costs and Cost-Effectiveness of Syphilis Diagnosis and Treatment during Pregnancy to Prevent Congenital Syphilis in Kalomo District of Zambia." *PLoS One* 9 (12): e113868. doi:10.1371/journal.pone.0113868.

Larsson, E. C., A. E. Thorson, G. Pariyo, P. Waiswa, D. Kadobera, and others. 2012. "Missed Opportunities: Barriers to HIV Testing during Pregnancy from a Population Based Cohort Study in Rural Uganda." *PLoS One* 7 (8): e37590.

Lee, M. J., R. J. Hallmark, L. M. Frenkel, and G. Del Priore. 1998. "Maternal Syphilis and Vertical Perinatal Transmission of Human Immunodeficiency Virus Type-1 Infection." *International Journal of Gynecology and Obstetrics* 63 (3): 247–52.

Levin, C. E., and E. Brouwer. 2014. "Saving Brains: Literature Review of Reproductive, Neonatal, Child and Maternal Health and Nutrition Interventions to Mitigate Basic Risk Factors to Promote Child Development." Working Paper Series, GCC 14-08.

Levin, C. E., M. Steele, D. Atherly, S. G. Garcia, F. Tinajeros, and others. 2007. "Analysis of the Operational Costs of Using Rapid Syphilis Tests for the Detection of Maternal Syphilis in Bolivia and Mozambique." *Sexually Transmitted Diseases* 34 (Suppl 7): S47–54.

LSHTM (London School of Hygiene and Tropical Medicine). 2011. *The Rapid Syphilis Test Toolkit: A Guide to Planning, Management and Implementation.* London: LSHTM. https://www.lshtm.ac.uk/itd/crd/research /rapidsyphilistoolkit/rapid_syphilis_test_toolkit.pdf.

Luzuriaga, K., and L. M. Mofenson. 2016. "Challenges in the Elimination of Pediatric HIV-1 Infection." *New England Journal of Medicine* 374: 761–71.

Mabey, D., R. W. Peeling, R. Ballard, A. S. Benzaken, E. Galban, and others. 2006. "Prospective, Multi-Centre Clinic-Based Evaluation of Four Rapid Diagnostic Tests for Syphilis." *Sexually Transmitted Infections* 82 (Suppl 5): v13–16.

Mabey, D. C., K. A. Sollis, H. A. Kelly, A. S. Benzaken, E. Bitarakwate, and others. 2012. "Point-of-Care Tests to Strengthen Health Systems and Save Newborn Lives: The Case of Syphilis." *PLoS Medicine* 9 (6): e1001233.

Malonza, I. M., B. A. Richardson, J. K. Kreiss, J. J. Bwayo, and G. C. Stewart. 2003. "The Effect of Rapid HIV-1 Testing on Uptake of Perinatal HIV-1 Interventions: A Randomized Clinical Trial." *AIDS* 17 (1): 113–18.

Marseille, E., J. G. Kahn, F. Mmiro, L. Guay, P. Musoke, and others. 2000. "The Cost Effectiveness of a Single-Dose Nevirapine Regimen to Mother and Infant to Reduce Vertical HIV-1 Transmission in Sub-Saharan Africa." *Annals of the New York Academy of Sciences* 918: 53–56.

Mofenson, L. M., and D. H. Watts. 2014. "Safety of Pediatric HIV Elimination: The Growing Population of HIV- and Antiretroviral-Exposed but Uninfected Infants." *PLoS Medicine* 11 (4): e1001636.

Mwapasa, V., S. J. Rogerson, J. J. Kwiek, P. E. Wilson, D. Milner, and others. 2006. "Maternal Syphilis Infection Is Associated with Increased Risk of Mother-to-Child Transmission of HIV in Malawi." *AIDS* 20 (14): 1869–77.

Namukwaya, Z., L. Barlow-Mosha, P. Mudiope, A. Kekitinwa, E. Matovu, and others. 2015. "Use of Peers, Community Lay Persons and Village Health Team (VHT) Members Improves Six-Week Postnatal Clinic (PNC) Follow-up and Early Infant HIV Diagnosis (EID) in Urban and Rural Health Units in Uganda: A One-Year Implementation Study." *BMC Health Services Research* 15 (1). doi:10.1186/ s12913-015-1213-5.

Newell, M. L., H. Coovadia, M. Cortina-Borja, N. Rollins, P. Gaillard, and others. 2004. "Mortality of Infected and

Uninfected Infants Born to HIV-Infected Mothers in Africa: A Pooled Analysis." *The Lancet* 364 (9441): 1236–43.

Newman, L., M. Kamb, S. Hawkes, G. Gomez, L. Say, and others. 2013. "Global Estimates of Syphilis in Pregnancy and Associated Adverse Outcomes: Analysis of Multinational Antenatal Surveillance Data." *PLoS Medicine* 10 (2): e1001396.

NIH (National Institutes of Health). 2014. "NIH-Sponsored Study Identifies Superior Drug Regimen for Preventing Mother-to-Child HIV Transmission." Press release, November 17. http://www.nih.gov/news/health/nov2014 /niaid-17.htm.

Obimbo, E. M., D. A. Mbori-Ngacha, J. O. Ochieng, B. A. Richardson, P. A. Otieno, and others. 2004. "Predictors of Early Mortality in a Cohort of Human Immunodeficiency Virus Type 1-Infected African Children." *Pediatric Infectious Disease Journal* 23 (6): 536–43.

Obimbo, E. M., D. Wamalwa, B. Richardson, D. Mbori-Ngacha, J. Overbaugh, and others. 2009. "Pediatric HIV-1 in Kenya: Pattern and Correlates of Viral Load and Association with Mortality." *Journal of Acquired Immune Deficiency Syndromes* 51 (2): 209–15.

Orlando, S., M. C. Marazzi, S. Mancinelli, G. Liotta, S. Ceffa, and others. 2010. "Cost-Effectiveness of Using HAART in Prevention of Mother-to-Child Transmission in the DREAM-Project Malawi." *Journal of Acquired Immune Deficiency Syndromes* 55 (5): 631–14.

Osoti, A. O., G. John-Stewart, J. Kiarie, B. Richardson, J. Kinuthia, and others. 2014. "Home Visits during Pregnancy Enhance Male Partner HIV Counselling and Testing in Kenya: A Randomized Clinical Trial." *AIDS* 28 (1): 95–103.

Owusu-Edusei, K. Jr., G. Tao, T. L. Gift, A. Wang, L. Wang, and others. 2014. "Cost-Effectiveness of Integrated Routine Offering of Prenatal HIV and Syphilis Screening in China." *Sexually Transmitted Diseases* 41 (2): 103–10.

Palmer, H. M., S. P. Higgins, A. J. Herring, and M. A. Kingston. 2003. "Use of PCR in the Diagnosis of Early Syphilis in the United Kingdom." *Sexually Transmitted Infections* 79 (6): 479–83.

Peeling, R. W., D. Mabey, D. W. Fitzgerald, and D. Watson-Jones. 2004. "Avoiding HIV and Dying of Syphilis." *The Lancet* 364 (9445): 1561–63.

Reece, M., A. Hollub, M. Nangami, and K. Lane. 2010. "Assessing Male Spousal Engagement with Prevention of Mother-to-Child Transmission (PMTCT) Programs in Western Kenya." *AIDS Care: Psychological and Socio-Medical Aspects of AIDS/HIV* 22 (6): 743–50.

Robberstad, B., and B. Evjen-Olsen. 2010. "Preventing Mother to Child Transmission of HIV with Highly Active Antiretroviral Treatment in Tanzania—A Prospective Cost-Effectiveness Study." *Journal of Acquired Immune Deficiency Syndromes* 55 (3): 397–403.

Rydzak, C. E., and S. J. Goldie. 2008. "Cost Effectiveness of Rapid Point-of-Care Prenatal Syphilis Screening in Sub-Saharan Africa." *Sexually Transmitted Diseases* 35 (9): 775–84.

Saeed, A., M. H. Kim, and E. J. Abrams. 2013. "Risks and Benefits of Lifelong Antiretroviral Treatment for Pregnant and Breastfeeding Women: A Review of the Evidence for

the Option B+ Approach." *Current Opinion in HIV and AIDS* 8 (5): 474–89.

Sanchez, P. J., G. D. Wendel Jr., E. Grimprel, M. Goldberg, M. Hall, and others. 1993. "Evaluation of Molecular Methodologies and Rabbit Infectivity Testing for the Diagnosis of Congenital Syphilis and Neonatal Central Nervous System Invasion by *Treponema pallidum*." *Journal of Infectious Diseases* 167 (1): 148–57.

Schackman, B. R., C. P. Neukermans, S. N. Fontain, C. Nolte, P. Joseph, and others. 2007. "Cost-Effectiveness of Rapid Syphilis Screening in Prenatal HIV Testing Programs in Haiti." *PLoS Medicine* 4 (5): e183.

Schmid, G. P., B. P. Stoner, S. Hawkes, and N. Broutet. 2007. "The Need and Plan for Global Elimination of Congenital Syphilis." *Sexually Transmitted Diseases* 34 (Suppl 7): S5–10.

Schulte, J. M., S. Burkham, D. Hamaker, M. E. St. Louis, J. M. Paffel, and others. 2001. "Syphilis among HIV-Infected Mothers and Their Infants in Texas from 1988 to 1994." *Sexually Transmitted Diseases* 28 (6): 315–20.

Shah, M., B. Johns, A. Abimiku, and D. G. Walker. 2011. "Cost-Effectiveness of New WHO Recommendations for Prevention of Mother-to-Child Transmission of HIV in a Resource-Limited Setting." *AIDS* 25 (8): 1093–102.

Shetty, A. K., C. Marangwanda, L. Stranix-Chibanda, W. Chandisarewa, E. Chirapa, and others. 2008. "The Feasibility of Preventing Mother-to-Child Transmission of HIV Using Peer Counselors in Zimbabwe." *AIDS Research and Therapy* 5: 17.

Shields, M., R. J. Guy, N. J. Jeoffreys, R. J. Finlayson, and B. Donovan. 2012. "A Longitudinal Evaluation of *Treponema pallidum* PCR Testing in Early Syphilis." *BMC Infectious Diseases* 12: 353.

Shroufi, A., E. Mafara, J. F. Saint-Sauveur, F. Taziwa, and M. C. Vinoles. 2013. "Mother to Mother (M2M) Peer Support for Women in Prevention of Mother to Child Transmission (PMTCT) Programmes: A Qualitative Study." *PLoS One* 8 (6): e64717.

Siegfried, N., L. van der Merwe, P. Brocklehurst, and T. T. Sint. 2011. "Antiretrovirals for Reducing the Risk of Mother-to-Child Transmission of HIV Infection." *Cochrane Database of Systematic Reviews* (7): CD003510.

Strasser, S., E. Bitarakwate, M. Gill, H. J. Hoffman, O. Musana, and others. 2012. "Introduction of Rapid Syphilis Testing within Prevention of Mother-to-Child Transmission of HIV Programs in Uganda and Zambia: A Field Acceptability and Feasibility Study." *Journal of Acquired Immune Deficiency Syndromes* 61 (3): e40–46.

Stringer, J. S., D. J. Rouse, S. H. Vermund, R. L. Goldenberg, M. Sinkala, and others. 2000. "Cost-Effective Use of Nevirapine to Prevent Vertical HIV Transmission in Sub-Saharan Africa." *Journal of Acquired Immune Deficiency Syndromes* 24 (4): 369–77.

Sutcliffe, C. G., J. H. van Dijk, F. Hamangaba, F. Mayani, and W. J. Moss. 2014. "Turnaround Time for Early Infant HIV Diagnosis in Rural Zambia: A Chart Review." *PLoS One* 9 (1): e87028.

Sweat, M. D., K. R. O'Reilly, G. P. Schmid, J. Denison, and I. de Zoysa. 2004. "Cost-Effectiveness of Nevirapine to Prevent

Mother-to-Child HIV Transmission in Eight African Countries." *AIDS* 18 (12): 1661–71.

Taha, T. E., D. R. Hoover, N. I. Kumwenda, S. A. Fiscus, G. Kafulafula, and others. 2007. "Late Postnatal Transmission of HIV-1 and Associated Factors." *Journal of Infectious Diseases* 196 (1): 10–14.

Teerawattananon, Y., T. Vos, V. Tangcharoensathien, and M. Mugford. 2005. "Cost-Effectiveness of Models for Prevention of Vertical HIV Transmission—Voluntary Counseling and Testing and Choices of Drug Regimen." *Cost Effectiveness and Resource Allocation* 3: 7.

Temmerman, M., F. Mohamedalf, and L. Fransen. 1993. "Syphilis Prevention in Pregnancy: An Opportunity to Improve Reproductive and Child Health in Kenya." *Health Policy and Planning* 8 (2): 122–27.

Terris-Prestholt, F., P. Vickerman, S. Torres-Rueda, N. Santesso, S. Sweeney, and others. 2015. "The Cost-Effectiveness of 10 Antenatal Syphilis Screening and Treatment Approaches in Peru, Tanzania, and Zambia." *International Journal of Gynecology and Obstetrics* 130 (Suppl 1): S73–80.

Terris-Prestholt, F., D. Watson-Jones, K. Mugeye, L. Kumaranayake, L. Ndeki, and others. 2003. "Is Antenatal Syphilis Screening Still Cost Effective in Sub-Saharan Africa." *Sexually Transmitted Infections* 79 (5): 375–81.

Townsend, C. L., M. Cortina-Borja, C. S. Peckham, and P. A. Tookey. 2007. "Antiretroviral Therapy and Premature Delivery in Diagnosed HIV-Infected Women in the United Kingdom and Ireland." *AIDS* 21 (8): 1019–26.

Townsend, C. L., P. A. Tookey, M. L. Newell, and M. Cortina-Borja. 2010. "Antiretroviral Therapy in Pregnancy: Balancing the Risk of Preterm Delivery with Prevention of Mother-to-Child HIV Transmission." *Antiviral Therapy* 15 (5): 775–83.

UNAIDS (Joint United Nations Programme on HIV/AIDS). 2011. Press Release: "World Leaders Launch Plan to Eliminate New HIV Infections Among Children by 2015." UNAIDS, Geneva. http://www.unaids.org/en/resources /presscentre/pressreleaseandstatementarchive/2011/june /20110609prglobalplanchildren.

———. 2013. *Global Report: UNAIDS Report on the Global AIDS Epidemic 2013*. Geneva: UNAIDS.

———. 2015. *2015 Progress Report on the Global Plan towards the Elimination of New HIV Infections among Children and Keeping Their Mothers Alive*. Geneva: UNAIDS. http://www.unaids.org/sites/default/files/media_asset /JC2774_2015ProgressReport_GlobalPlan_en.pdf.

———. 2016a. Core Epidemiology Slides. 23 June 2016. http://www.unaids.org/en/resources/documents/2016 /core-epidemiology-slides.

———. 2016b. *On the Fast-Track to an AIDS-Free Generation*. Geneva: UNAIDS. http://www.unaids.org/sites/default /files/media_asset/GlobalPlan2016_en.pdf

UNAIDS and World Bank. 2002. "National AIDS Councils: Monitoring and Evaluation Operations Manual." UNAIDS, Geneva. http://www.unaids.org/sites/default/files/media _asset/jc808-moneval_en_1.pdf.

Wamalwa, D. C., E. M. Obimbo, C. Farquhar, B. A. Richardson, D. A. Mbori-Ngacha, and others. 2010. "Predictors of Mortality in HIV-1 Infected Children on Antiretroviral Therapy in Kenya: A Prospective Cohort." *BMC Pediatrics* 10: 33.

Watson-Jones, D., J. Changalucha, B. Gumodoka, H. Weiss, M. Rusizoka, and others. 2002. "Syphilis in Pregnancy in Tanzania. I. Impact of Maternal Syphilis on Outcome of Pregnancy." *Journal of Infectious Diseases* 186 (7): 940–47.

Watson-Jones, D., B. Gumodoka, H. Weiss, J. Changalucha, J. Todd, and others. 2002. "Syphilis in Pregnancy in Tanzania. II. The Effectiveness of Antenatal Syphilis Screening and Single-Dose Benzathine Penicillin Treatment for the Prevention of Adverse Pregnancy Outcomes." *Journal of Infectious Diseases* 186 (7): 948–57.

Watson-Jones, D., M. Oliff, F. Terris-Prestholt, J. Changalucha, B. Gumodoka, and others. 2005. "Antenatal Syphilis Screening in Sub-Saharan Africa: Lessons Learned from Tanzania." *Tropical Medicine and International Health* 10 (9): 934–43.

Watts, D. H., M. Lu, B. Thompson, R. E. Tuomala, W. A. Meyer III, and others. 2009. "Treatment Interruption after Pregnancy: Effects on Disease Progression and Laboratory Findings." *Infectious Diseases in Obstetrics and Gynecology* 2009: 456717.

Werayingyong, P., N. Phanuphak, K. Chokephaibulkit, S. Tantivess, N. Kullert, and others. 2013. "Economic Evaluation of 3-Drug Antiretroviral Regimens for the Prevention of Mother-to-Child HIV Transmission in Thailand." *Asia-Pacific Journal of Public Health* 27 (2): NP866–76.

WHO (World Health Organization). 2006. "Prevention of Mother-to-Child Transmission of Syphilis: Integrated Management of Pregnancy and Childbirth." Standards for Maternal and Neonatal Care. WHO, Geneva. http:// www.who.int/reproductivehealth/publications/maternal _perinatal_health/prevention_mtct_syphilis.pdf.

———. 2010a. "Advancing MDGs 4, 5 and 6: Impact of Congenital Syphilis Elimination." Partner Brief. WHO, Geneva. http://apps.who.int/iris/bitstream/10665/70331/1 /WHO_RHR_HRP_10.01_eng.pdf.

———. 2010b. *WHO Recommendations on the Diagnosis of HIV Infection in Infants and Children*. Geneva: WHO. http://apps .who.int/iris/bitstream/10665/44275/1/9789241599085 _eng.pdf.

———. 2012a. *Measuring the Impact of National PMTCT Programs: Towards the Elimination of New HIV Infections among Children by 2015 and Keeping Their Mothers Alive*. Geneva: WHO.

———. 2012b. *Programmatic Update: Use of Antiretroviral Drugs for Treating Pregnant Women and Preventing HIV Infection in Infants*. HIV/AIDS Programme. Geneva: WHO. http://www .who.int/hiv/pub/mtct/programmatic_update2012/en/.

———. 2013. Global Health Estimates. Online Database. WHO, Geneva. http://www.who.int/healthinfo/global _burden_disease/en/.

———. 2014a. *Global Guidance on Criteria and Processes for Validation: Elimination of Mother-to-Child Transmission of HIV and Syphilis*. Geneva: WHO.

———. 2014b. *Report on Global Sexually Transmitted Infection Surveillance 2013*. Geneva: WHO. http://apps

.who.int/iris/bitstream/10665/112922/1/9789241507400 _eng.pdf?ua=1.

———. 2015. "WHO Validates Elimination of Mother-to-Child Transmission of HIV and Syphilis in Cuba." Press release, June 30, WHO, Geneva. http://www.who.int /mediacentre/news/releases/2015/mtct-hiv-cuba/en/.

Wilkinson, D., K. Floyd, and C. F. Gilks. 2000. "National and Provincial Estimated Costs and Cost Effectiveness of a Programme to Reduce Mother-to-Child HIV Transmission in South Africa." *South African Medical Journal* 90 (8): 794–98.

Woldesenbet, S. A., D. Jackson, A. E. Goga, S. Crowley, T. Doherty, and others. 2014. "Missed Opportunities for Early Infant HIV Diagnosis: Results of a National Study in South Africa." *Journal of Acquired Immune Deficiency Syndromes* 68 (3): e26–32.

Yeganegh, N., H. Watts, M. Camarca, G. Soares, E. Joao, and others. 2015. "Syphilis in HIV-Infected Mothers and Infants: Results from the NICHD/HPTN 040 Study." *Pediatric Infectious Disease Journal* 34 (3): e52–57.

Yin, Y. P., X. S. Chen, W. H. Wei, K. L. Gong, W. L. Cao, and others. 2013. "A Dual Point-of-Care Test Shows Good Performance in Simultaneously Detecting Nontreponemal and Treponemal Antibodies in Patients with Syphilis: A Multisite Evaluation Study in China." *Clinical Infectious Diseases* 56 (5): 659–65.

Zulliger, R., S. Black, D. R. Holtgrave, A. L. Ciaranello, L. G. Bekker, and others. 2014. "Cost-Effectiveness of a Package of Interventions for Expedited Antiretroviral Therapy Initiation during Pregnancy in Cape Town, South Africa." *AIDS and Behavior* 18 (4): 697–705.

Chapter 7

Cost-Effectiveness of Interventions to Prevent HIV Acquisition

Geoff P. Garnett, Shari Krishnaratne, Kate L. Harris,
Timothy B. Hallett, Michael Santos, Joanne E. Enstone,
Bernadette Hensen, Gina Dallabetta, Paul Revill,
Simon A. J. Gregson, and James R. Hargreaves

INTRODUCTION

Because of the severe health consequences of human immunodeficiency virus/acquired immune deficiency syndrome (HIV/AIDS) and the costs of lifelong treatment, inexpensive and effective HIV prevention is bound to be cost-effective. But what constitutes HIV prevention, and can it be affordable and effective? The use of condoms that cost a few cents and prevent a young adult from acquiring a chronic and fatal disease will, over time, be cost saving. Avoiding sex with someone who is infected with HIV/AIDS will be even more so. What can be done to get people to use condoms? What can be done to facilitate the avoidance of risky sexual encounters? Additional efficacious biomedical tools have become available, but similar questions persist: What can be done to get young women at risk to use oral truvada effectively as preexposure prophylaxis (PrEP) and to get young men at risk to be circumcised? The answers to these questions will determine what packages of prevention are essential, how much prevention programs should cost, and how cost-effective they can be. This chapter reviews current evidence about the efficacy, effectiveness, and costs of HIV/AIDS prevention products, programs, and approaches.

HISTORY OF THE HIV/AIDS PANDEMIC AND PREVENTION INITIATIVES

Clusters of fatal infectious and chronic diseases were first detected in 1981, leading to remarkably rapid identification of HIV; development of tests to identify persons infected; and mapping of the routes of transmission via sex, blood products, and sharing of injection equipment (Oppenheimer 1988). Unfortunately, it also became clear that over a long and variable period averaging about 12 years, everyone infected would develop AIDS and die (Brandt 1987). This awareness lent urgency to identifying ways of preventing and treating HIV. Restrictions on who could donate blood and HIV screening of blood products were found to close off transmission via blood products (Hoots 2001). The use of clean needles and syringes was found to stop transmission among people who injected drugs (Fuller, Ford, and Rudolph 2009). Consistent and correct use of condoms was found to stop sexual transmission of HIV (Steiner and others 2008). Lowering the number of sexual partners was found to reduce risks, with mutually monogamous couples protected from sexual transmission (May and Anderson 1987). Although too late for many, this new knowledge allowed many others to avoid

Corresponding author: Geoff P. Garnett, Bill & Melinda Gates Foundation, Seattle, Washington, United States; Geoff.Garnett@gatesfoundation.org.

acquiring HIV infection. However, it also required people to perceive the risk and to adopt and rigorously adhere to difficult and unappealing behaviors. HIV continued to spread (Anderson and others 1991).

Quantifying the impact of these interventions is difficult. It requires knowing what the incidence would be in their absence. Moreover, a concentrated epidemic with heterogeneous transmission and acquisition risks will become saturated (Anderson and May 1990). Thus, a drop in incidence and leveling off of prevalence are expected, even in the absence of prevention (Hallett and others 2006). Nonetheless, reported changes in risk behavior have reduced the spread of HIV in some populations, particularly among people who inject drugs (PWID) and men who have sex with men (MSM) in high-income countries (Fuller, Ford and Rudolph 2009), sex workers and their clients in Thailand (Nelson and others 1996), and the general population in Uganda and Zimbabwe (Gregson and others 2007; Stoneburner and Low-Beer 2004).

In 1996, combination antiretroviral treatment was reported to be efficacious in reducing viral replication and in reconstituting the immune system (Eron and Hirsch 2008). Effective treatment transformed the response to the epidemic, initially dramatically reducing AIDS deaths in high-income countries (Palella and others 1998). Major reductions in medication costs and increased investments from the U.S. President's Emergency Plan for AIDS Relief (PEPFAR); the Global Fund to Fight AIDS, Tuberculosis and Malaria (the Global Fund); and others led to widespread treatment in low- and middle-income countries (LMICs) (Ford and others 2013). Initially, the impact of treatment on HIV transmission and spread was unclear, but evidence from randomized controlled trials (RCTs) demonstrated that antiretroviral treatment was extremely efficacious in preventing transmission (Cohen and others 2011). This finding and the clinical benefits of early treatment led the World Health Organization (WHO) to recommend that all people living with HIV should receive treatment (WHO 2015b; Holmes and others 2017).

However, the number of infected people on treatment remains far below the total number infected, and further prevention is required. By the end of 2014, an estimated 36.9 million people were living with HIV globally, and 2 million new infections were occurring each year (UNAIDS 2015), even with more than 15 million people globally receiving treatment. With the global response becoming difficult to sustain, there is an urgent need not only to scale up treatment, but also to make available other affordable and effective packages of prevention. Further expansion of treatment will reduce the infectiousness of infected persons; targets have been set for treatment expansion (including prevention among HIV-negative persons) (Piot and others 2015). However, logistical and social barriers mean that some delays will occur between infection and treatment, and many will fail HIV treatment. Even in populations in which coverage of treatment has hit the 90 percent targets for diagnosis, initiation of treatment, and suppression of viral load, the disease continues to spread (Gaolathe and others 2016).

CHALLENGES IN REVIEWING THE EFFICACY AND EFFECTIVENESS OF HIV PREVENTION

Determining the causal impact of prevention activities in affecting outcomes of interest (that is, reducing HIV infections and ultimately preserving health) has proved much more challenging than for many other kinds of health care intervention. We explore reasons for this challenge related to difficulties in categorizing and defining prevention interventions, defining and measuring intervention endpoints, and designing studies of impact.

Categorizing and Defining HIV Prevention Interventions

HIV prevention interventions have been categorized as biomedical, behavioral, or structural. These categories are based on whether the intervention includes use of a biomedical product or procedure, involves people changing their risk behavior, or targets changes in the environment within which risk takes place (Merson and others 2008). Thinking of these approaches as separate and distinct ignores the requirements for interventions to be effective in the real world. HIV transmissibility needs to be reduced—either by a product used during exposure or by a reduction in exposure. We call these direct mechanisms. Getting these products to be used requires behavioral changes, for example using condoms, taking PrEP, or getting circumcised. Such changes are only possible when condoms are available; PrEP programs and circumcision are organized; and laws do not prevent people from accessing clean needles, condoms, circumcision, or oral PrEP. Holistic or combined approaches are required (Hankins and de Zalduondo 2010; Schwartländer and others 2011), and the trials to test interventions need to consider all three categories, each of which should be carefully described if they are to be replicated and scaled up (figure 7.1).

Such combination approaches have been promoted to prevent the spread of HIV (Hankins and de Zalduondo 2010; Schwärtlander and others 2011). However, combining the use of prevention products, each with evidence of biological efficacy, can also be thought of as

Figure 7.1 Elements of Discipline-Specific and Holistic Approaches to Intervention

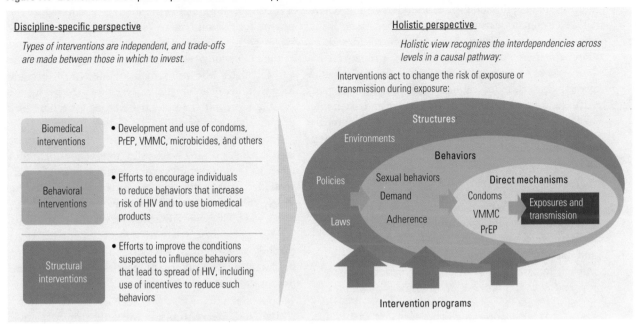

Note: HIV = human immunodeficiency virus; PrEP = preexposure prophylaxis; VMMC = voluntary medical male circumcision.

combination prevention, with a narrower perspective of which products are needed (Cremin and others 2013; Vermund and others 2013). It is simpler to standardize a prevention product and experimentally test whether that product has biological efficacy than to standardize the design of interventions to change the environment and behaviors (Hallett, White, and Garnett 2007; Lagakos and Gable 2008). Accordingly, with interventions requiring structural and behavioral components, there are major challenges in measuring the effects and costs of prevention because the interventions are rarely standardized and units of intervention are often unclear.

Defining and Measuring Intervention Endpoints

In addition to defining the interventions, it is important to define the endpoints of interest, which in studies are often intermediate variables instead of HIV incidence. Ultimately, the goal of prevention is to reduce incidence, but measuring incidence is difficult and expensive, especially where incidence is low (Hallett, White, and Garnett 2007). If reducing the number of partners or increasing the use of condoms could be assumed to decrease HIV incidence, then these intermediate measures would be reasonable endpoints for trials (Laga and others 2012). Alternatively, if correlated measures such as other acute sexually transmitted infections (STIs) or pregnancy share risks with HIV, they can be used to indicate a change in HIV risks. Unfortunately, the causal pathways are often not clear and

intermediate risks are not reliable measures of HIV risk, so the findings of studies using other endpoints—the majority of studies—have to be treated with caution (Garnett and others 2006).

Designing Studies of Impact

A third challenge pertains to the design of studies measuring the efficacy and effectiveness of HIV prevention interventions. For biomedical products intended to protect the individual, RCTs provide rigorous, causal evidence of efficacy (Lagakos and Gable 2008), but they do not guarantee impact at scale (Hallett, White, and Garnett 2007). Furthermore, some structural and behavioral elements of interventions need to be delivered to communities, not individuals—for example, education and communication campaigns or changes in policies. To have an impact, interventions often need to reach key individuals and to scale up what protects individuals so that the interventions protect communities. Such interventions can be evaluated in cluster or community randomized trials, but conducting such trials can be expensive and logistically challenging (Hallett, White, and Garnett 2007). When these trials find no impact, it is not clear whether the intervention was ineffective or the implementation in the trial was ineffective (Hallett, White, and Garnett 2007). RCTs are desirable if causality is to be established, the trials need to have a valid counterfactual with which to compare the effect of the intervention and should be randomized to distribute unmeasured confounding variables (Gertler and others 2011). Evaluation using methods other than RCTs can examine the delivery of programs at scale, trends in the incidence of infection and disease, qualitative data on risks and responses to interventions, and logical pathways by which interventions could have an impact. Analyses from such studies create a better understanding of the results of RCTs and yield plausibility arguments useful for improving implementation (Hargreaves and others 2016).

HIV PREVENTION CASCADES

Prevention cascades could be a powerful tool for analyzing how a prevention product should be delivered and identifying the steps required for it to have an impact. To date, in studying HIV interventions, cascades for treatment and prevention of mother-to-child transmission (PMTCT) have predominated (Gardner and others 2011; Mahendra and others 2007). The WHO has promoted a comprehensive approach to HIV, including prevention for those who are negative (WHO 2015a). A single, all-encompassing cascade is attractive. However, whether it can be populated with data and used successfully remains to be seen.

An alternative approach is to consider the different ways of preventing HIV and develop multiple cascades (Garnett and others 2016). This approach has the

disadvantage of thinking in programmatic siloes, but it is useful for illuminating the steps needed to reduce the risk of acquisition (figure 7.2). A hypothetical cascade starts with the number of individuals who would acquire infection or who are at risk over a period of time and calculates who will remain uninfected (or become infected) because of the intervention. Steps in the cascade represent the potential reasons for failure of a prevention intervention.

From the perspective of a policy maker or implementer, delivering a successful intervention requires targeting the population at risk, creating demand for prevention in that population, having a system in place to supply prevention, promoting adherence, and providing a direct and biologically efficacious prevention mechanism.

HIV prevention trials that focus on these aspects can be categorized. In a description of the literature, Krishnaratne and others (2016) classified reviews and primary studies under one of the following:

- **Demand interventions,** in which the principal aim is to influence behavior by targeting risk perception or strengthening awareness of, and positive attitudes toward, HIV prevention behaviors and technologies. These interventions could include providing information, education, and communication and aim to influence perceived norms through peer-based approaches.
- **Supply interventions,** in which the principal aim is to influence the supply of HIV prevention products and messages. These interventions include mass condom distribution, needle exchange initiatives, attempts to mainstream prevention within other services, and STI treatment strategies.
- **Use of or adherence to interventions,** in which the principal aim is to support adoption or maintenance of prevention behaviors, including the use of prevention technologies. They include interventions that provide risk counseling and target social determinants of behavior hypothesized to encourage or discourage access and adherence, such as conditional cash transfers or livelihood interventions.
- **Direct mechanisms for HIV prevention,** in which the principal aim is to stop transmission. These interventions include biomedical products or procedures, for example, microbicides or medical male circumcision (MMC).

SYSTEMATIC REVIEWS OF HIV PREVENTION

To understand the evidence available on prevention and address some of these challenges, Krishnaratne and others (2016) undertook three systematic reviews of prevention interventions. They then reviewed the original

Figure 7.2 HIV Prevention Cascade for a Single Intervention

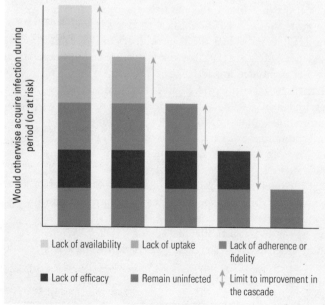

Legend:
- Lack of availability
- Lack of uptake
- Lack of adherence or fidelity
- Lack of efficacy
- Remain uninfected
- Limit to improvement in the cascade

Y-axis: Would otherwise acquire infection during period (or at risk)

Source: Garnett and others 2016.
Note: HIV = human immunodeficiency virus.

studies, reclassifying the interventions into a cascade framework, dissecting different endpoints, and grading the quality of evidence. The initial search identified 666 reviews of which 88 were eligible for inclusion. From these 88 reviews, 1,964 primary studies were identified, of which 292 were eligible for inclusion.

The division of studies within the cascade framework is notable for several reasons (figure 7.3). First, there were many more studies of demand interventions and direct mechanisms than studies of supply and use interventions. Most supply interventions were mass distribution of condoms and clean needles and syringes. The overwhelming majority of use interventions entailed counseling. With regard to study design, use and direct interventions were highly likely to be RCTs.

Two dimensions were used to summarize the evidence, following the scheme that Mavedzenge, Luecke, and Ross (2014) used to review HIV prevention interventions aimed at adolescents. The first dimension classifies the level of internal validity and replication, emphasizing proof of causation and generalizability. It does not include evidence of scalability, impact, or cost-effectiveness. The second dimension describes the direction of the effect.

Results from demand, supply, and use interventions could include intermediate variables, and Krishnaratne and others (2016) included condom use and HIV testing as endpoints. In addition, HIV prevalence could be compared between arms in a trial as a marker of past incidence, rather than directly assessing incidence by following up trial participants. For this reason, HIV prevalence was included as an endpoint. Table 7.1 summarizes the evidence from the review; the number of studies by type of intervention is shown with the number of RCTs in parentheses.

Of note, HIV incidence was most often an endpoint in trials of direct mechanisms, and some of these interventions were consistently found to be efficacious. Where the endpoint was HIV incidence, the evidence for demand, supply, and use interventions was either mixed or consistently ineffective; the single exception was a non-RCT of couples counseling. Demand interventions were ineffective in reducing HIV prevalence, whereas supplying condoms and clean needles and syringes was consistently associated with a decline in HIV prevalence but only in non-RCT studies. The majority of studies measured condom use and HIV testing rather than HIV incidence and prevalence. Across populations, there is good evidence of effectiveness in increasing condom use

Figure 7.3 Mapping HIV Prevention Studies to the HIV Prevention Cascade

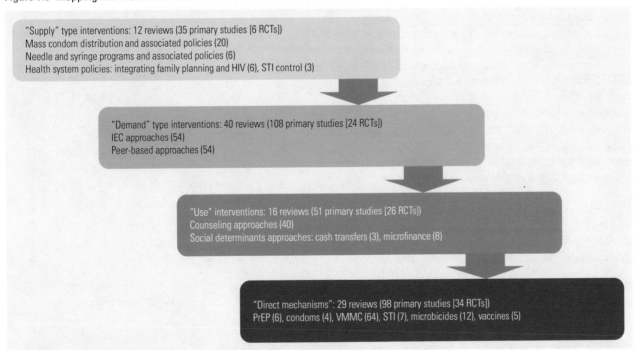

"Supply" type interventions: 12 reviews (35 primary studies [6 RCTs])
Mass condom distribution and associated policies (20)
Needle and syringe programs and associated policies (6)
Health system policies: integrating family planning and HIV (6), STI control (3)

"Demand" type interventions: 40 reviews (108 primary studies [24 RCTs])
IEC approaches (54)
Peer-based approaches (54)

"Use" interventions: 16 reviews (51 primary studies [26 RCTs])
Counseling approaches (40)
Social determinants approaches: cash transfers (3), microfinance (8)

"Direct mechanisms": 29 reviews (98 primary studies [34 RCTs])
PrEP (6), condoms (4), VMMC (64), STI (7), microbicides (12), vaccines (5)

Source: Based on a systematic review of HIV prevention studies in low- and middle-income countries by Krishnaratne and others 2016.

Note: HIV = human immunodeficiency virus; IEC = information, education, and communication; PrEP = preexposure prophylaxis; RCT = randomized controlled trial; STI = sexually transmitted infection; VMMC = voluntary medical male circumcision.

Table 7.1 Trials Assessing HIV Incidence and Prevalence, with Condom Use and Testing as Endpoints

Type of intervention	Incidence; number of studies (number of RCTs)	Incidence: QA rating	Prevalence; number of studies (number of RCTs)	Prevalence; QA rating	Condom use; number of studies (number of RCTs)	Condom use: QA rating	Testing; number of studies (number of RCTs)	Testing: QA rating
Demand-side interventions								
Impact of IEC interventions focused on youth	3 (1)	B4	1 (1)	B4	28 (7)	A3		
Impact of IEC interventions focused on men					9 (3)	A2	1 (0)	C1
Impact of IEC interventions focused on women					2 (2)	B3		
Impact of IEC interventions using mass media	1 (1)	B3			9 (1)	B4		
Impact of IEC interventions focused on PWUD					4 (3)	A1		
Impact of peer-based interventions focused on youth	1 (1)	B4			11 (0)	C2	2 (0)	C1
Impact of peer-based interventions focused on MSM					3 (1)	B1	1 (0)	C1
Impact of peer-based interventions focused on FSW	3 (1)	B4	4 (0)	C4	22 (3)	A2	3 (0)	C1
Impact of peer-based interventions focused on PWUD/alcohol	2 (2)	B4	1 (1)	B4	5 (2)	B3		
Impact of peer-based interventions with no population focus					10 (2)	B1	1 (0)	C1
Supply-side interventions								
Impact of interventions that integrate HIV services into routine care					1 (0)	C1	5 (0)	C1
Impact of clean needle and syringe programs	2 (0)	C3	6 (0)	C1				
Impact of condom distribution interventions			3 (0)	C1	20 (5)	A1		
Impact of community-level STI interventions	3 (3)	A4			1 (1)	B4		
Adherence interventions								
Impact of couples-based counseling	1 (0)	C1			9 (3)	A1	4 (3)	A3
Impact of HIV testing and counseling	1 (1)	B4			8 (1)	B2	3 (2)	B1
Impact of individual-level counseling	1 (1)	B3			12 (7)	A1	2 (1)	B3
Impact of HIV prevention counseling					7 (4)	A3		
Impact of microfinance interventions	1 (1)	B4			8 (4)	A3	1 (1)	B1
Impact of cash transfer interventions	2 (2)	B4	2 (2)	B1	1 (1)	B4		

table continues next page

Table 7.1 Trials Assessing HIV Incidence and Prevalence, with Condom Use and Testing as Endpoints (continued)

Type of intervention	Outcome							
	Incidence; number of studies (number of RCTs)	Incidence: QA rating	Prevalence; number of studies (number of RCTs)	Prevalence; QA rating	Condom use; number of studies (number of RCTs)	Condom use: QA rating	Testing; number of studies (number of RCTs)	Testing: QA rating
Direct mechanisms								
MMC heterosexual risk (female to male)	38 (3)	A1						
MMC heterosexual risk (male to female)	7 (1)	B3						
Male circumcision, MSM individual level	19 (0)	C3						
Condoms (heterosexual), individual level	4 (0)	C1						
Oral PrEP (overall), individual level	6 (6)	A2						
Microbicide prophylaxis, individual-level studies	12 (12)	A3						
STI treatment, individual-level studies	7 (7)	A4						
HIV vaccine, individual-level studies	5 (5)	A3						

Source: Krishnaratne and others 2016.

Note: Level of internal validity and replication available is defined as A (3 or more RCTs), B (1–2 RCTs), and C (no RCT). The direction of effectiveness is defined as 1 (consistently effective), 2 (mainly effective), 3 (mixed results), and 4 (consistently ineffective). FSW = female sex workers; HIV = human immunodeficiency virus; IEC = information, education, and communication; MMC = medical male circumcision; MSM = men who have sex with men; STI = sexually transmitted infection; PrEP = preexposure prophylaxis; PWUD = people who use drugs; QA = quality assessment; RCT = randomized controlled trial. Blank cells = not available.

and testing. Unfortunately, the impact of condom use depends on who is using the condoms and when, that is, in sexual acts where they would be exposed to the virus. The impact of HIV testing depends on changes in subsequent behavior, and there is scant evidence that this is a focus or product of HIV testing.

Cash transfers are an area of interest. An RCT found that cash transfers were associated with reduced HIV prevalence in young women in Malawi (Baird and others 2012). However, the effect was reversed when the transfers were withdrawn. Another study found no impact of cash transfers in a less resource constrained setting, where many girls stayed in school regardless of the intervention (HPTN 2015).

EFFICACY, EFFECTIVENESS, AND DURATION OF PROTECTION

The distinction between efficacy and effectiveness is crucial and somewhat opaque. By definition, trials measure the effect of an intervention in an artificial setting because the subjects have been recruited, have consented to take part, and are observed. Accordingly, there is a well-acknowledged distinction between effectiveness in a trial and in the real world, with real-world effectiveness expected to be lower than trial effectiveness.

To partly address this discrepancy, trials distinguish between participants that do and do not follow the intervention and trial protocol closely. Analysis of the effects according to protocol attempts to approximate the underlying biological effect of the product, while intention-to-treat analysis attempts to approximate its potential effectiveness in the real world. Unfortunately, the situation is much more complicated because there is very likely a difference between the efficacy observed in the according-to-protocol analysis of a trial and the biological effect of a product in reducing transmission. A trial compares the cumulative incidence of HIV among participants who potentially have multiple exposures. Biological efficacy is the reduction in risk for one exposure and is the parameter that would logically be used in models of HIV transmission (Jewell and others 2015).

To add to the confusion, a product could protect a fraction of individuals from all challenges (take-type efficacy) or all individuals from a fraction of challenges (degree-type efficacy) and have the same efficacy (Garnett 2005). Cumulatively as the number of challenges increases, take-type efficacy will fare better than degree-type efficacy because, in the former, the number of breakthrough infections will plateau as all those still at risk acquire infection. RCTs are not capable of distinguishing between these types of efficacy.

Likewise, effectiveness in the real world will depend on similarities in adherence and exposure in different settings with those found during the trial.

A further challenge is in estimating how long protection lasts. A trial will uncover whether protection is short lived, but if protection wanes over the medium or long term, assessing the duration of protection will be harder. The results of studies of the effectiveness of direct mechanisms of HIV prevention need to be considered, keeping these problems of interpretation in mind.

EVIDENCE OF EFFICACY OF DIRECT MECHANISMS OF HIV/AIDS PREVENTION

Barrier Methods

Male and female condoms that prevent HIV from crossing the barrier in vitro may prevent the acquisition of HIV (Steiner and others 2008). However, there is a problem in ethically and practically testing the effectiveness of condoms in RCTs. Observational studies need to consider whether condom use is consistent and correct and whether self-reported use is valid. Observed effectiveness will likely underestimate biological efficacy.

Good-quality studies on the effectiveness of condoms against HIV are lacking. Estimates of effectiveness in the past have been low. Weller (1993) concluded that condoms were only 69 percent effective in preventing acquisition of HIV. However, that study misaggregated some groups on condom use and did not compare "always" users with "never" users. Other researchers attempted to address this issue by exploring the direction of transmission. Pinkerton and Abramson (1997) concluded that condoms were 90 percent to 95 percent effective when used consistently. However, Davis and Weller (1999) criticized their paper for incorrectly categorizing "sometimes" users with never users and estimated effectiveness at 87 percent (as low as 60 percent or as high as 96 percent).

A meta-analysis by Weller and Davis (2002) concluded that condoms reduced HIV seroconversion approximately 80 percent, comparing always users with never users; their analysis used the difference between the two pooled rates to estimate effectiveness.

None of the reviews identified HIV effectiveness data for female condoms. However, one systematic review of the effectiveness of female-controlled barrier methods in preventing STI and HIV transmission concluded that RCTs provide evidence that female condoms confer as much protection from STIs as male condoms (Minnis and Padian 2005). However, this finding was based on results for chlamydia, gonorrhea, syphilis, and trichomoniasis rather than for HIV.

No trials found that the use of diaphragms affords significant protection. Marrazzo and Cates (2011) compared protection using a diaphragm and condom versus using a condom alone and found that using both provided no additional protection. They concluded that diaphragms should not be relied on for protection against STIs or HIV.

Medical Male Circumcision

Early in the study of heterosexually transmitted HIV infection in Sub-Saharan Africa, an association was observed at both the national (Bongaarts and others 1989) and individual (Cameron and others 1989) levels between circumcision status and HIV risk. Subsequent data collection repeatedly showed a protective effect of circumcision, with a systematic review and meta-analysis of 27 studies showing a 48 percent lower risk without controlling for other variables, and a meta-analysis of 15 studies showing a reduced risk of 58 percent that did account for confounding (Weiss, Quigley, and Hayes 2000).

Despite this observational evidence, two major questions remained:

- Could uncontrolled confounding related to the characteristics and behaviors of men from cultural groups that circumcise explain the observed protective effect?
- Would an intervention providing adult male circumcision provide the same protection as infant circumcision?

These questions required clinical trials using randomization to avoid uncontrolled confounding. The first trial in South Africa was stopped early because circumcision was found to be protective, with 20 HIV infections in circumcised men and 49 in uncircumcised men. Calculated rates of 0.85 per 100 person years in circumcised men and 2.1 per 100 person years in uncircumcised men meant that this was a 60 percent reduction in risk (Auvert and others 2005). In Kenya, 22 circumcised men and 47 uncircumcised men acquired HIV, representing a 53 percent reduction in risk (Bailey and others 2007). In Uganda, 0.66 cases of HIV per 100 person years in circumcised men and 1.3 cases per 100 person years in uncircumcised men represented a 55 percent reduction in risk (Gray and others 2007). These three rigorous trials provided definitive evidence of the protective effect of adult MMC in protecting men from heterosexual acquisition of HIV infection over time.

There is little evidence that MMC directly reduces the risk of HIV in women through vaginal intercourse: the one RCT that included this outcome measure was stopped early with some infections acquired by women whose partners acquired infection before the wound from the circumcision had healed (Wawer and others 2009). However, the fact that male circumcision reduces the incidence of HIV in men will indirectly benefit women by lessening their exposure to HIV. Male circumcision has also been shown to reduce rates of genital ulcers in men, as well as bacterial vaginosis and trichomoniasis in female partners of circumcised men (Tobian, Kacker, and Quinn 2014).

For MSM, the evidence of protection via circumcision is weak. A meta-analysis of observational studies concluded that there was insufficient evidence that circumcision provided protection for MSM (Millett and others 2008). In a subgroup analysis by sexual role in the relationship, 7 of 21 studies indicated that male circumcision is more protective among MSM who have a mainly insertive role (Wiysonge and others 2011).

Oral Preexposure Prophylaxis

The effectiveness of oral PrEP using either truvada (tenofovir plus emtricitabine) or tenofovir alone has been studied in trials of MSM and of men and women in HIV-discordant couples (figure 7.4).

Analyses accounting for adherence have shown greater effectiveness with high adherence and no significant effectiveness with poor adherence (Marrazzo and others 2015; Van Damme and others 2012).

A study of on-demand PrEP in MSM found 86 percent effectiveness (Molina and others 2015); a trial

comparing immediate PrEP to PrEP deferred for one year found a similar 86 percent relative effectiveness (McCormack and others 2016). In both cases, infections occurred among those who ceased taking the drug. Subsequent WHO guidelines, based on a meta-analysis showing 51 percent effectiveness across reviewed trials, included a strong recommendation for offering oral PrEP to persons with a high risk of acquiring HIV (WHO 2015b).

Vaginal or Rectal Microbicides

A wide range of topical products to prevent HIV acquisition has been studied. A review by Obiero and others (2012) of 13 trials for vaginal microbicides conducted between 1996 and 2011 found no evidence of a significant reduction in risk of HIV in a pooled analysis, but one proof-of-concept trial of tenofovir gel and a placebo gel conducted in South Africa found a significant reduction in the risk of acquisition (Abdool Karim and others 2010). Two further phase 3 studies of tenofovir gel showed no significant effectiveness: one found only a 14.5 percent lower incidence of HIV infection in the tenofovir arm (Marrazzo and others 2015) and one found no difference (Rees and others 2015).

Work on longer-acting topical delivery of an antiviral agent through a vaginal ring was tested in women in two trials. One found 27 percent effectiveness (Baeten and others 2016), and one found 31 percent effectiveness (IPM 2016). In both cases, effectiveness was higher in women older than age 21 years, with continuous

Figure 7.4 Effectiveness of Oral PrEP in Randomized Controlled Trials, by Order of Increasing Effectiveness

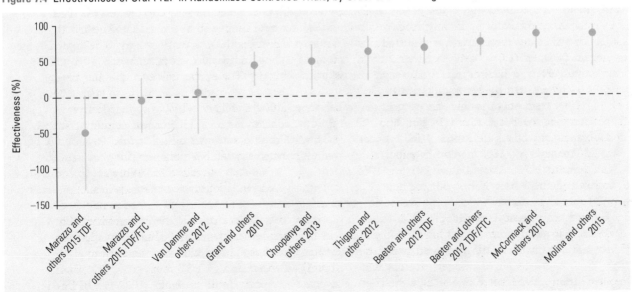

Sources: Baeten and others 2012; Marrazzo and others 2015.

Note: FTC = emtricitabine; PrEP = preexposure prophylaxis; TDF = tenofovir.

use of the ring needed to prevent HIV acquisition. Whether this effectiveness is sufficient to warrant launch of a product remains to be seen.

Vaccines

Systematic reviews of vaccines were included in broader reviews of HIV prevention measures (Marrazzo and Cates 2011; Padian and others 2010). Of four trials, only one (a double-blind, placebo-controlled trial conducted in more than 16,000 adults in Thailand) found a protective effect. In a modified intention-to-treat analysis, the combination of a vaccine plus a booster was 31 percent effective (Rerks-Ngarm and others 2009).

SEXUALLY TRANSMITTED INFECTION TREATMENT AS HIV PREVENTION

HIV acquisition is correlated with the presence of other STIs, and it has been hypothesized that the presence of these other infections could increase the transmissibility of HIV. Genital ulceration associated with chancroid; syphilis; herpes simplex virus (HSV) type 1 or 2; or inflammation associated with chlamydia, gonorrhea, trichomoniasis, or human papillomavirus may increase risks of HIV (Røttingen, Cameron, and Garnett 2001). Unfortunately, because of the common routes of transmission and the impossibility of measuring the complete sexual network, observational studies will always have unmeasured confounding.

To determine the effect of controlling STIs on HIV incidence, community randomized trials provided enhanced STI control in intervention communities. The first of these trials, conducted in Mwanza, Tanzania, using syndromic management of STIs found a 40 percent reduction in HIV incidence (Grosskurth and others 1995). This finding was not replicated in further trials of syndromic management or mass treatment of the population (Gregson and others 2007; Kamali and others 2003; Wawer and others 1999). This discrepancy was explained by the importance of symptoms to HIV risk and stage of the HIV epidemic. Padian and others (2010) reviewed nine STI treatment trials, only one of which was effective in preventing HIV acquisition. Three RCTs assessed the impact on HIV acquisition of suppressing HSV-2 with acyclovir. None of the trials found a protective effect. Adherence was reportedly mixed between the trials, and good prevention services were available to the control group, which may have affected behavior in all arms. The strength of the HSV-2 regimen also might have influenced susceptibility to HIV.

MEASURING THE HIV PREVENTION CASCADE TO EXPLORE IMPACT

From a population-based study in rural Zimbabwe, HIV prevention cascades were constructed to determine the effectiveness of HIV prevention and gaps in preventing infection (Garnett and others 2016). Figure 7.5 shows two cascades. The cascade in panel a is for male circumcision in 2009–11, where the cascade is applied to a population of men at risk of HIV. The initial step depends on whether there is a provider of voluntary medical male circumcision within 20 kilometers. Where there is, the next step includes persons who report having been circumcised; because adherence does not apply to circumcision, there is no drop-off at this step. The next drop-off is where circumcision is not efficacious. Finally, persons on the right were protected by circumcision.

The cascade in panel b is for HIV testing and counseling (HTC), with a reduction in the number of partners as the direct mechanism for protecting women from infection. The cascade is shown for women in two periods, 2009–11 and 2012–13. The first step is small because most women have access to testing services, but many do not use them; this situation improves over time. The greatest fall-off in protection occurs because the vast majority of women tested do not reduce the number of sexual partners, which suggests that HTC services will have little impact on HIV acquisition through this mechanism.

COSTS OF HIV PREVENTION

To understand the cost-effectiveness of HIV prevention interventions and how to budget for them, the costs of delivering the interventions have to be known. A literature search yielded 2,151 references, of which 66 were relevant. These papers varied in the interventions costed, the types of costing undertaken, the analyses performed, and the ability to link cost to effectiveness. Finding comparable, well-documented costing of interventions linked to outcomes is challenging. Walker (2003) found that many interventions were not covered, costs were inadequately described, and impact was rarely measured. In another systematic review, Galárraga and others (2009) found that HIV prevention was extremely cost-effective compared with treatment, but effectiveness was rarely measured, there was a gap in examining bundles of prevention interventions, and synergies were not included.

Avenir Health maintains a database of HIV intervention costs from 1993 to the present (Avenir Health 2016). UNAIDS (Joint United Nations Programme on HIV/AIDS) uses this database to estimate resource needs

Figure 7.5 Prevention Cascades from Rural Zimbabwe

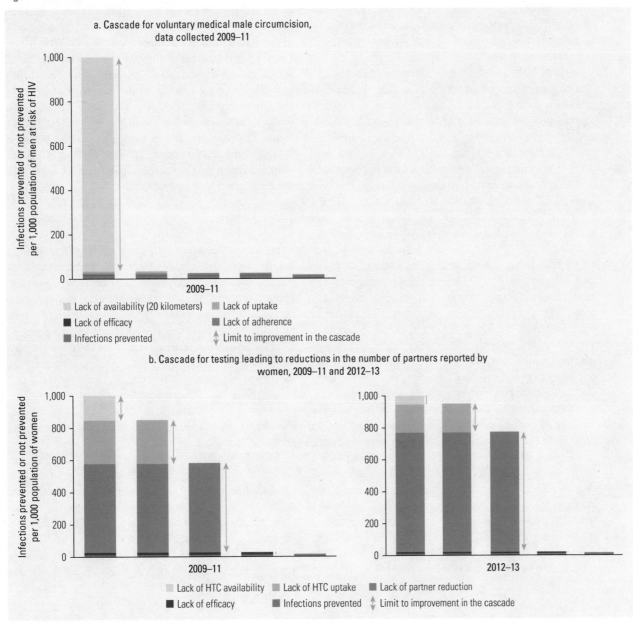

a. Cascade for voluntary medical male circumcision, data collected 2009–11

Infections prevented or not prevented per 1,000 population of men at risk of HIV

2009–11

- ▨ Lack of availability (20 kilometers)
- ▨ Lack of uptake
- ■ Lack of efficacy
- ▨ Lack of adherence
- ▨ Infections prevented
- ↕ Limit to improvement in the cascade

b. Cascade for testing leading to reductions in the number of partners reported by women, 2009–11 and 2012–13

Infections prevented or not prevented per 1,000 population of women

2009–11

2012–13

- ▨ Lack of HTC availability
- ▨ Lack of HTC uptake
- ▨ Lack of partner reduction
- ■ Lack of efficacy
- ▨ Infections prevented
- ↕ Limit to improvement in the cascade

Source: Garnett and others 2016.
Note: HTC = HIV (human immunodeficiency virus) testing and counseling.

(Hecht and others 2010). A large fraction of the costs in the database was gathered from regional experts in a series of workshops. The interventions reporting costs tend to be delivered in health facilities—PMTCT, VMMC, and HTC. This last intervention, HTC, is mostly geared toward diagnosing HIV-infected individuals; however, if testing and counseling attempt to reduce risky behaviors, the intervention could be considered preventive. The evidence suggests that persons who are HIV-positive do alter their behaviors, while those who are HIV-negative do not (Hallett and others 2009).

Other findings are that India has the most data on costs of HIV prevention, costs are often given per person reached, costs are generally for specific programs rather than the whole system, and costs decline over time (Avenir Health 2016).

Two international studies costing HIV prevention nearly a decade apart had similar findings: extreme heterogeneity in unit costs across sites and possibility of economies of scale in delivery (Bautista-Arrendondo and others 2015; Marseille and others 2007). One study examined the costs of voluntary counseling and testing;

male circumcision; PMTCT; risk reduction for people who inject drugs; risk reduction for sex workers; treatment of STIs; information, education, and communication; condom social marketing; and school curricula in India, Mexico, the Russian Federation, South Africa, and Uganda in 2003 and 2004 (Marseille and others 2004). The majority of costs measured were for "people reached," except for voluntary counseling and testing and for circumcision. Costs for the former varied 40-fold in Uganda and 2.5-fold in South Africa without adequate explanation. Programs showed efficiencies of scale, but the proportion of variation differed greatly between countries.

The other study examined the costs of HTC, PMTCT, and VMMC in Kenya, Rwanda, South Africa, and Zambia between 2011 and 2013 (Bautista-Arrendondo and others 2015; Sosa-Rubí and others 2015). For facilities carrying out HTC, a 10 percent increase in scale was associated with a 5.8 percent reduction in costs. For facilities carrying out VMMC, a 10 percent increase in procedures was associated with a 41 percent reduction in costs, and an increase in procedures was positively correlated with quality as measured in exit interviews. The main focus of both studies was efficiency. However, measuring the quality and impact of services is difficult, but necessary to determine efficiency, since lower costs could otherwise be offset by reduced effectiveness.

Extensive costing of HIV prevention service delivery was carried out between 2004 and 2008 as part of the Bill & Melinda Gates Foundation's Avahan Program in India. In this program, costs of prevention services depended on the scale of support provided to nongovernmental organizations, extent of community involvement, and organization of clinical services (Lépine and others 2016). A model-derived estimate of impact found a mean incremental cost of US$785 per HIV infection averted and US$46 per disability adjusted life-year (DALY) averted (Vassall and others 2014).

Based on RCT results for adult male circumcision, the WHO promoted the scale-up of circumcision programs in 14 Sub-Saharan African countries, leading to more than 9 million circumcisions (WHO 2015c). The circumcision programs allowed costs to be estimated across countries and across models of circumcision, including shifting tasks from doctors to nurses, using models to improve client flow, and using circumcision devices. In six countries, Bollinger and others (2014) found that the cost per circumcision varied between US$22 and US$70 (table 7.2). This finding is in line with estimated cost per circumcision used in exploring the cost-effectiveness of VMMC.

Cost-Effectiveness Analysis

In the Avahan program, the number of HIV infections averted was derived by comparing observed prevalence with a modeled counterfactual representing HIV spread without the intervention and self-reported increase in condom use among sex workers (Vassall and others 2014). Often the modeled effectiveness of interventions compares modeled incidence with and without the intervention; this is especially true of interventions using products in development and before scale-up. For prevention interventions, effectiveness is best established for VMMC and PrEP, the direct mechanisms with the most meaningful cost-effectiveness analyses.

Models were used to demonstrate that circumcision would be a cost-saving intervention where circumcision rates are low and HIV incidence is high. In a systematic review of circumcision cost-effectiveness, costs per HIV infection averted varied from US$174 to US$2,808 (Uthman and others 2010). In a subsequent analysis, Njeuhmeli and others (2011) found that circumcision would generate net savings, with predicted costs per

Table 7.2 Costs of Adult Male Circumcision in Six Sub-Saharan African Countries

Country	Period	Number of facilities	Number of circumcisions per facility	Average costs, 2012 US$ PPP
All		99	750 (average)	$49
Kenya	March 2010	29	743	$38
Namibia	April–May 2006	8	35	$31
South Africa	April 2008–March 2009	9	3,828	$22
Tanzania	2010–11	18	1,914	$70
Uganda	June–July 2009	26	286	$30
Zambia	2010	9	308	$61

Source: Bollinger and others 2014.
Note: PPP = purchasing power parity.

infection averted over the period 2011–25 varying from US$442 in Lesotho to US$4,096 in Rwanda.

The cost-effectiveness of oral PrEP in models is much less clear because it depends on assumptions made about HIV incidence, costs of the program, and coverage of the PrEP. In a systematic review of models of oral PrEP, the cost per infection averted in a generalized HIV epidemic varied from cost saving to US$39,900 (Gomez and others 2013).

Other cost-effectiveness analyses are of dubious validity because they depend upon assumed effectiveness. Topical PrEP (since found ineffective) was estimated to cost between US$18 and US$181 per DALY averted and between US$1,800 and US$2,700 per life year saved, with the major differences being due to assumptions about costs. Subsequent analyses for tenofovir gel estimated a cost of less than US$300 per DALY averted (Terris-Prestholt and others 2014), assuming effectiveness. Similarly, the incremental cost-effectiveness for an HIV vaccine, also assuming effectiveness, was US$43 per DALY averted (Moodley, Gray, and Bertram 2016). A study of female condom program modeling found a low of US$107 per DALY averted in Zimbabwe and a high of US$303 per DALY averted in Mozambique, assuming that condoms would be used and would be effective (Mvundura and others 2015).

Expenditure Analyses

The unit costs assumed in models and estimated from programs are substantially different from the resources expended on programs.

Analyses of expenditure indicate what programs are costing and what interventions are being prioritized by policy makers. PEPFAR has made expenditures available online, but expenditure by one donor does not describe the full expenditure on a program in a country. An estimated US$4.5 billion was spent on HIV prevention in low- and middle-income countries in 2012, with PEPFAR providing US$1.6 billion of this from its total expenditure of US$4.5 billion (UNAIDS 2015). Figure 7.6 shows the distribution of PEPFAR expenditures for HIV prevention in fiscal year 2013, excluding treatment as prevention. The largest fraction of spending was on PMTCT and HTC.

With the addition of country spending, we can focus on one country with complete expenditure data. Such data are rarely available, but have been compiled in Kenya (figure 7.7) and show that the majority of domestic HIV prevention resources (which excludes treatment as prevention) are deployed for HTC and PMTCT, and the proportion allocated to HTC and PMTCT was even greater than the proportion of all PEPFAR prevention expenditures in 19 countries on PMTCT and HTC.

Figure 7.6 PEPFAR Expenditure on HIV Prevention across Selected Countries, by Category of Prevention, 2014

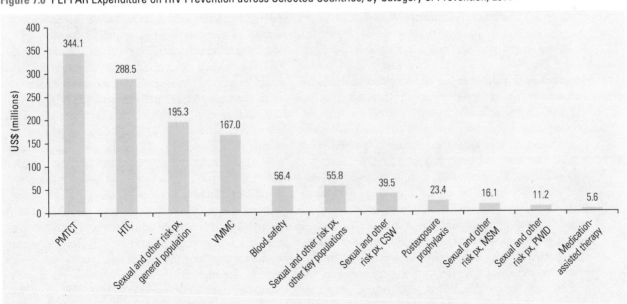

Source: PEPFAR (President's Emergency Plan for AIDS Relief) 2014, Data Dashboard, http://www.pepfar.gov/funding/c63793.htm, accessed March 31, 2015.
Note: CSW = commercial sex workers; HIV = human immunodeficiency virus; HTC = HIV testing and counseling; MSM = men who have sex with men; PEPFAR = President's Emergency Plan for AIDS Relief; PMTCT = prevention of mother-to-child transmission; PWID = persons who inject drugs; px = prevention; VMMC = voluntary medical male circumcision. Includes 17 countries in Sub-Saharan Africa, Haiti, and Vietnam.

Figure 7.7 Expenditure on HIV Prevention for Kenya, by Category of Prevention, 2012

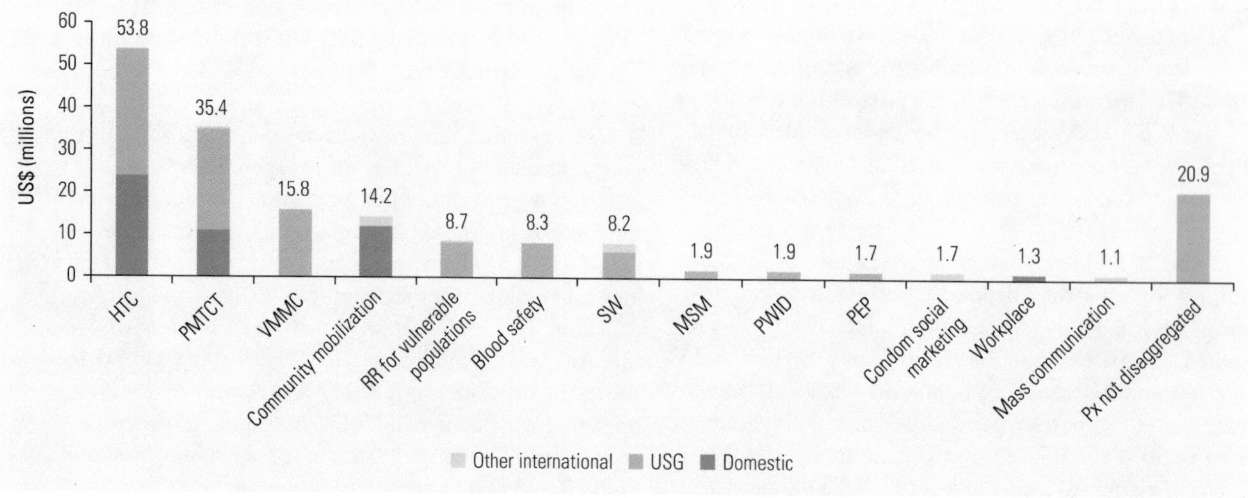

Sources: PEPFAR (President's Emergency Plan for AIDS Relief) 2014, Data Dashboard, http://www.pepfar.gov/funding/c63793.htm, accessed March 31, 2015; Kenya National AIDS Spending Assessment 2014, http://files.unaids.org/en/media/unaids/contentassets/documents/data-and-analysis/tools/nasa/20141017/kenya_2011_en.pdf, last accessed October 19, 2016.
Note: HIV = human immunodeficiency virus; HTC = HIV testing and counseling; MSM = men who have sex with men; PEP = postexposure prophylaxis; PMTCT = prevention of mother-to-child transmission; PWID = persons who inject drugs; Px = prevention; RR = risk reduction; SW = sex workers; USG = United States government; VMMC = voluntary medical male circumcision.

Because of the limited data on effectiveness for interventions other than PMTCT, VMMC, and oral PrEP (which has only recently been recommended), this expenditure may be appropriate. It does illustrate that few funds are being spent on the prevention interventions with a weak evidence base or even on those that are likely efficacious in preventing transmission and that the largest proportion of prevention funding is spent on HTC as an entry to treatment.

TARGETING HIV PREVENTION

The relationship between expenditure and health benefit is straightforward for treatment interventions. In comparison, the cost-effectiveness of interventions for prevention depends on the risk of acquiring infection and disease. This risk can vary across individuals and populations and over time, making a single measure of cost-effectiveness nonsensical. Simply viewed, prevention interventions will be more cost-effective the higher incidence would otherwise be. However, changes in individual- and population-level risk as a function of coverage and intensity greatly complicate the relationship between costs and benefits, especially with the cost-effectiveness of one intervention depending on the success of other interventions. This relationship has been challenging in modeling the impact of prevention, where if coverage of treatment as prevention is assumed to be high and effective, other prevention interventions have a smaller role to play (Stover and others 2014).

The more that prevention interventions can focus on persons who would otherwise acquire or spread infection, the more cost-effective they can be: targeting should increase cost-effectiveness. However, effectiveness is not the same as impact. As interventions target progressively fewer, higher-risk individuals, they may become more cost-effective but have less impact. Taking into account the full cost of developing and implementing programs, this lack of impact could lower the attractiveness of investments in programs to develop and use new prevention products.

This sequence can be illustrated by exploring what would be required to avert 20 percent of HIV infections using approximately 20 percent of the HIV prevention budget (figure 7.8). Assuming that there are 1.5 million new infections each year, US$4.5 billion is spent on prevention (UNAIDS 2015), the goal explored is to reduce new infections by 300,000, and the budget is US$0.9 billion, it is possible to explore, for different effectiveness, the relationship between incidence in the target population and the number of people who would have to be covered. To achieve a given impact goal with a budget, there is a trade-off between how well the intervention can be focused and the resources available per person reached; the higher the incidence, the more could be spent per person in the program. Figure 7.8a shows how many people at a given HIV incidence would need to be reached to avert 300,000 infections; figure 7.8b shows the cost per person reached with prevention allowable, if the cost per infection averted is to be US$3,000.

Figure 7.8 Isoclines Showing the Values Required to Achieve Target Reductions in HIV Infections and Costs of Infection Averted

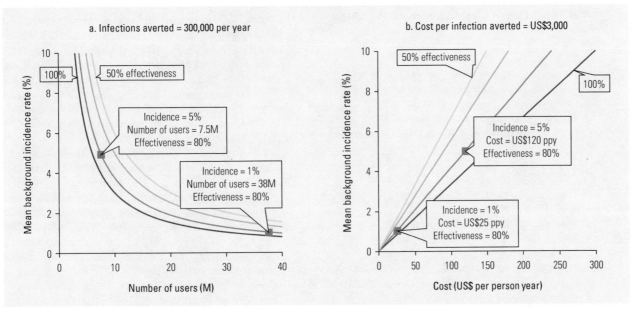

Note: HIV = human immunodeficiency virus; M = millions; ppy = per person year. In panel a, to avert 300,000 infections, the lines show effectiveness of 50, 60, 80, and 100 percent for direct mechanisms of prevention; the number of users in millions; and a given incidence of infection. In panel b, to achieve a cost per infection averted of US$3,000, the lines show effectiveness of 50, 60, 80, and 100 percent for direct mechanisms of prevention; the required cost per person year; and a given incidence of infection.

Better targeting of HIV prevention to persons with a high incidence of acquisition or transmission makes the intervention more cost-effective, but this invites the questions of how to target and what impact is possible.

CONCLUSIONS

Prevention has probably averted many millions of HIV infections, but it is impossible to be sure how many, given the difficulties of knowing what the scale of spread would have been in the absence of behavior changes among those at risk. Despite the scale-up of effective treatment, which can contribute to HIV prevention, other prevention interventions are needed, but which ones? HIV prevention should be a cost-effective intervention, but 35 years into the global HIV pandemic, large questions remain about which prevention programs are effective, how best to implement them, and how much should be spent on them. A fundamental problem is identifying those who are at risk and then ensuring that they adopt preventive behavior.

Large gaps are evident in the supply of prevention interventions. Furthermore, data on effectiveness are available for only a few direct mechanisms. Evidence of effectiveness exists for VMMC and oral PrEP, and it is logical that using condoms and having fewer partners will reduce risk. Costing data for HIV prevention, except for VMMC, are also unavailable. When appropriately targeted, HIV prevention will, at most thresholds, be cost-effective, but that cost-effectiveness will depend on the other interventions in use and the ability to target interventions appropriately.

What resources should be used for HIV prevention and what should they be used for? Two prevention products—VMMC and oral PrEP—conservatively should reduce HIV incidence by 50 percent; using condoms and having fewer partners could have similar effectiveness. However, products are not interventions. Interventions need to get people to use the products, and resources need to be directed to this effort.

An HIV infection costs either decades of lost life or decades of expense on treatment. If an infection causes 20 DALYs and averting 1 DALY is "worth" US$500, then an infection prevented is worth US$10,000. Alternatively, if treating someone for 20 years would cost US$500 per year, then treating an infection would cost US$10,000. So if it is possible to prevent half of the infections with current products and HIV incidence is 10 percent, we should be spending US$500 per person per year on prevention. If HIV incidence is 1 percent, we should be spending US$50 per person per year. If HIV incidence is 0.1 percent, we should be spending US$5 per person per year. Alternatively, if there are 2 million HIV infections per year, we should be spending at least US$5 billion per year. By any account, the world is falling well short of providing what is needed for HIV prevention.

NOTE

World Bank Income Classifications as of July 2014 are as follows, based on estimates of gross national income (GNI) per capita for 2013:

- Low-income countries (LICs) = US$1,045 or less
- Middle-income countries (MICs) are subdivided:
  (a) lower-middle-income = US$1,046 to US$4,125
  (b) upper-middle-income (UMICs) = US$4,126 to US$12,745
- High-income countries (HICs) = US$12,746 or more.

REFERENCES

Abdool Karim, Q., S. S. Abdool Karim, J. A. Frohlich, A. C. Grobler, C. Baxter, and others. 2010. "Effectiveness and Safety of Tenofovir Gel, an Antiretroviral Microbicide, for the Prevention of HIV Infection in Women." *Science* 329 (5996): 1168–74.

Anderson, R. M., and R. M. May. 1990. *Infectious Diseases of Humans: Dynamics and Control.* Oxford, U.K.: Oxford University Press.

Anderson, R. M., R. M. May, M.-C. Boily, G. P. Garnett, and J. T. Rowley. 1991. "The Spread of HIV-1 in Africa: Sexual Contact Patterns and the Predicted Demographic Impact of AIDS." *Nature* 352 (6336): 581–89.

Auvert, B., D. Taljaard, E. Lagarde, J. Sobngwi-Tambekou, R. Sitta, and others. 2005. "Controlled Intervention Trial of Male Circumcision for Reduction of HIV Infection Risk: The ANRS 1265 Trial." *PLoS Medicine* 2 (11): e298.

Avenir Health. 2016. "Unit Cost Repository." Avenir Health, London. http://www.avenirhealth.org/policytools/UC/.

Baeten, J. M., D. Donnell, P. Ndase, M. R. Mugo, J. D. Campbell, and others. 2012. "Antiretroviral Prophylaxis for HIV Prevention in Heterosexual Men and Women." *New England Journal of Medicine* 367 (5): 399–410.

Baeten, J. M., T. Palanee-Phillips, E. R. Brown, K. Schwartz, L. E. Soto-Torres, and others. 2016. "Use of a Vaginal Ring Containing Dapivirine for HIV-1 Prevention in Women." *New England Journal of Medicine* February 22. doi:10.1056/NEJMoa1506110.

Bailey, R. C., S. Moses, C. B. Parker, K. Agot, I. Maclean, and others. 2007. "Male Circumcision for HIV Prevention in Young Men in Kisumu, Kenya: A Randomised Controlled Trial." *The Lancet* 369 (9562): 643–56.

Baird, S. J., R. S. Garfein, C. T. McIntosh, and B. Özler. 2012. "Effect of a Cash Transfer Programme for Schooling on Prevalence of HIV and Herpes Simplex Type 2 in Malawi: A Cluster Randomised Trial." *The Lancet* 379 (9823): 1320–29.

Bautista-Arrendondo, S., S. G. Sosa-Rubí, M. Opuni, A. Kwan, C. Chaumont, and others. 2015. "Efficiency of VMMC and Its Determinants: Results from the ORPHEA Study in Kenya, Rwanda, South Africa, and Zambia." Paper presented at the International AIDS Society Conference, Vancouver, July 19–22.

Bollinger, L., A. Adesina, S. Forsythe, R. Godbole, E. Reuben, and others. 2014. "Cost Drivers for Voluntary Medical Male Circumcision Using Primary Source Data from Sub-Saharan Africa." *PLoS One* 9 (5): e84701.

Bongaarts, J., P. Reining, P. Way, and F. Conant. 1989. "The Relationship between Male Circumcision and HIV Infection in African Populations." *AIDS* 3 (6): 373–77.

Brandt, A. M. 1987. *No Magic Bullet: A Social History of Venereal Disease in the United States since 1880.* Oxford, U.K.: Oxford University Press.

Cameron, W., J. N. Simonsen, L. J. D'Costa, A. R. Ronald, G. M. Maitha, and others. 1989. "Female to Male Transmission of Human Immunodeficiency Virus Type 1: Risk Factors for Seroconversion in Men." *The Lancet* 334 (8660): 403–7.

Choopanya, K., M. Martin, P. Suntharasamai, U. Sangkum, P. A. Mock, and others. 2013. "Antiretroviral Prophylaxis for HIV Infection in Injecting Drug Users in Bangkok, Thailand (the Bangkok Tenofovir Study): A Randomised, Double-Blind, Placebo-Controlled Phase 3 Trial." *The Lancet* 381 (9983): 2083–90.

Cohen, M. S., Y. Q. Chen, M. McCauley, T. Gamble, M. C. Hosseinipour, and others. 2011. "Prevention of HIV-1 Infection with Early Antiretroviral Therapy." *New England Journal of Medicine* 365 (6): 493–505.

Cremin, I., R. Alsallaq, M. Dybul, P. Piot, G. Garnett, and others. 2013. "The New Role of Antiretrovirals in Combination HIV Prevention: A Mathematical Modelling Analysis." *AIDS* 27 (3): 447–58.

Davis, K. R., and S. C. Weller. 1999. "The Effectiveness of Condoms in Reducing Heterosexual Transmission of HIV." *Family Planning Perspectives* 31 (6): 272–79.

Eron, J. J., Jr., and M. S. Hirsch. 2008. "Antiviral Therapy of Human Immunodeficiency Virus Infection." In *Sexually Transmitted Diseases*, 4th ed., edited by K. Holmes, P. F. Spirling, W. E. Stamm, P. Pilot, J. N. Wasserheit, and others. New York: McGraw-Hill.

Ford, N., M. Vitoria, G. Hirnschall, and M. Doherty. 2013. "Getting to Zero HIV Deaths: Progress, Challenges, and Ways Forward." *Journal of the International AIDS Society* 16 (1): 18927.

Fuller, C. M., C. Ford, and A. Rudolph. 2009. "Injection Drug Use and HIV: Past and Future Considerations for HIV Prevention and Interventions." In *HIV Prevention: A Comprehensive Approach*, edited by K. H. Meyer and H. F. Pizer. Amsterdam: Academic Press.

Galárraga, O., M. A. Colchero, R. G. Wamai, and S. M. Bertozzi. 2009. "HIV Prevention Cost-Effectiveness: A Systematic Review." *BMC Public Health* 9 (Suppl 1): S5.

Gaolathe, T., K. Wirth, M. Pretorius Holme, J. Makhema, S. Moyo, and others. 2016. "Botswana Is Close to Meeting UNAIDS 2020 Goals of 90-90-90 Coverage." Paper presented at the Conference on Retroviruses and Opportunistic Infections, Boston, MA, February 22–25.

Gardner, E. M., M. P. McLees, J. F. Steiner, C. Del Rio, and W. J. Burman. 2011. "The Spectrum of Engagement in HIV Care and Its Relevance to Test-and-Treat Strategies for Prevention of HIV Infection." *Clinical Infectious Diseases* 52 (6): 793–800.

Garnett, G. P. 2005. "The Role of Herd Immunity in Determining the Impact of Sexually Transmitted Disease

Vaccines." *Journal of Infectious Diseases* 191 (Suppl 1): S97–106.

Garnett, G. P., J. M. Garcia-Calleja, T. Rehle, and S. A. J. Gregson. 2006. "Behavioural Data as an Adjunct to HIV Surveillance Data." *Sexually Transmitted Infections* 82 (Suppl. 1): i57–i62.

Garnett, G. P., T. B. Hallett, A. Takaraza, J. Hargreaves, R. Rhead, and others. 2016. "Providing a Conceptual Framework for HIV Prevention Cascades and Assessing Feasibility of Empirical Measurement with Data from East Zimbabwe: A Case Study." *The Lancet HIV* 3 (7): e297–e306.

Gertler, P. J., S. Martinez, P. Premand, L. B. Rawlings, and C. M. Vermeersch. 2011. *Impact Evaluation in Practice.* Washington, DC: World Bank.

Gomez, G. B., A. Borquez, K. K. Case, A. Wheelock, A. Vassall, and others. 2013. "The Cost and Impact of Scaling Up Pre-Exposure Prophylaxis for HIV Prevention: A Systematic Review of Cost-Effectiveness Modelling Studies." *PLoS Medicine* 10 (3): e1001401.

Grant, R. M., J. R. Lama, P. L. Anderson, V. McMahan, A. Y. Liu, and others. 2010. "Preexposure Chemoprophylaxis for HIV Prevention in Men Who Have Sex with Men." *New England Journal of Medicine* 363 (27): 2587–99.

Gray, R. H., G. Kigozi, D. Serwadda, F. Makumbi, S. Watya, and others. 2007. "Male Circumcision for HIV Prevention in Men in Rakai, Uganda: A Randomised Trial." *The Lancet* 369 (9562): 657–66.

Gregson, S., S. Adamson, S. Papaya, T. Chimbadzwa, J. Mundondo, and others. 2007. "Impact and Process Evaluation of Integrated Community and Clinic-Based HIV-1 Control in Eastern Zimbabwe." *PLoS Medicine* 4 (3): e102.

Grosskurth, H., J. Todd, E. Mwijarubi, P. Mayaud, A. Nicoll, and others. 1995. "Impact of Improved Treatment of Sexually Transmitted Diseases on HIV Infection in Rural Tanzania: Randomised Controlled Trial." *The Lancet* 346 (8974): 530–36.

Hallett, T. B., J. Aberle-Grasse, G. Bello, L. M. Boulos, M. P. A. Cayemittes, and others. 2006. "Declines in HIV Prevalence Can Be Associated with Changing Sexual Behaviour in Uganda, Urban Kenya, Zimbabwe, and Urban Haiti." *Sexually Transmitted Infections* 82 (Suppl 1): i1–8.

Hallett, T. B., S. Dube, I. Cremin, B. Lopman, A. Mahomva, and others. 2009. "Testing and Counselling for HIV Prevention and Care in the Era of Scaling-up Antiretroviral Therapy." *Epidemics* 1 (2): 77–82.

Hallett, T. B., P. J. White, and G. P. Garnett. 2007. "The Appropriate Evaluation of HIV Prevention Interventions: From Experiment to Full-Scale Intervention." *Sexually Transmitted Infections* 83 (Suppl 1): i55–60.

Hankins, C. A., and B. O. de Zalduondo. 2010. "Combination Prevention: A Deeper Understanding of Effective HIV Prevention." *AIDS* 24 (Suppl 4): S70–80.

Hargreaves, J., S. Delaney-Moretlwe, T. B. Hallett, S. Johnson, S. Kapiga, and others. 2016. "The HIV Prevention Cascade: Integrating Theories of Epidemiological, Behavioural and Social Science into Programme Design and Monitoring." *The Lancet HIV* 3 (7): e318–e22.

Harris, K., T. Guthrie, R. Omban, and G. Garnett. Forthcoming. "Follow the Money: Assessing the Efficiency of HIV Prevention Expenditures." Submitted to *The Lancet HIV*.

Hecht, R., J. Stover, L. Bollinger, F. Muhib, K. Case, and others. 2010. "Financing of HIV/AIDS Programme Scale-up in Low-Income and Middle-Income Countries, 2009–31." *The Lancet* 376 (9748): 1254–60.

Holmes, C. B., T. B. Hallett, R. P. Walensky, T. Bärnighausen, Y. Pillay, and M. S. Cohen. 2017. "Effectiveness and Cost-Effectiveness of Treatment as Prevention for HIV." In *Disease Control Priorities* (third edition): Volume 6, *Major Infectious Diseases*, edited by K. K. Holmes, S. Bertozzi, B. R. Bloom, and P. Jha. Washington, DC: World Bank.

Hoots, W. K. 2001. "History of Plasma-Product Safety." *Transfusion Medical Reviews* 2 (Suppl 1): 3–10.

HPTN (HIV Prevention Trials Network). 2015. "Cash Transfers Conditional on Schooling Do Not Prevent HIV Infection among Young South African Women." http://www.hptn .org/network_information/hptnnews/15/068results_IAS .html.

IPM (International Partnership for Microbicides). 2016. "The Ring Study 2016." IPM, Silver Spring, MD. http://www .ipmglobal.org/the-ring-study.

Jewell, B. L., I. Cremin, M. Pickles, C. Celum, J. M. Baeten, and others. 2015. "Estimating the Cost-Effectiveness of Pre-Exposure Prophylaxis to Reduce HIV-1 and HSV-2 Incidence in HIV-Serodiscordant Couples in South Africa." *PLoS One* 10 (1): e0115511.

Kamali, A., M. Quigley, J. Nakiyingi, J. Kinsman, J. Kengeya-Kayondo, and others. 2003. "Syndromic Management of Sexually-Transmitted Infections and Behaviour Change Interventions on Transmission of HIV-1 in Rural Uganda: A Community Randomised Trial." *The Lancet* 361 (9358): 645–52.

Krishnaratne, S., B. Hensen, J. Cordes, J. Enstone, and J. R. Hargreaves. 2016. "Interventions to Strengthen the HIV Prevention Cascade: A Systematic Review of Reviews." *The Lancet HIV* 3 (7): e307–e317.

Laga, M., D. Rugg, G. Peersman, and M. Ainsworth. 2012. "Evaluating HIV Prevention Effectiveness: The Perfect as the Enemy of the Good." *AIDS* 26 (7): 779–83.

Lagakos, S., and A. R. Gable, eds. 2008. *Methodological Challenges in Biomedical HIV Prevention Trials.* Washington, DC: National Academies Press.

Lépine, A., S. Chandrashekar, G. Shetty, P. Vickerman, J. Bradley, and others. 2016. "What Determines HIV Prevention Costs at Scale? Evidence from the Avahan Programme in India." *Health Economics* 25 (Suppl 1): 67–82.

Mahendra, V. S., R. Mudoi, A. Oinam, V. Pakkela, A. Sarna, and others. 2007. *Continuum of Care for HIV-Positive Women Accessing Programs to Prevent Parent-to-Child Transmission: Findings from India.* Horizons Final Report. Washington, DC: Population Council.

Marrazzo, J. M., and W. Cates. 2011. "Interventions to Prevent Sexually Transmitted Infections, Including HIV Infection." *Clinical Infectious Diseases* 53 (Suppl 3): S64–78.

Marrazzo, J. M., G. Ramjee, B. A. Richardson, K. Gomez, N. Mgodi, and others. 2015. "Tenofovir-Based Preexposure Prophylaxis for HIV Infection among African Women." *New England Journal of Medicine* 372 (6): 509–18.

Marseille, E., L. Dandona, N. Marshall, P. Gaist, S. Bautista-Arredondo, and others. 2007. "HIV Prevention Costs and Program Scale: Data from the PANCEA Project in Five Low and Middle-Income Countries." *BioMed Central Health Services Research* 7: 108.

Marseille, E., L. Dandona, J. Saba, C. McConnel, B. Rollins, and others. 2004. "Assessing the Efficiency of HIV Prevention around the World: Methods of the PANCEA Project." *Health Services Research* 39 (6, pt 2): 1993–2012.

Mavedzenge, S. N., E. Luecke, and D. A. Ross. 2014. "Effective Approaches for Programming to Reduce Adolescent Vulnerability to HIV Infection, HIV Risk, and HIV-Related Morbidity and Mortality: A Systematic Review of Systematic Reviews." *Journal of Acquired Immune Deficiency Syndromes* 66 (Suppl 2): S154–69.

May, R. M., and R. M. Anderson. 1987. "Transmission Dynamics of HIV Infection." *Nature* 326 (6109): 137–42.

McCormack, S., D. T. Dunn, M. Desai, D. I. Dolling, M. Gafos, and others. 2016. "Pre-Exposure Prophylaxis to Prevent the Acquisition of HIV-1 Infection (PROUD): Effectiveness Results from the Pilot Phase of a Pragmatic Open-Label Randomised Trial." *The Lancet* 387 (10013): 53–60.

Merson, M., N. Padian, T. J. Coates, G. R. Gupta, S. M. Bertozzi, and others. 2008. "Combination HIV Prevention." *The Lancet* 372 (9652): 1805–6.

Millett, G. A., S. A. Flores, G. Marks, J. B. Reed, and J. H. Herbst. 2008. "Circumcision Status and Risk of HIV and Sexually Transmitted Infections among Men Who Have Sex with Men: A Meta-Analysis." *Journal of the American Medical Association* 300 (14): 1674–84.

Minnis, A. M., and N. S. Padian. 2005. "Effectiveness of Female Controlled Barrier Methods in Preventing Sexually Transmitted Infections and HIV: Current Evidence and Future Research Directions." *Sexually Transmitted Infections* 81 (3): 193–200.

Molina, J. M., C. Capitant, B. Spire, G. Pialoux, L. Cotte, and others. 2015. "On-Demand Preexposure Prophylaxis in Men at High Risk for HIV-1 Infection." *New England Journal of Medicine* 373 (23): 2237–46.

Moodley, N., G. Gray, and M. Bertram. 2016. "The Case for Adolescent HIV Vaccination in South Africa: A Cost-Effectiveness Analysis." *Medicine* 95 (4): e2528.

Mvundura, M., N. Nundy, M. Kilbourne-Brook, and P. S. Coffey. 2015. "Estimating the Hypothetical Dual Health Impact and Cost-Effectiveness of the Woman's Condom in Selected Sub-Saharan African Countries." *International Journal of Women's Health* 7: 271–77.

Nelson, K. E., D. D. Celentano, S. Eiumtrakol, D. R. Hoover, C. Beyrer, and others. 1996. "Changes in Sexual Behavior and a Decline in HIV Infection among Young Men in Thailand." *New England Journal of Medicine* 335 (5): 297–303.

Njeuhmeli, E., S. Forsythe, J. Reed, M. Opuni, L. Bollinger, and others. 2011. "Voluntary Medical Male Circumcision: Modeling the Impact and Cost of Expanding Male Circumcision for HIV Prevention in Eastern and Southern Africa." *PLoS Medicine* 8 (11): e1001132.

Obiero, J., P. G. Mwethera, G. D. Hussey, and C. S. Wiysonge. 2012. "Vaginal Microbicides for Reducing the Risk of Sexual Acquisition of HIV Infection in Women: Systematic Review and Meta-Analysis." *BMC Infectious Diseases* 12: 289.

Oppenheimer, G. M. 1988. "In the Eye of the Storm: The Epidemiological Construction of AIDS." In *AIDS, the Burdens of History*, edited by E. Fee and D. M. Fox. Berkeley: University of California Press.

Padian, N. S., S. I. McCoy, J. E. Balkus, and J. N. Wasserheit. 2010. "Weighing the Gold in the Gold Standard: Challenges in HIV Prevention Research." *AIDS* 24 (5): 621–35.

Palella, F. J., Jr., K. M. Delaney, A. C. Moorman, M. O. Loveless, J. Fuhrer, and others. 1998. "Declining Morbidity and Mortality among Patients with Advanced Human Immunodeficiency Virus Infection." *New England Journal of Medicine* 338 (13): 853–60.

Pinkerton, S. D., and P. R. Abramson. 1997. "Effectiveness of Condoms in Preventing HIV Transmission." *Social Science and Medicine* 44 (9): 1303–12.

Piot, P., S. S. Abdool Karim, R. Hecht, H. Legido-Quigley, K. Buse, and others. 2015. "Defeating AIDS: Advancing Global Health." *The Lancet* 386 (9989): 171–218.

Rees, H., S. A. Delany-Moretlwe, C. Lombard, D. Baron, R. Panchia, and others. 2015. "FACTS 001 Phase III Trial of Pericoital Tenofovir 1% Gel for HIV Prevention in Women." Paper presented at the Conference on Retroviruses and Opportunistic Infections (CROI), Seattle, WA, February 23–26.

Rerks-Ngarm, S., P. Pitisuttithum, S. Nitayaphan, J. Kaewkungwal, J. Chiu, and others. 2009. "Vaccination with ALVAC and AIDSVAX to Prevent HIV-1 Infection in Thailand." *New England Journal of Medicine* 361 (23): 2209–20.

Røttingen, J. A., D. W. Cameron, and G. P. Garnett. 2001. "A Systematic Review of the Epidemiological Interactions between Classical STDs and HIV." *Sexually Transmitted Diseases* 28 (10): 579–97.

Schwartländer, B., J. Stover, T. Hallett, R. Atun, C. Avila, and others. 2011. "Towards an Improved Investment Approach for an Effective Response to HIV/AIDS." *The Lancet* 377 (9782): 2031–41.

Sosa-Rubí, S. G., S. Bautista-Arredondo, M. Opuni, D. Contreras-Loya, I. Moreno, and others. 2015. "Efficiency of Facility-Based HTC and Its Determinants: Results from the ORPHEA Study in Kenya, Rwanda, South Africa, and Zambia." Paper presented at the eighth International AIDS Society conference, Vancouver, BC, July 19–22.

Steiner, M., L. Warner, K. M. Stone, and W. Cates Jr. 2008. "Condoms and Other Barrier Methods for Prevention of STD/HIV Infection and Pregnancy." In *Sexually Transmitted Diseases*, 4th ed., edited by K. K. Holmes, P. F. Spirling, W. E. Stamm, P. Pilot, J. N. Wasserheit, and others. New York: McGraw-Hill.

Stoneburner, R. L., and D. Low-Beer. 2004. "Population-Level HIV Declines and Behavioral Risk Avoidance in Uganda." *Science* 304 (5671): 714–18.

Stover, J., T. B. Hallett, Z. Wu, M. Warren, C. Gopalappa, and others. 2014. "How Can We Get Close to Zero? The Potential Contribution of Biomedical Prevention and the

Investment Framework towards an Effective Response to HIV." *PLoS One* 9 (11): e111956.

Terris-Prestholt, F., A. M. Foss, A. P. Cox, L. Heise, G. Meyer-Rath, and others. 2014. "Cost-Effectiveness of Tenofovir Gel in Urban South Africa: Model Projections of HIV Impact and Threshold Product Prices." *BMC Infectious Diseases* 14: 14.

Thigpen, M. C., P. M. Kebaabetswe, L. A. Paxton, D. K. Smith, C. E. Rose, and others. 2012. "Antiretroviral Preexposure Prophylaxis for Heterosexual HIV Transmission in Botswana." *New England Journal of Medicine* 367 (5): 423–34.

Tobian, A. A., S. Kacker, and T. C. Quinn. 2014. "Male Circumcision: A Globally Relevant but Under-Utilized Method for the Prevention of HIV and Other Sexually Transmitted Infections." *Annual Review of Medicine* 65: 293–306.

UNAIDS (Joint United Nations Programme on HIV/AIDS). 2015. "AIDS by the Numbers." UNAIDS, Geneva.

Uthman, O. A., T. A. Popoola, M. M. Uthman, and O. Aremu. 2010. "Economic Evaluations of Adult Male Circumcision for Prevention of Heterosexual Acquisition of HIV in Men in Sub-Saharan Africa: A Systematic Review." *PLoS One* 5 (3): e9628.

Van Damme, L., A. Corneli, K. Ahmed, K. Agot, J. Lombaard, and others. 2012. "Preexposure Prophylaxis for HIV Infection among African Women." *New England Journal of Medicine* 367 (5): 411–22.

Vassall, A., M. Pickles, S. Chandrashekar, M. C. Boily, G. Shetty, and others. 2014. "Cost-Effectiveness of HIV Prevention for High-Risk Groups at Scale: An Economic Evaluation of the Avahan Programme in South India." *The Lancet Global Health* 2 (9): e531–40.

Vermund, S. H., S. J. Fidler, H. Ayles, N. Beyers, and R. J. Hayes. 2013. "Can Combination Prevention Strategies Reduce HIV Transmission in Generalized Epidemic Settings in Africa? The HPTN 071 (PopART) Study Plan in South Africa and Zambia." *Journal of Acquired Immune Deficiency Syndrome* 63 (Suppl 2): S221–27.

Walker, D. 2003. "Cost and Cost-Effectiveness of HIV/AIDS Prevention Strategies in Developing Countries: Is There an Evidence Base?" *Health Policy and Planning* 18 (1): 4–17.

Wawer, M. J., F. Makumbi, G. Kigozi, D. Serwadda, S. Watya, and others. 2009. "Circumcision in HIV-Infected Men and Its Effect on HIV Transmission to Female Partners in Rakai, Uganda: A Randomised Controlled Trial." *The Lancet* 374 (9685): 229–37

Wawer, M. J., N. K. Sewankambo, D. Serwadda, T. C. Quinn, L. A. Paxton, and others. 1999. "Control of Sexually Transmitted Diseases for AIDS Prevention in Uganda: A Randomised Community Trial. Rakai Project Study Group." *The Lancet* 353 (9152): 525–35.

Weiss, H. A., M. A. Quigley, and R. J. Hayes. 2000. "Male Circumcision and Risk of HIV Infection in Sub-Saharan Africa: A Systematic Review and Meta-Analysis." *AIDS* 14 (15): 2361–70.

Weller, S. C. 1993. "A Meta-Analysis of Condom Effectiveness in Reducing Sexually Transmitted HIV." *Social Science and Medicine* 36 (12): 1635–44.

Weller, S. C., and K. Davis. 2002. "Condom Effectiveness in Reducing Heterosexual HIV Transmission." *Cochrane Database of Systematic Reviews* 1: CD003255.

WHO (World Health Organization). 2015a. "Consolidated Strategic Information Guidelines for HIV in the Health Sector." WHO, Geneva.

———. 2015b. "Guideline on When to Start Antiretroviral Therapy and on Pre-Exposure Prophylaxis for HIV." WHO, Geneva.

———. 2015c. "Voluntary Medical Male Circumcision for HIV Prevention in 14 Priority Countries in East and Southern Africa." Progress Brief, WHO, Geneva.

Wiysonge, C. S., E. J. Kongnyuy, M. Shey, A. S. Muula, O. B. Navti, and others. 2011. "Male Circumcision for Prevention of Homosexual Acquisition of HIV in Men." *Cochrane Database of Systematic Reviews* 6: CD007496.

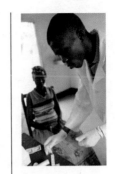

Chapter 8

Tailoring the Local HIV/AIDS Response to Local HIV/AIDS Epidemics

David Wilson and Jessica Taaffe

INTRODUCTION

In the 30 years since the global appearance of the human immunodeficiency virus/acquired immune deficiency syndrome (HIV/AIDS), we have come extraordinarily far in our fight against it. We know its physical routes of transmission and how to prevent infection at the individual level, and we have proven intervention strategies at the population level. Yet, despite global declines in modeled incidence, measured incidence remains high in cohort studies and is growing within certain demographic groups. This concerning trend underscores the need to thoroughly examine how local and national HIV/AIDS epidemics are sustained.

Knowledge of epidemic and transmission dynamics will help HIV/AIDS programs invest in the right interventions. Proven interventions exist for both concentrated and generalized epidemics. For example, simple targeted interventions for concentrated epidemics have been implemented at scale with considerable durability in numerous contexts. Targeting resources and interventions to the right people and the right places is also essential. More than one key population may drive a concentrated epidemic, and new infections within a generalized or mixed epidemic come from multiple demographic groups and behaviors within the general population. Geographic targeting and hotspot mapping can assist in identifying both geographic areas of elevated transmission and high-risk groups. Epidemic modeling

software, such as Optima, can help identify the right mix of interventions and financial allocations, resulting in cost-effective programming.[1]

This chapter reviews factors to consider when tailoring the local response to a local epidemic. It explores transmission dynamics in concentrated, generalized, and mixed epidemics, while acknowledging the complexity and variation within these distinctions. It also addresses interventions shown to work in different contexts and discusses how program science can assist in reaching the right people in the right places, providing examples of successful implementation. Finally, it elaborates on what Optima software is and how it can improve allocative and implementation efficiency.

KNOW YOUR EPIDEMIC: TRANSMISSION DYNAMICS

A thorough understanding of the heterogeneity of HIV transmission, between and within epidemics, is the first step in a targeted response. This understanding includes appreciating transmission dynamics at national and subnational levels, across geographic regions, and within different demographics, as well as the risk factors sustaining transmission.

Distinguishing between concentrated, generalized, and mixed epidemics is helpful for understanding transmission dynamics.

Corresponding author: David Wilson, Global Lead, Decision and Delivery Science; Program Director, Global HIV/AIDS Program, Health, Nutrition, and Population, World Bank; dwilson@worldbank.org.

- An epidemic is *concentrated* if "HIV has spread rapidly in one or more defined subpopulation but is not well established in the general population" (WHO 2013). In this context, protecting key populations, such as injecting drug users (IDUs), men who have sex with men (MSM), and sex workers, would significantly mitigate the epidemic.
- An epidemic is *generalized* if transmission at a level to sustain the epidemic would occur even if key populations were protected from infection, as when "HIV infection is firmly established in the general population" (WHO 2013).
- An epidemic is *mixed* if transmission would be sustained by both key populations and the general population and would continue even if transmission in either population were stopped. Mixed epidemics are essentially one or more concentrated epidemics within a generalized epidemic.

Previously, concentrated and generalized epidemics were distinguished from one another based on HIV prevalence in key populations or the general population. Prevalence of more than 5 percent in key populations and

less than 1 percent in the general population (prevalence in pregnant women as a proxy) indicated a concentrated epidemic, whereas prevalence of more than 1 percent in the general population indicated a generalized epidemic (UNAIDS/WHO Working Group on Global HIV/AIDS and STI Surveillance 2000). While this approach is a simple numerical way of defining epidemics, it does not address what the transmission dynamics are, how these epidemics are sustained, where the majority of new infections are occurring, and where target prevention activities are in place. For example, Wilson and Challa (2009) demonstrate that three African epidemics have HIV prevalence of more than 1 percent in the general population, but they are not all considered generalized because of the source of new infections.

Most epidemics are concentrated (map 8.1). However, the global burden of HIV/AIDS is heaviest in Sub-Saharan Africa, where 24.7 million people live with the disease and 1.5 million new infections occur each year (more than 70 percent of the global total for existing and new infections) (UNAIDS 2014b). Most HIV/AIDS epidemics in Sub-Saharan Africa are generalized or mixed transmission (Wilson and Halperin 2008).

Map 8.1 Global HIV Transmission Dynamics

IBRD 42331 | DECEMBER 2016

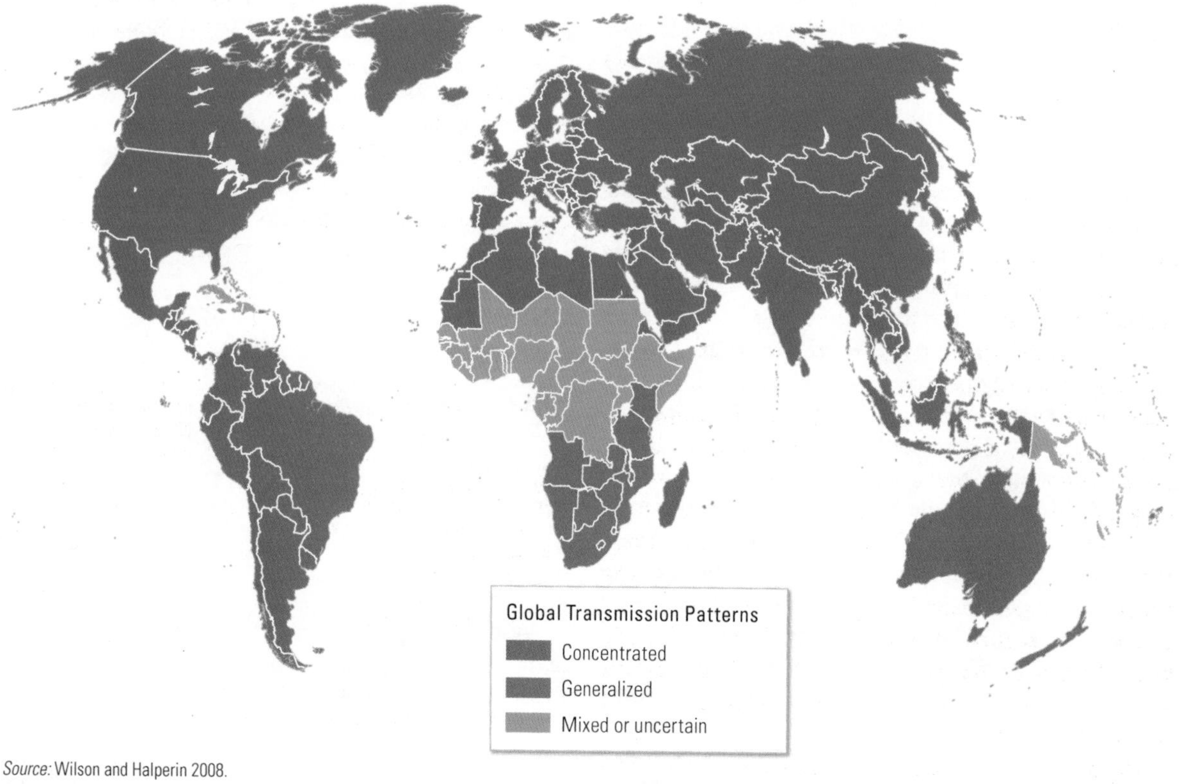

Global Transmission Patterns

- Concentrated
- Generalized
- Mixed or uncertain

Source: Wilson and Halperin 2008.
Note: HIV = human immunodeficiency virus.

Concentrated Epidemics

Concentrated HIV/AIDS epidemics are occurring primarily in Asia; Australasia; Europe; the Middle East; and North, Central, and South America. They are sustained through key populations, which are at much higher risk for infection (figure 8.1). A targeted approach acknowledges and addresses the factors and behaviors that are putting these key populations at increased risk.

Sex Workers

Female sex workers have a risk of HIV infection that is 13.5 times higher than that of the general population (Baral and others 2012). Globally, HIV prevalence is higher among sex workers than among the general population. It is 12 times higher in 110 countries with available data and at least 50-fold higher in 4 countries (UNAIDS 2014b). In 16 Sub-Saharan African countries, female sex workers have a pooled HIV prevalence of 37 percent (Kerrigan and others 2013); these countries include Swaziland, where as many as 70 percent of sex workers are living with HIV/AIDS (figure 8.2).

Biological, behavioral, and structural factors put sex workers at greater risk of contracting HIV and other sexually transmitted infections (STIs). Compared with the general population, sex workers have more sexual partners and more concurrent sexual partners, are more likely to use injection drugs (Johnston and Corceal 2013; Lau and others 2008; Needle and others 2008; UNAIDS 2006; Zohrabyan and others 2013), and are more often subject to violence (Decker and others 2014; Deering and others 2013). It is common practice for police to arrest individuals because they are carrying condoms and then to confiscate them, further compromising the ability of sex workers to protect themselves (Ireri 2012; Maseko and Ndlovu 2012; Open Society Foundations 2012; WHO 2012). Furthermore, discrimination and stigma discourage sex workers from seeking health services, including HIV testing (King and others 2013; Scorgie and others 2011).

The spectrum of sex work is especially complex in Sub-Saharan Africa, where sexual transactions often occur in the context of poverty and inequality. Sex work involves both those who identify themselves as professionals and those who do not but who do engage in informal sex work and transactional sex. In Burkina Faso, some nonprofessional sex workers (bar waitresses and mobile traders) have higher HIV prevalence than some professional sex workers (roamers), despite fewer reported sexual partners (2.6 and 3.3 clients per week for waitresses and traders, respectively, versus 18.6 for professional roamers) (Nagot and others 2002).

Figure 8.1 HIV Risk in Key Populations Relative to the General Population

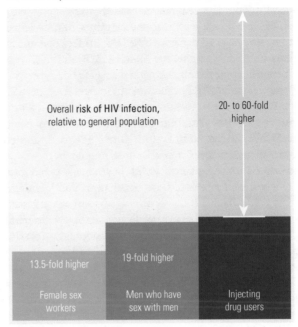

Sources: Baral and others 2012; UNAIDS 2014b.
Note: HIV = human immunodeficiency virus.

Figure 8.2 Prevalence of HIV among Sex Workers versus General Population

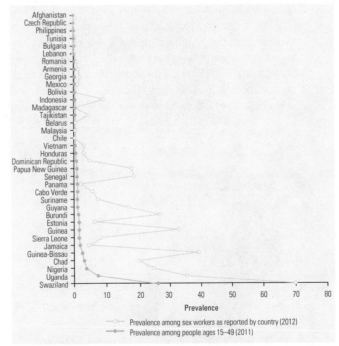

Source: UNAIDS (Joint United Nations Programme on HIV/AIDS). 2012. *UNAIDS Report on the Global AIDS Epidemic 2012.* Geneva.
Note: HIV = human immunodeficiency virus.

Men Who Have Sex with Men

MSM is another key population in concentrated epidemics. They are 19 times more likely to be living with HIV/AIDS than the general population, with prevalence of 6 percent to 15 percent (UNAIDS 2014b). Epidemics have been spreading among MSM in many settings, even in high-income settings with good coverage of antiretroviral treatment (ART) (Sullivan and others 2009). MSM account for the largest share of new infections in Latin America and the Caribbean (33 percent in the Dominican Republic, 56 percent in Peru) (figure 8.3) and for a substantial percentage of new infections in other parts of the world (Gouws and Cuchi 2012). In Ghana, 8 percent to 18 percent of new infections occur in MSM (UNAIDS and World Bank 2012).

Biological and behavioral factors multiply the risk among MSM at both individual and population levels. The estimated risk of acquiring HIV is 18 times greater through anal than through vaginal sex (Grulich and Zablotska 2010). Frequent casual sex with multiple partners is relatively common among MSM. In larger networks, as the number of partners increases, so does the incidence of unprotected sex (Choi, Gibson, and others 2004; Choi, McFarland, and others 2004; Kelly and others 2010). In these situations, acute infections may be more prevalent, driving higher incidence, because acutely infected individuals have higher viral loads and are more infectious.

Sexual and other risk factors also play a role. MSM may have sex with both men and women (and may even be in long-term heterosexual marriages or partnerships, especially in the global South). Drug use is also associated with riskier sexual practices. In Bangkok, HIV prevalence among MSM rose from 2009 to 2011 with the use of amphetamine-type stimulants (Colfax and others 2010; Freeman and others 2011; van Griensven and others 2009).

Injecting Drug Users

An estimated 13 percent of the 12.7 million IDUs worldwide are infected with HIV; IDUs have, on average, 28 times greater HIV prevalence than the general population, ranging from 1.3 to 2,000 times greater in 74 countries (UNAIDS 2014b). Outside of Sub-Saharan Africa, an estimated 30 percent of new infections come from IDUs; in many countries in Asia, Eastern Europe, and the Middle East, IDUs are driving the national epidemic (Mathers and others 2008; UNAIDS 2014b). In the Islamic Republic of Iran, more than two-thirds of new infections occur in IDUs and their sexual partners (figure 8.4).

IDU-driven epidemics exhibit much heterogeneity. In 30 countries reporting gender-specific data, HIV prevalence is higher among female than among male IDUs (UNAIDS 2014b). This enhanced risk may be due to high rates of sex work among female IDUs (Blouin and others 2013). IDUs under age 25 are also at comparatively high risk for HIV infection, with a prevalence of 5.2 percent.

Shared needles are a main risk factor for infection, although sexual transmission between IDUs and their non-IDU partners can play a small to major role depending on context. Modeling of epidemics for the period 2010–15 showed that HIV infection due to unprotected sex among and with IDUs was 5 percent of total HIV incidence in Nairobi, Kenya, and Karachi, Pakistan, but 15 percent to 45 percent in Odessa, Ukraine (Strathdee and others 2010).

Generalized Epidemics

Generalized epidemics were previously defined as epidemics in which more than 1 percent of the general population was infected. Recent definitions focus on transmission dynamics, and generalized epidemics are now defined as epidemics that are sustained by heterosexual transmission in the general population.

The distinction between concentrated and generalized epidemics is important: interventions in a concentrated epidemic should address specific key populations (Wilson and Halperin 2008), whereas interventions in a generalized epidemic should address the broader, general population, while also focusing on high risk subgroups within it. As heterogeneous as community norms and sexual values and practices can be in the general population, so, too, are the sources of infection. For example, in KwaZulu-Natal, South Africa's most HIV/AIDS-afflicted region, most infections are transmitted through heterosexual sex (figure 8.5). However, key populations and their sexual partners also play a large role.

Figure 8.3 Sources of New HIV Infections in Peru

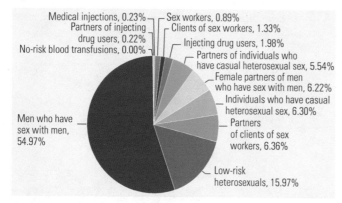

Source: UNAIDS and OPS 2009.
Note: HIV = human immunodeficiency virus.

Casual sex is highly prevalent in countries experiencing severe generalized epidemics. In Lesotho and Swaziland, where HIV prevalence was 23 percent and 27 percent, respectively, in 2013 (UNAIDS 2014b), casual sex, as opposed to commercial sex, is highly prevalent among men who work as soldiers, police, miners, drivers, guards, and seasonal workers (Family Health International and others 2002; Swaziland Ministry of Health and Social Welfare 2002).

HIV prevalence also varies across gender and age groups. In Swaziland, more than half of females ages 30–34 and nearly half of men ages 35–39 are living with HIV/AIDS. For people ages 18–29, prevalence is at least twice as high in women as in men (Swaziland Ministry of Health 2012).

Mixed Epidemics

Mixed epidemics are characterized by both concentrated and generalized transmission, often in the same area, as in much of West Africa. Transmission can also change, moving from concentrated to generalized. In mixed epidemics that are changing from concentrated to generalized transmission, bridge populations, such as paying and nonpaying partners of sex workers and bisexual MSM, transmit HIV to the general population.

Epidemics of mixed transmission can also be geographically mixed, with concentrated epidemics occurring in some areas and generalized epidemics occurring in others. In most provinces in Indonesia, the epidemic is concentrated and sustained in key populations of IDUs and MSM, especially transgender (*waria*) and male sex workers. However, in the Indonesian provinces of Papua and West Papua, the epidemic is driven largely by heterosexual transmission, both by sex workers and by the general population, and HIV prevalence is much higher than in the rest of the country, at 2.40 percent in Papua and 0.27 percent in West Papua (Indonesian National AIDS Commission 2012).

According to projections for 2000–20, the epidemic in Jakarta began with male IDUs but quickly spread to MSMs, who soon became the largest source of transmission. The epidemic in Papua spread steadily through females in the general population (figure 8.6).

TAILOR THE HIV/AIDS RESPONSE

Tailoring the local response to a local epidemic requires more than just knowledge of transmission dynamics. It also requires the use of proven interventions that target the right people and that are applied effectively in the right places.

Figure 8.4 Sources of New HIV Infections in the Islamic Republic of Iran

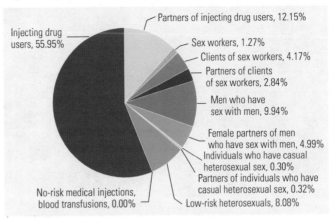

Source: Nasirian 2011.
Note: HIV = human immunodeficiency virus.

Figure 8.5 Sources of New HIV Infections in KwaZulu-Natal, South Africa

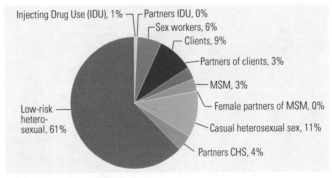

Source: SACEMA 2009.
Note: CHS = individuals who have casual heterosexual sex; HIV = human immunodeficiency virus; MSM = men who have sex with men.

Invest in the Right Interventions

Several biomedical and sociobehavioral interventions have been effective at preventing infection and transmission at the individual and population levels. All are important in any comprehensive response, but specific interventions have been proven to be most effective in certain epidemic contexts. Prioritizing the right interventions based on epidemic context is essential.

Interventions for Concentrated Epidemics

Effective targeted interventions for concentrated epidemics have six core components:

- Behavior-change communication
- Condom programs and needle and syringe programs (NSPs)
- Sexual health and harm-reduction services, including opioid substitution therapy (OST)

Figure 8.6 Projected Transmission Dynamics of the Mixed HIV Epidemic in Jakarta and Papua, Indonesia, 2000–20

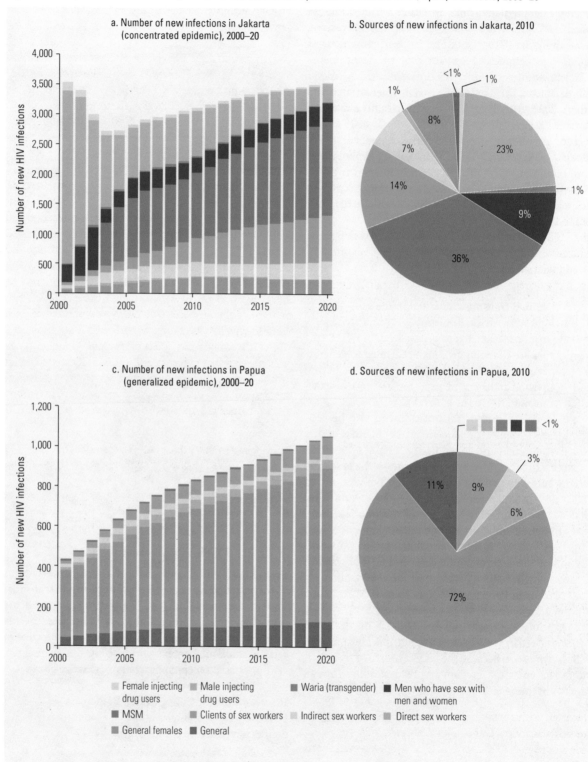

a. Number of new infections in Jakarta (concentrated epidemic), 2000–20

b. Sources of new infections in Jakarta, 2010

c. Number of new infections in Papua (generalized epidemic), 2000–20

d. Sources of new infections in Papua, 2010

Female injecting drug users · Male injecting drug users · Waria (transgender) · Men who have sex with men and women · MSM · Clients of sex workers · Indirect sex workers · Direct sex workers · General females · General

Source: Modeling by Kirby Institute, University of South Wales.

Note: HIV = human immunodeficiency virus; MSM = men who have sex with men.

- HIV testing, counseling, and treatment (ART)
- Solidarity and community empowerment
- Supportive local and national legal and policy environments.

The World Health Organization (WHO), the United Nations Joint Programme on HIV/AIDS (UNAIDS), and the United Nations Office on Drugs and Crime promote a comprehensive package of HIV interventions for IDUs, including three priority interventions: NSPs, OST, and ART. In a study of 99 cities, those with NSPs saw a 19 percent reduction in prevalence per year, while those without NSPs experienced an 8 percent increase over approximately one decade (MacDonald and others 2003). Among other effects, OST programs have been shown to reduce HIV incidence among IDUs (MacArthur and others 2012; van den Berg and others 2007). ART has reduced transmission by reducing infectiousness (Cohen and others 2011; Quinn and others 2000; Wood and others 2009).

Community empowerment, often leading to community mobilization, has been effective in programs targeting sex workers. Community empowerment and mobilization has led to increased condom use, lower risk for STIs, and increased HIV testing in India (Beattie and others 2014; Blanchard and others 2013; Fonner and others 2014) and Africa (Chersich and others 2013). In Asia, social programs marketing condoms have increased condom use (Lipovsek and others 2010; Ngoc and others 2011; USAID 2011). Along with promoting the use of condoms, other interventions to address sexual health, including reducing the incidence of and treating STIs, have also been associated with a reduction in HIV prevalence in sex-worker populations (Ghys and others 2001; Ghys and others 2002; Laga and others 1994; Rojanapithayakorn and Hanenberg 1996). One of the most successful interventions has been India's Avahan Program, which is supported by the Bill & Melinda Gates Foundation. A large-scale, cost-effective program promoting all of the core components of interventions for concentrated epidemics, the Avahan Program averted an estimated 42 percent of HIV infections in 4 years and an estimated 57 percent in 10 years (Pickles and others 2013; Vassall and others 2014).

Condom promotion; HIV testing, counseling, and treatment; and behavior change to reduce risky sexual practices are important interventions for MSM. In the 1980s, behavior change on a large scale, including a decrease in the number of sexual partners and an increase in the use of condoms, helped to curb the epidemic in MSM in Australia and the United States (Kippax and Race 2003; Winkelstein and others 1987). However,

in randomized clinical trials, behavioral interventions had a minimal effect on reducing incidence of HIV among MSM.

Solid evidence exists for the use of specific interventions in concentrated epidemics, but coverage and implementation are lacking in many programs. UNAIDS (2012) reports that 86 percent of countries have low or no coverage of NSPs, and more than 85 percent of people who inject drugs lack access to NSP, OST, or ART services (Stoicescu 2012). MSM and sex workers are poorly represented in prevention programs, with 70 percent and 75 percent of countries reporting very low or no coverage for these populations, respectively (UNAIDS 2012). The inadequate coverage of sex workers is especially disconcerting, since the bulk of new infections come from this group in many concentrated epidemics.

Finally, preexposure prophylaxis (PrEP) is a promising new biomedical tool for use in key populations and is recommended by the WHO for individuals at "substantial risk" of HIV (WHO 2015). The WHO made the recommendation based on evaluations of PrEP effectiveness in a number of studies among serodiscordant couples, heterosexual men, women, MSM, IDU, and transgender women, especially when adherence was high. For example, PrEP reduced HIV incidence by 44 percent among MSM and by 90 percent among fully adherent MSM in a multicountry study (Grant and others 2010). PrEP has been shown to prevent infection in IDUs, resulting in a 49 percent reduction of HIV incidence in PrEP groups compared with placebo groups (Choopanya and others 2013). Overall, across studies in different at-risk populations, a meta-analysis of 10 randomized controlled trials found a 51 percent reduction in infection risk among PrEP users versus those who took a placebo (Fonner and others 2016). Many studies show PrEP efficacy, but success outside the context of clinical trials will not be easy. Adherence may be lower in real-life implementation scenarios, challenging the effectiveness of PrEP. In these settings, implementation of adherence-support programs will be very important in combination with PrEP. Also, achieving success in developing countries will be much more difficult because fewer programs in low- and middle-income countries reach key populations such as MSM and IDUs.

Interventions for Generalized Epidemics
Various interventions have been tested for generalized epidemics, including those that have been effective in concentrated epidemics. However, randomized controlled trials using HIV incidence endpoints have found only VMMC, ART-based prevention, and financial

incentives to be consistently effective (figure 8.7). Of the cash transfer trials, one used STIs, not HIV specifically, as an endpoint, and another used prevalence as a proxy for incidence.

ART-based prevention, such as TasP, has been proven to reduce transmission. In clinical trials, TasP can reduce risk by more than 96 percent (Cohen and others 2011). Outside of clinical trials, it is still effective but less so. In KwaZulu-Natal, South Africa, infection was 34 percent lower in areas with 30 percent to 40 percent ART coverage than in areas with less than 10 percent coverage (Tanser and others 2013). In China, infection was 26 percent lower in serodiscordant couples in which the infected partner received ART than in couples in which the infected partner did not (Jia and others 2013). In Swaziland, where about 85 percent of persons with CD4 cell counts of less than 350 are on ART, measured annual HIV/AIDS incidence was 2.4 percent on top of 26 percent adult prevalence (Swaziland Ministry of Health and Social Welfare 2002). Because of TasP's proven prevention benefits, the WHO now recommends a universal TasP strategy. Under the test-and-treat strategy, all individuals living with HIV/AIDS are eligible for ART, regardless of CD4 count, and catching and treating HIV infection earlier may prevent new infections within the community. As more programs adopt and implement this strategy, more information will be available on the effectiveness of TasP at the population level. In addition, randomized clinical trials are under way in several African field sites (Botswana, Kenya, South Africa, Uganda, and Zambia) to evaluate changes in incidence as a result of TasP and other interventions.

VMMC is extraordinarily effective at reducing HIV incidence in generalized epidemics. In clinical trials, the protective effect of VMMC was 60 percent (Auvert and others 2005; Bailey and others 2007; Gray and others 2007); the long-term effect may be even higher. Longer-term follow-up suggested that incidence in persons who were circumcised, compared with those who were not, was 67 percent lower over 4.5 years in Kenya, 73 percent lower over 2.8 years in Uganda, and 76 percent lower over 3.0 years in South Africa (Auvert and others 2013; Bailey and others 2010; Gray and others 2012). In 13 countries, projections suggest that 80 percent implementation of VMMC (20 million circumcisions) and sustaining this level of coverage could avert 3.4 million new infections through 2025 (Njeuhmeli and others 2011). This target has not yet been met; at the end of 2015, only 11.6 million circumcisions had been performed (UNAIDS 2016).

Randomized controlled trials with STI and HIV endpoints conducted by the World Bank and others show that financial incentives, including conditional cash transfers, can reduce HIV and other STIs (figure 8.8). The premise behind financial incentives is that the income effect on sexual behavior may mitigate sexually risky behavior, such as when impoverished young girls seek out older males (who are more likely to be infected) for gifts and financial assistance or engage in transactional sex. In Tanzania, individuals who received up to US$60 annually to stay STI-free had 25 percent lower STI prevalence (de Walque and others 2012). In Malawi, girls whose families received up to US$15 a month to stay in school had 70 percent lower prevalence, compared with the control group, members of which received no payment (Baird and others 2012). Adolescents in Lesotho who received a lottery ticket to win up to US$50 or US$100 every four months if they stayed STI- and HIV-free had 25 percent lower HIV incidence, with even greater reductions among girls (33 percent) and in the group receiving US$100 (31 percent).

Although promising, these initial studies represent only early efforts to determine whether financial incentives can and should be included in HIV prevention programs. The Tanzania study assessed the impact on STIs other than HIV, although reducing STI risk may also reduce HIV risk; the Lesotho study found only a small statistically significant effect. The Malawi study used cumulative HIV prevalence among young women as a

Figure 8.7 Effectiveness of Interventions for Preventing Infections in Generalized HIV/AIDS Epidemics

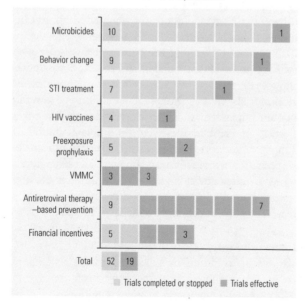

□ Trials completed or stopped   ■ Trials effective

Sources: Baeten and others 2012; Marrazzo and others 2015; Padian and others 2010; Peterson and others 2007; Thigpen and others 2012; Van Damme and others 2012; Weiss and others 2008.
Note: HIV/AIDS = human immunodeficiency virus/acquired immune deficiency syndrome; STI = sexually transmitted infection; VMMC = voluntary medical male circumcision.

Figure 8.8 Effect of Financial Incentives on Reducing HIV and STIs in Lesotho, Malawi, and Tanzania

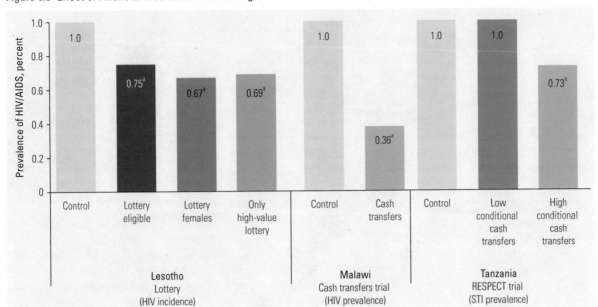

Sources: Baird and others 2012; de Walque and others 2012; Nyqvist and others 2015.
Note: HIV = human immunodeficiency virus; RESPECT = Rewarding STI Prevention and Control in Tanzania; STIs = sexually transmitted infections.
a. Statistically significant effect.

proxy for incidence, and there was no baseline or randomization. Furthermore, to the disappointment of the HIV-prevention field, the most recent evaluations of cash transfer interventions in South Africa's generalized epidemic have not shown the same success as the studies in Lesotho, Malawi, and Tanzania, and were challenged by study design and context issues (HPTN 2015; Karim and others 2015). Further studies are needed to evaluate the effectiveness of financial incentives for prevention, whether they are scalable and affordable, and whether their outcomes are durable.

For the general population and in generalized epidemics, limited data exist on the effectiveness of promoting condom use and of behavior-change programs, and a Cochrane review found no clear evidence that community interventions promoting condom use reduce HIV or STI transmission (Moreno and others 2014). However, these interventions need to be supported as part of the overall HIV/AIDS response, as they absorb a small share of the budget.

Tailor the Response for the Right People in the Right Places

It is important not only to invest in context-appropriate interventions, but also to reach the right people with these interventions and to apply them in the right places.

While an epidemic may be classified as generalized, concentrated, or mixed at the national level, there may be much heterogeneity at the subnational level. For example, Vietnam's concentrated epidemic is sustained by high prevalence in MSM, male IDUs, and female sex workers, but considerable regional variation is evident in the number of infections and persons infected (map 8.2).

Two approaches are useful for identifying and reaching the right people in the right places: (1) program science, and (2) geographic targeting and hotspot mapping.

Right People: Program Science Approach

Program science is the "systematic application of theoretical and empirical scientific knowledge to improve the design, implementation, and evaluation of public health programmes" (Blanchard and Aral 2011, 1). Program science is useful for tailoring the response to local epidemics and has three core components:

- *Program intelligence*: Data collection and information gathering on modes of transmission, optimal resource allocation, local epidemic appraisal, and ethnographic-linked interventions
- *Program implementation*: Design, development, and delivery of standard intervention packages,

Map 8.2 HIV/AIDS Burden and Sources of New Infections in Vietnam, by Region, 1990 and 2014

IBRD 42332 | DECEMBER 2016

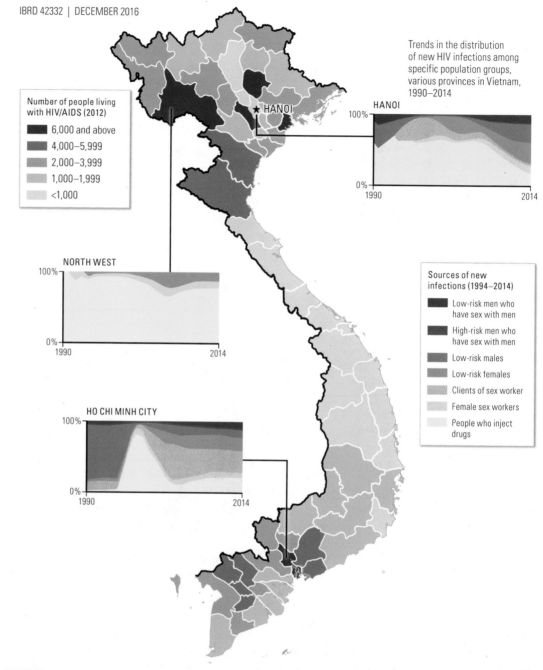

Trends in the distribution of new HIV infections among specific population groups, various provinces in Vietnam, 1990–2014

Number of people living with HIV/AIDS (2012)
- 6,000 and above
- 4,000–5,999
- 2,000–3,999
- 1,000–1,999
- <1,000

Sources of new infections (1994–2014)
- Low-risk men who have sex with men
- High-risk men who have sex with men
- Low-risk males
- Low-risk females
- Clients of sex worker
- Female sex workers
- People who inject drugs

HANOI

NORTH WEST

HO CHI MINH CITY

Source: UNAIDS 2014a.
Note: HIV/AIDS = human immunodeficiency virus/acquired immune deficiency syndrome.

implementation manuals, quality assurance guidelines, support and training for coordinated program implementation, and knowledge exchange
- *Program evaluation*: Real-time program management data and impact evaluation.

Program science has been used to assess and design the response to the epidemic in Nigeria, which is the world's most diverse and second-largest epidemic by numbers infected. The transmission dynamics are mixed: 42 percent of new infections occur in low-risk heterosexual individuals within the general population, although key populations—only 1 percent of the total population—account for 23 percent of new infections (Blanchard and Aral 2011; NACA 2014). In Cross River State, more than 50 percent of transmission is from key populations and their partners (Prudden and others 2013) (figure 8.9). Prevalence is equally varied, with the highest prevalence concentrated in four states and the lowest (well under the 3 percent of the national average) in nine states (map 8.3).

Program intelligence, gathered through biological and behavioral surveillance and through local epidemic appraisals conducted initially in eight states, provided additional information on populations at risk in Nigeria. HIV/AIDS prevalence is high in key populations, specifically IDUs (42 percent), MSM (17 percent), sex workers not in brothels (22 percent), and sex workers in brothels (27 percent) (NACA 2014). Local epidemic appraisals mapped out key population hotspots and estimated their size. Female sex workers were the largest key population: there were 10,581 female sex workers, compared with 447 IDUs and 495 MSM (NACA 2013). Sex workers by state were enumerated and, in some cases, geospatially mapped out (map 8.4). An assessment of the venues most frequented by individuals seeking new sexual partners revealed that bars, clubs, and restaurants were the primary locations in which both sexes sought out sexual partners (figure 8.10).

The information gathered through program intelligence provided the basis for the design of a strategy that targeted key populations and that ranged from national- to local-level planning. This strategy entailed the following steps (NACA 2013):

- Specify the target population, for example, female sex workers, and develop the rationale for selection.
- Define the intervention package, segmented by population group.
- Set coverage targets at the macro level; for example, cover 60 percent of estimated female sex workers.
- Set specific objectives for project reach at the micro level; for example, reach 80 percent of female sex workers using peer education.
- Set outcome objectives; for example, obtain consistent condom use of 80 percent.
- Plan and implement a scaled program, including a scaling-up strategy.

The final component of program science is evaluation. The Nigerian government has indicated that it plans to conduct an evaluation using a combination of dose-response behavioral and biological data and mathematical modeling.

Figure 8.9 Example of Heterogeneity of Sources of New HIV Infections in Cross River State, Nigeria

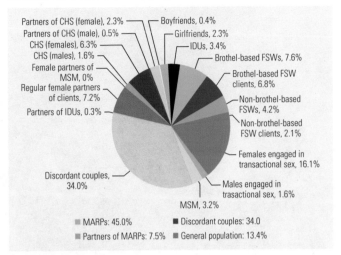

Source: Prudden and others 2013.
Note: CHS = individuals who have casual heterosexual sex; FSW = female sex worker; HIV = human immunodeficiency virus; IDU = injecting drug user; MARP = most-at-risk population; MSM = men who have sex with men.

Right Places: Geographic Targeting and Hotspot Mapping

Hotspot mapping can help locate key populations in a concentrated epidemic and help determine the optimal allocation of national resources, based on the size of the epidemic across regions.

Geographic targeting can reveal locations where epidemics are concentrated. For example, more than 70 percent of India's HIV/AIDS burden began in four southern states (Andhra Pradesh, Karnataka, Maharashtra, and Tamil Nadu) and four northeastern states (Bihar, Gujarat, Uttar Pradesh, and West Bengal) and spread from there (NACO 2013; World Bank 2012).

Hotspot targeting can also help locate key populations. Pakistan has a severe epidemic in its IDU population, 69 percent of whom live in four cities (Faisalabad, Hyderabad, Karachi, and Lahore) that account for 19 percent of the total population.[2] HIV is also growing among female and transgender sex workers: 72 percent of female sex workers are in five cities (Faisalabad, Hyderabad, Karachi, Lahore, and Multan), and 64 percent of transgender sex workers are in three cities (Karachi, Lahore, and Multan) (Blanchard 2012; Reza and others 2013) (map 8.5).[3]

Average national HIV prevalence masks subnational variations. An analysis of 20 Sub-Saharan African countries revealed spatial clustering of infections, in which 14 percent of the population lives in high-prevalence clusters and 16 percent lives in low-prevalence clusters,

Map 8.3 Prevalence of HIV/AIDS in Nigeria, by Region

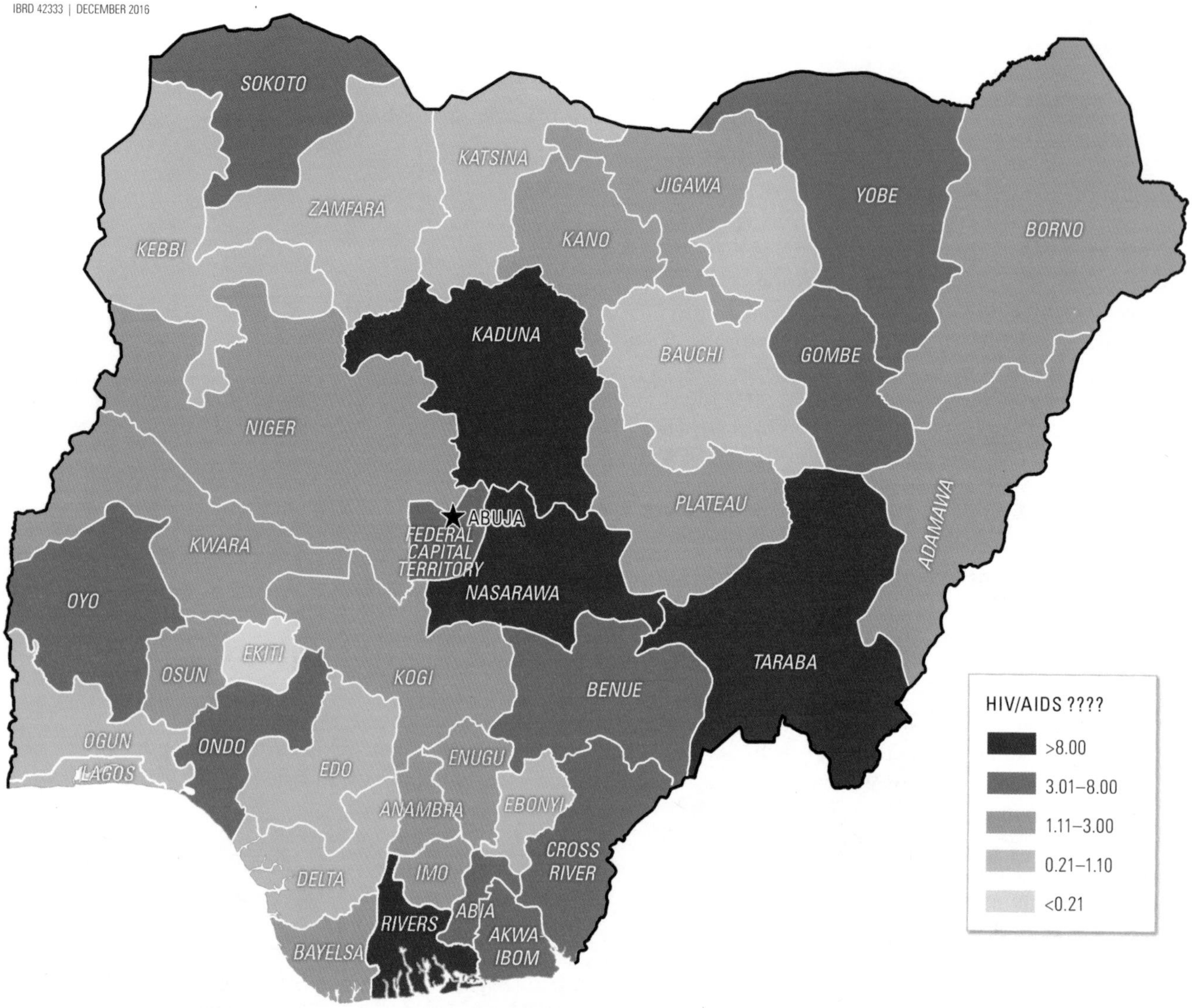

IBRD 42333 | DECEMBER 2016

HIV/AIDS ????	
	>8.00
	3.01–8.00
	1.11–3.00
	0.21–1.10
	<0.21

Source: NACA 2014. "Global AIDS Response Country Progress Report: Nigeria GARPR 2014." NACA, Abuja.
Note: HIV/AIDS = human immunodeficiency virus/acquired immune deficiency syndrome.

the difference potentially due to behavioral or biological factors (Cuadros, Awad, and Abu-Raddad 2013). Islands of high or low prevalence, due to intense clustering, can serve as prime targets for a focused response.

Hotspot mapping can also guide targeted prevention efforts. In Thailand, 70 percent of new infections occur in 33 of the country's 76 provinces (National AIDS Management Center 2013); in Kenya, nine counties with the highest burden account for 54 percent of new infections but account for only 24 percent of the Kenyan population (Government of Kenya 2013).[4] It makes sense to allocate the majority of prevention resources to

these high-burden regions while scaling back resources for the eight lowest-burden counties, which account for less than 2 percent of new infections (Government of Kenya 2013).

Geographic targeting and hotspot mapping are relatively new and need to be tested rigorously for feasibility and utility. Ideally, this time- and resource-intensive approach would reveal epidemic dynamics adhering to the 80:20 rule, where 80 percent of a parameter (prevalence, new infections, risk, transmission dynamics) can be attributed to 20 percent of a larger group (population, region). This outcome may be obtained

Map 8.4 Number of Sex Workers in Nigerian Hotspots

IBRD 42334 | DECEMBER 2016

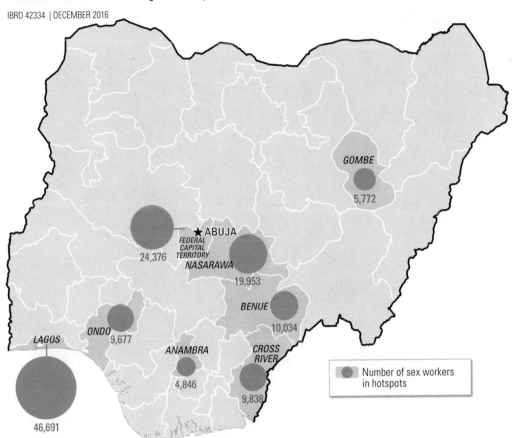

Source: NACA (National Agency for the Control of AIDS). 2013. "HIV Epidemic Appraisals in Nigeria: Evidence for Prevention Programme Planning and Implementation: Data from the First Eight States." NACA, Abuja.

Figure 8.10 Popularity of Venues Where Individuals Seek New Sexual Partners in Nigeria

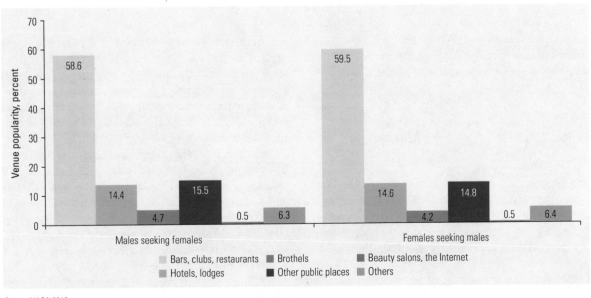

Source: NACA 2013.

Map 8.5 Population Density (per 1,000 Adult Males) of Key HIV/AIDS Populations in City Hotspots in Pakistan

IBRD 42335 | DECEMBER 2016

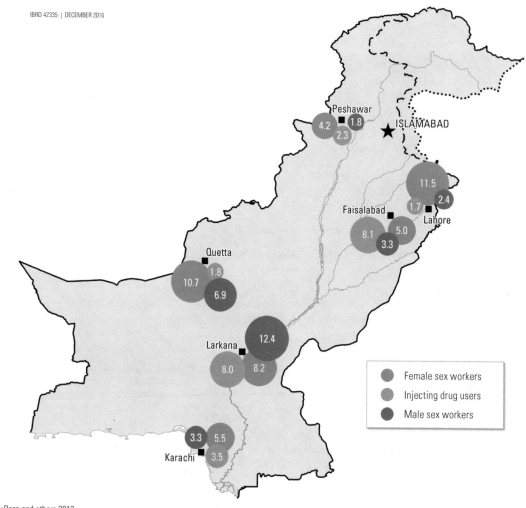

Source: Reza and others 2013.

more typically in concentrated epidemics, but even generalized epidemics exhibit varying degrees of geographic and population-level concentration of infections.

OPTIMIZE ALLOCATIVE EFFICIENCY FOR COST-EFFECTIVE PROGRAMMING: THE RIGHT MIX

In all epidemics, the response is more effective and more cost-effective if it is tailored to the local transmission dynamics. To achieve maximum impact per expenditure, prioritizing and optimizing the allocation of resources are crucial; that is, the right mix of interventions must be applied.

The use of Optima—an epidemic- and cost-modeling software—can facilitate the effort to apply the right

mix of interventions. Developed by the Kirby Institute at the University of New South Wales with input from the World Bank, Optima is a mathematical model of transmission dynamics and disease progression integrated with an economic and financial analysis framework. Its highly flexible structure can accommodate country-specific inputs. It can divide the population into subgroups and characterize them by demographics, HIV risk, disease, and clinical and treatment status, including changes in health states and population groups. The model uses a range of inputs (demographic, epidemiological, behavioral, clinical, and financial) to generate the most appropriate ratio of interventions at different spending levels. Although not all parameters have to be entered, the more data points in the model, the more reliable the analysis.

The result is a set of analyses showing outcomes based on a range of programmatic allocations and financial investments in comparison with current allocations and investments. For example, an Optima analysis for Belarus suggests that current allocations would have to be restructured if the number of new HIV infections is to be reduced by 2020. The optimal programmatic structure would shift funds from the general population to key populations, specifically increasing NSP spending until saturation is reached, and tripling and doubling spending on condom programs targeting MSM and female sex workers, respectively. To minimize new infections, the results suggest that Belarus should substantially increase ART coverage (figure 8.11).

Optima can produce optimal allocations for a range of budget scenarios. In the tightest budget scenario, Belarus should focus on prevention in key populations

and gradually add counseling, testing, and treatment services as the budget increases. Only when spending exceeds the current budget will investments in prevention be warranted for low-risk populations.

Optima can also indicate ways to maximize the impact of current spending. By spending the same amount of money differently, Belarus could reduce the number of new infections by 27 percent, and a 2014 analysis projected halving the number of new infections in Swaziland by 2016. This improvement in allocative and technical efficiency in Swaziland would cost only an additional US$8 million, as compared with 10 times that amount based on current allocations (figure 8.12). Table 8.1 lists the costs associated with scaling up specific interventions in Swaziland, including the incremental cost-effectiveness ratio for infections averted.

The use of Optima for Belarus is an excellent example of how shifting allocations can maximize the impacts of

Figure 8.11 Optima-Projected Results for Belarus: Current and Optimal Allocation of Resources for HIV/AIDS Programs

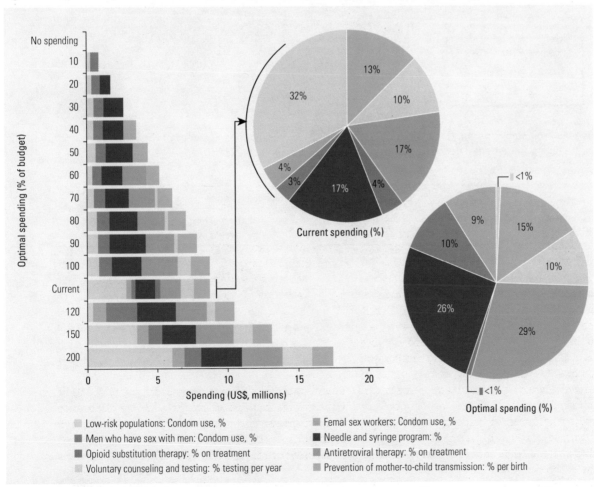

Legend:
- Low-risk populations: Condom use, %
- Men who have sex with men: Condom use, %
- Opioid substitution therapy: % on treatment
- Voluntary counseling and testing: % testing per year
- Femal sex workers: Condom use, %
- Needle and syringe program: %
- Antiretroviral therapy: % on treatment
- Prevention of mother-to-child transmission: % per birth

Source: Wilson and others 2013.

Note: HIV/AIDS = human immunodeficiency virus/acquired immune deficiency syndrome.

Figure 8.12 Allocative and Technical Efficiency Gains and Costs Associated with Halving the Number of New HIV Infections in Swaziland by 2016

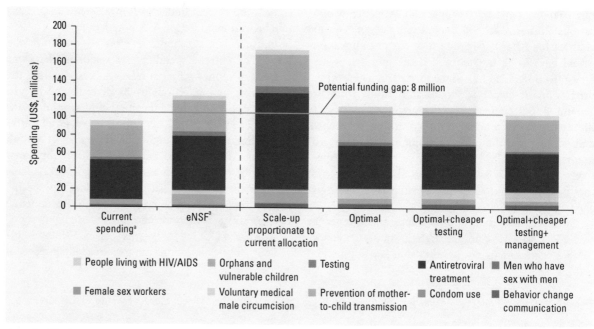

Source: Unpublished data from Wilson and Kerr.

Note: eNSF= Extended National Strategic Framework; HIV = human immunodeficiency virus.

a. The Optima model projects that incidence will decline by 13 percent by 2018 under current spending, and by 35 percent under the eNSF.

Table 8.1 Optima-Projected Program Costs of Moderate Scale-up of Interventions, Number of New Infections and Deaths Averted, and Resulting Incremental Cost-Effectiveness Ratios in Swaziland by 2030

US$ unless otherwise noted

Moderate scale-up of interventions	Unit costs (US$ per person per year)	Discounted cost of program[a]*	Infections averted		AIDS-related deaths averted	
			Number	Incremental cost-effectiveness ratio	Number	Incremental cost-effectiveness ratio
All interventions	—	74,205,074	27,355	2,713	7,413	10,010
Antiretroviral therapy	131.70	13,654,653	7,452	1,832	4,254	3,210
Voluntary medical male circumcision	130.70 (per male age 10–49)	2,475,488	13,291	186	1,334	1,856
CCTs	76.56[a] (per female age 15–24)	45,031,793	9,895	4,551	1,033	43,608
Prevention of mother-to-child transmission of HIV	186.00 (per pregnant woman)	767,735	1,164	659	221	3,480
TB and HIV/AIDS co-treatment	247.00[b]	37,669,429	—	—	1,220	30,883

Source: Kelly and others 2014.

Note: * = Discounted cost is today's dollar equivalent of future costs. CCT = conditional cash transfer; TB = tuberculosis; — = not applicable.

a. It was assumed that only 29 percent of the costs for the CCT program would be allocated to the HIV program, as there are multiple benefits to this intervention (see Remme and others 2014, table 3); therefore, the HIV program would not be expected to fund the full cost of the CCT program, which is US$264 per girl or young woman age 15–24 per year.

b. It was assumed that the cost of the TB/HIV program would increase proportionately to the increased TB/HIV coverage over time to meet targets. As well, since it was reported that "the prevalence of HIV among TB patients is 79.6 percent, therefore 79.6 percent of total expenditure on TB was captured as TB/HIV treatment expenditure" (UNAIDS, n.d.), it follows that only 80 percent of the TB/HIV spending was allocated to the HIV program.

Figure 8.13 Optima Analysis Findings in Eastern Europe and Central Asia

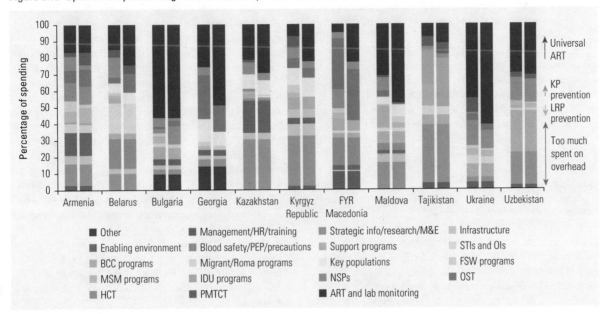

Source: David Wilson, personal communication.

Note: ART = antiretroviral therapy; BCC = behavioral change communication; FSW = female sex worker; HCT = HIV counseling and testing; HR = human resources; KP = key population; LRP = low-risk population; M&E = monitoring and evaluation; MSM = men who have sex with men; NSP = needle and syringe program; OI = opportunistic infection; OST = opioid substitution therapy; PEP = postexposure prophylaxis; PMTCT = prevention of mother to child transmission; PWID = people who inject drugs; STI = sexually transmitted infection.

current and future spending in a concentrated epidemic. The opportunity to increase allocative efficiency is modest in generalized epidemics, such as in Swaziland, because transmission is not highly concentrated and resources are not grossly misallocated. It is difficult to determine what programs or interventions could be assigned a lower priority or given up. Nevertheless, Optima is an important first step in painstaking hands-on work that focuses on intracategory analyses and the interplay between allocative and implementation efficiency, keeping in mind the heterogeneity and uniqueness of each epidemic at national and subnational levels. However, some general conclusions can be made from looking at a range of Optima analyses performed in Eastern Europe and Central Asia. Across the board, optimal allocations include larger investments in ART for all populations and in HIV programs for key populations. Fewer resources could be spent on programs for low-risk populations, and the analyses reveal that far too much is spent on overhead and program administration (figure 8.13).

CONCLUSIONS

Financing of HIV/AIDS programs is subject to numerous competing priorities. To make better use of existing resources, a greater understanding of the heterogeneity, transmission dynamics, and geographic variation of epidemics is needed, together with the use of proven interventions. Greater targeting of the right interventions for the right people in the right places at the right times will improve the efficiency and effectiveness of the global response. The HIV/AIDS epidemic will not end without an effective vaccine or cure. In the meantime, greater understanding of transmission dynamics and more efficient implementation and delivery of prevention, detection, and treatment programs can prevent a substantial proportion of new infections.

NOTES

World Bank Income Classifications as of July 2014 are as follows, based on estimates of gross national income (GNI) per capita for 2013:

- Low-income countries (LICs) = US$1,045 or less
- Middle-income countries (MICs) are subdivided:
  (a) lower-middle-income = US$1,046 to US$4,125
  (b) upper-middle-income (UMICs) = US$4,126 to US$12,745
- High-income countries (HICs) = US$12,746 or more.

1. For more a more detailed discussion on the use of models to inform decision making regarding resource allocation for HIV program planning, please refer to chapter 9 of this volume (Kahn and others 2017).

2. Calculations based on 2010 and 2011 data from City Mayors.com (http://citymayors.com/statistics/largest-cities -mayors-mr2.html) and Knoema.com (http://knoema .com/atlas/Pakistan/Population).

3. Calculations based on 2010 and 2011 data from City Mayors.com (http://citymayors.com/statistics/largest -cities-mayors-mr2.html) and Knoema.com (http:// knoema.com/atlas/Pakistan/Population).

4. Calculations based on 2010 data from Kenya National Bureau of Statistics (http://www.knbs.or.ke/index.php ?option=com_content&view=article&id=176&Itemid=645).

REFERENCES

Auvert, B., D. Taljaard, E. Lagarde, J. Sobngwi-Tambekou, R. Sitta, and others. 2005. "Randomized, Controlled Intervention Trial of Male Circumcision for Reduction of HIV Infection Risk: The ANRS 1265 Trial." *PLoS Medicine* 2 (11): e298.

Auvert, B., D. Taljaard, D. Rech, P. Lissouba, B. Singh, and others. 2013. "Association of the ANRS-12126 Male Circumcision Project with HIV Levels among Men in a South African Township: Evaluation of Effectiveness Using Cross-Sectional Surveys." *PLoS Medicine* 10 (9): e1001509.

Baeten, J. M., D. Donnell, P. Ndase, N. R. Mugo, J. D. Campbell, and others. 2012. "Antiretroviral Prophylaxis for HIV Prevention in Heterosexual Men and Women." *New England Journal of Medicine* 367 (5): 399–410.

Bailey, R. C., S. Moses, C. B. Parker, K. Agot, I. Maclean, and others. 2007. "Male Circumcision for HIV Prevention in Young Men in Kisumu, Kenya: A Randomised Controlled Trial." *The Lancet* 369 (9562): 643–56.

———. 2010. "The Protective Effect of Adult Male Circumcision against HIV Acquisition Is Sustained for at Least 54 Months: Results from the Kisumu, Kenya Trial." XVIII International AIDS Conference, Vienna.

Baird, S. J., R. S. Garfein, C. T. McIntosh, and B. Ozler. 2012. "Effect of a Cash Transfer Programme for Schooling on Prevalence of HIV and Herpes Simplex Type 2 in Malawi: A Cluster Randomised Trial." *The Lancet* 379 (9823): 1320–29.

Baral, S., C. Beyrer, K. Muessig, T. Poteat, A. L. Wirtz, and others. 2012. "Burden of HIV among Female Sex Workers in Low-Income and Middle-Income Countries: A Systematic Review and Meta-Analysis." *The Lancet Infectious Diseases* 12 (7): 538–49.

Beattie, T. S., H. L. Mohan, P. Bhattacharjee, S. Chandrashekar, S. Isac, and others. 2014. "Community Mobilization and Empowerment of Female Sex Workers in Karnataka State, South India: Associations with HIV and Sexually Transmitted Infection Risk." *American Journal of Public Health* 104 (8): 1516–25.

Blanchard, A. K., H. L. Mohan, M. Shahmanesh, R. Prakash, S. Isac, and others. 2013. "Community Mobilization, Empowerment, and HIV Prevention among Female Sex Workers in South India." *BMC Public Health* 13: 234.

Blanchard, J. 2012. "Global Program Science Initiatives." Paper prepared for the National STD Prevention Conference, Minneapolis, March 12.

Blanchard, J., and S. O. Aral. 2011. "Program Science: An Initiative to Improve the Planning, Implementation, and Evaluation of HIV/Sexually Transmitted Infection Prevention Programmes." *Sexually Transmitted Infections* 87 (1): 2–3.

Blouin, K., P. Leclerc, C. Morissette, É. Roy, C. Blanchette, and others. 2013. "P3.099 Sex Work as an Emerging Risk Factor for HIV Seroconversion among Injection Drug Users in the SurvUDI Network." *Sexually Transmitted Infections* 89 (Suppl 1): A178.

Chersich, M. F., S. Luchters, I. Ntaganira, A. Gerbase, Y. R. Lo, and others. 2013. "Priority Interventions to Reduce HIV Transmission in Sex Work Settings in Sub-Saharan Africa and Delivery of These Services." *Journal of the International AIDS Society* 16 (1): 17980.

Choi, K. H., D. R. Gibson, L. Han, and Y. Guo. 2004. "High Levels of Unprotected Sex with Men and Women among Men Who Have Sex with Men: A Potential Bridge of HIV Transmission in Beijing, China." *AIDS Education and Prevention* 16 (1): 19–30.

Choi, K. H., W. McFarland, T. B. Neilands, S. Nguyen, B. Louie, and others. 2004. "An Opportunity for Prevention: Prevalence, Incidence, and Sexual Risk for HIV among Young Asian and Pacific Islander Men Who Have Sex with Men, San Francisco." *Sexually Transmitted Diseases* 31 (8): 475–80.

Choopanya, K., M. Martin, P. Suntharasamai, U. Sangkum, P. A. Mock, and others. 2013. "Antiretroviral Prophylaxis for HIV Infection in Injecting Drug Users in Bangkok, Thailand (The Bangkok Tenofovir Study): A Randomised, Double-Blind, Placebo-Controlled Phase 3 Trial." *The Lancet* 381 (9883): 2083–90.

Cohen, M. S., Y. Q. Chen, M. McCauley, T. Gamble, M. C. Hosseinipour, and others. 2011. "Prevention of HIV-1 Infection with Early Antiretroviral Therapy." *New England Journal of Medicine* 365 (6): 493–505.

Colfax, G., G. M. Santos, P. Chu, E. Vittinghoff, A. Pluddemann, and others. 2010. "Amphetamine-Group Substances and HIV." *The Lancet* 376 (9739): 458–74.

Cuadros, D. F., S. F. Awad, and L. J. Abu-Raddad. 2013. "Mapping HIV Clustering: A Strategy for Identifying Populations at High Risk of HIV Infection in Sub-Saharan Africa." *International Journal of Health Geographics* 12: 28.

Decker, M. R., A. L. Crago, S. K. Chu, S. G. Sherman, M. S. Seshu, and others. 2014. "Human Rights Violations against Sex Workers: Burden and Effect on HIV." *The Lancet* 385 (9963): 186–99.

Deering, K. N., T. Lyons, C. X. Feng, B. Nosyk, S. A. Strathdee, and others. 2013. "Client Demands for Unsafe Sex: The Socioeconomic Risk Environment for HIV among Street and Off-Street Sex Workers." *Journal of Acquired Immune Deficiency Syndromes* 63 (4): 522–31.

de Walque, D., W. H. Dow, R. Nathan, R. Abdul, F. Abilahi, and others. 2012. "Incentivising Safe Sex: A Randomised Trial of Conditional Cash Transfers for HIV and Sexually

Transmitted Infection Prevention in Rural Tanzania." *BMJ Open* 2: e000747.

Family Health International, the Lesotho Ministry of Health, LAPCA (Lesotho AIDS Programme Co-ordinating Authority), Sechaba Consultants, and USAID (U.S. Agency for International Development). 2002. "HIV/AIDS Behavioral Surveillance Survey: Lesotho 2002; Summary Technical Report—Round 1." USAID, Washington, DC.

Fonner, V. A., S. L. Dalglish, C. E. Kennedy, R. Baggaley, K. R. O'reilly, and others. 2016. "Effectiveness and Safety of Oral HIV Pre-Exposure Prophylaxis (PrEP) for All Populations: A Systematic Review and Meta-Analysis." *AIDS*.

Fonner, V. A., D. Kerrigan, Z. Mnisi, S. Ketende, C. E. Kennedy, and others. 2014. "Social Cohesion, Social Participation, and HIV Related Risk among Female Sex Workers in Swaziland." *PLoS One* 9 (1): e87527.

Freeman, P., B. C. Walker, D. R. Harris, R. Garofalo, N. Willard, and others. 2011. "Methamphetamine Use and Risk for HIV among Young Men Who Have Sex with Men in 8 U.S. Cities." *Archives of Pediatrics and Adolescent Medicine* 165 (8): 736–40.

Ghys, P. D., M. O. Diallo, V. Ettiegne-Traore, K. Kale, O. Tawil, and others. 2002. "Increase in Condom Use and Decline in HIV and Sexually Transmitted Diseases among Female Sex Workers in Abidjan, Côte d'Ivoire, 1991–1998." *AIDS* 16 (2): 251–58.

Ghys, P. D., M. O. Diallo, V. Ettiegne-Traore, G. A. Satten, C. K. Anoma, and others. 2001. "Effect of Interventions to Control Sexually Transmitted Disease on the Incidence of HIV Infection in Female Sex Workers." *AIDS* 15 (11): 1421–31.

Gouws, E., and P. Cuchi. 2012. "Focusing the HIV Response through Estimating the Major Modes of HIV Transmission: A Multi-Country Analysis." *Sexually Transmitted Infections* 88 (Suppl 2): i76–85.

Government of Kenya. 2013. "Kenya HIV Investment Case Summary." Government of Kenya, Nairobi.

Grant, R. M., J. R. Lama, P. L. Anderson, V. McMahan, A. Y. Liu, and others. 2010. "Preexposure Chemoprophylaxis for HIV Prevention in Men Who Have Sex with Men." *New England Journal of Medicine* 363 (27): 2587–99.

Gray, R. H., G. Kigozi, X. Kong, V. Ssempiija, F. Makumbi, and others. 2012. "The Effectiveness of Male Circumcision for HIV Prevention and Effects on Risk Behaviors in a Posttrial Follow-up Study." *AIDS* 26 (5): 609–15.

Gray, R. H., G. Kigozi, D. Serwadda, F. Makumbi, S. Watya, and others. 2007. "Male Circumcision for HIV Prevention in Men in Rakai, Uganda: A Randomised Trial." *The Lancet* 369 (9562): 657–66.

Grulich, A. E., and I. Zablotska. 2010. "Commentary: Probability of HIV Transmission through Anal Intercourse." *International Journal of Epidemiology* 39 (4): 1064–65.

HPTN (HIV Prevention Trials Network). 2015. "Cash Transfers Conditional on Schooling Do Not Prevent HIV Infection among Young South African Women." Presentation at the 8th International AIDS Society Conference on HIV Pathogenesis, Treatment, and Prevention, Vancouver, Canada, July 19–22.

Indonesian National AIDS Commission. 2012. "Country Report on the Follow-Up to the Declaration of Commitment on HIV/AIDS." Indonesian National AIDS Commission, Jakarta.

Ireri, A. W. 2012. "Police Discrimination against Commercial Sex Workers' Possession of Condoms." Paper prepared for the 19th International AIDS Conference, Washington, DC, July 22–27.

Jia, Z., Y. Mao, F. Zhang, Y. Ruan, Y. Ma, and others. 2013. "Antiretroviral Therapy to Prevent HIV Transmission in Serodiscordant Couples in China (2003–11): A National Observational Cohort Study." *The Lancet* 382 (9899): 1195–203.

Johnston, L. G., and S. Corceal. 2013. "Unexpectedly High Injection Drug Use, HIV, and Hepatitis C Prevalence among Female Sex Workers in the Republic of Mauritius." *AIDS and Behavior* 17 (2): 574–84.

Kahn, J. G., L. A. Bollinger, J. Stover, and E. Marseille. 2017. "Improving the Efficiency of the HIV/AIDS Policy Response: A Guide to Resource Allocation Modeling." In *Disease Control Priorities* (third edition): Volume 6, *Major Infectious Diseases*, edited by K. K. Holmes, S. Bertozzi, B. R. Bloom, and P. Jha. World Bank: Washington, DC.

Karim, Q. A., K. Leask, A. Kharsany, H. Humphries, and others. 2015. "Impact of Conditional Cash Incentives on HSV-2 and HIV Prevention in Rural South African High School Students: Results of the CAPRISA 007 Cluster Randomized Controlled Trial." Presentation at the 8th International AIDS Society Conference on HIV Pathogenesis, Treatment, and Prevention, Vancouver, Canada, July 19–22.

Kelly, J. A., Y. A. Amirkhanian, D. W. Seal, C. M. Galletly, W. Difranceisco, and others. 2010. "Levels and Predictors of Sexual HIV Risk in Social Networks of Men Who Have Sex with Men in the Midwest." *AIDS Education and Prevention* 22 (6): 483–95.

Kelly, S., A. Shattock, C. C. Kerr, T. Gama, N. Nhlabatsi, and others. 2014. *HIV Mathematical Modelling to Support Swaziland's Development of Its HIV Investment Case*. Final Report. Washington, DC: World Bank.

Kerrigan, D., A. Wirtz, S. Baral, M. Decker, L. Murray, and others. 2013. *The Global HIV Epidemics among Sex Workers*. Directions in Development. Washington, DC: World Bank.

King, E. J., S. Maman, J. M. Bowling, K. E. Moracco, and V. Dudina. 2013. "The Influence of Stigma and Discrimination on Female Sex Workers' Access to HIV Services in St. Petersburg, Russia." *AIDS and Behavior* 17 (8): 2597–603.

Kippax, S., and K. Race. 2003. "Sustaining Safe Practice: Twenty Years On." *Social Science and Medicine* 57 (1): 1–12.

Laga, M., M. Alary, N. Nzila, A. T. Manoka, M. Tuliza, and others. 1994. "Condom Promotion, Sexually Transmitted Diseases Treatment, and Declining Incidence of HIV-1 Infection in Female Zairian Sex Workers." *The Lancet* 344 (8917): 246–48.

Lau, J. T. F., H. Y. Tsui, Y. Zhang, F. Cheng, L. Zhang, and others. 2008. "Comparing HIV-Related Syringe-Sharing Behaviors among Female IDU Engaging versus Not Engaging in Commercial Sex." *Drug and Alcohol Dependence* 97 (1–2): 54–63.

Lipovsek, V., A. Mukherjee, D. Navin, P. Marjara, A. Sharma, and others. 2010. "Increases in Self-Reported Consistent Condom Use among Male Clients of Female Sex Workers Following Exposure to an Integrated Behaviour Change Programme in Four States in Southern India." *Sexually Transmitted Infections* 86 (Suppl 1): i25–32.

MacArthur, G. J., S. Minozzi, N. Martin, P. Vickerman, S. Deren, and others. 2012. "Opiate Substitution Treatment and HIV Transmission in People Who Inject Drugs: Systematic Review and Meta-Analysis." *British Medical Journal* 345: e5945.

MacDonald, M., M. Law, J. Kaldor, J. Hales, and G. J. Dore. 2003. "Effectiveness of Needle and Syringe Programmes for Preventing HIV Transmission." *International Journal of Drug Policy* 14 (5): 353–57.

Marrazzo, J. M., G. Ramjee, B. A. Richardson, K. Gomez, N. Mgodi, and others. 2015. "Tenofovir-Based Preexposure Prophylaxis for HIV Infection among African Women." *New England Journal of Medicine* 372 (6): 509–18. doi:10.1056/NEJMoa1402269.

Maseko, S., and S. Ndlovu. 2012. "Condoms as Evidence: Police, Sex Workers, and Condom Confiscation in Zimbabwe." Paper prepared for the 19th International AIDS Conference, Washington, DC, July 22–27.

Mathers, B. M., L. Degenhardt, B. Phillips, L. Wiessing, M. Hickman, and others. 2008. "Global Epidemiology of Injecting Drug Use and HIV among People Who Inject Drugs: A Systematic Review." *The Lancet* 372 (9651): 1733–45.

Moreno, R., H. Y. Nababan, E. Ota, W. M. Wariki, S. Ezoe, and others. 2014. "Structural and Community-Level Interventions for Increasing Condom Use to Prevent the Transmission of HIV and Other Sexually Transmitted Infections." *Cochrane Database of Systematic Reviews* 7: CD003363. doi:10.1002/14651858.CD003363.pub3.

NACA (National Agency for the Control of AIDS). 2013. "HIV Epidemic Appraisals in Nigeria: Evidence for Prevention Programme Planning and Implementation; Data from the First Eight States." NACA, Abuja.

———. 2014. "Global AIDS Response: Country Progress Report; Nigeria GARPR 2014." NACA, Abuja.

NACO (National AIDS Control Organisation). 2013. "HIV Sentinel Surveillance 2012–13: A Technical Brief." Ministry of Health and Family Welfare, New Delhi.

Nagot, N., A. Ouangre, A. Ouedraogo, M. Cartoux, P. Huygens, and others. 2002. "Spectrum of Commercial Sex Activity in Burkina Faso: Classification Model and Risk of Exposure to HIV." *Journal of Acquired Immune Deficiency Syndromes* 29 (5): 517–21.

Nasirian, Maryam. 2011. *Modeling of New HIV Infections Based on Exposure Groups in Iran: Predictions for Planning.* Saarbrucken, Germany: Lambert Academic Publishing.

National AIDS Management Center. 2013. *Ending AIDS in Thailand.* Bangkok: Ministry of Public Health.

Needle, R., K. Kroeger, H. Belani, A. Achrekar, C. D. Parry, and S. Dewing. 2008. "Sex, Drugs, and HIV: Rapid Assessment of HIV Risk Behaviors among Street-Based Drug Using Sex Workers in Durban, South Africa." *Social Science and Medicine* 67 (9): 1447–55.

Ngoc, K. V., G. Mundy, Y. Madan, J. Ayers, D. Sherard, and others. 2011. "Using Formative Research to Promote Behavior Change among Male Clients of Female Sex Workers in Vietnam." *Cases in Public Health Communication and Marketing* 5 (Proceedings): 27–47.

Njeuhmeli, E., S. Forsythe, J. Reed, M. Opuni, L. Bollinger, and others. 2011. "Voluntary Medical Male Circumcision: Modeling the Impact and Cost of Expanding Male Circumcision for HIV Prevention in Eastern and Southern Africa." *PLoS Medicine* 8 (11): e1001132.

Nyqvist, M. B., L. Corno, D. de Walque, and J. Svensson. 2015. "Using Lotteries to Incentivize Safer Sexual Behavior: Evidence from a Randomized Controlled Trial on HIV Prevention." Policy Research Working Paper 7215, World Bank, Washington, DC.

Open Society Foundations. 2012. "Criminalizing Condoms: How Policing Practices Put Sex Workers and HIV Services at Risk in Kenya, Namibia, Russia, South Africa, the United States, and Zimbabwe." Sexual Health and Rights Project, Open Society Foundations, New York.

Padian, N. S., S. I. McCoy, J. E. Balkus, and J. N. Wasserheit. 2010. "Weighing the Gold in the Gold Standard: Challenges in HIV Prevention Research." *AIDS* 24 (5): 621–35.

Peterson, L., D. Taylor, R. Roddy, G. Belai, P. Phillips, and others. 2007. "Tenofovir Disoproxil Fumarate for Prevention of HIV Infection in Women: A Phase 2, Double-Blind, Randomized, Placebo-Controlled Trial." *PLoS Clinical Trials* 2 (5): e27.

Pickles, M., M. C. Boily, P. Vickerman, C. M. Lowndes, S. Moses, and others. 2013. "Assessment of the Population-Level Effectiveness of the Avahan HIV-Prevention Programme in South India: A Preplanned, Causal-Pathway-Based Modelling Analysis." *The Lancet Global Health* 1 (5): e289–99.

Prudden, H. J., C. H. Watts, P. Vickerman, N. Bobrova, L. Heise, and others. 2013. "Can the UNAIDS Modes of Transmission Model Be Improved? A Comparison of the Original and Revised Model Projections Using Data from a Setting in West Africa." *AIDS* 27 (16): 2623–35.

Quinn, T. C., M. J. Wawer, N. Sewankambo, D. Serwadda, C. Li, and others. 2000. "Viral Load and Heterosexual Transmission of Human Immunodeficiency Virus Type 1." *New England Journal of Medicine* 342 (13): 921–29.

Remme, M. I., A. Vassall, B. Lutz, and C. Watts. 2014. "Financing Structural Interventions: Going beyond HIV-Only Value for Money Assessments." *AIDS* 28 (3): 425–34.

Reza, T., D. Y. Melesse, L. A. Shafer, M. Salim, A. Altaf, and others. 2013. "Patterns and Trends in Pakistan's Heterogeneous HIV Epidemic." *Sexually Transmitted Infections* 89 (Suppl 2): ii4–10.

Rojanapithayakorn, W., and R. Hanenberg. 1996. "The 100% Condom Program in Thailand." *AIDS* 10 (1): 1–7.

SACEMA (South African Centre for Epidemiological Modelling and Analysis). 2009. "The Modes of Transmission of HIV in South Africa." SACEMA, Stellenbosch.

Scorgie, F., S. Nakato, D. O. Akoth, M. Netshivhambe, P. Chakuvinga, and others. 2011. "*I Expect to Be Abused and I Have Fear*":

Sex Workers' Experiences of Human Rights Violations and Barriers to Accessing Healthcare in Four African Countries; Final Report. Cape Town: African Sex Worker Alliance.

Stoicescu, Claudia, ed. 2012. *The Global State of Harm Reduction 2012: Towards an Integrated Response*. London: Harm Reduction International.

Strathdee, S. A., T. B. Hallett, N. Bobrova, T. Rhodes, R. Booth, and others. 2010. "HIV and Risk Environment for Injecting-Drug Users: The Past, Present, and Future." *The Lancet* 376 (9737): 268–84.

Sullivan, P. S., A. Carballo-Diéguez, T. Coates, S. M. Goodreau, I. McGowan, and others. 2012. "Successes and Challenges of HIV Prevention in Men Who Have Sex with Men." *The Lancet* 380 (9839): 388–99.

Sullivan, P. S., O. Hamouda, V. Delpech, J. E. Geduld, J. Prejean, and others. 2009. "Reemergence of the HIV Epidemic among Men Who Have Sex with Men in North America, Western Europe, and Australia, 1996–2005." *Annals of Epidemiology* 19 (6): 423–31.

Swaziland Ministry of Health. 2012. *Swaziland HIV Incidence Measurement Survey (SHIMS): First Findings Report*. Mbabane: Ministry of Health.

Swaziland Ministry of Health and Social Welfare. 2002. "Swaziland Behavioral Surveillance Survey (BSS)." Ministry of Health and Social Welfare, Mbabane.

Tanser, F., T. Bärnighausen, E. Grapsa, J. Zaidi, and M. L. Newell. 2013. "High Coverage of ART Associated with Decline in Risk of HIV Acquisition in Rural KwaZulu-Natal, South Africa." *Science* 339 (6122): 966–71.

Thigpen, M. C., P. M. Kebaabetswe, L. A. Paxton, D. K. Smith, C. E. Rose, and others. 2012. "Antiretroviral Preexposure Prophylaxis for Heterosexual HIV Transmission in Botswana." *New England Journal of Medicine* 367 (5): 423–34. doi: 10.1056/NEJMoa1110711.

UNAIDS (Joint United Nations Programme on HIV/AIDS). 2006. *UNAIDS Report on the Global AIDS Epidemic 2006*. Geneva: UNAIDS.

———. 2012. *UNAIDS Report on the Global AIDS Epidemic 2012*. Geneva: UNAIDS. http://www.unaids.org/sites/default/files/media_asset/20121120_UNAIDS_Global_Report_2012_with_annexes_en_1.pdf.

———. 2014a. *Local Epidemics Issue Brief*. Geneva: UNAIDS.

———. 2014b. *UNAIDS GAP Report 2014*. Geneva: UNAIDS.

———. n.d. "National AIDS Spending Assessment 2007–2010: The Kingdom of Swaziland." UNAIDS, Geneva.

———. 2016. *Prevention Gap Report*. Geneva: UNAIDS. http://www.unaids.org/sites/default/files/media_asset/2016-prevention-gap-report_en.pdf.

UNAIDS and OPS (Organización Panamericana de la Salud). 2009. "Modos de transmisión del VIH en America Latina: Resultados de la aplicación del modelo." OPS, Lima.

UNAIDS/WHO Working Group on Global HIV/AIDS and STI Surveillance. 2000. *Guidelines for Second Generation HIV Surveillance*. Geneva: World Health Organization and Joint United Nations Programme on HIV/AIDS.

UNAIDS and World Bank. 2012. "New HIV Infections by Mode of Transmission in West Africa: A Multicountry Analysis, 2010." UNAIDS and World Bank, Dakar.

USAID (U.S. Agency for International Development). 2011. "Condom Social Marketing: Rigorous Evidence; Usable Results." *Research to Prevention* 5, USAID, New York.

Van Damme, L., A. Corneli, K. Ahmed, K. Agot, J. Lombaard, and others. 2012. "Preexposure Prophylaxis for HIV Infection among African Women." *New England Journal of Medicine* 367 (5): 411–22. doi:10.1056/NEJMoa1202614.

van den Berg, C., C. Smit, G. Van Brussel, R. Coutinho, and M. Prins. 2007. "Full Participation in Harm Reduction Programmes Is Associated with Decreased Risk for Human Immunodeficiency Virus and Hepatitis C Virus: Evidence from the Amsterdam Cohort Studies among Drug Users." *Addiction* 102 (9): 1454–62.

van Griensven, F., A. Varangrat, W. Wimonsate, S. Tanpradech, K. Kladsawad, and others. 2009. "Trends in HIV Prevalence, Estimated HIV Incidence, and Risk Behavior among Men Who Have Sex with Men in Bangkok, Thailand, 2003–2007." *Journal of Acquired Immune Deficiency Syndromes* 53 (2): 234–39.

Vassall, A., M. Pickles, S. Chandrashekar, M.-C. Boily, G. Shetty, and others. 2014. "Cost-Effectiveness of HIV Prevention for High-Risk Groups at Scale: An Economic Evaluation of the Avahan Programme in South India." *The Lancet Global Health* 2 (9): e531–40.

Weiss, H. A., J. N. Wasserheit, R. V. Barnabas, R. J. Hayes, and L. J. Abu-Raddad. 2008. "Persisting with Prevention: The Importance of Adherence for HIV Prevention." *Emerging Themes in Epidemiology* 5 (8): PMC2507711.

WHO (World Health Organization). 2012. "Prevention and Treatment of HIV and Other Sexually Transmitted Infections for Sex Workers in Low- and Middle-Income Countries: Recommendations for a Public Health Approach." Department of HIV/AIDS, WHO, Geneva.

———. 2013. "Consolidated ARV Guidelines." WHO, Geneva. http://www.who.int/hiv/pub/guidelines/arv2013/intro/keyterms/en/.

———. 2014. "WHO Progress Brief: Voluntary Medical Male Circumcision for HIV Prevention in Priority Countries of East and Southern Africa." Progress Brief, WHO, Geneva. http://www.who.int/hiv/topics/malecircumcision/male-circumcision-info-2014/en/.

———. 2015. "Guideline on When to Start Antiretroviral Therapy and on Pre-Exposure Prophylaxis for HIV." WHO, Geneva.

Wilson, D., and S. Challa. 2009. "HIV Epidemiology: Recent Trends and Lessons." In *The Changing HIV/AIDS Landscape*, edited by E. L. Lule, R. M. Seifman, and A. C. David, 474. Washington, DC: World Bank.

Wilson, D., and D. T. Halperin. 2008. "'Know Your Epidemic, Know Your Response': A Useful Approach, If We Get It Right." *The Lancet* 372 (9637): 423–26.

Wilson, D. P., A. Yakusik, C. Kerr, and C. Avila. 2013. "HIV Resource Needs, Efficient Allocation, and Resource Mobilization for the Republic of Belarus." UNAIDS, Geneva.

Winkelstein, W. Jr., M. Samuel, N. S. Padian, J. A. Wiley, W. Lang, and others. 1987. "The San Francisco Men's Health Study: III; Reduction in Human Immunodeficiency Virus Transmission among Homosexual/Bisexual Men,

1982–86." *American Journal of Public Health* 77 (6): 685–89.

Wood, E., T. Kerr, B. D. L. Marshall, K. Li, R. Zhang, and others. 2009. "Longitudinal Community Plasma HIV-1 RNA Concentrations and Incidence of HIV-1 among Injecting Drug Users: Prospective Cohort Study." *British Medical Journal* 338: b1649.

World Bank. 2012. "HIV/AIDS in India." World Bank, Washington, DC.

Zohrabyan, L., L. G. Johnston, O. Scutelniciuc, A. Iovita, L. Todirascu, and others. 2013. "Determinants of HIV Infection among Female Sex Workers in Two Cities in the Republic of Moldova: The Role of Injection Drug Use and Sexual Risk." *AIDS and Behavior* 17 (8): 2588–96.

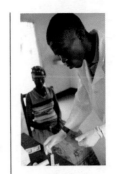

Chapter **9**

Improving the Efficiency of the HIV/AIDS Policy Response: A Guide to Resource Allocation Modeling

James G. Kahn, Lori A. Bollinger, John Stover,
and Elliot Marseille

INTRODUCTION

Resources devoted to combating the human immuno-deficiency virus and acquired immune deficiency syndrome (HIV/AIDS) have increased dramatically since 2005 (Dieleman and others 2014). However, the rate of increase has slowed in recent years, even though the commitment required to serve all of those in need and to reverse the epidemic has not been reached (Schwärtlander and others 2011; UNAIDS 2013, 2014; WHO 2013). In addition, new recommendations to start treatment earlier in the disease course mean that more resources will be needed than previously estimated. Many of the countries with the highest prevalence of HIV/AIDS have low incomes and carry a heavy burden of other diseases, and it is particularly important to deploy resources judiciously. Finally, efficiency is an even greater imperative in the current era of transition away from funding dominated by international donor aid toward a funding model in which the national governments in affected countries bear a larger portion of the costs; this is especially so since, by some metrics, national governments are failing to increase their own contributions rapidly enough (Resch, Ryckman, and Hecht 2015).

Ensuring that available resources are allocated to the most-cost-effective activities is essential to pursuing the aspirational "Getting to Zero" goals of the Joint United Nations Programme on HIV/AIDS (UNAIDS): zero new infections, zero AIDS-related deaths, and zero discrimination. Similar challenges also face global efforts to control tuberculosis and malaria—resources fall short of ambitious prevention and treatment targets.

Various effectiveness, cost-effectiveness, and resource allocation models have been developed to evaluate the costs and outcomes of the choices facing HIV/AIDS policy makers at national and international levels. This chapter presents an overview—including features, uses, and limitations—of the small subset of models that explores the allocation of HIV/AIDS resources across many intervention options and purposes. It does not assess the more numerous models that analyze the cost-effectiveness of one or a few interventions for one purpose. Accordingly, it assesses the set of software tools that portray a wide range of interventions and combinations of interventions in different settings with the goal of providing broad guidance for improved resource allocation.

Corresponding author: James G. Kahn, University of California, San Francisco Institute for Health Policy Studies, San Francisco, California, United States; jgkahn@ucsf.edu.

GENERAL OVERVIEW OF THE ROLE OF MODELS

What Are Models?

Three types of models are relevant to determining the cost-effectiveness of interventions. Epidemic and disease models use mathematics to describe the dynamics of disease acquisition or progression within individuals. Cost-effectiveness models combine epidemic and disease models with a quantitative description of one or more intervention activities typically aimed at altering a specific undesirable event (such as mother-to-child HIV transmission), estimating each intervention's cost and effectiveness in reducing morbidity or mortality. Finally, resource allocation models consider multiple interventions and health events simultaneously and in various configurations to guide the division of effort and funding among different strategies. Often, those disparate health events are translated into a common disease burden metric, disability-adjusted life years (DALYs).[1]

This chapter focuses on the third type, resource allocation models, for several reasons.

- First, in the field of global health, the most useful models for decision makers provide information that is organized and presented to help them choose courses of action that result in better population health outcomes. Resource allocation models are designed explicitly for this purpose.
- Second, they incorporate the two other types of models or practical simplifications of them. For policy makers, it is not essential to understand the individual intervention models because they often examine narrow technical issues that do not contribute meaningfully to more rational resource allocation across multiple interventions.
- Finally, limiting this chapter to resource allocation is practical. Considering the far more numerous epidemic, disease, and cost-effectiveness models and explaining their incompatibilities would be overwhelming for authors and readers alike. Table 9.1 provides a brief comparison of the models reviewed in this chapter.

Strengths and Weaknesses of Models

Resource allocation models, if thoughtfully structured and populated with sound, current data, are able to quantify and logically assemble diverse factors relevant to program decisions in ways that would otherwise be impossible. They highlight and integrate policy-relevant data and dynamics from a complex world,

ignoring myriad contextual factors that do not have an important effect on the decision at hand. They can also portray outcomes that are not empirically measurable because of technical or time constraints, such as long-term health outcomes and costs. Finally, they offer a more explicit and rational alternative to other approaches to decision making, such as guesses, inertia, political expedience, or ideology.

The limitations of models reflect the challenge of analyzing a decision with imperfect information. The best models are parsimonious enough to be understandable and buildable, yet adequately realistic to be policy relevant. They are technically sophisticated but easy to use. These competing demands confront modelers with trade-offs that are sometimes difficult to navigate wisely. This is the art of modeling. Despite best efforts, the technical details of models are opaque to all but the most sophisticated users and sometimes even to them. This opacity can be mitigated with clear documentation. Finally, values for the required inputs can be imprecise or biased. For example, efficacy data may be derived from programs in different settings or with modified implementation. To understand the importance of these uncertainties, models rely extensively on sensitivity analyses, that is, assessments of how results change with different input values. Fortunately, the basic findings of models are often robust to input uncertainties.

COMPARISON OF HIV/AIDS RESOURCE ALLOCATION MODELS

HIV/AIDS resource allocation models include the OneHealth Tool, which contains the Goals model and the Resource Needs Model (RNM) by Avenir Health; Optima HIV (part of the suite of Optima models) by the Burnet Institute and the World Bank; the AIDS Epidemic Model (AEM) by the East-West Center; Epidemiological Modeling (EMOD) by the Institute for Disease Modeling; and Global Health Decisions (GHD) by the University of California, San Francisco. Each model is best used as follows:

- *Goals* and *RNM* are widely used and supported by United Nations (UN) agencies and linked with the OneHealth Tool and other disease models for broad health sector planning. The process is moderately intensive, although the models can be adapted to specific purposes in easy-to-use formulations.
- *Optima HIV* is widely used, supported by the World Bank, and consistent with the Goals model. It uses an algorithm to optimize resource allocation across interventions and geography for a given

Table 9.1 Comparison of Models

	Goals, AIDS Impact Model (AIM), and Resource Needs Model (RNM) in Spectrum/OneHealth Tool	Optima HIV	AIDS Epidemic Model (AEM)	Epidemiological Modeling (EMOD)	Global Health Decisions
Institutional home	Avenir Health (www.avenirhealth.org /software-spectrum.php)	Optima Consortium for Decision Science (www.optimamodel.com)	East-West Center (http://www .eastwestcenter.org/research /research-projects/hiv-policy -analysis-research-and-training)	Institute for Disease Modeling (www.idmod.org)	University of California, San Francisco (www .globalhealthdecisions.org)
Disease scope	HIV/AIDS; Spectrum also includes family planning, STIs, tuberculosis, malaria, NCDs, maternal and child health, and OneHealth (health systems).	HIV/AIDS. Optima Consortium has models for TB; malaria; HCV; nutrition; and others.	HIV/AIDS	HIV/AIDS; other EMOD models address tuberculosis, airborne respiratory infections (especially TB), vector-borne diseases (especially malaria), and waterborne diseases (especially polio).	HIV/AIDS
Main use	Widely used across all epidemic types, supported by United Nations agencies; used in partnership with in-country stakeholders to support national strategic planning; linked with OneHealth Tool for broad health sector planning. Automatic optimization of resources across interventions is available. More intensive process for full model, but simplified version is newly available.	Widely used across all epidemic types; in partnership with in-country stakeholders to support national strategic planning. Is one of models supported by World Bank and PEPFAR for use in operations and technical support to governments. Core feature is algorithm to optimize resources across interventions and geography toward strategic objective, subject to specified constraints. More intensive process for full model, but simplified version available.	Used primarily in Asia to model concentrated epidemics; used in partnership with in-country stakeholders to support national strategic planning. Automatic optimization of resources across interventions is available.	Used primarily for research; generalized, concentrated-FSW-based (but not MSM or IDV yet), or mixed epidemics; fully implemented for limited countries. Models MTCT and sexual transmission based on partnership patterns. Simulates impact and cost-effectiveness of scaling-up, targeting, and varied intervention implementation. Automatic user-defined optimization across interventions.	Not widely used at country-level; most appropriate for generalized epidemics. Simplified use and easy interface to explore impact and costs of intervention combinations, implementation scales, and delivery modalities. Manual optimization of resources across interventions.

table continues next page

Table 9.1 Comparison of Models (continued)

	Goals, AIDS Impact Model (AIM), and Resource Needs Model (RNM) in Spectrum/OneHealth Tool	Optima HIV	AIDS Epidemic Model (AEM)	Epidemiological Modeling (EMOD)	Global Health Decisions
Interventions	**Prevention:** Condom promotion/marketing; STI treatment, PMTCT, blood safety, behavior change programs, interventions for high-risk groups (for example, FSW, IDU), voluntary medical male circumcision, PrEP, vaccines				
	Treatment and support: antiretroviral therapy, retention in care, opportunistic infection prophylaxis, support to people living with HIV/AIDS				
	Evolving as recommendations change.	Includes interventions listed immediately above and also innovative user-specified interventions, including complementary service modalities, targeted and cross-sectoral interventions, and treatment retention.	Based on user-defined local best-practice prevention packages for key populations (FSW, MSM, PWID, FSW who inject, transgendered populations) and population-specific antiretroviral therapy, which often reflects standard intervention list above.	Targeting by age, gender, location, time, risk, accessibility, sociodemographics. Individual-level variation over time in intervention participation and efficacy.	Subset only.
Geography	National, subnational, or any level for which necessary data are available.	National, subnational, or any level for which necessary data are available.	National and subnational.	National, subnational, and smaller. Allows age- and gender-stratified migration between geographic locations and populations.	National, subnational, or any level for which necessary data are available.
Population groups	Adults 15–49 divided into subpopulations by gender, sexual behavior (eg FSW, clients, MSMs), and injecting drug use. Also by HIV disease and treatment status. Perinatally infected children.				
	Standard groups.	Default standard risk and age groups. Users may define unlimited number of population groups as targets of chosen interventions.	Above plus transgender populations. Not children.	Users define groups via traits of individuals, for example, risks (sex behavior, condom use, concurrent partnerships) and health care access (use of ART). Trait intensity can vary by individual within group.	Standard groups.
Time frame	100 years; by year as desired.	Specified by user, by year as desired.	1975 to 2050, by year.	Specified by user; typically monthly or yearly reporting from start of epidemic until 2050.	20 years, by year.
Type of model	**Compartmental deterministic**	**Compartmental deterministic**		**Individual stochastic**	**Compartmental deterministic**
	• Divides population into groups, outcomes reflect movement between groups each time period.			• Each person is portayed, outcomes reflect random chance of change each time period.	
	• Modest flexibility, low computational requirements.			• Maximum flexibility, high computational requirements.	

table continues next page

Table 9.1 Comparison of Models (continued)

	Goals, AIDS Impact Model (AIM), and Resource Needs Model (RNM) in Spectrum/OneHealth Tool	Optima HIV	AIDS Epidemic Model (AEM)	Epidemiological Modeling (EMOD)	Global Health Decisions
Software	• Data entry and storage: Spectrum software in Windows; data can be copied from other software, for example, Excel. • Parameters are specified within Spectrum. • Calculations within Spectrum.	• Microsoft Excel for data entry with background calculations in Python. • Cloud-based graphical user interface.	• Data entry and storage: Excel 2013 or 2016. • Interventions specified in Excel workbook. • Custom Java interface for user interaction; custom Java code for computation.	• Data entry: JSON or Excel. • Database: COMPS platform (http://comps.idmod.org). • Operation: clickable run file or command line, calculation in C++.	• Data entry: prepopulated, adjust in web interface. • Intevention specified with JAVA graphical web interface. • Computation: Google Go.
User inputs	**Demographics:** (population sizes by age range, gender, major HIV risks; birth & mortality rates); **Disease prevalence:** (HIV, AIDS, STI); **Risk behaviors:** (partnerships, condom use); **HIV program coverage** and **cost**				
	Relevant variables for 7 risk categories. Defaults available for 100 countries.	Flexible population groups defined by user. Defaults available for most countries. If resource allocation analyses then program-related cost functions.	Historical trends for prevalence and behaviors, program effectiveness, and cost by key populations.	Fine detail by age/gender /year. Migration between pairs of geographic locations. Risk and health care access stratification. Health care process flow to define health care intervention access /update/drop-out/re-initiation. Selection of output units and strata.	Default values set for selected countries; calibration available; values modifiable by user. Intevention coverage by delivery model and risk group.
Access	Online (free); training courses are available and support is provided.		Available in conjunction with trainings.	Online (free). Extensive support /collaboration required. Source code (www.github.com /InstituteForDiseaseModeling /EMOD), tutorials and parameters (www.idmod.org /idmdoc), installer (www.idmod.org/software), and database linked to cloud computing resources (http://comps.idmod .org).	Online (free); coordinate with contact person to determine applicability for intended use and request support.
Users	National, local, and international planners (including government), researchers; and monitoring and evaluation officers.			Planners propose model settings and scenarios to be implemented by IDM team or research collaborators.	Planners, researchers, monitoring and evaluation officers.

table continues next page

Table 9.1 Comparison of Models (continued)

	Goals, AIDS Impact Model (AIM), and Resource Needs Model (RNM) in Spectrum/OneHealth Tool	Optima HIV	AIDS Epidemic Model (AEM)	Epidemiological Modeling (EMOD)	Global Health Decisions
Training	Workshops lasting several days.		Normally 3 workshops focused on data needs and collection; preliminary model building; and scenario building for policy and program planning.	Tutorials and demonstration files online, half-day introductory trainings in university classes and conferences; 1-4 weeks of on-site training for detailed projects; and 4-8 weeks to calibrate a new country or setting.	Ten-minute video to use with default values; further guidance required to change input values.
Technical assistance	Minor TA is free, major TA support funded via various mechanisms (UN agencies, bilateral agencies, foundations, national government, and so forth).			By arrangement (free).	By arrangement (free).
Initial set-up time	Default values often available. Otherwise, 3-5 days for data collation and entry.		Normally done as a national process, including extensive review of historical sources of information. As such, generally several months for data collation and trend analysis, then projections and scenarios prepared in about 3 days, normally with vetting by national experts. Updates typically done in less than a week.	Three-hour workshop or webinar; inputs for new setting 2 months; modified inputs for existing setting minutes.	Some default values available. Otherwise, 2-3 days for data collation and entry.
User manuals	Technical documentation: http://avenirhealth.org/software-spectrum.php. Tutorials: https://www.youtube.com/user/spectrummodel	Available at: optimamodel.com/user-guide	Available with training or email request.	• Online at http://idmod.org/idmdoc/—Technical documentation, topic-specific tutorials, parameter definitions, and output file "data dictionary."	Online intro video http://fast.wistia.net/embed/iframe/h08v1rkpvf?wvideo=h08v1rkpvf. No written manual.
Analysis time	Run time 1-3 minutes. Calibration several hours (if needed).		Run time 1-3 minutes. Calibration several days.	Days to months, depending on complexity, from conception of modeling question to results. Some standard analyses run in <1 hour.	Run time < 1 min. Calibration hours.

table continues next page

Table 9.1 Comparison of Models (continued)

	Goals, AIDS Impact Model (AIM), and Resource Needs Model (RNM) in Spectrum/OneHealth Tool	Optima HIV	AIDS Epidemic Model (AEM)	Epidemiological Modeling (EMOD)	Global Health Decisions
Outputs	All outputs overall and by population group, by year & cumulative. By intervention scenario. Number in group, deaths, HIV/AIDS new cases and prevalence; ART prevalence by CD4 count and stage of treatment. DALYs or QALYs. Intervention participation; Costs by interventions/care. Cost-effectiveness ratios. Optimal allocations.			Same as Goals and Optima models, plus health care use; relationship and transmission network over time; biomarkers such as CD4. Outputs also available as distributions.	Same as Goals and Optima models.
Sample outputs	Sample outputs are available online at www.avenirhealth.org.	Sample outputs are available online at www.optimamodel.com.	Sample outputs are available online at www.eastwestcenter.org/research/research-projects/hiv-policy-analysis-research-and-training.	Sample input and output files and graphing/analysis scripts available online at www.idmod.org/software.	Sample outputs are available online at www.globalhealthdecisions.org.
Special features	Integrated into OneHealth Tool, permitting cost and impact comparisons across many health sectors; Goals Express offers a simpler version.	Constrained optimization of resource envelopes using algorithms. Flexible group and intervention definition. Modeling of multiple diseases, allowing cost and impact comparison. Optima Lite has simpler preloaded and calibrated projects.	Customized fit of behavioral trends to observed epidemiologic trends by adjusting transmission probabilities and cofactors; use of local data on program effectiveness.	Maximum flexibility to portray individual variation. Users can specify health system and care flow.	User-friendly graphical user interface, direct intervention scenario comparisons.
Limitations	Only one adult age group (15–49) in Goals although outputs are available by five-year age group in AIM.	As with all compartmental models, individual-level data included in aggregated form and homogeneity assumptions apply within specified modeled groups.	Only concentrated epidemics; aggregate age structure based on age pattern of new male and female infections.	Not yet implemented: viral load testing and relationship between VL, age, and survival; evolution and transmission of antiretroviral drug resistance; transmission among MSM and IDU.	No PrEP or vaccines; calibration to countries limited to date. No formal rollout.
Contacts	John Stover (Jstover@AvenirHealth.org)	David Wilson (info@optimamodel.com)	Tim Brown (tim@hawaii.edu)	Anna Bershteyn (abershteyn@idmod.org), Daniel Klein (dklein@idmod.org)	Jim Kahn (jgkahn@gmail.com)

Note: AIDS = acquired immune deficiency syndrome; ART = antiretroviral treatment; DALY = disability-adjusted life year; FSW = female sex worker; HCV = hepatitis C virus; HIV = human immunodeficiency virus; IDM = Institute for Disease Modeling; IDU = injecting drug user; MSM = men who have sex with men; MTCT = mother-to-child transmission; NCD = noncommunicable diseases; PEPFAR = U.S. President's Emergency Plan for AIDS Relief; PMTCT = prevention of mother to child transmission; PrEP = preexposure prophylaxis; PWID = people who inject drugs; QALY = quality-adjusted life year; STI = sexually transmitted infection; TA = technical assistance; TB = tuberculosis; UN = United Nations.

objective, subject to budgetary, logistical, ethical, and political constraints.

- *AEM* is used for studying concentrated epidemics, especially in Asia. The task of calibrating and populating the model is intensive, and exploring the various available packages encourages stakeholders to understand local epidemics and the effectiveness of past, present, and potential future responses.

- *EMOD* is used to examine policy issues involving the interplay of demographics, risks, disease progression, and health care. Individual-based modeling captures heterogeneity and permits a nuanced portrayal—for example, HIV/AIDS transmission is based on independent risk per sex act within partnerships that evolve over time, and disease progression depends on age. Health system dynamics (for example, cycles of antiretroviral use) reflect factors such as age, gender, geography, and risk. Of the models reviewed, it is the most computationally intensive and has the most sophisticated population portrayal and calibration.

- *GHD* is relatively simple to use, with an interface that makes exploring the costs and effects of various combinations of interventions and delivery modalities easy. It is not in widespread use, but is available for appropriate applications by arrangement with the owners. GHD and Optima are exploring a collaboration to incorporate key GHD features into Optima HIV.

The choice of model for a specific user depends on the user's needs and the models' intended uses, strengths, and limitations. As presented in table 9.1, some models are uniquely well suited to specific purposes, such as EMOD for detailed simulation of how individuals' characteristics affect use of health care, and Avenir Health's OneHealth Tool for placing HIV/AIDS programming in the context of the broader health system. When models serve similar purposes, such as Avenir Health's and Optima's resource allocations across HIV/AIDS interventions, users may want to consult the contacts for each model to discuss how comprehensively and efficiently each model can address users' needs. Annex 9A provides a list of country applications for the models.

A more technical comparison and assessment conducted in early 2015 by the HIV Modeling Consortium (HIV Modeling Consortium 2015) was used to inform this review, although it is now slightly outdated because of ongoing model improvements.

Avenir Health Models

Over the past 40 years, Avenir Health, formerly known as the Futures Institute, has led the development of models across many areas of the health sector. Most of these models are assembled within Spectrum, a suite of integrated software models that provides policy makers with an analytical tool to support the decision-making process; it is also widely known by its overlay, the OneHealth Tool. Many of the models also exist as Excel-based models and web-based tools. This chapter focuses on models useful for resource allocation for HIV/AIDS: the AIDS Impact Model (AIM), Goals, and RNM, in particular.

Spectrum is a system of policy models that support analysis, planning, and advocacy for health programs.[2] The models are used to project future needs and examine the effects of policy choices, including the impact of taking actions now rather than later, evaluating the costs and benefits of a particular policy, examining the interrelatedness of different policy decisions, and evaluating how a change in age and sex distribution can affect a wide range of social indicators.

The central impact model in Spectrum is DemProj, which projects the population for an entire country or region by age and gender based on assumptions about fertility, mortality, and migration. A full set of demographic indicators can be displayed for up to 100 years into the future; urban and rural projections can also be prepared. Default data needed to project population are provided from the estimates produced by the Population Division of the United Nations. Models not related to HIV/AIDS include FamPlan, which projects family planning requirements; Resources for the Awareness of Population Impacts on Development, which projects the social and economic consequences of high fertility and rapid population growth; Tuberculosis Impact Model and Estimates, which performs epidemiological and cost-effectiveness analysis of tuberculosis control strategies; Lives Saved Tool, which estimates the cost and impact of scaling up child and maternal health interventions on mortality; and NonCommunicable Diseases, which calculates the impact of scaling up interventions on populations affected by noncommunicable diseases.

The four models related to HIV/AIDS interact with one another. AIM uses the Estimation and Projection Package (EPP) module developed by the East-West Center to fit prevalence and incidence trends to surveillance and survey data and then calculates the consequences of these trends for key indicators such as new infections, deaths, need for treatment, and number of orphans. RNM calculates the costs associated with HIV-related interventions. Goals simulates HIV/AIDS incidence on the basis of behaviors and estimates the epidemiological effects of biomedical interventions and behavioral interventions (using an impact matrix) to calculate infections averted and cost-effectiveness ratios. The Lives Saved Tool evaluates the cost and impact of child and maternal health interventions, including HIV/AIDS and malaria, using inputs from AIM.

AIM

AIM began as a relatively simple Excel-based tool developed in 1991 in collaboration with Family Health International under the AIDS Technical Support and AIDS Control and Prevention projects funded by the U.S. Agency for International Development (USAID). The program has been revised several times since then in collaboration with the UNAIDS Reference Group on Estimates, Models, and Projections. Since 2009, it has been maintained and updated with support from the Bill & Melinda Gates Foundation and UNAIDS. It has evolved to become a comprehensive model within Spectrum used to estimate the impact of the HIV/AIDS epidemic. Several years ago, the Estimation and Projection Package (EPP) was incorporated into Spectrum. Both incidence and prevalence curves are now estimated within AIM, which then projects the consequences of the epidemic, including the number of people living with HIV/AIDS, new infections, and deaths by age and gender, as well as the number of new cases of tuberculosis and the number of orphans. Many of these results are then used in other models in Spectrum. UNAIDS uses AIM to make the national and regional estimates it releases every two years.

The major inputs and outputs of AIM are as follows: Demographic projections are based on user inputs or projections prepared by the United Nations Population Division. The projections start with an estimate and projection of adult HIV/AIDS incidence, which is combined with information on the age and gender distribution of incidence and progression to death to estimate the number of new infections in adults, by age and gender. New infections in infants are estimated from prevalence among pregnant women and the rate of mother-to-child transmission, which is dependent on infant feeding practices and the coverage of prevention with antiretroviral agents. New infections progress to lower CD4 cell counts and are subject to HIV/AIDS-related mortality. Persons who receive first-line antiretroviral therapy (ART), second-line ART, or both live longer than those who do not. People at any stage are subject to other-cause mortality at the same rates as people who are not infected. Adult deaths result in orphans.

In addition to estimating the epidemic and projecting its impacts, AIM has other features, including the ability to validate its estimates by comparing AIM outputs with other data sources, to perform uncertainty analyses for certain output variables, and to aggregate projections, for example, a series of subnational projection files.

The model is continuously updated to reflect the most recent research.

RNM

RNM grew out of efforts developed in 2001 for the first United Nations General Assembly Special Session on HIV/AIDS to estimate the global resources required to combat HIV/AIDS (Schwartländer and others 2001); the estimates are referred to as the Global Resource Needs Estimates (GRNE). Although that first Excel-based model was calculated at the individual country level, it was a global model and not appropriate for country-level use. After the first few rounds of the GRNE, in 2007 UNAIDS initiated a consultative process with countries with high burdens of HIV/AIDS to validate their country-specific portions of the GRNE, which required adapting the global model to the country level. By 2009, the consultative process reached 60 countries, and countries began to use RNM (still in Excel) for their own planning purposes. Because of this, RNM gradually migrated over to Spectrum and now is used to calculate the funding required to expand national responses to HIV/AIDS. It estimates the costs of implementing HIV/AIDS programs, including the costs of care and treatment, prevention, and policy and program support.

RNM projects the costs of various interventions, given assumptions about the size of various population groups, unit costs of interventions, and coverage targets (figure 9.1). Costs can be calculated from any perspective, including provider, public, patient, and societal, depending on the perspective of the data that are provided. A significant portion of the model application process, described in more detail below, involves obtaining reliable cost data. RNM's projections can then be used to enhance knowledge of HIV/AIDS among policy makers and to build support for effective prevention, treatment, care, and mitigation. The projection results are usually transferred to software, such as PowerPoint, for presentation to leadership audiences.

RNM estimates the number of people receiving each service by multiplying the number of people needing the service by the coverage rate (percentage of persons needing the service who actually receive it). The resources needed are then estimated by multiplying the number of people receiving the service by the unit cost of providing it. Before RNM can be used, both a demographic and an HIV/AIDS projection must be prepared. The epidemiology section of AIM calculates the number of HIV/AIDS infections, persons needing treatment, and orphans. This information is used in the treatment section to calculate the costs of treatment for preventing mother-to-child transmission, HIV/AIDS, and associated tuberculosis and opportunistic infections and can be

Figure 9.1 Structure of RNM: DemProj and AIM

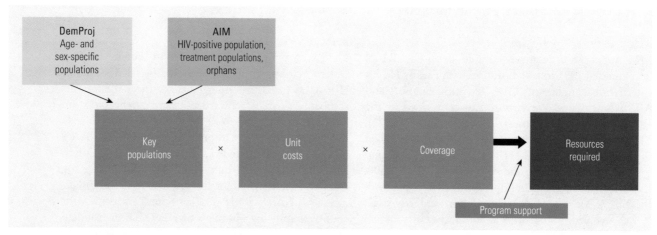

Note: AIM = AIDS Impact Model; RNM = Resource Needs Model; DemProj = central model in Spectrum.

used in the mitigation section to calculate the cost of providing services for orphans. AIM modifies the demographic projection through HIV/AIDS deaths and the impact of HIV/AIDS on fertility.

Goals

The Goals model supports efforts to respond to the HIV/AIDS epidemic by showing how the amount and allocation of funding is related to the achievement of national goals, such as the reduction of prevalence and expansion of care and support. It also explores the impact of potential vaccines. The Goals model evolved out of an effort to identify what program managers need to plan effectively. Stover and Bollinger (2002) surveyed 14 national program managers and learned that their most challenging issue was using cost-effectiveness information in their countries' key priority-setting exercise, the National Strategic Plan. The model was developed to be used in that process.

The Goals model is intended to support strategic planning at the national level by providing a tool to link program goals and funding. It can help answer several key questions:

- How much funding is required to achieve the goals of the strategic plan?
- What goals can be achieved with the available resources?
- What effect do alternate patterns of resource allocation have on the achievement of program goals?

The Goals model does not provide all the answers. It is intended to assist planners in understanding the effects of funding levels and allocation patterns on program impact. The model can help planners understand how funding levels and patterns can lead to lower

incidence and prevalence and improved coverage of treatment, care, and support programs. It does not calculate the optimum pattern of allocation or recommend a specific allocation of resources between prevention, care, and mitigation, although an optimization routine is available. Sexual mixing is random within risk groups. Mixing between risk groups is limited to low-risk adults who can have partners from higher-risk groups. Extensive literature underlies both the impact matrix coefficients and other model parameters; these sources are well documented in the manual. The Goals model underwent an external validity check comparing 12 mathematical models; results were basically consistent, particularly in the short term (Eaton and others 2013). A recently formed Models for Policy Planning Reference Group, led by the HIV Modelling Consortium (http://www .hivmodelling.org), will be providing ongoing internal and external validity checks.

The Goals model is a compartmentalized model, modeling heterogeneity by dividing the adult population ages 15–49 years by gender and risk group: not sexually active, low-risk stable couples, medium-risk people engaging in casual sex, sex workers and clients, men who have sex with men, and people who inject drugs (figure 9.2). The model calculates new infections by sex and risk group as a function of behaviors and epidemiological factors such as prevalence among partners and stage of infection. The risk of transmission is determined by behaviors (number of partners, number of contacts per partner, and condom use) and biomedical factors (use of antiretroviral agents, male circumcision, prevalence of other sexually transmitted infections). Interventions can change any of these factors and affect the future course of the epidemic. Interventions with either a behavioral or biomedical effect on HIV/AIDS

Figure 9.2 Structure of the Goals Model

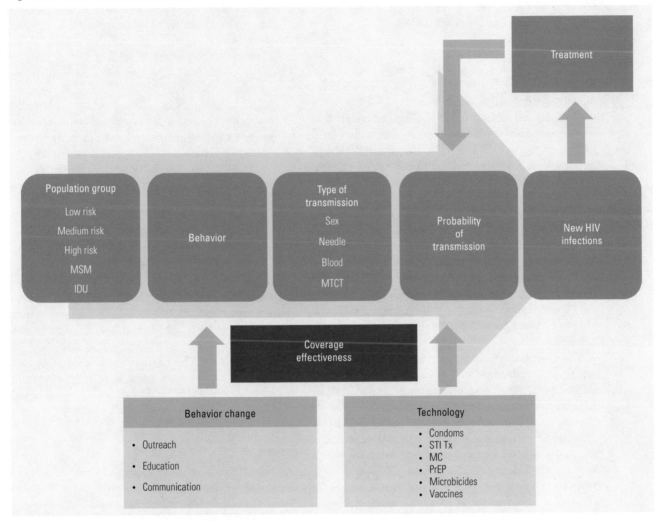

Source: Avenir Health. http://avenirhealth.org/software-spectrum.php.
Note: IDU = injecting drug user; MC = male circumcision; MSM = men who have sex with men; MTCT = mother-to-child transmission; PrEP = preexposure prophylaxis; STI Tx = sexually transmitted infection treatment.

transmission are modeled, including behavior change through outreach; education and communication interventions; and biomedical interventions such as condom distribution, voluntary medical male circumcision (VMMC), ART, preexposure prophylaxis, microbicides, and vaccines.

The effect of interventions on behaviors is modeled through an impact matrix that summarizes the impact literature to describe changes in behavior by risk group as a result of exposure to behavior change interventions (Bollinger 2008). The Goals model is then linked to the AIM module in Spectrum to calculate the effects on children (ages 0–14 years) and adults older than age 49 years. The AIM module also includes the effects on pediatric infections of programs to prevent mother-to-child transmission.

The Goals model has been used to assess the impact of prevention and treatment at the global level (Eaton and others 2013; Schwartländer and others 2011; Stover and others 2006) and for more than 30 applications at the country level (see annex 9A for a list of countries).

DMPPT

One of the Excel-based tools developed by Avenir Health is a two-part cost and impact tool available for examining the effects of VMMC; the most recent version of the impact model is called Decision Makers' Program Planning Tool (DMPPT) 2.0 (http://www.malecircumcision.org). The first DMPPT was used to estimate the costs and impact of VMMC in many countries for adult males ages 15–49 years. When experience showed that most VMMC clients were under age 25 years, a second version of the model was developed to evaluate the impact of targeted coverage of VMMC services (Stover and Kripke 2014). This tool is being developed for the web.

OneHealth Tool

The OneHealth Tool is a series of modules overlaid on the impact models of Spectrum. It is intended for medium-term strategic health planning (3–10 years) at the national and subnational levels. The OneHealth Tool was developed by a group of UN agencies, the World Bank, and the World Health Organization (WHO) in response to requests made during a 2008 technical consultation in Senegal by countries looking for standardized costing tools. The model builds on the International Health Partnership and Joint Assessment of National Health Strategies and Plans framework, and experts in costing from all participating UN agencies contributed both fund and staff time to the technical development of the model. The project also received funds from the Global Fund to Fight AIDS, Tuberculosis, and Malaria; the Global Health Workforce Alliance; and the Health Metrics Network, as well as from bilateral development agencies.

The OneHealth Tool was developed because most costing tools at the time took a disease-specific approach rather than a health systems approach (figure 9.3). In addition to covering public sector health interventions at both national and subnational levels, it incorporates coverage of private sector interventions and includes selected nonhealth interventions that may have health impacts. It is a unified tool for planning, costing, impact analysis, and financial space analysis performed jointly and can be implemented at either the health system or program level. The OneHealth Tool provides a way to estimate the cost and impact of interventions for HIV/AIDS, tuberculosis, and malaria simultaneously, as well as other diseases, and to examine the resource requirements from the health system. Default costs from a variety of sources are available, but should be validated and can be subsequently modified by the user. Sources of cost data include the Management Sciences for Health International Drug Price Indicator Guide; the UNAIDS Global Price Reporting Mechanism; Gavi, the Vaccine Alliance; and UNICEF.

The OneHealth Tool includes the following modules:

- *Human resources.* The human resources module allows salaries, benefits, and incentives for health service providers and health management and support personnel to be costed, along with preservice training and nonspecific in-service training.
- *Infrastructure.* The infrastructure model deals with planning and costing functions for all facilities providing medical interventions, as well as for most facilities offering support functions. It also includes planning functions for equipment, furniture, vehicles, and communications.
- *Governance.* The governance module includes costing templates for assessing the costs of governance activities.
- *Logistics.* The logistics module allows for the planning of warehouses and vehicles needed to move commodities or drugs and supplies from central warehouses to the endpoints of a logistics system.
- *Health financing.* The health financing module is used to estimate the costs of implementing health financing programs such as vouchers, subsidies, or cash transfers.
- *Health information systems.* The health information systems module includes templates for assessing the costs of implementing a health information system.
- *Budget mapping.* The budget mapping module can be used to allocate intervention and health system costs across budget categories established by the user, to match country or international institution cost categories.
- *Financial space.* The financial space module is used to analyze the financial space, including both public and private health expenditures, within which health plans are expected to be executed.

Optima

Optima HIV is a software package and modeling tool developed by the Optima Consortium for Decision Science in collaboration with the World Bank. It is one of a suite of models for different disease areas that have been developed by the Optima Consortium, all of which are designed to help national decision makers, program managers, and funding partners achieve allocative efficiency and plan for financial sustainability. This is done by applying the Optima approach, a framework for informing public health investment choices that consists of the following core steps:

- **Assess the burden of disease** over time, for each population group, and for each disease sequelae or state through data synthesis and epidemiological modeling.
- **Specify the efficacy and effectiveness of interventions** (including different modes of delivery) that have the potential to reduce incidence, morbidity, and mortality.
- **Assess the costs required to deliver services** at different levels of coverage, including through different service modalities and implementation or efficiency options.

Figure 9.3 Structure of the OneHealth Tool

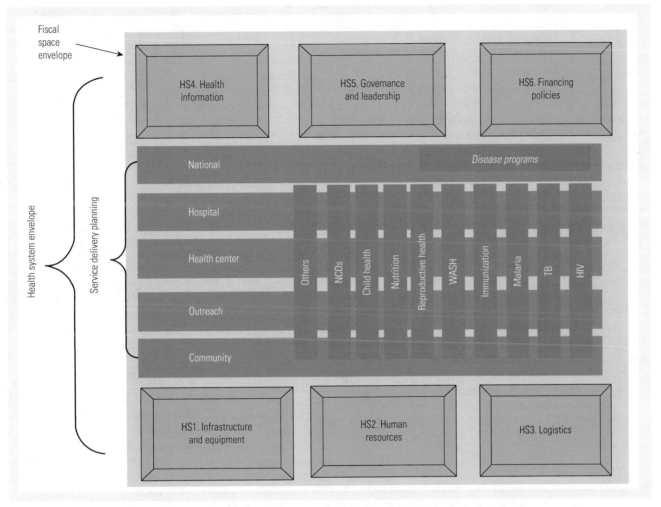

Source: World Health Organization (http://www.who.int/choice/onehealthtool/OneHealth_Tool_Supporting_integrated_strategic_health_planning.pdf?ua=1).
Note: HIV = human immunodeficiency virus; HS = health system; NCD = noncommunicable diseases; TB = tuberculosis; WASH = Water, Sanitation, and Hygiene for All.

- *Define strategic objectives and national priority targets*—as well as the *budgetary, logistical, ethical, and political constraints* related to achieving these objectives—across the entire population and by disease.
- *Use a formal mathematical optimization algorithm* around the constructs from the previous steps to assess the optimal allocation of a given level of resources to reduce disease burden, subject to the defined constraints.

Optima HIV is a software package designed to implement the steps listed above. It consists of a mathematical model of disease transmission and progression, a module for defining interventions and cost functions, and a mathematical optimization module that integrates the epidemic, programmatic, and cost data in order to determine

an optimal allocation of HIV investments. Optima HIV is the only quantitative tool currently available in the HIV field that includes a formal mathematical optimization routine, real-world budgetary, logistical, and political constraints, and economics of scaling up intervention programs and responses.

Optima HIV is intended to address various policy questions:

- *How close is achievement of the National Strategic Plan targets under current funding?* Over the strategic plan period, how close will the country get to its disease-related targets (a) with the current volume of funding allocated according to current expenditure and (b) with the current volume of funding allocated optimally?
- *How much funding is required to achieve the National Strategic Plan targets?* Over the strategic plan period

or over a longer period, according to current program implementation practices and costs, how much total funding is required to meet the targets, and how is this funding optimally allocated between programs?

- *What benefits can be achieved with more efficient implementation?*
- *What impacts have past programs had?* How would the country's HIV/AIDS trajectory have changed if investment had not occurred in different programs, and what is the estimated cost-effectiveness of the past response?
- *What is the expected future impact of policy or program implementation scenarios?* What is the projected future trajectory of the country's epidemic with and without investment in specific programs or with and without attaining program-specific targets?

Optima HIV extends allocative efficiency analyses to (a) include geographic prioritization and (b) integrate technical efficiency within allocative efficiency, considering the various modalities of service delivery for different programs. As such, it addresses the following questions: Which service delivery modalities and mechanisms should be implemented in which geographic areas? How should the HIV/AIDS response prioritize investment across population groups and geographic areas, and which service delivery modalities and mechanisms should be implemented and to what extent in each area, to get as close as possible to national targets with available resources? Additional descriptions of the uses of Optima HIV for planning a national response are available in chapter 8 of this volume (Wilson and Taaffe 2017).

AIDS Epidemic Model

The AEM, developed in the early 1990s, is patterned after the HIV/AIDS situation in countries with concentrated epidemics, primarily in Asia. It allows countries to build locally tuned models that accurately represent their epidemiological situations. These models can then be used with a set of analytic tools—the AEM workbooks (baseline, intervention, and impact analysis)—to prepare scenarios that analyze alternative responses to the epidemic, assess the impact of these responses, and estimate the cost of implementation.

These scenarios provide essential inputs into national strategic planning processes, help countries allocate their resources more efficiently, and help countries identify weaknesses that must be addressed to strengthen their responses. Using the AEM is an intensive process that builds stakeholder involvement in and ownership of the planning process.

Epidemiological Modeling (EMOD)

The Institute for Disease Modeling[3] developed the EMOD software primarily for use by disease modelers, researchers, epidemiologists, and public health professionals seeking to simulate infectious disease conditions and evaluate the effectiveness of eradication or mitigation approaches. The model is agent based, that is, portraying each individual rather than aggregate group behavior; in discrete time, that is, calculating transmission risk and other processes in small but noncontinuous time steps; and using a Monte Carlo simulator to predict populations, that is, drawing many random samples from a specified probability distribution for each input. This agent-based approach is computationally intensive as opposed to the fast speeds normally achieved with compartmental models (whether dynamic [using differential and integral equations] or in discrete time steps). The advantage is the ability to portray individual characteristics and transitions over time much more precisely. For example, the risk of infection can reflect a large set of person-specific risk factors, such as type of risk behavior and frequency, type of protective behavior and consistency, geographic location, and interactions with other individuals in the same and other risk groups—all of which can and do vary over time. The complex overall EMOD architecture provides disease transmission projections for environmental, sexual, vector-based, and airborne diseases and may be adapted to support additional infectious diseases. The binary software or source files are available for download. Data and training requirements are substantial.

Global Health Decisions

The GHD model was developed by the University of California, San Francisco, to provide an HIV/AIDS resource allocation model with a sophisticated and flexible user interface prepopulated with epidemiologic and programmatic data. The goal was to permit relatively rapid but nuanced allocation of resources across populations and interventions.

A website allows users to specify a country from among those implemented, verify the default input values (for HIV/AIDS prevalence and use of ART, for example), alter the values as needed, and then run a series of tailored intervention scale-up scenarios. The results of each scenario are incidence, prevalence, deaths, and costs, by risk group, over time. These scenario results are stored and can be named and compared graphically.

The back end is a deterministic compartmental model with five risk groups (general population female, general population male, sex workers, drug users, and men who have sex with men), implemented in Google Go. Given a set of predictions for treatment and prevalence in future years, the model uses simulated annealing—a stepwise statistical sampling approach—to align model predictions with these benchmark projections.

The model provides tiered access to functionality, including the use of country-specific defaults for input values (for example, demography, epidemiology, interventions, and costs), real-time adjustment of intervention portfolios, and manipulation of input values by more technically informed users. Policy makers have not used GHD.

WHAT WORKS REVIEWS

A central function of policy modeling is to convey the impact of interventions on health and economic outcomes. This means that resource allocation models need to incorporate the latest evidence on intervention efficacy in changing risks and risk behaviors. Systematic reviews of efficacy are now commonplace, but overwhelming in number and complexity. A distilled review that conveys efficacy and associated strength of evidence can be helpful for informing modeling and educating decision makers about the evidence. Thus, the GHD project initiated an activity called What Works Reviews (WWR) in 2010 to address a perceived gap in the availability of information about intervention efficacy for policy discussions and models.

WWR translates empirical evidence on the effects of interventions into a quantitative synthesis that is technically accurate while being concise and accessible to nontechnical audiences. Each estimate of efficacy is accompanied by a strength-of-evidence rating that reflects the quantity and type of underlying studies. WWR examines both prevention and treatment for each health condition, with a focus on data with the most potential relevance for policy and an emphasis on health outcomes (for example, deaths and disease incidence) rather than process measures (for example, satisfaction with services or adherence).

WWR includes nearly 50 categories of interventions for HIV/AIDS, including some found to be ineffective.[4]

Methods

WWR proceeds in explicit and small steps from existing systematic reviews and important new studies to key findings (figure 9.4).

- The first step is to search for systematic reviews and pivotal new studies. Most reviews come from the

Cochrane Library, with others identified through PubMed and other sources. The evidence at this level is massive, diverse in form, and technically complex.

- The second step is to select potentially relevant reviews based on whether the information could affect major decisions on policy or funding, such as whether and at what scale to support a particular intervention. Important but narrower questions, such as drug dosing or comparisons between very similar intervention designs, are usually excluded, as are universally accepted practices. All of these decisions are documented.

- The third step is to extract information from the selected comparisons, including context (for example, country and type of population), research methods (for example, study design and outcome measures), and quantitative findings on efficacy.

- The fourth step is to rate the strength of evidence based on the quantity and type of studies, as well as the precision of findings, that is, the width of the relative risk confidence interval. The result is a summary table that presents the intervention comparisons, findings (for example, mortality and incidence), relative risk reduction, and strength of evidence for each review and study.

- The next step, which is critical, is to combine evidence by intervention type where possible. For example, if different insecticides for environmental control of a disease vector (for example, a mosquito) all work with similar efficacy, the findings are combined into a single row. All summary data are linked to original extractions to allow review of the aggregation decisions.

- The last step is to consult with subject area experts to review provisional findings. This step may result in the addition of new reviews or studies or adjustment of the interpretation of existing evidence.

Figure 9.4 Structure of the What Works Reviews Process

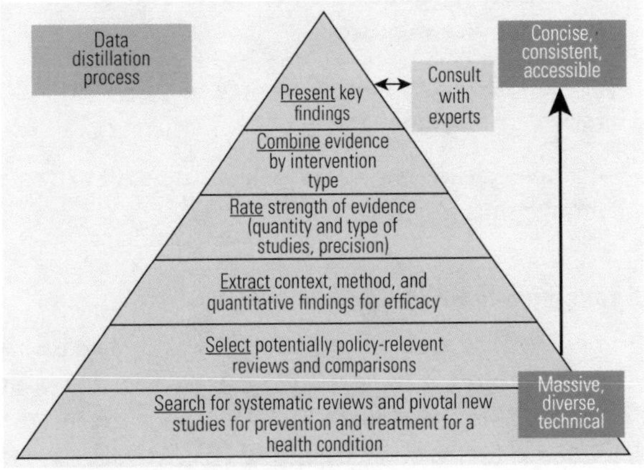

Source: What Works Reviews (http://globalhealthdecisions.org/wwr/).

The key outcome is relative risk reduction. This is a standardized metric, designed to put diverse outcome metrics (for example, odds ratio, means) onto a consistent footing (Mirzazadeh, Malekinejad, and Kahn 2015). It equals the percentage reduction in the risk of negative health outcomes and can be used for mortality, morbidity, and indirect health indicators.

Findings are presented in three parts:

- A key findings table has a row for each type of intervention, with the relative risk reduction and strength of evidence for mortality, morbidity, and other indicators.
- An overview reviews the health condition, epidemiology, key findings, and future directions.
- A logic model graphically represents modes of disease acquisition and progression as well as the location of intervention opportunities.

Strength of Evidence

WWR rates strength of evidence on a scale of 0–6 (visually represented by bars). The score is based on the extent and type of studies (for example, randomized controlled trials [RCTs]), quality of available systematic reviews, and precision (that is, narrowness of uncertainty bounds). The following is the typical evidence associated with each score:

6 = three or more RCTs, well reviewed, good precision (very strong)

5 = three or more RCTs, minor problems with review or precision (strong)

4 = two RCTs, good review and precision (moderate strength)

3 = one RCT or multiple non-RCTs, good review and precision (moderate strength)

2 = one RCT or multiple non-RCTs, problems with review or precision (weak)

1 = one or more non-RCTs, serious problems with review or precision (very weak)

0 = no evidence, because of lack of studies or extreme imprecision.

Application to HIV/AIDS

The HIV/AIDS component of WWR was updated with new literature searches and extractions between December 2015 and January 2016. Figure 9.5 presents the logic model for the broad context of HIV/AIDS intervention. Key findings for all intervention types are presented

in annex 9B. To illustrate results, this section summarizes the findings for biological prevention strategies.

Circumcision of adult males is 70 percent effective in reducing transmission from females to males based on three RCTs, other studies, and long follow-up (very strong evidence). Evidence for men who have sex with men and transgender individuals suggests little if any protection from male circumcision (strong evidence). Treatment of sexually transmitted infections has been examined in eight studies, with a 12 percent non–statistically significant reduction in incidence and a wide confidence interval, including a negative effect (−49 percent to 48 percent), with lower incidence of sexually transmitted infections and risk behaviors (16 percent to 23 percent, moderate strength evidence). Nonoxynol-9 and microbicides failed to reduce HIV/AIDS incidence. Data on microbicides containing an antiretroviral drug suggest a 37 percent reduction in HIV/AIDS incidence (weak evidence). Vaccines did not work, with exception of one trial with 30 percent efficacy, and neither did the latex diaphragm. Preexposure prophylaxis (PrEP) with the antiretroviral combination tenofovir plus emtricitabine reduced HIV/AIDS transmission in several RCTs by 47 percent (very strong evidence). Two trials found no effect, due to low sample size and adherence. Use of antiretrovirals reduced incidence by 96 percent in serodiscordant couples in a large RCT in Africa, with similar results from several earlier non-RCTs (strong evidence). The female condom reduced the nonuse of condoms.

FIELD EXPERIENCE WITH MODELS INFLUENCING POLICY DECISIONS

A typical model application associated with developing a National Strategic Plan must be integrated across a number of different dimensions: models used, stakeholders involved, capacity building, and dissemination activities. When an application begins, the first step should be to establish a stakeholder group that will provide input throughout the process. Evaluating the current status of data available is necessary to inform and design the process to be undertaken; some countries may have facility-based costing information for certain interventions, such as HIV/AIDS counseling and testing or ART, but not for other interventions.

The models to be applied then need to be ascertained; many of the models described in this chapter are integral and required in the National Strategic Plan. For the Spectrum models, a country in

Figure 9.5 Logic Model for the HIV/AIDS Component of What Works Reviews

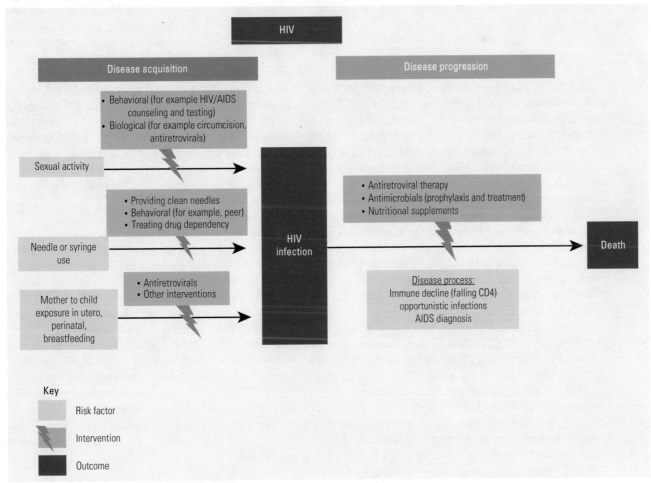

Source: Global Health Decisions (http://globalhealthdecisions.org/wwr/hivaids/hivaids-key-findings/).
Note: HIV/AIDS = human immunodeficiency virus; acquired immune deficiency syndrome.

Sub-Saharan Africa would need to apply the AIM model (to estimate the need for treatment and prevention of mother-to-child-transmission services), the RNM (to estimate the resources required to scale up from current coverage to future levels of desired coverage), and the Goals model (to estimate the impact of various scale-up and resource allocation strategies). The resources required for universal access are compared with an assessment of the resources likely to be available based on National AIDS Spending Assessments, to assess the size of the gap.

Alternative resource allocation strategies can then be developed that prioritize different goals—prevention, treatment, and mitigation. These alternative strategies can be discussed at stakeholder meetings to reach a consensus on the best approach to allocating available resources. The steps include the following:

• Identify and meet with national planning officials and local consultants and perform situation analysis.
• Collect facility-based data and other data.
• Set up models.
• Present initial results to national planning team
• Revise initial analysis, as required.
• Present results to stakeholders and conduct prioritization discussions.
• Prepare the final analysis and report.

Several of the models described in this chapter have been influential in policy making. However, models not only can be influential in changing policy and the policy-making process, but also the interaction of that process can change the models and affect their evolution.

DMPPT

One model that both changed policy and itself was changed through the policy-making process is the DMPPT, developed by the USAID Health Policy Initiative in collaboration with UNAIDS, to inform decision makers about the potential cost and impact of options for scaling up VMMC. When the RCT results for the effect of VMMC on HIV/AIDS transmission were first announced, no publicly accessible, flexible, and supported models were available to estimate the costs and impact of providing VMMC services. In 2007, a large consultative meeting was held by UNAIDS and the WHO, at which consensus was reached to prioritize VMMC in countries with high prevalence of HIV/AIDS and low prevalence of male circumcision (UNAIDS, WHO, and SACEMA Expert Group 2009).

After the model was developed, model applications were performed for 14 Sub-Saharan African countries using readily available data. Based on the results, a series of briefs were written, one for each country and a summary brief for the region as a whole (Njeuhmeli and others 2011). The U.S. President's Emergency Plan for AIDS Relief (PEPFAR) used the briefs heavily to persuade countries either to further investigate the potential cost and impact of VMMC based on primary source data, or simply to adopt a VMMC policy based on the initial results. The briefs were extremely useful in showing the magnitude of those results so clearly.

The original model targeted males ages 15–49 years. Since then, evidence on VMMC began to show that males under age 25 years were most likely to use VMMC services. Because of this finding, a new version of the model, DMPPT 2.0, was developed to estimate the impact of targeting VMMC services by five-year age groups (Stover and Kripke 2014). Several applications of the new DMPPT are under way; new applications of the costing tool are sometimes included to update previous cost estimates based on older technology.

GRNE

Another example of how a model can affect policy is the development and use of the GRNE. The first estimates were developed at the request of UNAIDS to establish a global price tag for the estimated funding required for a comprehensive response to the HIV/AIDS epidemic. Those results were influential in setting the agenda for HIV/AIDS, including the establishment of the Global Fund to Fight AIDS, Tuberculosis, and Malaria.

As both the epidemic and the GRNE evolved, each iteration added various interventions in response to perceived needs. For example, since the original estimates, interventions such as postexposure prophylaxis, safe injection, community mobilization, and prevention for people living with HIV/AIDS were added. Health system considerations began to be included, including health systems strengthening, training, incentives, and infrastructure. A separate effort to estimate the resources needed to support orphans and vulnerable children was spawned and then fed into the existing estimates (Stover and others 2007).

By 2010, the GRNE had expanded to contain many interventions and the total price tag had grown commensurately, while the growth in financial resources had begun to flatten out. In response to these policy issues, the next round of estimates underwent an extensive consultative process to devise a more targeted and strategic approach, identifying interventions that would have relatively higher impact, known as the Investment Framework (Schwartländer and others 2011). Since then, many countries and donors have adopted this approach and developed investment cases to illustrate the validity of the choice of strategy. Throughout this process, models have informed policy making, and the models have evolved and adapted to changes in the policy environment.

AEM

The typical process for the AEM is collaborative. Normally AEM is applied in an in-country process, organized around three initial in-country meetings:

- The first meeting discusses data needs and inputs, how to extract epidemiological and behavioral trends, and sources of data. This meeting is followed by an intensive period of in-country collation of relevant data and extraction of the required AEM inputs.
- The second meeting reviews and uses these extracted trends to build an initial model and then validate it against numerous other data sources, including male/female ratios, results of incidence studies, and early HIV/AIDS trends and more recent ART trends. The resulting model is then normally vetted by various in-country experts, who review both the inputs and outputs and recommend changes where necessary. Based on their input, any required adjustments are made to generate a final national baseline model.

In the third workshop, key stakeholders are convened to develop scenarios using the intervention and analysis workbooks to explore the epidemic impacts of different resource allocations for prevention and treatment programs, identify differing levels of resource availability, and determine optimal use of available resources under prevailing epidemic conditions.

These workshops are generally held in-country to maximize the engagement of all key stakeholders, ranging from behavioral scientists, epidemiologists, and public health specialists, to program managers, affected communities, and key decision makers. This approach helps increase understanding of what the data are saying about the epidemic, build a common understanding of the forces behind the epidemic, and inform decision makers about which choices will maximize their progress in reversing the epidemic.

Several countries, for example, Bangladesh, Indonesia, Myanmar, and the Philippines, have developed their own in-country AEM teams that work closely with national counterparts to ensure the models produced meet their policy and advocacy needs. AEM helps countries determine where best to focus their prevention dollars to maximize return on investment. Many Asian countries have used AEM as the basis for revising their national plans, to help them in preparing concept notes for the Global Fund, and for national advocacy for more effective responses and expanded resources. In the Philippines, AEM scenarios are being used to actively advocate for expanded HIV/AIDS resources. In Thailand, AEM was instrumental in promoting ART for all by demonstrating substantial downstream savings from removing thresholds for ART access. AEM also formed the basis for the analyses of the Commission on AIDS in Asia, emphasizing the need for responses focused on key populations and high-impact interventions given existing resource constraints rather than trying to cover everybody.

ROLE FOR MULTIPLE MODELS VERSUS CONVERGENCE

With the availability of multiple cost-effectiveness models, often addressing similar policy territory, the issue that arises is the relative merits of multiple models versus convergence on a single model. The following presents some of the advantages and disadvantages of each approach.

- *Complementary substantive areas of focus.* Different models may vary in areas of focus. For example, one model may consider the general features of ART, while another may highlight differences among regimens or monitoring strategies. Thus, policy makers may determine an allocation for ART overall based on one model and allocations for specific activities within an antiretroviral program based on another. The downside is the lack of an integrated assessment and the need to use an extra model. Misalignment of two models may create confusion. If one model considers options A, B, and C, but another model considers B, C, and D, users may become frustrated.
- *Differing level of technical engagement by users.* Some users prefer simpler but less flexible engagement with a model, whereas others prefer more complex and flexible engagement. Policy makers may fall in the former camp, and epidemiologists and other academics may fall in the latter. Although some models offer choice in level of engagement, obviating this distinction, they may excel in either the simpler or the more detailed level of engagement.
- *Competition.* Having multiple models may provide the impetus to improve model design to build a user base through quality improvement.
- *Confirmation and confidence building.* When different models yield substantially similar results, confidence in the validity of the findings is stronger (Hankins, Forsythe, and Njeuhmeli 2011). When results diverge, the attempt to resolve differences can illuminate variations in assumptions or data values that would not otherwise have come under scrutiny.
- *Efficiency.* Perhaps the strongest argument for convergence is efficiency: interested parties can focus efforts on one model, building consensus on methods and inputs. A rigorous review process is essential to provide the quality control that would otherwise arise from competition and comparison.

In 2016, there are two dominant models and other less widely used models. Avenir Health's system of models is widely used in countries and global agencies for policy-making discussions. The Optima HIV model has been used in dozens of countries and for global health agency decisions. Other models are used in more limited settings in specific countries and published in academic journals. They have served many of the quality control functions that might otherwise arise from more balanced competition.

FRONTIERS OF MODELING: WHERE IS ADDED VALUE POSSIBLE?

Unit Cost Resources

All cost-effectiveness models for HIV/AIDS, tuberculosis, and other diseases suffer from a significant gap in required input data—the unit cost of delivering interventions. Although costing studies for many interventions are available, they have several serious limitations: many interventions or important variations in intervention delivery have not been formally costed; many geographic settings are poorly represented in costing studies overall or for specific interventions; and costing methods are inconsistent across studies. The Global Health Cost Consortium, funded by the Bill & Melinda Gates Foundation, is developing a strategy for standardizing existing cost data to improve comparability, extrapolate to new geographic settings, strategically fill gaps in existing data, and improve the efficiency and quality of collecting and analyzing cost data. These data will improve the reach of and confidence in cost-effectiveness models.

Model Comparisons

The multiple HIV/AIDS resource allocation models offer important choices for potential users, with preferences based on the policy questions being examined and the availability of detailed local data. Comparing model results is highly desirable to ensure that estimates are comparable and valid. Comparisons have been made for general predictions, male circumcision (Hankins, Forsythe, and Njeuhmeli 2011), and ART as prevention (Eaton and others 2013) but not for detailed resource allocation issues, despite a comparison of model structure and features (HIV Modelling Consortium 2015). A structured output comparison would be valuable, and may be forthcoming from the HIV Modelling Consortium in late 2016.

External Validity

It has long been recognized that efficacy data collected from research projects, often in atypically well-resourced situations, may not accurately portray the results that could be expected in typical operating programs; the research findings thus have low external validity. However, efforts to describe and enumerate the challenges to external validity vastly outnumber the efforts to improve or even measure external validity. The GHD project has taken initial steps to assess how well research results might be replicated in actual practice settings. Six external indicators were associated with the effect of HIV/AIDS testing on condom use: number of implementation sites, financial incentives, mobile mode of delivering testing and counseling, female sex workers as the target, requirement that clients return to receive test results, and indeterminate or positive HIV/AIDS test results. These results are limited and preliminary, and the analysis needs to be repeated for other interventions. Further progress in developing methods to measure external validity would increase users' knowledge of the accuracy of resource allocation models and their utility as an aid to decision making.

Implementation Approaches

The bulk of massive recent spending on HIV/AIDS services has been vertical: programs focused entirely on prevention, treatment, or care, with no resources for other diseases and largely separate operational structures. Yet various factors highlight the need to consider horizontal implementation: control of the disease, meaning that infected individuals live long enough to experience other illnesses; the ability to identify infected individuals in other service settings, such as reproductive health; and renewed interest in health system strengthening, such as highlighted in *The Lancet* Global Health 2035 Commission on Investing in Health (Jamison and others 2013). Current resource allocation models permit limited examination of implementation approaches, but not comprehensively (the OneHealth Tool comes closest, with explicit consideration of system costs); future modeling would do well to build in more specific options. Analysis of other implementation issues, such as facility- versus community-based service delivery, with or without demand generation, and geographically targeted to high-risk or high-need areas, would be valuable; such analysis is likely to be possible in several of the reviewed models.

Interactions

HIV/AIDS interacts with other diseases in several ways. It co-occurs in certain populations, such as with hepatitis C among persons who inject drugs. The pathophysiologies interact; for example, hepatitis C progression is sped by HIV/AIDS, and CD4 decline accelerates with episodes of malaria. Therapy for HIV/AIDS affects (usually reduces) the risk of other diseases, such as tuberculosis. Capturing these interactions and their potential implications for intervention opportunities and health impact will more accurately portray the relative merits of alternative investment strategies.

Behavioral Economics

Increasingly, behavioral economics—the use of cognitive psychology to influence economically relevant behaviors such as taking risks and seeking care—is gaining traction in health. Cost-effectiveness models can start to incorporate behavioral economics strategies known to be effective. The evidence relevant for infectious and maternal-child disease is in the process of being reviewed by a team at the University of California, San Francisco. In addition, cost-effectiveness analysis can potentially benefit from the insights of behavioral economics. Behavioral economics and its underlying prospect theory note that individuals are more averse to loss than attracted to equivalent gains. Perhaps users of a model will be more influenced if the presentation is framed as *missed* opportunities to avert infections rather than as *new* opportunities to avert infections.

New Cost-Effectiveness Analysis Outcomes

Cost-effectiveness analysis traditionally compares average incremental health impact and cost. It does not consider the effects on financial solvency of high expenditures, nor does it address equity. Extended cost-effectiveness analysis assesses three important considerations for policy makers:

- Household out-of-pocket private expenditures
- Financial risk protection (number of cases of poverty averted)
- Distributional consequences per socioeconomic status or geographic setting (Verguet, Laxminarayan, and Jamison 2014).

An example is provided in *Disease Control Priorities*, third edition, volume 2, chapter 19 on health gains and financial risk protection (Verguet and others 2016).

CONTROVERSIES IN MODELING

The use of models to inform health policy in general and cost-effectiveness models in particular has stimulated debate and controversy.

One of the objections is that cost-effectiveness modeling tacitly reflects ethical judgments about which thoughtful people can disagree. For example, in any comparison of outcomes that uses life years, such as quality-adjusted life years or DALYs, a life-saving intervention will, all else equal, favor younger rather than older people. Most people accept the utilitarian principle on which this rests—as a society, we prefer to save more life years than fewer; others perceive it as a systematic bias against older people. Similarly, and perhaps more controversial, cost-effectiveness analysis puts no greater value on identified lives, such as particular people who are eligible for treatment, than on anonymous, statistical lives that might be saved through, for example, prevention activities. Trading off identified and statistical lives challenges, even offends, the ethical values of some people.

Another area of controversy concerns a central question in cost-effectiveness modeling: the determination of whether an evaluated option is or is not cost-effective, for example, by calculating whether the incremental cost-effectiveness ratio is above or below a threshold. The most widely adopted threshold was initially promoted by the Commission on Macroeconomics and Health and adopted by the WHO and by WHO-CHOICE. This threshold links per capita gross domestic product with returns on investments in health to define the characteristics of cost-effective and very cost-effective interventions (Hutubessy, Chisholm, and Edejer 2003; WHO 2002; WHO-CHOICE 2014).

Many published cost-effectiveness analyses of health interventions in low-resource countries explicitly refer to these WHO criteria as the standard for determining cost-effectiveness. This approach is extremely easy to apply and reflects the fact that willingness to pay for health care depends in part on national income. However, critics argue that these criteria have at least four major limitations:

1. They have little theoretical justification.
2. They skirt the difficult but necessary ranking of the relative values of locally applicable interventions.
3. They omit any consideration of affordability.
4. Finally, the thresholds set such a low bar for cost-effectiveness that very few interventions with evidence of efficacy can be ruled out.

An alternative, if more labor-intensive approach, would be to compare the cost-effectiveness of an intervention being analyzed with the cost-effectiveness of as many locally relevant interventions as possible (Marseille and others 2015).

Other controversies are rooted in methodological concerns. For example, health-state utility is difficult to measure, and results vary for the same disease or condition according to which of a number of accepted methods is used to determine it.

In addition, the related concept of disability weight does not vary by setting for any chosen disease or condition. The disability weights for mobility, visual, or hearing impairment are the same regardless of the economic status of the country or region in which the analyses are being applied. Yet the practical effect on peoples' lives of the same disability is likely to be greater in poorer countries where, for example, roads are more difficult to navigate and fewer aids are available to assist persons with disabilities.

Other concerns pertain to the fact that the data used in models are rarely perfectly suited to the setting or population being studied. Some critics believe that, in view of these and other limitations, undue reliance is placed on the results of models, they are treated as more reliable than they actually are, and they are used to address consequential policy questions for which they are unsuitably designed or parameterized.

CONCLUSIONS

The foregoing tour of HIV/AIDS resource allocation models presents a robust set of options. The models we describe are able to support the flexible examination of the most critical policy questions:

- What will be the cost and health outcomes of investing in different combinations of prevention and treatment interventions?
- How will those outcomes vary according to local factors such as epidemiology, ongoing interventions, and costs?

The models do require some initial setup, although less with the newer streamlined versions than has been the case in the past. More nuanced questions, such as the experience of individuals with particular traits, can be examined, albeit with substantially more investment of effort.

The relative abundance of resource allocation models now available, each with its own particular focus, strengths, and weaknesses, has two sides. Users can choose a model that fits their particular goals and purposes; however, assessing which model is most fit-for-purpose requires more investigation than would be necessary in a world of fewer options. One purpose of this chapter is to serve as a starting point for making such an assessment.

A long-term challenge for models is keeping up with an ever-evolving set of prevention and treatment approaches, and with fine-grained strategies such as micro-targeting of interventions to disease hotspots. The models are constantly improving to reflect these innovations as well as new analytic techniques made possible by enhanced computing power and the advent of "big data" that can help inform model parameters. We believe that resource allocation models will continue to provide up-to-date assistance to HIV/AIDS policy makers, program designers, and other users. Furthermore, the technology is adaptable to health areas outside HIV—some modeling techniques are already being applied to other diseases and more are anticipated.

ANNEXES

The annexes to this chapter are as follows. They are available at http://www.dcp-3.org/infectiousdiseases.

- Annex 9A. List of Countries with Model Applications
- Annex 9B. What Works Reviews

NOTES

World Bank Income Classifications as of July 2014 are as follows, based on estimates of gross national income (GNI) per capita for 2013:

- Low-income countries (LICs) = US$1,045 or less
- Middle-income countries (MICs) are subdivided:
  (a) lower-middle-income = US$1,046 to US$4,125
  (b) upper-middle-income (UMICs) = US$4,126 to US$12,745
- High-income countries (HICs) = US$12,746 or more.

1. https://www.youtube.com/watch?v=Exce4gy7aOk.
2. Spectrum was developed with funding from the U.S. Agency for International Development's Health Policy Project, the Bill & Melinda Gates Foundation, Johns Hopkins University, the U.S. Fund for the United Nations Children's Fund, UNAIDS, the World Health Organization, the Global Health Workforce Alliance, and the United Nations Population Fund.
3. See the Institute for Disease Modeling, Bellevue, Washington, at http://idmod.org.
4. WWR can be found at http://globalhealthdecisions.org /wwr/.

REFERENCES

Bollinger, L. A. 2008. "How Can We Calculate the 'E' in 'CEA'?" *AIDS* 22 (Suppl 1): S51–57.

Dieleman, J., C. Graves, T. Templin, E. Johnson, R. Baral, and others. 2014. "Global Health Development Assistance Remained Steady in 2013 but Did Not Align with Recipients' Disease Burden." *Health Affairs* 33: 878–86.

Eaton, J. W., N. A. Menzies, J. Stover, V. Cambiano, L. Chindelevitch, and others. 2013. "Health Benefits, Costs, and Cost-Effectiveness of Earlier Eligibility for Adult Antiretroviral Therapy and Expanded Treatment Coverage: A Combined Analysis of Twelve Mathematical Models." *The Lancet Global Health* 2 (1): 23–34.

Hankins, C., S. Forsythe, and E. Njeuhmeli. 2011. "Voluntary Medical Male Circumcision: An Introduction to the Cost, Impact, and Challenges of Accelerated Scaling Up." *PLoS Medicine* 8 (11): e1001127.

HIV Modelling Consortium. 2015. "Allocative Efficiency Tools and Methods to Support Country HIV Programme Budget Allocation." Imperial College, London.

Hutubessy, R., D. Chisholm, and T. T. Edejer. 2003. "Generalized Cost-Effectiveness Analysis for National-Level Priority-Setting in the Health Sector." *Cost-Effectiveness and Resource Allocation* 1 (1): 8.

Jamison, D. T., L. H. Summers, G. Alleyne, K. J. Arrow, S. Berkley, and others. 2013. "Global Health 2035: A World Converging within a Generation." *The Lancet* 382 (9908): 1898-1955.

Marseille, E., B. Larson, D. S. Kazi, J. G. Kahn, and S. Rosen. 2015. "Thresholds for the Cost-Effectiveness of Interventions: Alternative Approaches." *Bulletin of the World Health Organization* 93: 118–24.

Mirzazadeh, A., M. Malekinejad, and J. G. Khan. 2015. "Relative Risk Reduction Is Useful Metric to Standardize Effect Size for Public Health Interventions for Translational Research." *Journal of Clinical Epidemiology* 68 (3): 317–23.

Njeuhmeli, E., S. Forsythe, J. Reed, M. Opuni, L. Bollinger, and others. 2011. "Voluntary Medical Male Circumcision: Modeling the Impact and Cost of Expanding Male Circumcision for HIV Prevention in Eastern and Southern Africa." *PLoS* 9 (11): e1001132.

Resch, S., T. Ryckman, and R. Hecht. 2015. "Funding AIDS Programmes in the Era of Shared Responsibility: An Analysis of Domestic Spending in 12 Low-Income and Middle-Income Countries." *The Lancet Global Health* 3 (1): e52–61.

Schwartländer, B., J. Stover, T. Hallett, R. Atun, C. Avila, and others. 2011. "Towards an Improved Investment Approach for an Effective Response to HIV/AIDS." *The Lancet* 377 (9782): 2031–41.

Schwartländer, B., J. Stover, N. Walker, L. Bollinger, J. P. Gutierrez, and others. 2001. "Resource Needs for HIV/AIDS." *Science* 292 (5526): 2434–36.

Stover, J., S. Bertozzi, J. P. Gutierrez, N. Walker, K. A. Stanecki, and others. 2006. "The Global Impact of Scaling-up HIV/AIDS Prevention Programs in Low- and Middle-Income Countries." *Science* 311 (5766): 1474–76.

Stover, J., and L. Bollinger. 2002. "Resource Allocation within HIV/AIDS Programs." In *State of the Art: AIDS and Economics*, edited by S. Forsythe. Washington, DC: POLICY Project, Futures Group.

Stover, J., L. Bollinger, N. Walker, and R. Monasch. 2007. "Resource Needs to Support Orphans and Vulnerable Children in Sub-Saharan Africa." *Health Policy and Planning* 22 (1): 21–27.

Stover, J., and K. Kripke. 2014. "Estimating the Effects of Targeting Voluntary Medical Male Circumcision (VMMC) Programs to Different Age Groups: The Decision Makers Program Planning Toolkit (DMPPT 2.0)." Paper presented at the International AIDS Society biannual meeting, Melbourne, July 20–25.

UNAIDS (Joint United Nations Programme on HIV/AIDS). 2013. "Treatment 2015." UNAIDS, Geneva. http://www.unaids.org/sites/default/files/media_asset/JC2484_treatment-2015_en_1.pdf.

———. 2014. *Fasttrack: Ending the AIDS Epidemic by 2030.* Geneva, Switzerland: UNAIDS. http://www.unaids.org/sites/default/files/media_asset/JC2686_WAD2014report_en.pdf.

UNAIDS, WHO (World Health Organization), and SACEMA (South African Centre for Epidemiological Modelling and Analysis) Expert Group on Modelling the Impact and Cost of Male Circumcision for HIV Prevention. 2009. "Male Circumcision for HIV Prevention in High HIV Prevalence Settings: What Can Mathematical Modelling Contribute to Informed Decision Making?" *PLoS Medicine* 6 (9): e1000109.

Verguet, S., R. Laxminarayan, and D. T. Jamison. 2014. "Universal Public Finance of Tuberculosis Treatment in India: An Extended Cost-Effectiveness Analysis." *Health Economics* 24: 318–22.

Verguet, S., C. Pecenka, K. A. Johansson, S. T. Memirie, I. K. Friberg, and others. 2016. "Health Gains and Financial Risk Protection Afforded by Treatment and Prevention of Diarrhea and Pneumonia in Ethiopia: An Extended Cost-Effectiveness Analysis." In *Disease Control Priorities* (third edition): Volume 2, *Reproductive, Maternal, Newborn, and Child Health*, edited by R. Black, R. Laxminarayan, M. Temmerman, and N. Walker. Washington, DC: World Bank.

Wilson, D., and J. Taaffe. 2017. "Tailoring the Local HIV/AIDS Response to the Local HIV/AIDS Epidemic." In *Disease Control Priorities* (third edition): Volume 6, *Major Infectious Diseases*, edited by K. K. Holmes, S. Bertozzi, B. R. Bloom, and P. Jha. Washington, DC: World Bank.

WHO (World Health Organization). 2002. *World Health Report 2002: Reducing Risks, Promoting Healthy Life.* Geneva: WHO.

———. 2013. *Consolidated Guidelines on General HIV Care and the Use of Antiretroviral Drugs for Treating and Preventing HIV Infection: Recommendations for a Public Health Approach.* Geneva: WHO. http://www.who.int/hiv/pub/guidelines/arv2013/download/en.

WHO-CHOICE (Choosing Interventions That Are Cost-Effective). 2014. "Cost-Effectiveness Results for Malaria." WHO, Geneva. http://www.who.int/choice/results/mal_afrd/en/.

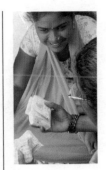

Chapter **10**

Sexually Transmitted Infections: Impact and Cost-Effectiveness of Prevention

Harrell W. Chesson, Philippe Mayaud, and Sevgi O. Aral

INTRODUCTION

Sexually transmitted infections (STIs) impose major health and economic burdens globally. More than 35 bacterial, viral, and parasitic pathogens have been identified as sexually transmissible. An estimated 498.9 million new cases of four of the curable STIs occurred among adults ages 15–49 years in 2008, an increase of 11.3 percent from the estimated 448.3 million new cases in 2005 (WHO 2012a). In 2008, these cases included 105.7 million new cases of chlamydia, 106.1 million new cases of gonorrhea, 10.6 million new cases of syphilis, and 276.4 million new cases of trichomoniasis (WHO 2012a). Males accounted for 266.1 million (53 percent) new cases. At any point in 2008, an estimated 100.4 million adults were infected with chlamydia, 36.4 million with gonorrhea, 36.4 million with syphilis, and 187.0 million with trichomoniasis (WHO 2012a).

The incidence and prevalence of these curable STIs varies remarkably across World Health Organization (WHO) regions, as shown in map 10.1, figure 10.1, and table 10.1. In general, low- and middle-income countries (LMICs) have higher estimated burdens of STIs than do high-income countries (HICs) (WHO 2012a). However, comparing income and STI burden by region can be challenging because income can vary substantially across countries within a given region. For example, the Americas include two relatively wealthy countries—Canada and the United States—yet the overall prevalence of these four curable STIs is higher in this than in

any other region. The highest estimated prevalence and incidence rates of chlamydia and trichomoniasis occur in the Americas, while the highest rates of gonorrhea and syphilis are in Sub-Saharan Africa (figures 10.2 and 10.3) In general, trichomoniasis is the most prevalent STI across regions, with the exception of Europe and the Western Pacific, where chlamydia is more prevalent.

A great deal of uncertainty surrounds the global and regional estimates of the incidence and prevalence of these four STIs (WHO 2012a). Relative to the size of the population in each region, the Americas has the highest annual incidence rate of these four curable STIs (0.264), followed by Africa (0.241), Western Pacific (0.130), Europe (0.104), Eastern Mediterranean (0.085), and South-East Asia (0.083). However, given heterogeneity in the quality of STI surveillance across regions, it is difficult to make cross-regional comparisons.

The incidence of STIs can vary substantially within, as well as across, regions according to the WHO's Global Health Observatory Data Repository. In 2010, the proportion of antenatal care attendees who were positive for syphilis was 0.2 percent in Côte d'Ivoire and 10.0 percent in the Central African Republic; the proportion of sex workers with active syphilis was 1.5 percent in Honduras and 17.5 percent in El Salvador; and the proportion with active syphilis among men who have sex with men (MSM) was 1.1 percent in Vietnam and 18.4 percent in Singapore. The incidence of STIs in a given country can vary substantially over time. For example, the percentage

Corresponding author: Harrell W. Chesson, Centers for Disease Control and Prevention, Atlanta, Georgia, United States; Hbc7@cdc.gov.

Map 10.1 Estimated Incidence of Four Curable STIs in Adults

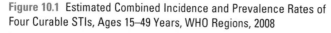

European Region
46.8 million

Western
Pacific Region
128.2 million

Eastern
Mediterranean
Region
26.4 million

Region of the Americas
125.7 million

South-East
Asia Region
78.5 million

African Region
92.6 million

Global total
498.9 million

Source: WHO 2012a.
Note: STI = sexually transmitted infection.

Figure 10.1 Estimated Combined Incidence and Prevalence Rates of Four Curable STIs, Ages 15–49 Years, WHO Regions, 2008

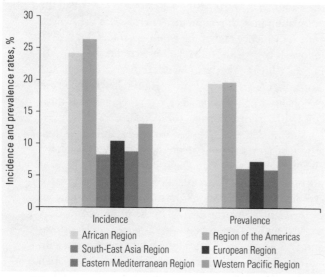

Source: WHO 2012a.
Note: STI = sexually transmitted infection; WHO = World Health Organization. Calculated based on the estimated number of incidence cases and prevalence cases of four curable STIs (chlamydia, gonorrhea, syphilis, and trichomoniasis) and the estimated population ages 15–49 years as estimated by WHO (2012a). The combined rates were calculated by summing the number of estimated cases and dividing by the population size.

of MSM with active syphilis in Indonesia ranged from 4.0 percent in 2008 to 21.9 percent in 2012.[1] Differences in the burden of STIs across regions, and within regions over time, preclude the identification of feasible programs and policies that can successfully reduce the burden of STIs in a cost-effective manner in all settings.

HEALTH AND ECONOMIC BURDEN OF STIs

If left untreated, common STIs may cause complications, including pelvic inflammatory disease, ectopic pregnancy, postpartum endometriosis, infertility, and chronic abdominal pain in women; adverse pregnancy outcomes, including abortion, intrauterine death, and premature delivery; neonatal and infant infections and blindness; urethral strictures and epididymitis in men; genital malignancies; proctitis, colitis, and enteritis in MSM; arthritis secondary to gonorrhea and chlamydia; liver failure and liver cancer secondary to hepatitis B virus (HBV); myelopathy and lymphoma or leukemia due to human T-cell lymphotropic virus type 1; and central nervous system disease or meningoencephalitis secondary to syphilis or herpes simplex virus (HSV)

Table 10.1 Estimated Annual Incidence and Prevalence of Four Curable STIs, Ages 15–49 Years, by WHO Region, 2008

	WHO region (number of countries in region)						
Indicator	Africa (46)	Americas (35)	South-East Asia (11)	Europe (53)	Eastern Mediterranean (23)	Western Pacific (37)	All regions
Population (millions)	384.4	476.9	945.2	450.8	309.6	986.7	3,553.6
Chlamydia							
Incidence cases (millions)	8.3	26.4	7.2	20.6	3.2	40.0	105.7
Prevalence cases (millions)	9.1	25.2	8.0	17.3	3.0	37.8	100.4
Incidence (%)	2.2	5.5	0.8	4.6	1.0	4.1	3.0
Prevalence (%)	2.4	5.3	0.8	3.8	1.0	3.8	2.8
Gonorrhea							
Incidence cases (millions)	21.1	11.0	25.4	3.4	3.1	42.0	106.1
Prevalence cases (millions)	8.2	3.6	9.3	1.0	1.0	13.3	36.4
Incidence (%)	5.5	2.3	2.7	0.8	1.0	4.3	3.0
Prevalence (%)	2.1	0.8	1.0	0.2	0.3	1.3	1.0
Syphilis							
Incidence cases (millions)	3.4	2.8	3.0	0.2	0.6	0.5	10.6
Prevalence cases (millions)	14.3	6.7	12.3	0.3	1.6	1.2	36.4
Incidence (%)	0.9	0.6	0.3	0.0	0.2	0.1	0.3
Prevalence (%)	3.7	1.4	1.3	0.1	0.5	0.1	1.0
Trichomoniasis							
Incidence cases (millions)	59.7	85.4	42.9	22.6	20.2	45.7	276.4
Prevalence cases (millions)	42.8	57.8	28.7	14.3	13.2	30.1	187.0
Incidence (%)	15.5	17.9	4.5	5.0	6.5	4.6	7.8
Prevalence (%)	11.1	12.1	3.0	3.2	4.3	3.1	5.3
Four STIs combined							
Incidence cases (millions)	92.6	125.7	78.5	46.8	26.4	128.2	498.9
Prevalence cases (millions)	74.4	93.3	58.3	32.9	18.8	82.4	360.2
Incidence (%)	24.1	26.4	8.3	10.4	8.5	13.0	14.0
Prevalence (%)	19.4	19.6	6.2	7.3	6.1	8.4	10.1

Source: WHO 2012a.
Note: STI = sexually transmitted infection; WHO = World Health Organization.

infection (Aral and others 2006; Holmes and Aral 1991; van Dam, Dallabetta, and Piot 1999).

STI sequelae disproportionately affect women and children. STIs are one of the leading causes of morbidity and mortality, as measured by disability-adjusted life years (DALYs) for reproductive-age women (Kamb and others 2007) in LMICs. Moreover, the health burden of STIs is often greatly underestimated. Although most cervical cancers are caused by human papillomaviruses (HPVs), the millions of DALYs caused by cervical cancer are not included in estimates of mortality and morbidity due to STIs; they

are typically listed in estimates of cancer (Low and others 2006).

The global burden of cervical and other cancers attributable to HPV is substantial. Of the estimated 610,000 HPV-attributable cancer cases worldwide in 2008, 490,000 occurred in LMICs, where 88 percent of cervical cancer deaths also occurred (Forman and others 2012). Similarly, HBV-related chronic hepatitis, liver failure, and liver cancer attributable to sexual, perinatal, or injection drug use transmission are seldom included in estimates of morbidity attributable to STIs.

Figure 10.2 Estimated Incidence Rates of Four Curable STIs, Ages 15–49 Years, by WHO Region, 2008

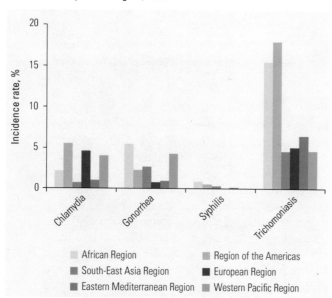

Source: WHO 2012a.
Note: STI = sexually transmitted infection; WHO = World Health Organization. Calculated based on the estimated incidence of four curable STIs and the estimated population ages 15–49 years as estimated by WHO (2012a).

Figure 10.3 Estimated Prevalence Rates of Four Curable STIs, Ages 15–49 Years, by WHO Region, 2008

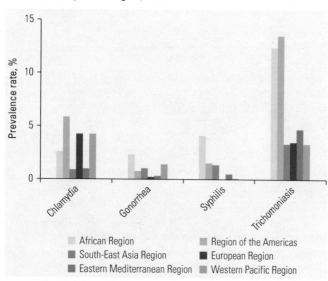

Source: WHO 2012a.
Note: STI = sexually transmitted infection; WHO = World Health Organization. Calculated based on the estimated prevalence of four curable STIs and the estimated population ages 15–49 years, as estimated by the WHO (2012a).

Delayed and Inadequate Diagnosis

Delayed or inadequate diagnosis and treatment of STIs in LMICs result in high rates of complications. To a large extent, inadequacies in health service provision and health care seeking are responsible for the high levels of STIs and the high rates of complications and sequelae in LMICs (Aral, Hogben, and Wasserheit 2008). STI care is provided by a variety of health care providers, many of whom are poorly trained in STI case management, and the quality of care is often inadequate (Mayaud and Mabey 2004). Health care seeking for STIs is often delayed and inadequate, particularly among women, as a result of the asymptomatic nature of many STIs; low levels of awareness of sexual health; stigma associated with genital symptoms; and tendency to seek care through traditional healers, home remedies (Mayaud and Mabey 2004; Moses and others 1994; van Dam 1995), and pharmacies where drugs are dispensed by workers not trained in STI treatment.

Factors Affecting Duration and Burden in LMICs

In resource-poor settings, variables that affect the duration of infectiousness include adequacy of health worker training, attitudes of health workers toward marginalized groups, patient loads at health centers, availability of drugs and clinic supplies, and cost of care (Moses and others 2002). Improvements in these factors would greatly improve STI-related services, reduce the duration of infectiousness, and decrease the incidence of STIs (Aral 2002). However, in many LMICs, worsening economic conditions; increasing burden of human immunodeficiency virus/acquired immune deficiency syndrome (HIV/AIDS); and occasional health crises, such as natural disasters, refugee situations, or epidemics like the recent Ebola outbreak in West Africa, can adversely affect these variables (Nam and Blanchet 2014).

Sociocultural, economic, and political contexts also affect sexual behaviors that contribute to the STI burden in LMICs. Changes have included rising inequality in income and other factors within countries, growing inequality among countries, increased globalization, higher proportions of persons living outside of their cultures, increased numbers of unemployed people, and larger proportions of people living in postconflict societies (Aral 2002; Aral and others 2006). All of these changes are associated with increases in multipartner sexual activity. Furthermore, changes in technology, including the widespread use of cell phones and the Internet, can facilitate the formation of short-term sexual partnerships (Bull and McFarlane 2000). These technological changes, concurrent with changes in norms and attitudes, have led to the expansion of transactional and commercial sex that increases sexual exposure (Aral and Ward 2014).

Direct medical costs for eight major STIs have been estimated at US$16.7 billion in the United States (Owusu-Edusei, Chesson, Gift, and others 2013). This estimate includes costs in the United States in 2008 for gonorrhea, chlamydia, syphilis, trichomoniasis, hepatitis B, diseases associated with sexually transmitted HPV, genital HSV-2 infections, and HIV infection. The total direct medical cost for each of these STIs in 2008 was computed as the estimated number of new cases in 2008 multiplied by the estimated discounted lifetime cost per case, adjusted to 2012 U.S. dollars. The estimated costs totaled US$16.7 billion (range of US$11.8 billion to US$22.1 billion) when including HIV. Total costs excluding HIV infections were US$3.2 billion. Although few estimates exist for LMICs, the direct medical costs of STIs are undoubtedly substantial given the high prevalence of these and other STIs in these settings. STIs also impose extensive productivity costs that can often exceed the direct medical costs (Owusu-Edusei, Chesson, Gift, and others 2013). Productivity costs are particularly burdensome in LMICs at both the individual and the community levels, especially for populations in which most people are under age 40 years (World Bank 2007). The youthful age composition in these countries contributes to the high prevalence and the direct costs of STIs. The economic burden of STIs in LMICs is so high that the treatment of curable STIs is considered one of the most cost-effective ways to improve health worldwide (World Bank 2007).

STIs can impose a considerable financial burden on those infected. For example, the cost of drugs is equivalent to several days' wages in most LMICs (Terris-Prestholt and others 2006). The direct costs associated with medical treatment of STI sequelae in LMICs have not been well defined, and the indirect costs associated with lost productivity due to STIs or STI sequelae are not known.

CHANGES IN SEXUAL BEHAVIORS AND PRACTICES, EPIDEMIOLOGY, AND PREVENTION

Significant changes have occurred in sexual behaviors and practices, epidemiology, and prevention. Technological advances, political conflicts, the economic downturn experienced in many HICs, and natural and health crises all have had important effects.

Sexual Behaviors and Practices

Most of the data on sexual behaviors and practices come from HICs. However, the increased volume of travel, sex tourism, transactional and commercial sex, and role of technology in establishing these connections have expanded sexual networks beyond national boundaries (Aral and Ward 2014; Ward and Aral 2006).

Moreover, population displacement in LMICs often affects sexual networks, for example, by allowing or forcing sexual mixing among groups that did not mix before the displacement (Hankins and others 2002).

Where available, systematically collected data on representative samples of the general population reflect increases in a number of risky behaviors, including the following: large numbers of sex partners, indiscriminate choice of sex partners, short periods between the time two people meet each other and the initiation of sexual activity, short time spent during the sexual encounter, lack or short duration of social links between sex partners, short duration of gaps between consecutive sex partners and sexual encounters, and a tendency for both partners to recruit each other for sex. These trends are observed particularly among younger cohorts. Moreover, sexual behaviors have been changing more rapidly for women than for men (Aral and Ward 2014; Mercer and others 2013).

Sexual practices have also been changing. Recent data from the United Kingdom and the United States suggest trends toward initiation of sex at a younger age, greater frequency of same-sex and bisexual behaviors, and greater frequency of oral and anal sex (Aral and Ward 2014). Although increases in oral sex began with the generation born between 1946 and 1964, increases in anal sex began with the generations born between 1965 and 2000 (Aral and Ward 2014).

These changes may result from temporal trends in demographic and social patterns. Marriage rates have declined, and divorce rates have risen in the Organisation for Economic Co-operation and Development countries and the United States (Aral and Ward 2014; International Futures Program 2011; Stevenson and Wolfers 2007). Globally, people who marry are doing so at older ages than before (Aral and Ward 2014). Because of these trends, many people spend a higher percentage of their adult lives outside of marriage (Aral and Ward 2014), which probably increases the number of sex partners.

Data collected in LMICs over the past two decades have revealed the importance of sex work to the spread of STIs (Baral and others 2012) and the presence (and considerable prevalence) of MSM among sex workers (Baral and others 2007). These key populations have high prevalence of STIs, including HIV/AIDS, and play an important role in spreading STIs to the general population.

Epidemiology

The understanding of STI epidemiology in LMICs has been shaped by the reemergence and escalation of gonorrhea and congenital syphilis; recognition of sexual transmission as a key factor in the spread of other STIs; emergence of MSM as key populations in transmission; emergence and impact of HIV/AIDS mortality; and patterns of STI spread, such as clustering and globalization. Although these issues can be difficult problems globally, they are especially daunting to monitor, control, and prevent in LMICs.

Gonococcal Antimicrobial Resistance

Widespread, high-level gonococcal antimicrobial resistance has been observed in Africa, South-East Asia, and the Western Pacific (Bala and others 2013; Lahra, Lo, and Whiley 2013; Ndowa and others 2013). In addition to resistance to penicillin, tetracycline, and quinolones, decreased susceptibility to third-generation cephalosporins has been reported. Decreased susceptibility to treatment has been associated with increased gonorrhea incidence at the population level in the United States (Chesson and others 2014). These trends highlight the importance of sustaining and enhancing surveillance to monitor the spread and threat of antimicrobial resistance (Lahra, Lo, and Whiley 2013).

Congenital Syphilis and Other Complications of Syphilis in Pregnancy

Syphilis in pregnancy can lead to a wide range of adverse outcomes, including stillbirth, fetal loss, neonatal death, premature and low-birthweight infants, and infection or disease in newborns (John-Stewart and others 2017; Kahn and others 2014; Newman and others 2013; WHO 2012b). Even though these adverse outcomes could be prevented through antenatal screening programs, syphilis in pregnancy imposes a substantial global burden each year, resulting in 692,000–1,530,000 adverse outcomes annually (Kamb and others 2010). As measured by DALYs, the global burden of disease due to syphilis during pregnancy is comparable to that of mother-to-child transmission of HIV (Kahn and others 2014; Kamb and others 2010; WHO 2012b).

LMICs bear a disproportionate share of the global health and economic burden of syphilis in pregnancy (Kamb and others 2010). In the Mwanza Region of Tanzania, from 1998 to 2000, maternal syphilis accounted for more than 50 percent of all stillbirths and 17 percent of all adverse pregnancy outcomes among unscreened women (Watson-Jones and others 2002).

AIDS Mortality

The probable impact of AIDS mortality, before the advent of effective antiretroviral therapy (ART), on the declining incidence of bacterial STIs was substantial.

Empirical and model-based studies in HICs suggest that AIDS mortality contributed to declines in bacterial STIs through two main mechanisms:

- Behavioral responses to the HIV/AIDS epidemic, such as increased condom use and smaller number of partners
- AIDS mortality among those at highest risk of acquiring and transmitting STIs (Becker and Joseph 1988; Boily and Brunham 1993; Boily and others 2004; Chesson, Dee, and Aral 2003; Kault 1992).

However, a few years after effective ART became available in 1996, STI incidence increased in subpopulations most affected by HIV/AIDS. Syphilis outbreaks among MSM have been observed in metropolitan areas worldwide since the late 1990s, in large part because of decreased fear of HIV/AIDS and increased survival of persons with HIV/AIDS (Chesson and Gift 2008; Stolte and others 2004).

The availability of ART has increased greatly in LMICs. At the end of 2009, 5.25 million people in these settings were receiving ART, compared with 4 million at the end of 2008 (WHO 2010). Peterman and Furness (2015) report notable declines in syphilis in some parts of Africa and attribute these declines in part to syndromic treatment of genital ulcers and possibly the impact of AIDS mortality. Building on experience acquired during the syphilis resurgence among MSM in HICs, researchers have cautioned that an increase in STIs is possible in LMICs as a result of the increased availability of ART, particularly in areas with high coverage (Kenyon, Osbak, and Chico 2014; Kenyon and others 2014).

Key Populations

The role of key populations in the epidemiology of STIs in LMICs has become increasingly clear (Baral and others 2007; Baral and others 2012). In particular, MSM are understudied and underserved in these countries. Patterns of sexual networks linking MSM and the general population warrant future research so that appropriate responses can be developed.

Clustering, Social Determinants, and Globalization

Three additional patterns have influenced and enhanced understanding of STI epidemiology in LMICs:

- Geographic clustering and concentration of risk behaviors and infections
- Importance of context, social determinants, and structural drivers
- Globalization.

Nonuniform distribution and clustering of risk—both in behaviors and infections—have been reported for the epidemiologies of both HIV and other STIs (Chesson 2010a, 2010b; Leichliter and others 2010). More recent attention has been drawn to geographic concentration (Tanser and others 2009) and to the critical role of local context in the epidemiology of STIs. The Priorities for Local AIDS Control Efforts method can identify sites where people with high rates of partner change can receive STI prevention services (Weir and others 2003). Similarly, the Situational Analysis of Sexual Health method can identify specific locations where vulnerable and at-risk people can receive STI prevention services (Benzaken and others 2012). Insight into variations in STI epidemiology has important implications for prevention and control, including targeting of interventions and allocation of resources (Aral and Cates 2013).

In the past two decades, the importance of social determinants of sexual health and structural drivers for STI epidemiology have received increasing recognition. Examples of social determinants include low socioeconomic status and poor access to quality health care (Hogben and Leichliter 2008). Underlying social, economic, legal, and political structures have a notable influence on sexual behaviors (Hogben and Leichliter 2008; Parkhurst 2014). Moreover, these factors affect the formation, evolution, and persistence of STIs in key populations. Finally, globalization shapes and connects sexual behaviors, practices, and networks around the world (Aral, Bernstein, and Torrone 2015; Aral and Ward 2005, 2014; Ward and Aral 2006).

Current developments in methodological approaches promise to have an impact on the study and understanding of STI epidemiology in all settings. Two developments are particularly remarkable: (1) the increasing use of sophisticated geographic mapping methodologies (Tanser and others 2009) and (2) phylogenetic analyses combined with social epidemiology (Avila and others 2014), specifically, phylogenetic and network analyses. When combined, these approaches provide powerful explanations of transmission dynamics within and between groups; if used in conjunction with geo-mapping, they may enhance the understanding of aspects of STI prevention science, such as subgroup targeting.

Prevention

Important changes in the approach to STI prevention have been influenced by the HIV epidemic. During the 1980s and 1990s, behavioral prevention dominated the HIV world and gained prominence in the STI domain. However, since the turn of the century, there has been increasing recognition that behavioral interventions have not brought sustainable decreases in incidence (Aral 2011; Kippax and Stephenson 2012). Concurrently, remarkable progress has been made in biomedical approaches to preventing HIV/AIDS, including male circumcision, preexposure prophylaxis (PrEP), and ART (Baeten and others 2012; Dodd, Garnett, and Hallett 2010; Grant and others 2010; Katz and Wright 2008; Pretorius and others 2010; Thigpen and others 2012). Given the success of biomedical approaches to the prevention of HIV/AIDS, the field of STI prevention is drawing increasingly on biomedical interventions, reinforced by development of effective biomedical interventions for preventing STIs other than HIV. More specifically, the HPV and HBV vaccines, point-of-care diagnostic tests for syphilis and dual tests for syphilis and HIV, and an understanding of the preventive effects of circumcision for certain STIs are beginning to show promise in preventing specific STIs other than HIV.

STI prevention has also been influenced by other insights. Prevention activities have increasingly sought to achieve impact at the population level. In addition to protecting individuals, the focus has turned to decreasing population incidence. This shift has brought several other changes given that it requires system-level thinking, planning, and evaluation. It is important to take into account how interventions may have additive, synergistic, or antagonistic effects (Aral 2011; Aral and Douglas 2007; Parkhurst 2014). The social and epidemiological context and interactions between interventions and context have also emerged as important issues (Aral and Cates 2013; Parkhurst 2014).

More attention is being given to the elements of complex systems (mixing patterns, networks, clustering, and hot spots) and to social, economic, legal, and sexual structures (Blanchard and Aral 2010; Parkhurst 2014). The need for new approaches to designing prevention programs is now widely recognized (Aral and Blanchard 2012; Blanchard and Aral 2011; Parkhurst 2014).

With the reality of limited and declining resources, emphasis has been placed on accountability, resource allocation, efficiency, prioritization, and return on investment (Over and Aral 2006). These developments are changing the STI prevention field in important ways. The hope is that the next decade will bring significantly greater prevention for the money in LMICs, where health systems are often weak (Mills 2014). Reforming and strengthening of health care infrastructure may be needed before the recent advances in STI prevention science can be successfully implemented in these contexts.

EFFECTIVENESS OF STI PREVENTION INTERVENTIONS: LITERATURE REVIEW

Over the past 20 years, many STI prevention interventions have been rigorously evaluated for effectiveness. In a review of STI prevention interventions evaluated by randomized controlled trials (RCTs) in HICs and LMICs, Wetmore, Manhart, and Wasserheit (2010) found that 44 of 75 interventions (59 percent) significantly reduced the risk of acquiring at least one STI. Interventions were organized according to modality, including behavior change, vaginal microbicides, male circumcision, partner services, treatment, and vaccines. The percentage of trials in which a statistically significant reduction in the risk of a laboratory-confirmed STI was observed in the intervention arm (compared with the control arm) was highest for treatment, vaccines, and male circumcision, followed by behavioral interventions, partner services, and vaginal microbicides. These findings are consistent with those of Manhart and Holmes (2005), in which 54 percent of the trials led to a significant reduction in STI acquisition, transmission, or complications.

For this section, a literature search was conducted to identify studies of the impact of STI prevention interventions in LMICs. The search was conducted from January 2014 to April 2014, and the following databases were used: Cochrane Library, Database of Abstracts of Reviews of Effects, MEDLINE, and Embase. The MEDLINE search terms used to identify the relevant literature are listed in annexes 10A and 10B, and these search terms were amended as necessary to search the other databases. This search was supplemented with additional sources, such as the bibliographies of articles obtained in the search and previous reviews of the impact of STI prevention interventions (Manhart and Holmes 2005; Mayaud and Mabey 2004; Wetmore, Manhart, and Wasserheit 2010). Although this review and that of Wetmore, Manhart, and Wasserheit (2010) overlap, there are four key differences. First, this review was not systematic—no specific inclusion or exclusion criteria were applied. Instead, studies were selected to highlight key aspects of the evidence, focusing on studies that use biological outcomes rather than changes in attitudes or behaviors. Second, the search was not limited to RCTs, but also considered cohort and cross-sectional studies. Third, this review focused on interventions that were evaluated in LMICs. Finally, it included more recent articles, published from January 2000 to July 2014, than the earlier review, which included articles published through December 2009.

In this summary of the literature, interventions were organized according to intervention modality using a structure adapted from Mayaud and Mabey (2004).

Specifically, interventions were organized as primary prevention (behavioral interventions, male circumcision, vaccines, and microbicides), STI case management, partner notification and management, targeted interventions and periodic presumptive treatment (PPT), mass treatment, and community-level and structural interventions.

Primary Prevention

Table 10.2 summarizes selected studies of the impact of primary prevention interventions, categorized as behavior change interventions, male circumcision, vaccines, and microbicides.

Behavior Change Interventions

Promotion of condom use, STI and HIV education, and knowledge and skill building are common behavior change interventions. Interventions to increase condom use are generally effective in reducing STI incidence in high-risk populations (Celentano and others 2000; Feldblum and others 2005; Patterson and others 2008), although promotion of male and female condoms is likely of modest benefit in populations already exposed to interventions promoting male condoms (Hoke and others 2007). However, Fontanet and others (1998) found that female sex workers in Thailand who had the option of using female condoms in situations where male condoms were not used had STI incidence rates that were 24 percent lower than those using male condoms only.

Male Circumcision

Male circumcision has a protective effect against HSV-2, HPV, and *Mycoplasma genitalium* in circumcised men (Auvert and others 2009; Mehta and others 2012; Tobian and others 2009) and against trichomoniasis and bacterial vaginosis in their female partners (Gray and others 2009). Effects of male circumcision on trichomoniasis were mixed (Mehta and others 2009; Sobngwi-Tambekou and others 2009); no protective effect was observed against gonorrhea, chlamydia, or syphilis (Mehta and others 2009; Sobngwi-Tambekou and others 2009; Tobian and others 2009). Although the trials of male circumcision found no significant impact on chlamydia, Castellsague and others (2002) and Castellsague and others (2005) present evidence that women with uncircumcised partners have a higher prevalence of chlamydia than women with circumcised partners.

HPV Vaccines: HSV, HPV, and HBV

An HSV-2 glycoprotein-D–adjuvant vaccine administered to persons with no serological evidence of previous

Table 10.2 Selected Evaluations of the Effectiveness of Primary STI Prevention Interventions, with a Focus on Interventions in Low- and Middle-Income Countries

Type of intervention and study	Description of intervention	Setting	Key results
Behavior change interventions			
Ford and others 2000	Peer education program addressing topics such as STIs and HIV, condom use, and condom negotiation	Female sex workers in Bali, Indonesia	Gonorrhea prevalence was lower in clusters with a peer educator versus clusters without.
Celentano and others 2000	Institution-based, 15-month intervention to promote consistent and proper condom use, reduce alcohol consumption, and reduce brothel patronage	Men in Royal Thai Army	Relative risk of STI infection (gonorrhea, syphilis, chancroid, nongonococcal urethritis) was 0.15 for those in intervention group versus those in control group.
Feldblum and others 2005	Male condom promotion intervention, comparing clinic-based counseling and peer promotion to peer promotion only	Female sex workers in Madagascar	Odds ratios for aggregate STI prevalence (chlamydia, gonorrhea, trichomoniasis) were significantly lower for group with clinic plus peer versus peer alone.
Hoke and others 2007	Male and female condom promotion intervention, comparing clinic-based counseling and peer promotion to peer promotion only among those already exposed to intensive male condom promotion	Female sex workers in Madagascar	STI prevalence (chlamydia, gonorrhea, trichomoniasis) did not differ significantly by study arm.
Jewkes and others 2008	A 50-hour program to build knowledge and skills	Men and women ages 15–26 years in Eastern Cape Province, South Africa	A 33 percent reduction in incidence of HSV-2 occurred in the intervention group.
Patterson and others 2008	Brief condom promotion intervention	Female sex workers in Mexico	A 40 percent decline in cumulative STI incidence (HIV, syphilis, gonorrhea, chlamydia) occurred in the intervention group.
Chong and others 2013	Online education program addressing topics such as sexual rights, contraception, condom use and STIs and HIV, empowerment, and violence prevention	Adolescents attending Colombian public schools	Among those sexually active at baseline, the intervention group had a 5 percent reduction in self-reported STIs (including chlamydia, gonorrhea, trichomoniasis, and syphilis).
Male circumcision			
Mehta and others 2009	Randomized trial of circumcision to prevent HIV and other STIs	Men ages 18–24 years in Kisumu, Kenya	No significant impact of circumcision on incidence of gonorrhea, chlamydia, or trichomoniasis was noted.
Sobngwi-Tambekou and others 2009	Randomized trial of circumcision to prevent HIV and other STIs	Men ages 15–29 years in Orange Farm, South Africa	Male circumcision reduced trichomoniasis, but no effect on gonorrhea and chlamydia was noted.
Auvert and others 2009	Randomized trial of circumcision to prevent HIV and other STIs	Men ages 15–29 years in Orange Farm, South Africa	Male circumcision reduced prevalence of high-risk HPV types in men.
Tobian and others 2009	Randomized trial of circumcision to prevent HIV and other STIs	Men ages 15–29 years in Rakai, Uganda	Statistically significant lower rates of HSV-2 seroconversion and HPV prevalence were noted among circumcised males; no significant impact on syphilis incidence was noted.

table continues next page

Table 10.2 Selected Evaluations of the Effectiveness of Primary STI Prevention Interventions, with a Focus on Interventions in Low- and Middle-Income Countries (continued)

Type of intervention and study	Description of intervention	Setting	Key results
Gray and others 2009	Randomized trial of circumcision to prevent HIV and other STIs	Men ages 15–29 years in Rakai, Uganda, and their wives or long-term consensual partners	Male circumcision reduced the risk of genital ulceration, trichomoniasis, and bacterial vaginosis in female partners.
Mehta and others 2012	Randomized trial of circumcision to prevent HIV and other STIs	Men ages 18–24 years in Kisumu, Kenya	Circumcision nearly halved the odds of urogenital *Mycoplasma genitalium*.
Vaccines			
Stanberry and others 2002	Randomized trial of safety and efficacy of genital herpes vaccine	Men and women ages 18 years and older in Australia, Canada, Italy, and the United States	Among women with no serological evidence of previous HSV-1 infection, vaccine offered partial protection; no efficacy was noted for women seropositive for HSV-1 at baseline or for men regardless of their HSV serologic status.
Harper and others 2004	Randomized trial of safety, immunogenicity, and efficacy of bivalent HPV vaccine	Women ages 15–25 years at enrollment in Brazil, Canada, and the United States	Vaccine protected against HPV 16 and 18 infection and associated cervical lesions, with evidence of cross-protection against other HPV types.
Villa and others 2006	Randomized trial of safety, immunogenicity, and efficacy of quadrivalent HPV vaccine	Women ages 16–23 years in Brazil, Nordic countries, and the United States	Vaccine protected against HPV 6, 11, 16, and 18 infection and associated cervical lesions and genital warts.
Garland and others 2007	Randomized trial of safety, immunogenicity, and efficacy of quadrivalent HPV vaccine	Women ages 16–24 years in Asia-Pacific, Europe, Latin America, and North America	Vaccine protected against external anogenital, vaginal, and cervical lesions associated with HPV 6, 11, 16, and 18.
Future II Study Group 2007	Randomized trial of safety, immunogenicity, and efficacy of quadrivalent HPV vaccine	Women ages 15–26 years in Asia-Pacific, Europe, Latin America, and North America	Vaccine protected against HPV 16– and 18– associated cervical intraepithelial neoplasia grade 2 or worse.
Muñoz and others 2009	Randomized trial of safety, immunogenicity, and efficacy of quadrivalent HPV vaccine	Women ages 24–45 years in Colombia, France, Germany, the Philippines, Spain, Thailand, and the United States	Vaccine protected against HPV 6, 11, 16, and 18 infection and associated disease.
Paavonen and others 2009	Randomized trial of safety, immunogenicity, and efficacy of bivalent HPV vaccine	Women ages 15–25 years from 14 countries in Asia-Pacific, Europe, Latin America, and North America	Vaccine protected against HPV 16– and 18– associated cervical intraepithelial neoplasia grade 2 or worse, with some protection against HPV 31, 33, and 45.
Giuliano and others 2011	Randomized trial of safety, immunogenicity, and efficacy of quadrivalent HPV vaccine	Men ages 16–26 years in Africa, Asia-Pacific, Europe, Latin America, and North America	Vaccine protected against HPV 6, 11, 16, and 18 infection and associated external genital lesions.
Palefsky and others 2011	Randomized trial of safety, immunogenicity, and efficacy of quadrivalent HPV vaccine	MSM ages 16–26 years in Australia, Brazil, Canada, Croatia, Germany, Spain, and the United States	Vaccine protected against anal intraepithelial neoplasia in MSM.
Joura and others 2015	Randomized trial of immunogenicity and efficacy of nonavalent HPV vaccine	Women ages 16–26 years in 18 countries	Vaccine protected against high-grade cervical, vulvar, and vaginal disease and persistent infection related to HPV 31, 33, 45, 52, and 58 and generated antibody response to HPV 6, 11, 16, and 18 that was noninferior to that of the quadrivalent HPV vaccine.

table continues next page

Table 10.2 Selected Evaluations of the Effectiveness of Primary STI Prevention Interventions, with a Focus on Interventions in Low- and Middle-Income Countries (continued)

Type of intervention and study	Description of intervention	Setting	Key results
Microbicides, suppressive therapy, and barrier methods			
Richardson and others 2001	Randomized trial of nonoxynol-9 gel for STI prevention	Female sex workers in Mombasa, Kenya	Intervention group had higher gonorrhea incidence than control group; no differences for other STIs.
Roddy and others 2002	Randomized trial of nonoxynol-9 gel for STI prevention	Women in Cameroon	Gel provided no protective effect against urogenital gonococcal or chlamydial infection.
Corey and others 2004	Suppressive therapy (once-daily valacyclovir) to reduce HSV transmission	HSV-2–discordant couples in Australia, Canada, Europe, Latin America, and the United States	Suppressive therapy reduced HSV transmission to the susceptible partner by about 75 percent.
Ramjee and others 2008	Randomized trial of diaphragm, lubricant gel, and condoms versus condoms alone to prevent STIs	Women in southern Africa	STI incidence (chlamydia, gonorrhea) did not differ significantly by study arm. Among consistent users, persons in the diaphragm arm had a lower risk of acquiring gonorrhea.
Karim and others 2010	Randomized trial of 1 percent vaginal gel formulation of tenofovir for HIV prevention	Women in KwaZulu-Natal, South Africa	There was a 39 percent reduction in HIV acquisition (54 percent among those with high adherence) and a 51 percent reduction in HSV-2 acquisition.
Bukusi and others 2011	Randomized trial of topical penile microbicide (62 percent alcohol in gel) to prevent bacterial vaginosis in sex partners	Heterosexual couples in Kenya	The hazard ratio of diagnosis of bacterial vaginosis was 1.44 in intervention arm versus control arm.
Guffey and others 2014	Randomized trial of microbicides BufferGel and 0.5 percent PRO 2000 for prevention of nonulcerative STIs	Women in Malawi, South Africa, Zambia, Zimbabwe, and the United States	Candidate microbicides did not protect against gonorrhea, chlamydia, or trichomoniasis.

Note: HIV = human immunodeficiency virus; HPV = human papillomavirus; HSV = herpes simplex virus; MSM = men who have sex with men; STI = sexually transmitted infection.

HSV-1 infection partially protected women, but not men, from acquiring genital herpes disease, with efficacy of about 75 percent across two trials (Stanberry and others 2002). In contrast, the bivalent, quadrivalent, and nonavalent HPV vaccines have shown remarkably high efficacy in preventing infection and disease, and the bivalent and quadrivalent vaccines may also offer some cross-protection against other types of HPV (Malagon and others 2012). These safe and effective vaccines could reduce the burden of cervical cancer and potentially other cancers, such as vulvar, vaginal, penile, anal, and oropharyngeal cancers (Markowitz and others 2014). In HICs with routine HPV vaccination programs, reductions in the prevalence of HPV and incidence of HPV-associated health outcomes, such as genital warts and cervical precancers, have been observed at the population level (Drolet and others 2015; Fairley and others 2009; Flagg, Schwartz, and Weinstock 2013; Hariri and others 2013; Markowitz and others 2013; Tabrizi and others 2012).

The HBV vaccine has been available for many years and is increasingly used in infants in many countries; vaccine programs are also now available in some countries for adolescents and young adults who did not receive the vaccine as infants. However, many adults at risk today have never received the HBV vaccine. For example, in an Internet survey conducted in the United States in 2010, 42.4 percent of HIV-negative MSM older than age 31 years reported never having received the HBV vaccine (Matthews, Stephenson, and Sullivan 2012). A cross-sectional survey of MSM in Beijing, China, in 2012 found that only 38.9 percent had received the HBV vaccination (Wang and others 2012).

Microbicides

Randomized trials have found that PrEP with antiretrovirals can reduce HIV acquisition among heterosexual men and women in serodiscordant couples (Baeten and others 2012; Thigpen and others 2012) and in MSM

(Grant and others 2010). A randomized trial of couples serodiscordant for HSV-2 in Australia, Canada, Europe, Latin America, and the United States found that once-daily valacyclovir for suppressive therapy reduced transmission of HSV-2 to the seronegative partner by about 75 percent (Corey and others 2004). However, an RCT in HIV-discordant couples in which the partner with HIV was also infected with HSV-2 found that daily acyclovir did not reduce the risk of HIV transmission to the HIV-negative partner (Celum and others 2010).

Karim and others (2010) and Karim and Baxter (2013) report that a 1 percent vaginal gel formulation of tenofovir reduced the risk of HIV and HSV-2 acquisition in a randomized trial involving women in KwaZulu-Natal, South Africa. Specifically, it reduced HIV acquisition by 39 percent (54 percent among those with high adherence) and HSV-2 acquisition by 51 percent. However, in a randomized, placebo-control trial of tenofovir-based PrEP in women in South Africa, Uganda, and Zimbabwe (the VOICE study), none of the drug regimens reduced HIV-1 acquisition rates in the intent-to-treat analysis (Marrazzo and others 2015). Similarly, the FACTS 001 trial in more than 2,000 women in nine sites in South Africa found that pericoital vaginal application of tenofovir 1 percent gel was not effective in preventing HIV acquisition (Rees and others 2015). In both the VOICE and the FACTS 001 studies, low rates of adherence to the drug regimen were considered a primary reason for this result.

An RCT involving sexually active women in southern Africa at risk for STIs found that providing condoms alone (control) was as effective as providing a diaphragm and lubricant gel in addition to condoms (intervention) in preventing chlamydia and gonorrhea (Ramjee and others 2008). However, consistent use of a diaphragm could be protective given that the incidence of gonorrhea among women in the intervention arm was significantly lower among those who reported always using a diaphragm.

STI Case Management

Pettifor and others (2000) review the literature on the effectiveness of syndromic management of STIs. Their review includes 5 studies of WHO algorithms for management of urethral discharge, 5 for genital ulcers, and 13 for vaginal discharge. Overall, the literature suggests that algorithms for urethral discharge, vaginal discharge, and genital ulcer disease can be effective. For example, La Ruche, Lorougnon, and Digbeu (1995) reported therapeutic success rates of 92 percent for male urethritis, 87 percent for vaginal discharge, and 100 percent for genital ulcer disease. The studies reviewed in Pettifor and others (2000) also show that

the algorithms to detect cervical infection can be improved by incorporating risk scores based on factors such as sexual history. Other studies also provide evidence that risk scores can improve the efficiency of syndromic management algorithms (Cornier and others 2010). Pettifor and others (2000) conclude that, although syndromic management can be effective for managing STIs, affordable, rapid, and effective diagnostic techniques to improve detection are urgently needed in resource-poor settings.

Although evidence is limited, widespread implementation of syndromic management as an approach to STI case management likely has reduced the burden of STIs, particularly in resource-poor settings (Aral and others 2006). A community randomized trial in Mwanza, Tanzania, found that syndromic treatment of STIs resulted in a 40 percent reduction in HIV incidence and a reduction in symptomatic urethritis in men and prevalence of syphilis seroreactivity (Grosskurth and others 1995; Mayaud and others 1997). Prevalence rates of other STIs were lower in the intervention communities as well, although the differences were not statistically significant for all indicators. A community randomized trial in Masaka, Uganda, offers evidence that the syndromic management of STIs reduced the incidence of curable STIs but not HIV (Kamali and others 2003). In a cluster randomized trial in Eastern Zimbabwe, an intervention that included syndromic management of STI had no impact over time on the incidence of STI symptoms, although male patients in the intervention communities were significantly more likely than those in the control communities to report cessation of symptoms (Gregson and others 2007). An RCT comparing enhanced syndromic management and PPT among hotel-based sex workers in Bangladesh found that both strategies were effective for STI control (McCormick and others 2013). A randomized trial involving men in Malawi with urethritis found that the addition of metronidazole to the syndromic management of male urethritis can reduce trichomoniasis infection in men (Price and others 2003).

Partner Notification and Management

Alam and others (2010) conducted a systematic literature review of the feasibility and acceptability of partner notification for STIs in low-resource settings and summarized the evidence that partner notification interventions can yield positive outcomes. An RCT in Harare, Zimbabwe, involving men and women with a syndromically diagnosed STI found that a partner referral intervention (client-centered, private session with a trained counselor) significantly increased the likelihood that at least one partner would be reported, compared with standard care in which the treating clinician discussed partner referral (Moyo and others 2002). A randomized trial in Kampala, Uganda, involving men and women with a syndromically diagnosed STI found that a significantly higher percentage of partners were treated using patient-delivered partner medication compared with patient-based partner referral (Nuwaha and others 2001).

Although no published evaluations are available of the impact of partner services on STI incidence in LMICs, evidence is available from trials conducted in HICs. Studies from the United States, for example, have shown that the administration of suppressive therapy to partners infected with HSV-2 in serodiscordant couples can reduce the incidence of HSV-2 seroconversion in uninfected partners (Corey and others 2004) and that expedited partner treatment (including patient-delivered therapy to a partner) can reduce the risk of persistence or reoccurrence of gonococcal or chlamydial infection in the index patient (Golden and others 2005). Golden and others (2015) conducted a community-level stepped-wedge RCT of a public health intervention to increase the uptake of expedited partner therapy. The intervention increased the percentage of persons receiving patient-delivered partner therapy and those receiving partner services. The investigators estimated that the intervention was associated with reductions of about 10 percent in chlamydia positivity and gonorrhea incidence, although these reductions were not statistically significant, perhaps as a result of inadequate statistical power and of state-financed uptake of parts of the intervention in control communities. Further trials are needed to assess the impact on STIs and cost-effectiveness of partner notification interventions in LMICs (Alam and others 2010; Ferreira and others 2013).

The potential benefits of partner notification strategies for STIs in LMICs are supported by encouraging results for HIV in LMICs. For example, Henley and others (2013) found that only 3.2 index cases needed to be interviewed, on average, to identify one additional person with HIV in Cameroon. Similarly, an RCT in Malawi found that 51 percent of partners returned for counseling and testing in the provider referral group in which health care providers notified partners, compared with 24 percent in the passive referral group in which patients were responsible for notifying their partners (Brown and others 2011). The health impact and cost-effectiveness of partner notification could be improved substantially by integrating HIV testing into STI clinics and providing HIV testing to partners of STI clinic patients. Furthermore, this integration could improve the diagnostics part of the HIV treatment continuum.

Targeted Interventions and Periodic Presumptive Treatment

Interventions commonly target groups at high risk of STI acquisition and transmission. These interventions can include the provision of PPT, which is the systematic treatment of people at high risk with a combination of drugs targeting the prevalent curable STIs. As shown by four rigorous evaluations, PPT interventions can be highly effective in reducing the STI burden within targeted groups. In an RCT among female sex workers in Kenya, the provision of monthly prophylaxis substantially reduced the incidence of gonorrhea, chlamydia, and trichomoniasis, but not of HIV (Kaul and others 2004). Reductions of about 45 percent in the prevalence of cervical infection with gonorrhea and chlamydia were observed among commercial sex workers in the Lao People's Democratic Republic after monthly PPT over a three-month period (O'Farrell and others 2006). Substantial reductions in STIs were also observed among hotel-based sex workers in Bangladesh following the provision of monthly PPT over a nine-month period (McCormick and others 2013). PPT with vaginal suppositories containing metronidazole and miconazole among HIV-negative women with one or more vaginal infections in Kenya and in Birmingham, Alabama, significantly reduced the prevalence of bacterial vaginosis among women during 12 months of follow-up, compared with women receiving a placebo (McClelland and others 2015). Steen, Chersich, and de Vlas (2012) noted that reductions in gonorrhea and chlamydia on the order of 50 percent were common across the 15 studies included in their review of PPT of curable STIs among sex workers.

The WHO (2008) reviewed the effectiveness of presumptive treatment, finding that PPT can lead to rapid, short-term reductions in STI prevalence among high-risk groups and that ongoing STI services help sustain these reductions. However, research is needed regarding the use of PPT in high-risk populations and the impact of PPT on the emergence of antimicrobial resistance in sexually transmitted and other pathogens.

Reducing STI prevalence among core groups (for example, sex workers) through PPT can have notable public health effects (such as prevention of STIs in the clients of sex workers), although the evidence is limited. An intervention of PPT plus STI prevention education targeted to high-risk women in a South African mining community was found to reduce the prevalence of gonorrhea and chlamydia not only in the women in the intervention but also in the miner population (Steen and others 2000). In contrast, a cluster randomized trial of PPT conducted among female sex workers in Benin and Ghana found substantial reductions in gonorrhea but not in chlamydia among sex workers themselves after nine months, and no impact on the prevalence of gonorrhea or chlamydia among their clients (Labbe and others 2012).

Although PPT can be effective, interventions targeting high-risk groups do not have to include PPT to be effective. For example, Avahan, the India AIDS Initiative, offers combination interventions for high-risk groups that include activities such as peer-based education, clinical services for STIs, condom promotion and distribution, and community mobilization. Among female sex workers in Maharashtra, India, Avahan led to significant declines in the prevalence of syphilis, chlamydia, and gonorrhea (Mainkar and others 2011). It also led to reductions in syphilis among high-risk MSM and male-to-female transgender persons (Subramanian and others 2013). Peer-mediated interventions have also shown promise among female sex workers in Mombasa, Kenya, where peer-based STI and HIV education and condom promotion among female sex workers increased consistent condom use with clients, but these interventions did not have a statistically significant impact on STI acquisition (Luchters and others 2008).

Mass Treatment

A community RCT in Rakai, Uganda, evaluated the efficacy of repeated mass treatment of STIs. The prevalence of syphilis seropositivity and trichomoniasis infection in women was significantly lower in intervention communities than in control communities, but there was no significant reduction in the prevalence of other STIs. However, in a subanalysis of pregnant women, the prevalence of trichomoniasis, bacterial vaginosis, gonorrhea, and chlamydia was significantly lower in communities that received mass treatment.

Although rigorous evaluations of the population-level impact of mass treatment strategies in LMICs are rare, mathematical modeling exercises suggest that mass treatment combined with sustained syndromic management could be an effective STI control strategy and substantially reduce STI-attributable HIV incidence (Korenromp and others 2000). This model suggests that the impact of a single round of mass treatment on STI incidence would be temporary without continued rounds of mass treatment or a sustained complementary intervention, such as syndromic management.

In general, however, mass treatment is discouraged because of its cost, adverse effects, promotion of resistance, and other factors (Mayaud and Mabey 2004). For example, a targeted mass treatment program to provide azithromycin to more than 4,000 at-risk persons in British Columbia

resulted in a temporary decrease in syphilis rates, but rates rebounded rapidly and soon exceeded previous levels (Pourbohloul, Rekart, and Brunham 2003; Rekart and others 2003). The intervention might have contributed to the rebound by increasing the number of people susceptible to infection (Pourbohloul, Rekart, and Brunham 2003). Emergence of azithromycin-resistant *Treponema pallidum* occurred during the intervention (Mabey 2009). The impact on azithromycin resistance of other bacteria was not studied. For these and other reasons, researchers have cautioned that mass treatment interventions should not be undertaken routinely (Pourbohloul, Rekart, and Brunham 2003; Rekart and others 2003).

Community and Structural Interventions

STI prevention interventions can be implemented at the individual, risk group, or community level. Although this literature review is stratified by intervention modality and not by level of implementation, most of the interventions reviewed thus far were targeted to individuals or high-risk groups.

The MEMA kwa Vijana ("good things for young people") intervention, a random community intervention in the Mwanza Region of Tanzania, examined the impact of a multipronged intervention that included school-based sexual and reproductive health education, youth-friendly health services, peer condom promotion, and community activities. Although the intervention increased knowledge and decreased reported risk behaviors, it had no apparent effect on HIV or HSV-2 seroincidence, incidence of other STIs, or pregnancy outcomes at the end of the trial (Hayes and others 2005), and no effect on HIV after about 10 years (Doyle and others 2010).

Community-based interventions have also been used to improve the quality of syndromic management of STIs. A district RCT in Lima, Peru, examined an intervention to improve the recognition and management of STI syndromes by pharmacy workers (Garcia and others 2003). The intervention was found to improve STI recognition and management, as well as STI and HIV risk-reduction counseling. A subsequent trial that chose 20 cities throughout Peru to receive or not receive this intervention resulted in substantial and significant improvements in STI syndromic management at pharmacies in the intervention cities but not in the control cities. The community trial in Peru (Peru PREVEN Study) combined four intervention modalities:

- Provision of training, workshops, and educational materials to pharmacy workers and clinicians
- STI screening and treatment for female sex workers by mobile outreach teams

- Provision of PPT using metronidazole to female sex workers with bacterial vaginosis
- Condom promotion among female sex workers by mobile outreach teams and among the general population by social marketing of low-cost condoms (Garcia and others 2012).

Adjusted for baseline prevalence, among 12,930 young adults ages 18–29 years there was a nonsignificant reduction in chlamydia, trichomoniasis, and gonorrhea infection and in syphilis seroreactivity. However, significant reductions were noted in certain subgroups, specifically young adult women and female sex workers in intervention cities.

Randomized trials at the clinic level offer comparable findings in Pakistan (Shah and others 2007) and South Africa (Harrison and others 2000). A cluster randomized trial in rural Vietnam showed that educational programs with interactive training can increase STI-related knowledge and practices of health care providers such as pharmacists, doctors, and nurses (Lan and others 2014).

Structural (or environmental) interventions to prevent STIs, including HIV, seek to change the physical and social environments in which risky sexual behavior takes place, with a focus on making healthy options the default choice (Frieden 2010; Kerrigan and others 2006). Government policies and regulations are a common example of structural interventions. A government policy in Puerto Plata, the Dominican Republic, requiring condom use between sex workers and clients (with penalties for violations incurred by owners of sex establishments), combined with a community-solidarity intervention, was associated with a 50 percent reduction in STI prevalence among female sex workers (Kerrigan and others 2006). This reduction was more substantial than that observed in Santo Domingo, the Dominican Republic, which received the community-solidarity intervention alone.

Although not evaluated through an RCT or comparative effectiveness design, the Thai government's response to prevention of HIV in the late 1980s and early 1990s provides compelling evidence of the potential impact of structural interventions. The response included three main components: the provision of condoms to commercial sex venues, the imposition of sanctions on commercial sex venues not adhering to the 100 percent condom use policy, and a mass advertising campaign advising men to use condoms with commercial sex workers (Hanenberg and others 1994). Within four years, condom use in commercial sex acts increased to 94 percent from 14 percent; STIs in males declined about 80 percent, with notable reductions in HIV incidence as well (Hanenberg and others 1994; Punpanich, Ungchusak, and Detels 2004).

Charania and others (2011) concluded that structural interventions to increase the availability of condoms do increase condom use, based on their review of 21 published studies. However, a Cochrane Review of nine RCTs of structural and community-level interventions to increase condom use found no evidence that these interventions reduced HIV or STIs (Moreno and others 2014). These findings are not necessarily contradictory, given key differences in their approaches. For example, unlike the review by Moreno and others (2014), the review by Charania and others (2011) focused exclusively on structural interventions, was not limited to RCTs, and examined behavioral outcomes (condom use) rather than health outcomes (STI or HIV incidence).

A cash transfer program was tested in a trial of never-married women ages 13–22 years in Zomba District of Malawi (Baird and others 2012). The provision of cash was intended to increase household income and sustain school enrollment in an attempt to offset two possible risk factors for HIV and STIs: poverty and lack of education. The cash transfer program was shown to reduce HIV and HSV-2 incidence, indicating high effectiveness in a low-income setting (Baird and others 2012).

Alcohol control policies (alcohol taxation and restrictions on advertising) have been proposed to reduce STIs and HIV/AIDS in Sub-Saharan Africa (Chersich and others 2009), given research linking alcohol consumption to risky sexual behaviors. In HICs, alcohol control policies have been associated with substantial declines in alcohol-related health outcomes, such as motor vehicle fatalities and homicides (Cook and Durrance 2013). They have also been shown to reduce risky sexual behaviors and STI incidence and to improve sexual health (Chesson, Harrison, and Kassler 2000; Cohen and others 2006; Dee 2001; Grossman, Kaestner, and Markowitz 2005; Sen and Luong 2008; Staras and others 2014). Grossman, Kaestner, and Markowitz (2005) found that a 10 percent increase in the state excise taxes on beer was associated with lower gonorrhea rates among males ages 15–24 years in the United States. Dee (2001) estimated that establishing a minimum legal drinking age of 21 years in the United States reduced childbearing by about 6 percent among black teenagers.

COST-EFFECTIVENESS OF STI PREVENTION INTERVENTIONS: LITERATURE REVIEW

The cost-effectiveness of STI prevention interventions depends in part on the degree to which reductions in STIs other than HIV might influence the HIV epidemic. In general, the estimated cost-effectiveness of STI prevention interventions is much higher if the potential benefits of preventing STI-attributable HIV transmission or acquisition are included. Modeling exercises have suggested that syndromic management of STIs can have a substantial influence on HIV incidence in LMICs and be cost saving in many scenarios (White and others 2008). However, given the scientific debate regarding the effects on HIV of STI treatment and prevention, some experts have advised assessing the cost-effectiveness of STI prevention interventions without considering the potential impacts on HIV (Galarraga and others 2009). This section focuses on studies that assess the cost-effectiveness of STI prevention in its own right, without regard to the potential effects on HIV.

A literature search was conducted to identify studies of the cost-effectiveness of STI prevention interventions in LMICs. The search was conducted through July 2014 using the same databases as those listed for the literature search on effective STI prevention interventions. Search terms used to identify the relevant literature are provided in annexes 10A and 10B. This search was supplemented with additional sources, such as the bibliographies of articles obtained in the search. Costs and cost-effectiveness ratios have been updated to 2012 U.S. dollars. The cost-effectiveness of programs to prevent syphilis during pregnancy and HIV/AIDS are not included in this review because this topic is addressed in chapter 6 of this volume (John-Stewart and others 2017). Table 10.3 summarizes selected studies of the cost-effectiveness of prevention interventions.

Table 10.3 Selected Cost-Effectiveness Analyses of Primary STI Prevention Interventions in Low- and Middle-Income Countries

Type of intervention and study	Description of intervention evaluated	Setting of intervention	Key cost-effectiveness results (2012 U.S. dollars unless noted otherwise)
Behavior change interventions			
Chong and others 2013	Online education program addressing topics such as sexual rights, contraception, condom use and STIs and HIV, empowerment, and violence prevention.	Adolescents attending Colombian public schools	Cost per STI averted ranged from $95 to $824, depending on assumptions regarding duration of intervention's effect.
HPV vaccination			
Goldie and others 2008; Levin and others 2015; Natunen and others 2013	HPV vaccination of females, either alone or in combination with cervical cancer screening.	LMICs eligible for support from Gavi, the Vaccine Alliance	HPV vaccination of females can be highly cost-effective even in the poorest countries.
STI case management			
Sahin-Hodoglugil and others 2003	Three protocols for diagnosing and treating gonorrhea and chlamydia: "gold-standard" care, syndromic management, and mass treatment.	Women in Africa	Cost-effectiveness of each protocol varied by locale. Syndromic management had two key advantages: low program costs and relative ease of implementation.
Adams and others 2003	Training pharmacists in syndromic management of urethral discharge and genital ulcer disease in males and vaginal discharge and pelvic inflammatory disease in females.	Peru	Intervention was cost saving from the societal perspective.
Colvin and others 2006	Provided syndromic management packets (including an information leaflet and appropriate antibiotics) to primary care clinics.	Durban, South Africa	A savings of US$2.39 occurred per additional patient appropriately managed for urethral discharge in males and vaginal discharge and lower abdominal pain in females.
Vickerman, Ndowa, and Mayaud 2008	Modification in STI treatment guidelines for syndromic management of genital ulcer disease that incorporated antiviral treatment for HSV-2 in certain situations.	LMICs	Although the incorporation of HSV-2 treatment could increase program costs, it could potentially increase the proportion of herpetic ulcers treated, while reducing the cost per ulcer appropriately treated.

table continues next page

Table 10.3 Selected Cost-Effectiveness Analyses of Primary STI Prevention Interventions in Low- and Middle-Income Countries (continued)

Type of intervention and study	Description of intervention evaluated	Setting of intervention	Key cost-effectiveness results (2012 U.S. dollars unless noted otherwise)
Targeted interventions and periodic presumptive treatment			
Borghi and others 2005	Voucher scheme to increase STI services for high-risk groups, including sex workers and their clients.	Managua, Nicaragua	Average cost per STI cured was US$140.17.
Carrara and others 2005	Providing STI clinical services and outreach to female sex workers and their male clients through nongovernmental organizations, with a focus on the management of genital discharge syndrome and genital ulcer syndrome.	Cambodia	Average cost per syndrome cured or improved was about US$84.35–US$154.34 for men and US$89.73–US$154.34 for women.
Marseille and others 2001	Distribution of 6,000 female condoms to female sex workers and to women with at least one casual partner per year.	Rural South Africa	The intervention was estimated to have averted 6 HIV infections, 33 gonorrhea infections, and 38 syphilis infections and to pay for itself in averted HIV and STI treatment costs.
Lafort and others 2010	Establishing a dedicated clinic specifically for high-risk populations (female sex workers and long-distance truck drivers).	Northern Mozambique	Cost per clinic visit was US$4.76.
Mass treatment			
Sahin-Hodoglugil and others 2003	Mass treatment compared with syndromic management.	Women in Africa	Mass treatment offered relative advantages in number and percentage of cases cured, but relative disadvantages in overall program costs and costs associated with overtreatment.
Community and structural interventions			
Sweat and others 2004	Structural intervention was a system of sanctions levied on sex establishment owners for failing to follow government policies requiring condom use during sex work; administered in conjunction with an environmental intervention that included community mobilization, peer education, and distribution of educational materials and promotional items.	Dominican Republic	The cost per DALY averted was US$1,468.94 with the environmental intervention alone. When the structural intervention was included along with the environmental intervention, the estimated number of HIV infections averted more than doubled and the cost per DALY averted was US$566.02.

Note: DALY = disability-adjusted life year; HIV = human immunodeficiency virus; HPV = human papillomavirus; HSV = herpes simplex virus; LMICs = low- and middle-income countries; STI = sexually transmitted infection.

Primary Prevention

Behavior Change Interventions

Although several studies have examined the cost-effectiveness of behavioral interventions to prevent HIV in LMICs (McCoy, Kangwende, and Padian 2010; Townsend, Mathews, and Zembe 2013), the literature search yielded only one study of the cost-effectiveness of behavioral interventions to prevent other STIs. The study assessed the cost-effectiveness of an online education program for adolescents attending public schools in Colombia (Chong and others 2013). The intervention addressed topics such as sexual rights, contraception, condom use and STIs and HIV, empowerment, and violence prevention. The findings suggested a cost per STI averted of US$95–US$824, depending on assumptions about the duration of the intervention's effect (table 10.3).

Male Circumcision

Adult male circumcision is a cost-effective and potentially cost-saving intervention for preventing heterosexual acquisition of HIV in men, according to a review of published studies (Uthman and others 2010). The cost-effectiveness of male circumcision to prevent STIs (other than HIV) has not been analyzed and is not of vital importance given that preventing HIV is the main goal of adult male circumcision.

HPV Vaccination

Although HPV vaccination is a relatively new intervention, a substantial body of research examines its cost-effectiveness in LMICs. Levin and others (2015) and Natunen and others (2013) reviewed the cost-effectiveness of HPV vaccination in LMICs with high rates of cervical cancer. Goldie and others (2008) assessed the cost-effectiveness of HPV vaccination in 72 countries eligible for support from Gavi, the Vaccine Alliance. Two key themes emerge from this literature. First, HPV vaccination of females (either alone or in combination with cervical cancer screening) can be highly cost-effective even in the poorest countries. Second, despite favorable cost-effectiveness, HPV vaccine programs will likely not be affordable in many countries. Gavi has helped address the affordability issue, making HPV vaccine available at less than US$5 per dose to Gavi-eligible countries as of 2014, compared with more than US$100 per dose in HICs.[2]

Microbicides

A modeling study suggested that a hypothetical microbicide with 55 percent efficacy in preventing male-to-female HIV transmission would be highly cost-effective in LMICs with generalized epidemics, but it likely would be less cost-effective in HICs (Verguet and Walsh 2010). In another modeling study, Terris-Prestholt and others (2014) calculated per act efficacy against HIV and HSV-2 consistent with the overall efficacy of the 1 percent vaginal gel formulation of tenofovir, as reported in the CAPRISA trial (Karim and others 2010). Results indicate that the gel could be cost-effective or cost saving in LMICs, depending on its price. However, subsequent trials have not confirmed that the gel reduces HIV/AIDS acquisition. The literature search yielded no cost-effectiveness analyses of using microbicides strictly to prevent STIs other than HIV/AIDS.

STI Case Management

Sahin-Hodoglugil and others (2003) used a decision tree model to examine the cost-effectiveness of three protocols for diagnosing and treating gonorrhea and chlamydia in women in Sub-Saharan Africa: gold-standard care (use of the best available yet expensive diagnostic tests), syndromic management, and mass treatment. They found that the cost-effectiveness of each strategy varied by locale, depending on STI prevalence, program coverage, and health-seeking behavior. Syndromic management had two key advantages—low program costs and relative ease of implementation—which likely explains why it is often used in resource-poor settings. This finding is consistent with a systematic review of the costs of treating curable STIs in LMICs (Terris-Prestholt and others 2006), which found that syndromic management had lower costs than other management strategies. However, syndromic management had a lower estimated impact on the percentage of chlamydia and gonorrhea cases cured than the gold-standard or mass treatment options (Sahin-Hodoglugil and others 2003).

Three studies examined the cost-effectiveness of strategies to improve the quality of syndromic management:

- An intervention in Peru that trained pharmacists in syndromic management of urethral discharge and genital ulcer disease in males and vaginal discharge and pelvic inflammatory disease in females was found to be cost saving from the societal perspective (Adams and others 2003).
- An intervention in Durban, South Africa, that provided syndromic management packets (including an information leaflet and appropriate antibiotics) to primary care clinics was found to cost US$2.39 per additional patient appropriately managed for urethral discharge in males and vaginal discharge and lower abdominal pain in females (Colvin and others 2006).
- Vickerman, Ndowa, and Mayaud (2008) examined the cost-effectiveness of a modification in the 2003 WHO guidelines for syndromic management of genital ulcer disease that incorporated antiviral treatment for HSV-2 in certain situations, such as in populations with HSV-2 prevalence of 30 percent or more. Although the incorporation of HSV-2 treatment could increase program costs, it could potentially increase the proportion of herpetic ulcers treated while reducing the cost per ulcer appropriately treated.

Incorporating HSV-2 treatment could be an affordable and cost-effective strategy in certain situations, depending on factors such as the cost of HSV-2 therapy. Perhaps more important, the implementation of syndromic management for genital ulcers that includes treatment for chancroid, in accordance with the WHO guidelines (WHO 2003), has been credited with major reductions in or even elimination of chancroid in many parts of the world (Ryan, Kamb, and Holmes 2008; Spinola 2008; Steen 2001). To the extent that chancroid is an important risk factor for HIV transmission, syndromic management to reduce its incidence may be exceptionally cost-effective (Makasa, Buve, and Sandøy 2012).

Partner Notification and Management

The literature search yielded no cost-effectiveness analyses of partner notification and partner management strategies for STIs other than HIV in LMICs. However, partner management strategies for HIV illustrate the potential for such strategies to be cost-effective for STIs. For example, Rutstein and others (2014) found that, in Sub-Saharan Africa, the incremental cost per HIV transmission averted was US$3,014.93 for "contract" notification, in which there is an agreement that the provider will attempt to notify partners if the index patient fails to do so within one week, compared with passive referral in which the index patient is encouraged to notify partners. Furthermore, partner notification is regarded as an efficient approach to identifying HIV-positive individuals in need of therapy and also identifies HIV-negative partners who may benefit from PrEP.

Targeted Interventions and Periodic Presumptive Treatment

Borghi and others (2005) examined the cost-effectiveness of a voucher scheme implemented in Managua, Nicaragua, to increase STI services for high-risk groups, including sex workers and their clients. The vouchers covered free STI services from a range of providers. The analysis focused on the cost of treating four STIs, and the incremental cost per STI cured by the voucher intervention was US$140.17.

Carrara and others (2005) examined the cost-effectiveness of providing STI clinical services and outreach to female sex workers and their male clients in Cambodia through nongovernmental organizations. The analysis focused on the management of genital discharge syndrome and genital ulcer syndrome; the average cost per syndrome cured or improved was about US$84.35 to US$154.34 for men and US$89.73 to US$154.34 for women.

Marseille and others (2001) examined the cost-effectiveness of an intervention to distribute female condoms to female sex workers and to women with at least one casual partner per year. The distribution of 6,000 female condoms was expected to avert 6 HIV infections, 33 gonorrhea infections, and 38 syphilis infections and to pay for itself in averted HIV and STI treatment costs.

Increasing access to STI prevention services by establishing a dedicated clinic specifically for high-risk populations could be a cost-effective strategy in LMICs. A study of the costs and use of a nighttime clinic in northern Mozambique for high-risk populations (female sex workers and long-distance truck drivers) found a cost per clinic visit of about US$4.76, based on a monthly

clinic cost of US$2,233.02 and treatment of 475 clients per month (Lafort and others 2010). Expanding the hours of operation, widening the geographic coverage of the clinic, and targeting additional risk groups could reduce the cost per client served.

Mass Treatment

Only one cost-effectiveness analysis of mass treatment strategies in LMICs was found (Sahin-Hodoglugil and others 2003). Their decision tree analysis suggested that mass treatment offered relative advantages over gold-standard care and syndromic management in number and percentage of cases cured, but relative disadvantages in overall program costs and costs associated with overtreatment. The decision trees used in the analysis did not account for the potential for mass treatment to promote antimicrobial resistance or for the potential adverse effects on persons treated unnecessarily.

Community and Structural Interventions

Sweat and others (2006) examined the cost-effectiveness of environmental and structural interventions to prevent HIV among female sex workers in the Dominican Republic. The environmental intervention consisted of activities such as community mobilization, peer education, and distribution of educational materials and promotional items. The structural intervention was a system of sanctions levied on sex establishment owners for failing to follow government policies requiring condom use during sex work. Accordingly, the structural intervention consisted of holding the establishment owners—not the commercial sex workers—responsible for ensuring that condoms were used consistently in all commercial sex transactions in the establishment. The cost per DALY averted was US$1,468.94 with the environmental intervention alone. When the structural intervention was included along with the environmental intervention, the estimated number of HIV infections averted more than doubled and the cost per DALY averted was reduced to US$566.02. Although the cost-effectiveness ratios were sensitive to various assumptions, the inclusion of the structural intervention consistently resulted in more favorable cost-effectiveness estimates (Sweat and others 2006).

Studies of the cost-effectiveness of structural interventions to prevent STIs in LMICs are rare, but structural interventions could yield substantial and lasting impacts at relatively low cost. For example, in a review of HIV prevention interventions in the United States, alcohol taxation ranked as one of the most cost-effective of all available interventions (Cohen, Wu, and Farley 2004).

KEY ISSUES REGARDING IMPACT AND COST-EFFECTIVENESS

HIV-Related Benefits of Preventing STIs Other than HIV

Few published studies examine the cost-effectiveness of interventions to control and prevent STIs other than HIV in LMICs. The review focused primarily on studies of the cost-effectiveness of prevention programs for specific STIs other than HIV that did not include costs averted and health benefits gained by preventing STI-attributable HIV infections. The inclusion of potential HIV prevention benefits could substantially alter the estimated cost-effectiveness of STI control and prevention programs (Chesson and Pinkerton 2000), particularly those targeted to high-risk populations. To the extent that prevention or control of STIs reduces the incidence of HIV, any effective STI intervention would be expected to be cost-effective, provided that the intervention itself is not excessively costly and that its effect on HIV is not too small. Furthermore, STI-related interventions can sometimes be cost-effective by reducing the progression of HIV in people infected with both HIV and another STI. For example, Vickerman and others (2011) found that suppressive therapy for HSV-2 in women with HSV-2 and HIV could be a cost-effective public health intervention based on the benefits of reducing the progression of HIV and improving the retention of women in care, a potential benefit of HSV-2 therapy suggested by Baggaley and others (2009).

To the extent that a variety of interventions targeting curable STIs might also reduce the risk of potentially fatal, incurable, and chronic STIs other than HIV such as sexually transmitted HPV, HBV, and HSV, the cost-effectiveness of such interventions would be more favorable when these additional benefits are included.

Conversely, certain HIV prevention interventions might also reduce other STIs. However, their cost-effectiveness is generally not as sensitive to the inclusion of other STI-related benefits as the reverse. For example, circumcision is a highly cost-effective (and potentially cost-saving) intervention for the prevention of HIV acquisition in men (Uthman and others 2010). Because it is cost-effective when considering HIV-related benefits alone, there is little need to include the potential benefits of preventing other STIs, at least in settings where prevention of other STIs is not the primary goal of circumcision.

Screening and Treatment for Syphilis in Pregnancy

The prevention of mother-to-child transmission of HIV and syphilis is addressed in chapter 6 of this volume (John-Stewart and others 2017). However, screening and treatment for syphilis in pregnancy warrants special mention here for several key reasons. First, the global burden of disease due to syphilis during pregnancy is comparable to that of mother-to-child transmission of HIV (WHO 2012b). Second, screening and treatment for syphilis in pregnancy is an inexpensive and highly cost-effective intervention (Blandford and others 2007; Hawkes and others 2011; Kahn and others 2014; Owusu-Edusei, Gift, and Ballard 2011; Rydzak and Goldie 2008; Schmid 2004; Terris-Prestholt and others 2003). However, despite their low cost and favorable cost-effectiveness, screening for and treatment of syphilis in pregnancy are vastly underutilized in LMICs today (WHO 2012b).

HPV and HBV Vaccination

Given the scarcity of published studies on the cost-effectiveness of interventions to prevent STIs in LMICs, the exceptionalism of HPV and HBV vaccination warrants mention. HPV vaccination is unique among STI prevention interventions in that its effectiveness has been demonstrated in RCTs, and its cost-effectiveness in LMICs has been analyzed extensively, as reviewed by Natunen and others (2013) and Levin and others (2015). Similar data exist for HBV vaccination (Kane 1995). However, young girls have limited access to HPV vaccine in poorer settings because of the high cost of the vaccine and other challenges associated with vaccinating (de Sanjosé and others 2012; Kane 2010). Nonetheless, Gavi's support for HPV vaccines is expected to increase access in LMICs and eventually reduce the disproportionate burden of HPV-associated cancers in these settings.

Income and Income Inequality

Aral and others (2006) examined the association between two economic measures—income and income inequality and STI burden—at the country level. For each country setting, income was measured using gross national income, and income inequality was measured using the Gini coefficient, which can range from 0 (complete equality) to 1 (complete inequality). The burden of STIs was negatively associated with income and positively associated with income inequality. Their analysis suggested that these two economic measures could explain almost half of the variation across countries in STI prevalence among low-risk groups (16 percent of the variation among high-risk groups).

These findings are consistent with other analyses in HICs. Bingham and others (2014) used the Gini coefficient to examine income inequality and gonorrhea incidence rates across 11 countries. Their analysis showed significant positive associations between income inequality and gonorrhea rates in women. Owusu-Edusei, Chesson, Leichliter, and others (2013) examined county-level data in the United States and found that racial disparities in income were associated with racial disparities in STI burden. One possible explanation is that racial income disparity contributes to residential segregation by race, which has been identified as a social determinant of STI risk (Hogben and Leichliter 2008; Owusu-Edusei, Chesson, Leichliter, and others 2013; Thomas and Gaffield 2003).

Research and Development Agenda

Aral and others (2006) provided the following list of priorities for global STI research, and they remain priorities today:

- Development, evaluation, and implementation of STI prevention and control interventions, including therapeutic interventions such as drug treatment and therapeutic vaccines, and primary prevention interventions such as prophylactic vaccines, structural interventions, and behavioral interventions
- Enhanced efforts to control the spread of drug-resistant strains of gonorrhea
- Development and evaluation of tools and methods for assessing the burden of STIs and STI-related sequelae and for allocating STI prevention resources efficiently to reduce this burden
- Development and evaluation of tools to promote early detection and treatment of STIs, particularly inexpensive and practical rapid diagnostic tests for gonorrhea and chlamydia
- Development and evaluation of strategies to identify persons at highest risk for STIs and to offer prevention services to reduce their risk of acquisition and transmission, especially to highly stigmatized populations (MSM, transgender persons, and sex workers)
- Promotion of health services research to inform the integration of practical and cost-effective prevention strategies or systems into the public health infrastructure
- Implementation of studies in support of global elimination programs, such as for syphilis and possibly cervical cancer
- Continued research on the importance of social determinants of STIs, with the goal of reducing racial and geographic disparities in sexual health.

CONCLUSIONS

STIs impose a considerable health and economic burden globally. Primary prevention and control of STIs in LMICs can be an efficient use of resources, although the impact and cost-effectiveness of interventions can vary substantially across settings. Furthermore, estimates of the cost-effectiveness of STI control in LMICs can be subject to considerable uncertainty and might not be generalizable across settings. The findings of this literature review should be considered in light of the limitations inherent in cost-effectiveness studies of STI control in LMICs, such as incomplete cost data and imprecise estimates of program impact.

Behavioral interventions can often lead to reductions in the risk of acquiring STIs, at least in the short term. In contrast, interventions with long-lasting effects—such as adult male circumcision and HPV and HBV vaccination—can have a more pronounced impact on disease burden at the individual and population levels. Given the challenges of providing STI prevention and treatment services in LMICs, structural interventions are needed to make it easier and more realistic for people to choose safer behaviors. Unfortunately, establishing that a given intervention is effective and cost-effective is not enough to ensure its delivery. Screening for syphilis in pregnancy remains vastly underutilized, even though it is relatively inexpensive, effective, and cost-effective. The underutilization of effective and cost-effective interventions highlights the need for more health services research and stronger health systems—not only to improve the delivery of STI prevention interventions in LMICs, but also to expand access to STI prevention services, especially among the most vulnerable populations.

ANNEXES

The annexes to this chapter are as follows. They are available at http://www.dcp-3.org/infectiousdiseases.

- Annex 10A. Search Terms Used to Identify Literature on the Impact of STI Prevention Interventions
- Annex 10B. Search Terms Used to Identify Literature on the Cost-Effectiveness of STI Prevention Interventions

NOTES

World Bank Income Classifications as of July 2014 are as follows, based on estimates of gross national income (GNI) per capita for 2013:

- Low-income countries (LICs) = US$1,045 or less

- Middle-income countries (MICs) are subdivided:
  (a) lower-middle-income = US$1,046–US$4,125
  (b) upper-middle-income (UMICs) = US$4,126–US$12,745
- High-income countries (HICs) = US$12,746 or more.

1. These numbers represent the WHO's best estimates, using indicators that aim for comparability across countries and time; they are updated as more recent or revised data become available or when changes occur in the methodology used. Visit the Global Health Observatory at http://apps.who.int/gho/data/?theme=main.
2. Visit the Gavi website at http://www.gavi.org.

REFERENCES

Adams, E. S., P. J. Garcia, G. P. Garnett, W. J. Edmunds, and K. K. Holmes. 2003. "The Cost-Effectiveness of Syndromic Management in Pharmacies in Lima, Peru." *Sexually Transmitted Diseases* 30 (5): 379–87.

Alam, N., E. Chamot, S. H. Vermund, K. Streatfield, and S. Kristensen. 2010. "Partner Notification for Sexually Transmitted Infections in Developing Countries: A Systematic Review." *BMC Public Health* 10: 19.

Aral, S. O. 2002. "Understanding Racial-Ethnic and Societal Differentials in STI." *Sexually Transmitted Infections* 78 (1): 2–4.

———. 2011. "Utility and Delivery of Behavioural Interventions to Prevent Sexually Transmitted Infections." *Sexually Transmitted Infections* 87 (Suppl 2): ii31–ii33.

Aral, S. O., K. Bernstein, and E. Torrone. 2015. "Geographical Targeting to Improve Progression through the Sexually Transmitted Infection/HIV Treatment Continua in Different Populations." *Current Opinion in HIV and AIDS* 10 (6): 477–82.

Aral, S. O., and J. F. Blanchard. 2012. "The Program Science Initiative: Improving the Planning, Implementation, and Evaluation of HIV/STI Prevention Programs." *Sexually Transmitted Infections* 88 (3): 157–59.

Aral, S. O., and W. Cates Jr. 2013. "Coverage, Context, and Targeted Prevention: Optimising Our Impact." *Sexually Transmitted Infections* 89 (4): 336–40.

Aral, S. O., and J. M. Douglas Jr., eds. 2007. *Behavioral Interventions for Prevention and Control of Sexually Transmitted Diseases.* New York: Springer Science+Business Media.

Aral, S. O., M. Hogben, and J. N. Wasserheit. 2008. "STD-Related Health Care Seeking and Health Service Delivery." In *Sexually Transmitted Diseases,* edited by K. K. Holmes, P. F. Sparling, W. E. Stamm, P. Piot, J. N. Wasserheit, and others. New York: McGraw-Hill.

Aral, S. O., M. Over, L. Manhart, and K. K. Holmes. 2006. "Sexually Transmitted Infections." In *Disease Control Priorities in Developing Countries,* second edition, edited by D. T. Jamison, J. G. Breman, A. R. Measham, G. Alleyne, M. Claeson, D. B. Evans, P. Jha, A. Mills, and P. Musgrove, 311–30. Washington, DC: World Bank and Oxford University Press.

Aral, S. O., and H. Ward. 2005. "Modern Day Influences on Sexual Behavior." *Infectious Disease Clinics of North America* 19 (2): 297–309.

———. 2014. "Behavioral Convergence: Implications for Mathematical Models of Sexually Transmitted Infection Transmission." *Journal of Infectious Diseases* 210 (Suppl 2): S600–04.

Auvert, B., J. Sobngwi-Tambekou, E. Cutler, M. Nieuwoudt, P. Lissouba, and others. 2009. "Effect of Male Circumcision on the Prevalence of High-Risk Human Papillomavirus in Young Men: Results of a Randomized Controlled Trial Conducted in Orange Farm, South Africa." *Journal of Infectious Diseases* 199 (1): 14–19.

Avila, D., O. Keiser, M. Egger, R. Kouyos, J. Boni, and others. 2014. "Social Meets Molecular: Combining Phylogenetic and Latent Class Analyses to Understand HIV-1 Transmission in Switzerland." *American Journal of Epidemiology* 179 (2): 1514–25.

Baeten, J. M., D. Donnell, P. Ndase, N. R. Mugo, J. D. Campbell, and others. 2012. "Antiretroviral Prophylaxis for HIV Prevention in Heterosexual Men and Women." *New England Journal of Medicine* 367 (5): 399–410.

Baggaley, R. F., J. T. Griffin, R. Chapman, T. D. Hollingsworth, N. Nagot, and others. 2009. "Estimating the Public Health Impact of the Effect of Herpes Simplex Virus Suppressive Therapy on Plasma HIV-1 Viral Load." *AIDS* 23 (8): 1005–13.

Baird, S. J., R. S. Garfein, C. T. McIntosh, and B. Ozler. 2012. "Effect of a Cash Transfer Programme for Schooling on Prevalence of HIV and Herpes Simplex Type 2 in Malawi: A Cluster-Randomised Trial." *The Lancet* 379 (9823): 1320–29.

Bala, M., M. Kakran, V. Singh, S. Sood, and V. Ramesh. 2013. "Monitoring Antimicrobial Resistance in *Neisseria gonorrhoeae* in Selected Countries of the WHO South-East Asia Region between 2009 and 2012: A Retrospective Analysis." *Sexually Transmitted Infections* 89 (Suppl 4): iv28–35.

Baral, S., C. Beyrer, K. Muessig, T. Poteat, A. L. Wirtz, and others. 2012. "Burden of HIV among Female Sex Workers in Low-Income and Middle-Income Countries: A Systematic Review and Meta-Analysis." *The Lancet Infectious Diseases* 12 (7): 538–49.

Baral, S., F. Sifakis, F. Cleghorn, and C. Beyrer. 2007. "Elevated Risk for HIV Infection among Men Who Have Sex with Men in Low- and Middle-Income Countries 2000–2006: A Systematic Review." *PLoS Medicine* 4 (12): e339.

Becker, M. H., and J. G. Joseph. 1988. "AIDS and Behavioral Change to Reduce Risk: A Review." *American Journal of Public Health* 78 (4): 394–410.

Benzaken, A., M. Sabido, E. Galban, D. L. Rodrigues Dutra, A. L. Leturiondo, and others. 2012. "HIV and Sexually Transmitted Infections at the Borderlands: Situational Analysis of Sexual Health in the Brazilian Amazon." *Sexually Transmitted Infections* 88 (4): 294–300.

Bingham, A. L., A. M. Kavanagh, C. K. Fairley, L. A. Keogh, R. J. Bentley, and others. 2014. "Income Inequality and *Neisseria gonorrhoeae* Notifications in Females: A Country-Level Analysis." *Sexual Health* 11 (6): 556–60.

Blanchard, J. F., and S. O. Aral. 2010. "Emergent Properties and Structural Patterns in Sexually Transmitted Infection and HIV Research." *Sexually Transmitted Infections* 86 (Suppl 3): iii4–9.

———. 2011. "Program Science: An Initiative to Improve the Planning, Implementation, and Evaluation of HIV/Sexually Transmitted Infection Prevention Programmes." *Sexually Transmitted Infections* 87 (1): 2–3.

Blandford, J. M., T. L. Gift, S. Vasaikar, D. Mwesigwa-Kayongo, P. Dlali, and others. 2007. "Cost-Effectiveness of On-Site Antenatal Screening to Prevent Congenital Syphilis in Rural Eastern Cape Province, Republic of South Africa." *Sexually Transmitted Diseases* 34 (Suppl 7): S61–66.

Boily, M. C., F. I. Bastos, K. Desai, and B. Masse. 2004. "Changes in the Transmission Dynamics of the HIV Epidemic after the Wide-Scale Use of Antiretroviral Therapy Could Explain Increases in Sexually Transmitted Infections: Results from Mathematical Models." *Sexually Transmitted Diseases* 31: 100–13.

Boily, M. C., and R. C. Brunham. 1993. "The Impact of HIV and Other STDs on Human Populations: Are Predictions Possible?" *Infectious Disease Clinics of North America* 7 (4): 771–92.

Borghi, J., A. Gorter, P. Sandiford, and Z. Segura. 2005. "The Cost-Effectiveness of a Competitive Voucher Scheme to Reduce Sexually Transmitted Infections in High-Risk Groups in Nicaragua." *Health Policy and Planning* 20 (4): 222–31.

Brown, L. B., W. C. Miller, G. Kamanga, N. Nyirenda, P. Mmodzi, and others. 2011. "HIV Partner Notification Is Effective and Feasible in Sub-Saharan Africa: Opportunities for HIV Treatment and Prevention." *Journal of Acquired Immune Deficiency Syndromes* 56 (5): 437–42.

Bukusi, E., K. K. Thomas, R. Nguti, C. R. Cohen, N. Weiss, and others. 2011. "Topical Penile Microbicide Use by Men to Prevent Recurrent Bacterial Vaginosis in Sex Partners: A Randomized Clinical Trial." *Sexually Transmitted Diseases* 38 (6): 483–89.

Bull, S. S., and M. McFarlane. 2000. "Soliciting Sex on the Internet: What Are the Risks for Sexually Transmitted Diseases and HIV?" *Sexually Transmitted Diseases* 27 (9): 545–50.

Carrara, V., F. Terris-Prestholt, L. Kumaranayake, and P. Mayaud. 2005. "Operational and Economic Evaluation of an NGO-Led Sexually Transmitted Infections Intervention: North-Western Cambodia." *Bulletin of the World Health Organization* 83 (6): 434–42.

Castellsague, X., F. X. Bosch, N. Muñoz, C. J. Meijer, K. V. Shah, and others. 2002. "Male Circumcision, Penile Human Papillomavirus Infection, and Cervical Cancer in Female Partners." *New England Journal of Medicine* 346 (15): 1105–12.

Castellsague, X., R. W. Peeling, S. Franceschi, S. de Sanjosé, J. S. Smith, and others. 2005. "*Chlamydia trachomatis* Infection in Female Partners of Circumcised and Uncircumcised Adult Men." *American Journal of Epidemiology* 162 (9): 907–16.

Celentano, D. D., K. C. Bond, C. M. Lyles, S. Eiumtrakul, V. F. Go, and others. 2000. "Preventive Intervention to Reduce Sexually Transmitted Infections: A Field Trial in the Royal Thai Army." *Archives of Internal Medicine* 160 (4): 535–40.

Celum, C., A. Wald, J. R. Lingappa, A. S. Magaret, R. S. Wang, and others. 2010. "Acyclovir and Transmission of HIV-1 from Persons Infected with HIV-1 and HSV-2." *New England Journal of Medicine* 362 (5): 427–39.

Charania, M. R., N. Crepaz, C. Guenther-Gray, K. Henny, A. Liau, and others. 2011. "Efficacy of Structural-Level Condom Distribution Interventions: A Meta-Analysis of U.S. and International Studies, 1998–2007 (Structured Abstract)." *AIDS and Behavior* 15 (7): 1283–97.

Chersich, M. F., H. V. Rees, F. Scorgie, and G. Martin. 2009. "Enhancing Global Control of Alcohol to Reduce Unsafe Sex and HIV in Sub-Saharan Africa." *Global Health* 5 (16).

Chesson, H. W., T. S. Dee, and S. O. Aral. 2003. "AIDS Mortality May Have Contributed to the Decline in Syphilis Rates in the United States in the 1990s." *Sexually Transmitted Diseases* 30 (5): 419–24.

Chesson, H. W., and T. L. Gift. 2008. "Decreases in AIDS Mortality and Increases in Primary and Secondary Syphilis in Men Who Have Sex with Men in the United States." *Journal of Acquired Immune Deficiency Syndromes* 47 (2): 263–64.

Chesson, H., P. Harrison, and W. J. Kassler. 2000. "Sex under the Influence: The Effect of Alcohol Policy on Sexually Transmitted Disease Rates in the United States." *Journal of Law and Economics* 43 (1): 215–38.

Chesson, H. W., R. D. Kirkcaldy, T. L. Gift, K. Owusu-Edusei Jr., and H. S. Weinstock. 2014. "Ciprofloxacin Resistance and Gonorrhea Incidence Rates in 17 Cities, United States, 1991–2006." *Emerging Infectious Diseases* 20 (4): 612–19.

Chesson, H. W., and S. D. Pinkerton. 2000. "Sexually Transmitted Diseases and the Increased Risk for HIV Transmission: Implications for Cost-Effectiveness Analyses of Sexually Transmitted Disease Prevention Interventions." *Journal of Acquired Immune Deficiency Syndromes* 24 (1): 48–56.

Chesson, H. W., M. Sternberg, J. S. Leichliter, and S. O. Aral. 2010a. "Changes in the State-Level Distribution of Primary and Secondary Syphilis in the USA, 1985–2007." *Sexually Transmitted Infections* 86 (Suppl 3): iii58–62.

———. 2010b. "The Distribution of Chlamydia, Gonorrhoea, and Syphilis Cases across States and Counties in the USA, 2007." *Sexually Transmitted Infections* 86 (Suppl 3): iii52–57.

Chong, A., M. Gonzalez-Navarro, D. Karlan, and M. Valdivia. 2013. "Effectiveness and Spillovers of Online Sex Education: Evidence from a Randomized Evaluation in Colombian Public Schools." Working Paper 18776, National Bureau of Economic Research, Cambridge, MA. http://www.nber.org/papers/w18776.

Cohen, D. A., B. Ghosh-Dastidar, R. Scribner, A. Miu, M. Scott, and others. 2006. "Alcohol Outlets, Gonorrhea, and the Los Angeles Civil Unrest: A Longitudinal Analysis." *Social Science and Medicine* 62 (12): 3062–71.

Cohen, D. A., S. Y. Wu, and T. A. Farley. 2004. "Comparing the Cost-Effectiveness of HIV Prevention Interventions." *Journal of Acquired Immune Deficiency Syndromes* 37 (3): 1404–14.

Colvin, M., M. O. Bachmann, R. K. Homan, D. Nsibande, N. M. Nkwanyana, and others. 2006. "Effectiveness and Cost-Effectiveness of Syndromic Sexually Transmitted

Infection Packages in South African Primary Care: Cluster-Randomised Trial." *Sexually Transmitted Infections* 82 (4): 290–94.

Cook, P. J., and C. P. Durrance. 2013. "The Virtuous Tax: Lifesaving and Crime-Prevention Effects of the 1991 Federal Alcohol-Tax Increase." *Journal of Health Economics* 32 (1): 261–67.

Corey, L., A. Wald, R. Patel, S. L. Sacks, S. K. Tyring, and others 2004. "Once-Daily Valacyclovir to Reduce the Risk of Transmission of Genital Herpes." *New England Journal of Medicine* 350 (1): 11–20.

Cornier, N., E. Petrova, P. Cavailler, R. Dentcheva, F. Terris-Prestholt, and others. 2010. "Optimising the Management of Vaginal Discharge Syndrome in Bulgaria: Cost-Effectiveness of Four Clinical Algorithms with Risk Assessment." *Sexually Transmitted Infections* 86 (4): 303–9.

Dee, T. S. 2001. "The Effects of Minimum Legal Drinking Ages on Teen Childbearing." *Journal of Human Resources* 36 (4): 823–38.

de Sanjosé, S., B. Serrano, X. Castellsague, M. Brotons, J. Muñoz, and others. 2012. "Human Papillomavirus (HPV) and Related Cancers in the Global Alliance for Vaccines and Immunization (GAVI) Countries: A WHO/ICO HPV Information Centre Report." *Vaccine* 30 (Suppl 4): 1–83.

Dodd, P. J., G. P. Garnett, and T. B. Hallett. 2010. "Examining the Promise of HIV Elimination by 'Test and Treat' in Hyperendemic Settings." *AIDS* 24 (5): 729–35.

Doyle, A. M., D. A. Ross, K. Maganja, K. Baisley, C. Masesa, and others. 2010. "Long-Term Biological and Behavioural Impact of an Adolescent Sexual Health Intervention in Tanzania: Follow-Up Survey of the Community-Based MEMA kwa Vijana Trial." *PLoS Medicine* 7 (6): e1000287.

Drolet, M., E. Benard, M. C. Boily, H. Ali, L. Baandrup, and others. 2015. "Population-Level Impact and Herd Effects Following Human Papillomavirus Vaccination Programmes: A Systematic Review and Meta-Analysis." *The Lancet Infectious Diseases* 15 (5): 565–80.

Fairley, C. K., J. S. Hocking, L. C. Gurrin, M. Y. Chen, B. Donovan, and others. 2009. "Rapid Decline in Presentations for Genital Warts after the Implementation of a National Quadrivalent Human Papillomavirus Vaccination Program for Young Women." *Sexually Transmitted Infections* 85 (7): 499–502.

Feldblum, P. J., T. Hatzell, K. Van Damme, M. Nasution, A. Rasamindrakotroka, and others. 2005. "Results of a Randomised Trial of Male Condom Promotion among Madagascar Sex Workers." *Sexually Transmitted Infections* 81 (2): 166–73.

Ferreira, A., T. Young, C. Mathews, M. Zunza, and N. Low. 2013. "Strategies for Partner Notification for Sexually Transmitted Infections, Including HIV." *Cochrane Database of Systematic Reviews* 10: CD002843.

Flagg, E. W., R. Schwartz, and H. Weinstock. 2013. "Prevalence of Anogenital Warts among Participants in Private Health Plans in the United States, 2003–2010: Potential Impact of HPV Vaccination." *American Journal of Public Health* 103 (8): 1428–35.

Fontanet, A. L., J. Saba, V. Chandelying, C. Sakondhavat, P. Bhiraleus, and others. 1998. "Protection against Sexually Transmitted Diseases by Granting Sex Workers in Thailand the Choice of Using the Male or Female Condom: Results from a Randomized Controlled Trial." *AIDS* 12 (14): 1851–59.

Ford, K., D. N. Wirawan, S. S. Suastina, B. D. Reed, and P. Muliawan. 2000. "Evaluation of a Peer Education Programme for Female Sex Workers in Bali, Indonesia." *International Journal of STD and AIDS* 11 (11): 731–33.

Forman, D., C. de Martel, C. J. Lacey, I. Soerjomataram, J. Lortet-Tieulent, and others. 2012. "Global Burden of Human Papillomavirus and Related Diseases." *Vaccine* 30 (Suppl 5): F12–23.

Frieden, T. R. 2010. "A Framework for Public Health Action: The Health Impact Pyramid." *American Journal of Public Health* 100 (4): 590–95.

Future II Study Group. 2007. "Quadrivalent Vaccine against Human Papillomavirus to Prevent High-Grade Cervical Lesions." *New England Journal of Medicine* 356 (19): 1915–27.

Galarraga, O., M. A. Colchero, R. G. Wamai, and S. M. Bertozzi. 2009. "HIV Prevention Cost-Effectiveness: A Systematic Review." *BMC Public Health* 9 (Suppl 1): S5.

Garcia, P., J. Hughes, C. Carcamo, and K. K. Holmes. 2003. "Training Pharmacy Workers in Recognition, Management, and Prevention of STDs: District-Randomized Controlled Trial." *Bulletin of the World Health Organization* 81 (11): 806–14.

Garcia, P. J., C. P. Carcamo, G. P. Garnett, P. E. Campos, and K. K. Holmes. 2012. "Improved STD Syndrome Management by a Network of Clinicians and Pharmacy Workers in Peru: The PREVEN Network." *PLoS One* 7 (10): e47750.

Garland, S. M., M. Hernandez-Avila, C. M. Wheeler, G. Perez, D. M. Harper, and others. 2007. "Quadrivalent Vaccine against Human Papillomavirus to Prevent Anogenital Diseases." *New England Journal of Medicine* 356 (19): 1928–43.

Giuliano, A. R., J. M. Palefsky, S. Goldstone, E. D. Moreira, M. E. Penny, and others. 2011. "Efficacy of Quadrivalent HPV Vaccine against HPV Infection and Disease in Males." *New England Journal of Medicine* 364 (5): 401–11.

Golden, M. R., R. P. Kerani, M. Stenger, J. P. Hughes, M. Aubin, and others. 2015. "Uptake and Population-Level Impact of Expedited Partner Therapy (EPT) on *Chlamydia trachomatis* and *Neisseria gonorrhoeae*: The Washington State Community-Level Randomized Trial of EPT." *PLoS Medicine* 12 (1): e1001777.

Golden, M. R., W. L. Whittington, H. H. Handsfield, J. P. Hughes, W. E. Stamm, and others. 2005. "Effect of Expedited Treatment of Sex Partners on Recurrent or Persistent Gonorrhea or Chlamydial Infection." *New England Journal of Medicine* 352 (7): 676–85.

Goldie, S. J., M. O'Shea, N. G. Campos, M. Diaz, S. Sweet, and S. Y. Kim. 2008. "Health and Economic Outcomes of HPV 16, 18 Vaccination in 72 GAVI-Eligible Countries." *Vaccine* 26 (32): 4080–93.

Grant, R. M., J. R. Lama, P. L. Anderson, V. McMahan, A. Y. Liu, and others. 2010. "Preexposure Chemoprophylaxis for HIV Prevention in Men Who Have Sex with Men." *New England Journal of Medicine* 363 (27): 2587–99.

Gray, R. H., G. Kigozi, D. Serwadda, F. Makumbi, F. Nalugoda, and others. 2009. "The Effects of Male Circumcision on Female Partners' Genital Tract Symptoms and Vaginal Infections in a Randomized Trial in Rakai, Uganda." *American Journal of Obstetrics and Gynecology* 200 (1): 42–47.

Gregson, S., S. Adamson, S. Papaya, J. Mundondo, C. A. Nyamukapa, and others. 2007. "Impact and Process Evaluation of Integrated Community and Clinic-Based HIV-1 Control: A Cluster-Randomised Trial in Eastern Zimbabwe." *PLoS Medicine* 4 (3): e102.

Grosskurth, H., F. Mosha, J. Todd, E. Mwijarubi, A. Klokke, and others. 1995. "Impact of Improved Treatment of Sexually Transmitted Diseases on HIV Infection in Rural Tanzania: Randomised Controlled Trial." *The Lancet* 346 (8974): 530–36.

Grossman, M., R. Kaestner, and S. Markowitz. 2005. "An Investigation of the Effects of Alcohol Policies on Youth STDs." *Advances in Health Economics and Health Services Research* 16: 229–56.

Guffey, M. B., B. Richardson, M. Husnik, B. Makanani, D. Chilongozi, and others. 2014. "HPTN 035 Phase II/IIb Randomised Safety and Effectiveness Study of the Vaginal Microbicides BufferGel and 0.5% PRO 2000 for the Prevention of Sexually Transmitted Infections in Women." *Sexually Transmitted Infections* 90 (5): 363–69.

Hanenberg, R. S., W. Rojanapithayakorn, P. Kunasol, and D. C. Sokal. 1994. "Impact of Thailand's HIV-Control Programme as Indicated by the Decline of Sexually Transmitted Diseases." *The Lancet* 344 (8917): 243–45.

Hankins, C. A., S. R. Friedman, T. Zafar, and S. A. Strathdee. 2002. "Transmission and Prevention of HIV and Sexually Transmitted Infections in War Settings: Implications for Current and Future Armed Conflicts." *AIDS* 16: 2245–52.

Hariri, S., L. E. Markowitz, E. F. Dunne, and E. R. Unger. 2013. "Population Impact of HPV Vaccines: Summary of Early Evidence." *Journal of Adolescent Health* 53 (6): 679–82.

Harper, D. M., E. L. Franco, C. Wheeler, D. G. Ferris, D. Jenkins, and others. 2004. "Efficacy of a Bivalent L1 Virus-Like Particle Vaccine in Prevention of Infection with Human Papillomavirus Types 16 and 18 in Young Women: A Randomized Trial." *The Lancet* 364 (9447): 1757–65.

Harrison, A., S. A. Karim, K. Floyd, C. Lombard, M. Lurie, and others. 2000. "Syndrome Packets and Health Worker Training Improve Sexually Transmitted Disease Case Management in Rural South Africa: Randomized Controlled Trial." *AIDS* 14 (17): 2769–79.

Hawkes, S., N. Matin, N. Broutet, and N. Low. 2011. "Effectiveness of Interventions to Improve Screening for Syphilis in Pregnancy: A Systematic Review and Meta-Analysis." *The Lancet Infectious Diseases* 11 (9): 684–91.

Hayes, R. J., J. Changalucha, D. A. Ross, A. Gavyole, J. Todd, and others. 2005. "The MEMA kwa Vijana Project: Design of a Community Randomised Trial of an Innovative Adolescent Sexual Health Intervention in Rural Tanzania." *Contemporary Clinical Trials* 26 (4): 430–42.

Henley, C., G. Forgwei, T. Welty, M. Golden, A. Adimora, and others. 2013. "Scale-Up and Case-Finding Effectiveness of an HIV Partner Services Program in Cameroon: An Innovative HIV Prevention Intervention for Developing Countries." *Sexually Transmitted Diseases* 40 (12): 909–14.

Hogben, M., and J. S. Leichliter. 2008. "Social Determinants and Sexually Transmitted Disease Disparities." *Sexually Transmitted Diseases* 35 (12): S13–18.

Hoke, T. H., P. J. Feldblum, K. V. Damme, M. D. Nasution, T. W. Grey, and others. 2007. "Randomised Controlled Trial of Alternative Male and Female Condom Promotion Strategies Targeting Sex Workers in Madagascar." *Sexually Transmitted Infections* 83 (6): 448–53.

Holmes, K. K., and S. O. Aral. 1991. "Behavioral Interventions in Developing Countries." In *Research Issues in Human Behavior and STD in the AIDS Era*, edited by J. Wasserheit, S. Aral, and K. Holmes, 318–44. Washington, DC: American Society of Microbiology Publications.

International Futures Program. 2011. *The Future of Families to 2030: A Synthesis Report.* Paris: OECD Publications.

Jewkes, R., M. Nduna, J. Levin, N. Jama, K. Dunkle, and others. 2008. "Impact of Stepping Stones on Incidence of HIV and HSV-2 and Sexual Behaviour in Rural South Africa: Cluster-Randomised Controlled Trial." *British Medical Journal* 337: a506.

John-Stewart, G., R. Peeling, C. Levin, P. J. Garcia, D. Mabey, and J. Kinuthia. 2017. "Prevention of Mother-to-Child Transmission of HIV and Syphilis." In *Disease Control Priorities* (third edition): Volume 6, *Major Infectious Diseases*, edited by K. K. Holmes, S. Bertozzi, B. R. Bloom, and P. Jha. Washington, DC: World Bank.

Joura, E. A., A. R. Giuliano, O. E. Iversen, C. Bouchard, C. Mao, and others. 2015. "A 9-Valent HPV Vaccine against Infection and Intraepithelial Neoplasia in Women." *New England Journal of Medicine* 372 (8): 711–23.

Kahn, J. G., A. Jiwani, G. B. Gomez, S. J. Hawkes, H. W. Chesson, and others. 2014. "The Cost and Cost-Effectiveness of Scaling up Screening and Treatment of Syphilis in Pregnancy: A Model." *PLoS One* 9: e87510.

Kamali, A., M. Quigley, J. Nakiyingi, J. Kinsman, J. Kengeya-Kayondo, and others. 2003. "Syndromic Management of Sexually Transmitted Infections and Behaviour Change Interventions on Transmission of HIV-1 in Rural Uganda: A Community Randomised Trial." *The Lancet* 361 (9358): 645–52.

Kamb, M. L., E. Lackritz, J. Mark, D. B. Jackson, and H. L. Andrews. 2007. "Sexually Transmitted Infections in Developing Countries: Current Concepts and Strategies on Improving STI Prevention, Treatment, and Control." Working Paper 42797, World Bank, Washington, DC.

Kamb, M. L., L. M. Newman, P. L. Riley, J. Mark, S. J. Hawkes, and others. 2010. "A Road Map for the Global Elimination of Congenital Syphilis." *Obstetrics and Gynecology International* 2010: 312798.

Kane, M. A. 1995. "Global Programme for Control of Hepatitis B Infection." *Vaccine* 13 (Suppl 1): S47–49.

———. 2010. "Global Implementation of Human Papillomavirus (HPV) Vaccine: Lessons from Hepatitis B Vaccine." *Gynecologic Oncology* 117 (Suppl 2): S32–35.

Karim, Q. A., and C. Baxter. 2013. "Microbicides for the Prevention of Sexually Transmitted HIV Infection." *Expert Review of Anti-Infective Therapy* 11 (1): 13–23.

Karim, Q. A., S. S. A. Karim, J. A. Frohlich, A. C. Grobler, C. Baxter, and others. 2010. "Effectiveness and Safety of Tenofovir Gel, an Antiretroviral Microbicide, for the Prevention of HIV Infection in Women." *Science* 329 (5996): 1168–74.

Katz, I. T., and A. A. Wright. 2008. "Circumcision: A Surgical Strategy for HIV Prevention in Africa." *New England Journal of Medicine* 359 (23): 2412–15.

Kaul, R., J. Kimani, N. J. Nagelkerke, K. Fonck, E. N. Ngugi, and others. 2004. "Monthly Antibiotic Chemoprophylaxis and Incidence of Sexually Transmitted Infections and HIV-1 Infection in Kenyan Sex Workers: A Randomized Controlled Trial." *Journal of the American Medical Association* 291 (21): 2555–62.

Kault, D. A. 1992. "Modelling the Effects of AIDS on Gonorrhea Epidemiology." *Mathematical and Computer Modelling* 16 (11): 3–14.

Kenyon, C. R., K. Osbak, J. Buyze, and R. M. Chico. 2014. "The Changing Relationship between Bacterial STIs and HIV Prevalence in South Africa: An Ecological Study." *International Journal of STD and AIDS* 26 (8).

Kenyon, C. R., K. Osbak, and R. M. Chico. 2014. "What Underpins the Decline in Syphilis in Southern and Eastern Africa? An Exploratory Ecological Analysis." *International Journal of Infectious Diseases* 29: 54–61.

Kerrigan, D., L. Moreno, S. Rosario, B. Gomez, H. Jerez, and others. 2006. "Environmental-Structural Interventions to Reduce HIV/STI Risk among Female Sex Workers in the Dominican Republic." *American Journal of Public Health* 96 (1): 120–25.

Kippax, S., and N. Stephenson. 2012. "Beyond the Distinction between Biomedical and Social Dimensions of HIV Prevention through the Lens of a Social Public Health." *American Journal of Public Health* 102 (5): 789–99.

Korenromp, E. L., V. C. Van, H. Grosskurth, A. Gavyole, C. P. Van der Ploeg, and others. 2000. "Model-Based Evaluation of Single-Round Mass Treatment of Sexually Transmitted Diseases for HIV Control in a Rural African Population." *AIDS* 14 (5): 573–93.

Labbe, A. C., J. Pepin, N. Khonde, A. Dzokoto, H. Meda, and others. 2012. "Periodical Antibiotic Treatment for the Control of Gonococcal and Chlamydial Infections among Sex Workers in Benin and Ghana: A Cluster-Randomized Placebo-Controlled Trial." *Sexually Transmitted Diseases* 39 (4): 253–59.

Lafort, Y., D. Geelhoed, L. Cumba, C. Lazaro, W. Delva, and others. 2010. "Reproductive Health Services for Populations at High Risk of HIV: Performance of a Night Clinic in Tete Province, Mozambique." *BMC Health Services Research* 10: 144.

Lahra, M. M., Y. R. Lo, and D. M. Whiley. 2013. "Gonococcal Antimicrobial Resistance in the Western Pacific Region." *Sexually Transmitted Infections* 89 (Suppl 4): iv19–23.

Lan, P., H. Phuc, N. Hoa, N. Chuc, and C. Lundborg. 2014. "Improved Knowledge and Reported Practice Regarding Sexually Transmitted Infections among Healthcare Providers in Rural Vietnam: A Cluster-Randomised Controlled Educational Intervention." *BMC Infectious Diseases* 14: 646.

La Ruche, G., F. Lorougnon, and N. Digbeu. 1995. "Therapeutic Algorithms for the Management of Sexually Transmitted Diseases at the Peripheral Level in Côte d'Ivoire: Assessment of Efficacy and Cost." *Bulletin of the World Health Organization* 73 (3): 305–13.

Leichliter, J. S., H. W. Chesson, M. Sternberg, and S. O. Aral. 2010. "The Concentration of Sexual Behaviours in the USA: A Closer Examination of Subpopulations." *Sexually Transmitted Infections* 86 (Suppl 3): iii45–51.

Levin, C. E., M. Sharma, Z. Olson, S. Verguet, J. F. Shi, and others. 2015. "An Extended Cost-Effectiveness Analysis of Publicly Financed HPV Vaccination to Prevent Cervical Cancer in China." In *Disease Control Priorities* (third edition): Volume 3, *Cancer*, edited by H. Gelband, P. Jha, R. Sankaranarayanan, and S. Horton. Washington, DC: World Bank.

Low, N., N. Broutet, Y. Adu-Sarkodie, P. Barton, M. Hossain, and S. Hawkes. 2006. "Global Control of Sexually Transmitted Infections." *The Lancet* 368 (9551): 1–16.

Luchters, S., M. F. Chersich, A. Rinyiru, M. S. Barasa, N. King'ola, and others. 2008. "Impact of Five Years of Peer-Mediated Interventions on Sexual Behavior and Sexually Transmitted Infections among Female Sex Workers in Mombasa, Kenya." *BMC Public Health* 8: 143.

Mabey, D. 2009. "Azithromycin Resistance in *Treponema pallidum*." *Sexually Transmitted Diseases* 36 (12): 777–78.

Mainkar, M. M., D. B. Pardeshi, J. Dale, S. Deshpande, S. Khazi, and others. 2011. "Targeted Interventions of the Avahan Program and Their Association with Intermediate Outcomes among Female Sex Workers in Maharashtra, India." *BMC Public Health* 11 (Suppl 6): S2.

Makasa, M., A. Buve, and I. F. Sandøy. 2012. "Etiologic Pattern of Genital Ulcers in Lusaka, Zambia: Has Chancroid Been Eliminated?" *Sexually Transmitted Diseases* 39 (10): 787–91.

Malagon, T., M. Drolet, M. C. Boily, E. L. Franco, M. Jit, and others. 2012. "Cross-Protective Efficacy of Two Human Papillomavirus Vaccines: A Systematic Review and Meta-Analysis." *The Lancet Infectious Diseases* 12 (10): 781–89.

Manhart, L. E., and K. K. Holmes. 2005. "Randomized Controlled Trials of Individual-Level, Population-Level, and Multilevel Interventions for Preventing Sexually Transmitted Infections: What Has Worked?" *Journal of Infectious Diseases* 191 (Suppl 1): S7–24.

Markowitz, L. E., E. F. Dunne, M. Saraiya, H. W. Chesson, C. R. Curtis, and others. 2014. "Human Papillomavirus Vaccination: Recommendations of the Advisory Committee on Immunization Practices (ACIP)." *Morbidity and Mortality Weekly Report. Recommendations and Reports* 63 (RR-05): 1–30.

Markowitz, L. E., S. Hariri, C. Lin, E. F. Dunne, M. Steinau, and others. 2013. "Reduction in Human Papillomavirus (HPV) Prevalence among Young Women Following HPV Vaccine Introduction in the United States, National Health and Nutrition Examination Surveys, 2003–2010." *Journal of Infectious Diseases* 208 (3): 385–93.

Marrazzo, J. M., G. Ramjee, B. A. Richardson, K. Gomez, N. Mgodi, and others. 2015. "Tenofovir-Based Preexposure Prophylaxis for HIV Infection among African Women." *New England Journal of Medicine* 372 (6): 509–18.

Marseille, E., J. G. Kahn, K. Billinghurst, and J. Saba. 2001. "Cost-Effectiveness of the Female Condom in Preventing HIV and STDs in Commercial Sex Workers in Rural South Africa." *Social Science and Medicine* 52 (1): 135–48.

Matthews, J. E., R. Stephenson, and P. S. Sullivan. 2012. "Factors Associated with Self-Reported HBV Vaccination among HIV-Negative MSM Participating in an Online Sexual Health Survey: A Cross-Sectional Study." *PLoS One* 7 (2): e30609.

Mayaud, P., and D. Mabey. 2004. "Approaches to the Control of Sexually Transmitted Infections in Developing Countries: Old Problems and Modern Challenges." *Sexually Transmitted Infections* 80 (3): 174–82.

Mayaud, P., F. Mosha, J. Todd, R. Balira, J. Mgara, and others. 1997. "Improved Treatment Services Significantly Reduce the Prevalence of Sexually Transmitted Diseases in Rural Tanzania: Results of a Randomized Controlled Trial." *AIDS* 11 (15): 1873–80.

McClelland, R. S., J. E. Balkus, J. Lee, O. Anzala, J. Kimani, and others. 2015. "Randomized Trial of Periodic Presumptive Treatment with High-Dose Intravaginal Metronidazole and Miconazole to Prevent Vaginal Infections in HIV-Negative Women." *Journal of Infectious Diseases* 211 (12): 1875–82.

McCormick, D. F., M. Rahman, S. Zadrozny, A. Alam, L. Ashraf, and others. 2013. "Prevention and Control of Sexually Transmissible Infections among Hotel-Based Female Sex Workers in Dhaka, Bangladesh." *Sexual Health* 10 (6): 478–86.

McCoy, S. I., R. A. Kangwende, and N. S. Padian. 2010. "Behavior Change Interventions to Prevent HIV Infection among Women Living in Low and Middle Income Countries: A Systematic Review." *AIDS and Behavior* 14 (3): 469–82.

Mehta, S. D., C. Gaydos, I. Maclean, E. Odoyo-June, S. Moses, and others. 2012. "The Effect of Medical Male Circumcision on Urogenital Mycoplasma Genitalium among Men in Kisumu, Kenya." *Sexually Transmitted Diseases* 39 (4): 276–80.

Mehta, S. D., S. Moses, K. Agot, C. Parker, J. O. Ndinya-Achola, and others. 2009. "Adult Male Circumcision Does Not Reduce the Risk of Incident *Neisseria gonorrhoeae*, *Chlamydia trachomatis*, or *Trichomonas vaginalis* Infection: Results from a Randomized, Controlled Trial in Kenya." *Journal of Infectious Diseases* 200 (3): 370–78.

Mercer, C. H., C. Tanton, P. Prah, B. Erens, P. Sonnenberg, and others. 2013. "Changes in Sexual Attitudes and Lifestyles in Britain through the Life Course and over Time: Findings from the National Surveys of Sexual Attitudes and Lifestyles (Natsal)." *The Lancet* 382 (9907): 1781–94.

Mills, A. 2014. "Health Care Systems in Low- and Middle-Income Countries." *New England Journal of Medicine* 370 (6): 552–57.

Moreno, R., H. Y. Nababan, E. Ota, W. M. Wariki, S. Ezoe, and others. 2014. "Structural and Community-Level Interventions for Increasing Condom Use to Prevent the Transmission of HIV and Other Sexually Transmitted Infections." *Cochrane Database of Systematic Reviews* 7: CD003363.

Moses, S., E. N. Ngugi, J. E. Bradley, E. K. Njeru, G. Eldridge, and others. 1994. "Health Care–Seeking Behavior Related to the Transmission of Sexually Transmitted Diseases in Kenya." *American Journal of Public Health* 84 (12): 1947–51.

Moses, S., E. N. Ngugi, A. Costigan, C. Kariuki, I. Maclean, and others. 2002. "Response of a Sexually Transmitted Infection Epidemic to a Treatment and Prevention Programme in Nairobi, Kenya." *Sexually Transmitted Infections* 78 (Suppl 1): i114.

Moyo, W., Z. M. Chirenje, J. Mandel, S. K. Schwarcz, J. Klausner, and others. 2002. "Impact of a Single Session of Counseling on Partner Referral for Sexually Transmitted Disease Treatment, Harare, Zimbabwe." *AIDS and Behavior* 6 (3): 237–43.

Muñoz, N., R. Manalastas Jr., P. Pitisuttithum, D. Tresukosol, J. Monsonego, and others. 2009. "Safety, Immunogenicity, and Efficacy of Quadrivalent Human Papillomavirus (Types 6, 11, 16, 18) Recombinant Vaccine in Women Aged 24–45 Years: A Randomised, Double-Blind Trial." *The Lancet* 373 (9679): 1949–57.

Nam, S. L., and K. Blanchet. 2014. "We Mustn't Forget Other Essential Health Services during the Ebola Crisis." *British Medical Journal* 349: g6837.

Natunen, K., T. A. Lehtinen, S. Torvinen, and M. Lehtinen. 2013. "Cost-Effectiveness of HPV-Vaccination in Medium or Low Income Countries with High Cervical Cancer Incidence—A Systematic Review." *Journal of Vaccines and Vaccination* 4: 172.

Ndowa, F. J., J. M. Francis, A. Machiha, H. Faye-Kette, and M. C. Fonkoua. 2013. "Gonococcal Antimicrobial Resistance: Perspectives from the African Region." *Sexually Transmitted Infections* 89 (Suppl 4): iv11–15.

Newman, L., M. Kamb, S. Hawkes, G. Gomez, L. Say, and others. 2013. "Global Estimates of Syphilis in Pregnancy and Associated Adverse Outcomes: Analysis of Multinational Antenatal Surveillance Data." *PLoS Medicine* 10: e1001396.

Nuwaha, F., F. Kambugu, P. S. Nsubuga, B. Hojer, and E. Faxelid. 2001. "Efficacy of Patient-Delivered Partner Medication in the Treatment of Sexual Partners in Uganda." *Sexually Transmitted Diseases* 28 (2): 105–10.

O'Farrell, N., R. Oula, L. Morison, and C. T. Van. 2006. "Periodic Presumptive Treatment for Cervical Infections in Service Women in 3 Border Provinces of Laos." *Sexually Transmitted Diseases* 33 (9): 558–64.

Over, A. M., and S. O. Aral. 2006. "The Economics of Sexually Transmitted Infections." *Sexually Transmitted Diseases* 33 (10): S79–83.

Owusu-Edusei, K., Jr., H. W. Chesson, T. L. Gift, G. Tao, R. Mahajan, and others. 2013. "The Estimated Direct Medical Cost of Selected Sexually Transmitted Infections in the United States, 2008." *Sexually Transmitted Diseases* 40 (3): 197–201.

Owusu-Edusei, K., Jr., H. W. Chesson, J. S. Leichliter, C. K. Kent, and S. O. Aral. 2013. "The Association between Racial Disparity in Income and Reported Sexually Transmitted Infections." *American Journal of Public Health* 103 (5): 910–16.

Owusu-Edusei, K., Jr., T. L. Gift, and R. C. Ballard. 2011. "Cost-Effectiveness of a Dual Non-Treponemal/Treponemal Syphilis Point-of-Care Test to Prevent Adverse Pregnancy

Outcomes in Sub-Saharan Africa." *Sexually Transmitted Diseases* 38 (11): 997–1003.

Paavonen, J., P. Naud, J. Salmeron, C. M. Wheeler, S. N. Chow, and others. 2009. "Efficacy of Human Papillomavirus (HPV)-16/18 AS04-Adjuvanted Vaccine against Cervical Infection and Precancer Caused by Oncogenic HPV Types (PATRICIA): Final Analysis of a Double-Blind, Randomised Study in Young Women." *The Lancet* 374 (9686): 301–14.

Palefsky, J. M., A. R. Giuliano, S. Goldstone, E. D. Moreira Jr., C. Aranda, and others. 2011. "HPV Vaccine against Anal HPV Infection and Anal Intraepithelial Neoplasia." *New England Journal of Medicine* 365 (17): 1576–85.

Parkhurst, J. O. 2014. "Structural Approaches for Prevention of Sexually Transmitted HIV in General Populations: Definitions and an Operational Approach." *Journal of the International AIDS Society* 17: 19052.

Patterson, T. L., B. Mausbach, R. Lozada, H. Staines-Orozco, S. J. Semple, and others. 2008. "Efficacy of a Brief Behavioral Intervention to Promote Condom Use among Female Sex Workers in Tijuana and Ciudad Juarez, Mexico." *American Journal of Public Health* 98 (11): 2051–57.

Peterman, T. A., and B. W. Furness. 2015. "Public Health Interventions to Control Syphilis." *Sexual Health* 12 (2): 126–34.

Pettifor, A., J. Walsh, V. Wilkins, and P. Raghunathan. 2000. "How Effective Is Syndromic Management of STDs? A Review of Current Studies." *Sexually Transmitted Diseases* 27 (7): 371–85.

Pourbohloul, B., M. L. Rekart, and R. C. Brunham. 2003. "Impact of Mass Treatment on Syphilis Transmission: A Mathematical Modeling Approach." *Sexually Transmitted Diseases* 30 (4): 297–305.

Pretorius, C., J. Stover, L. Bollinger, N. Bacaer, and B. Williams. 2010. "Evaluating the Cost-Effectiveness of Pre-Exposure Prophylaxis (PrEP) and Its Impact on HIV-1 Transmission in South Africa." *PLoS One* 5: e13646.

Price, M. A., D. Zimba, I. F. Hoffman, S. C. Kaydos-Daniels, W. C. Miller, and others. 2003. "Addition of Treatment for Trichomoniasis to Syndromic Management of Urethritis in Malawi: A Randomized Clinical Trial." *Sexually Transmitted Diseases* 30 (6): 516–22.

Punpanich, W., K. Ungchusak, and R. Detels. 2004. "Thailand's Response to the HIV Epidemic: Yesterday, Today, and Tomorrow." *AIDS Education and Prevention* 16 (Suppl 3A): 119–36.

Ramjee, G., A. van der Straten, T. Chipato, G. de Bruyn, K. Blanchard, and others. 2008. "The Diaphragm and Lubricant Gel for Prevention of Cervical Sexually Transmitted Infections: Results of a Randomized Controlled Trial." *PLoS One* 3 (10): e3488.

Rees, H., S. Delany-Moretlwe, D. Baron, C. Lombard, G. Gray, and others. 2015. "FACTS 001 Phase III Trial of Pericoital Tenofovir 1% Gel for HIV Prevention in Women." Paper presented at the Conference on Retroviruses and Opportunistic Infections (Abstract 26LB), Seattle, WA, February 23–26.

Rekart, M. L., D. M. Patrick, B. Chakraborty, J. J. Maginley, H. D. Jones, and others. 2003. "Targeted Mass Treatment for

Syphilis with Oral Azithromycin." *The Lancet* 361 (9354): 313–14.

Richardson, B. A., L. Lavreys, H. L. Martin Jr., C. E. Stevens, E. Ngugi, and others. 2001. "Evaluation of a Low-Dose Nonoxynol-9 Gel for the Prevention of Sexually Transmitted Diseases: A Randomized Clinical Trial." *Sexually Transmitted Diseases* 28 (7): 394–400.

Roddy, R. E., L. Zekeng, K. A. Ryan, U. Tamoufe, and K. G. Tweedy. 2002. "Effect of Nonoxynol-9 Gel on Urogenital Gonorrhea and Chlamydial Infection: A Randomized Controlled Trial." *Journal of the American Medical Association* 287 (9): 1117–22.

Rutstein, S. E., L. B. Brown, A. K. Biddle, S. B. Wheeler, G. Kamanga, and others. 2014. "Cost-Effectiveness of Provider-Based HIV Partner Notification in Urban Malawi." *Health Policy and Planning* 29 (1): 115–26.

Ryan, C. A., M. Kamb, and K. K. Holmes. 2008. "STI Care Management." In *Sexually Transmitted Diseases*, edited by K. K. Holmes, P. F. Sparling, W. E. Stamm, P. Piot, J. N. Wasserheit, and others, 855–75. New York: McGraw-Hill.

Rydzak, C. E., and S. J. Goldie. 2008. "Cost-Effectiveness of Rapid Point-of-Care Prenatal Syphilis Screening in Sub-Saharan Africa." *Sexually Transmitted Diseases* 35 (9): 775–84.

Sahin-Hodoglugil, N. N., R. Woods, A. Pettifor, and J. Walsh. 2003. "A Comparison of Cost-Effectiveness of Three Protocols for Diagnosis and Treatment of Gonococcal and Chlamydial Infections in Women in Africa." *Sexually Transmitted Diseases* 30 (5): 455–69.

Schmid, G. 2004. "Economic and Programmatic Aspects of Congenital Syphilis Prevention." *Bulletin of the World Health Organization* 82 (6): 402–9.

Sen, A., and M. Luong. 2008. "Estimating the Impact of Beer Prices on the Incidence of Sexually Transmitted Diseases: Cross-Province and Time Series Evidence from Canada." *Contemporary Economic Policy* 26 (4): 505–17.

Shah, S. A., S. Kristensen, M. A. Memon, H. L. White, and S. H. Vermund. 2007. "Syndromic Management Training for Non-Formal Care Providers in Pakistan Improves Quality of Care for Sexually Transmitted Diseases (STD) Care: A Randomized Clinical Trial." *South-East Asian Journal of Tropical Medicine and Public Health* 38 (4): 737–48.

Sobngwi-Tambekou, J., D. Taljaard, M. Nieuwoudt, P. Lissouba, A. Puren, and others. 2009. "Male Circumcision and *Neisseria gonorrhoeae*, *Chlamydia trachomatis*, and *Trichomonas vaginalis*: Observations after a Randomised Controlled Trial for HIV Prevention." *Sexually Transmitted Infections* 85 (2): 116–20.

Spinola, S. M. 2008. "Chancroid and *Haemophilus ducreyi*." In *Sexually Transmitted Diseases*, edited by K. K. Holmes, P. F. Sparling, W. E. Stamm, P. Piot, J. N. Wasserheit, and others, 689–99. New York: McGraw-Hill.

Stanberry, L. R., S. L. Spruance, A. L. Cunningham, D. I. Bernstein, A. Mindel, and others. 2002. "Glycoprotein-D–Adjuvant Vaccine to Prevent Genital Herpes." *New England Journal of Medicine* 347 (21): 1652–61.

Staras, S. A., M. D. Livingston, A. M. Christou, D. H. Jernigan, and A. C. Wagenaar. 2014. "Heterogeneous Population Effects of an Alcohol Excise Tax Increase on Sexually Transmitted Infections Morbidity." *Addiction* 109 (6): 904–12.

Steen, R. 2001. "Eradicating Chancroid." *Bulletin of the World Health Organization* 79 (9): 818–26.

Steen, R., M. Chersich, and S. J. de Vlas. 2012. "Periodic Presumptive Treatment of Curable Sexually Transmitted Infections among Sex Workers: Recent Experience with Implementation." *Current Opinion in Infectious Diseases* 25 (1): 100–6.

Steen, R., B. Vuylsteke, T. DeCoito, S. Ralepeli, G. Fehler, and others. 2000. "Evidence of Declining STD Prevalence in a South African Mining Community Following a Core-Group Intervention." *Sexually Transmitted Diseases* 27 (1): 1–8.

Stevenson, B., and J. Wolfers. 2007. "Marriage and Divorce: Changes and Their Driving Forces." Working Paper 1294, National Bureau of Economic Research, Cambridge, MA. http://www.nber.org/papers/w12944.

Stolte, I. G., N. H. Dukers, R. B. Geskus, R. A. Coutinho, and J. B. de Wit. 2004. "Homosexual Men Change to Risky Sex When Perceiving Less Threat of HIV/AIDS since Availability of Highly Active Antiretroviral Therapy: A Longitudinal Study." *AIDS* 18 (2): 303–9.

Subramanian, T., L. Ramakrishnan, S. Aridoss, P. Goswami, B. Kanguswami, and others. 2013. "Increasing Condom Use and Declining STI Prevalence in High-Risk MSM and TGs: Evaluation of a Large-Scale Prevention Program in Tamil Nadu, India." *BMC Public Health* 13: 857.

Sweat, M., D. Kerrigan, L. Moreno, S. Rosario, B. Gomez, and others. 2006. "Cost-Effectiveness of Environmental-Structural Communication Interventions for HIV Prevention in the Female Sex Industry in the Dominican Republic." *Journal of Health Communication* 11 (Suppl 2): 123–42.

Tabrizi, S. N., J. M. Brotherton, J. M. Kaldor, S. R. Skinner, E. Cummins, and others. 2012. "Fall in Human Papillomavirus Prevalence Following a National Vaccination Program." *Journal of Infectious Diseases* 206 (11): 1645–51.

Tanser, F., T. Bärnighausen, G. S. Cooke, and M. L. Newell. 2009. "Localized Spatial Clustering of HIV Infections in a Widely Disseminated Rural South African Epidemic." *International Journal of Epidemiology* 38 (4): 1008–16.

Terris-Prestholt, F., A. M. Foss, A. P. Cox, L. Heise, G. Meyer-Rath, and others. 2014. "Cost-Effectiveness of Tenofovir Gel in Urban South Africa: Model Projections of HIV Impact and Threshold Product Prices." *BMC Infectious Diseases* 14: 14.

Terris-Prestholt, F., S. Vyas, L. Kumaranayake, P. Mayaud, and C. Watts. 2006. "The Costs of Treating Curable Sexually Transmitted Infections in Low- and Middle-Income Countries: A Systematic Review." *Sexually Transmitted Diseases* 33 (10): S153–66.

Terris-Prestholt, F., D. Watson-Jones, K. Mugeye, L. Kumaranayake, L. Ndeki, and others. 2003. "Is Antenatal Syphilis Screening Still Cost-Effective in Sub-Saharan Africa." *Sexually Transmitted Infections* 79 (5): 375–81.

Thigpen, M. C., P. M. Kebaabetswe, L. A. Paxton, D. K. Smith, C. E. Rose, and others. 2012. "Antiretroviral Preexposure Prophylaxis for Heterosexual HIV Transmission in Botswana." *New England Journal of Medicine* 367 (5): 423–34.

Thomas, J. C., and M. E. Gaffield. 2003. "Social Structure, Race, and Gonorrhea Rates in the Southeastern United States." *Ethnicity and Disease* 13 (3): 362–68.

Tobian, A. A., D. Serwadda, T. C. Quinn, G. Kigozi, P. E. Gravitt, and others. 2009. "Male Circumcision for the Prevention of HSV-2 and HPV Infections and Syphilis." *New England Journal of Medicine* 360 (13): 1298–309.

Townsend, L., C. Mathews, and Y. Zembe. 2013. "A Systematic Review of Behavioral Interventions to Prevent HIV Infection and Transmission among Heterosexual, Adult Men in Low- and Middle-Income Countries." *Prevention Science* 14 (1): 88–105.

Uthman, O. A., T. A. Popoola, M. M. B. Uthman, and O. Aremu. 2010. "Economic Evaluations of Adult Male Circumcision for Prevention of Heterosexual Acquisition of HIV in Men in Sub-Saharan Africa: A Systematic Review." *PLoS One* 5 (3): e9628.

van Dam, C. J. 1995. "HIV, STD, and Their Current Impact on Reproductive Health: The Need for Control of Sexually Transmitted Diseases." *International Journal of Gynecology and Obstetrics* 50 (Suppl 2): S121–29.

van Dam, C. J., G. Dallabetta, and P. Piot. 1999. "Prevention and Control of Sexually Transmitted Diseases in Developing Countries." In *Sexually Transmitted Diseases*, edited by K. K. Holmes, P. F. Sparling, P. Mardh, S. M. Lemon, W. E. Stamm, and others, 1381–90. New York: McGraw-Hill.

Verguet, S., and J. A. Walsh. 2010. "Vaginal Microbicides Save Money: A Model of Cost-Effectiveness in South Africa and the USA." *Sexually Transmitted Infections* 86 (3): 212–16.

Vickerman, P., A. Devine, A. M. Foss, S. Delany-Moretlwe, P. Mayaud, and others. 2011. "The Cost-Effectiveness of Herpes Simplex Virus-2 Suppressive Therapy with Daily Aciclovir for Delaying HIV Disease Progression among HIV-1-Infected Women in South Africa." *Sexually Transmitted Diseases* 38 (5): 401–09.

Vickerman, P., F. Ndowa, and P. Mayaud. 2008. "Modelling the Cost per Ulcer Treated of Incorporating Episodic Treatment for HSV-2 into the Syndromic Algorithm for Genital Ulcer Disease." *Sexually Transmitted Infections* 84 (3): 243–48.

Villa, L. L., K. A. Ault, A. R. Giuliano, R. L. Costa, C. A. Petta, and others. 2006. "Immunologic Responses Following Administration of a Vaccine Targeting Human Papillomavirus Types 6, 11, 16, and 18." *Vaccine* 24 (27–28): 5571–83.

Wang, C., Y. Wang, X. Huang, X. Li, T. Zhang, and others. 2012. "Prevalence and Factors Associated with Hepatitis B Immunization and Infection among Men Who Have Sex with Men in Beijing, China." *PLoS One* 7 (10): e48219.

Ward, H., and S. O. Aral. 2006. "Globalisation, the Sex Industry, and Health." *Sexually Transmitted Infections* 82 (5): 345–47.

Watson-Jones, D., J. Changalucha, B. Gumodoka, H. Weiss, M. Rusizoka, and others. 2002. "Syphilis in Pregnancy in Tanzania. I. Impact of Maternal Syphilis on Outcome of Pregnancy." *Journal of Infectious Diseases* 186 (7): 940–47.

Weir, S. S., C. Pailman, X. Mahlalela, N. Coetzee, F. Meidany, and others. 2003. "From People to Places: Focusing AIDS Prevention Efforts Where It Matters Most." *AIDS* 17 (6): 895–903.

Wetmore, C. M., L. E. Manhart, and J. N. Wasserheit. 2010. "Randomized Controlled Trials of Interventions to Prevent Sexually Transmitted Infections: Learning from the Past to Plan for the Future." *Epidemiologic Reviews* 32 (1): 121–36.

White, R. G., K. K. Orroth, J. R. Glynn, E. E. Freeman, R. Bakker, and others. 2008. "Treating Curable Sexually Transmitted Infections to Prevent HIV in Africa: Still an Effective Control Strategy?" *Journal of Acquired Immune Deficiency Syndromes* 47 (3): 346–53.

WHO (World Health Organization). 2003. *Guidelines for the Management of Sexually Transmitted Infections.* Geneva: WHO.

————. 2008. *Periodic Presumptive Treatment for Sexually Transmitted Infections: Experience from the Field and Recommendations for Research.* Geneva: WHO.

————. 2010. *More Developing Countries Show Universal Access to HIV/AIDS Services Is Possible: Sustained Commitments Necessary to Secure Future Progress.* Geneva: WHO.

————. 2012a. *Global Incidence and Prevalence of Selected Curable Sexually Transmitted Infections: 2008.* Geneva: WHO.

————. 2012b. *Investment Case for Eliminating Mother-to-Child Transmission of Syphilis: Promoting Better Maternal and Child Health and Stronger Health Systems.* Geneva: WHO.

World Bank. 2007. "Sexually Transmitted Infections in Developing Countries." *Public Health at a Glance.* Washington, DC: World Bank. http://web.worldbank.org/archive /website01213/WEB/0__CO-54.HTM.

Chapter 11

Tuberculosis

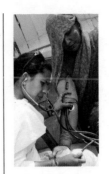

Barry R. Bloom, Rifat Atun, Ted Cohen, Christopher Dye,
Hamish Fraser, Gabriela B. Gomez, Gwen Knight,
Megan Murray, Edward Nardell, Eric Rubin,
Joshua Salomon, Anna Vassall, Grigory Volchenkov,
Richard White, Douglas Wilson, and Prashant Yadav

OVERVIEW

Despite 90 years of vaccination and 60 years of chemotherapy, tuberculosis (TB) remains the world's leading cause of death from an infectious agent, exceeding human immunodeficiency virus/acquired immune deficiency syndrome (HIV/AIDS) for the first time (WHO 2015b, 2016a). The World Health Organization (WHO) estimates that there are about 10.4 million new cases and 1.8 million deaths from TB each year. One-third of these new cases (about 3 million) remain unknown to the health system, and many are not receiving proper treatment.

Tuberculosis is an infectious bacterial disease caused by *Mycobacterium tuberculosis* (Mtb), which is transmitted between humans through the respiratory route and most commonly affects the lungs, but can damage any tissue. Only about 10 percent of individuals infected with Mtb progress to active TB disease within their lifetime; the remainder of persons infected successfully contain their infection. One of the challenges of TB is that the pathogen persists in many infected individuals in a latent state for many years and can be reactivated to cause disease. The risk of progression to TB disease after infection is highest soon after the initial infection and increases dramatically for persons co-infected with HIV/AIDS or other immune-compromising conditions.

Treatment of TB disease requires multiple drugs for many months. These long drug regimens are challenging for both patients and health care systems, especially in low- and middle-income countries (LMICs), where the disease burden often far outstrips local resources. In some areas, the incidence of drug-resistant TB, requiring even longer treatment regimens with drugs that are more expensive and difficult to tolerate, is increasing.

Diagnosis in LMICs is made primarily by microscopic examination of stained smears of sputum of suspected patients; however, smear microscopy is capable of detecting only 50–60 percent of all cases (smear-positive). More sensitive methods of diagnosing TB and detecting resistance to drugs have recently become available, although they are more expensive. The time between the onset of disease and when diagnosis is made and treatment is initiated is often protracted, and such delays allow the transmission of disease. Although bacille Calmette–Guérin (BCG) remains the world's most widely used vaccine, its effectiveness is geographically highly variable and incomplete. Modeling suggests that more effective vaccines will likely be needed to drive tuberculosis toward elimination in high-incidence settings.

The basic strategy to combat TB has been, for 40 years, to provide diagnosis and treatment to individuals

Corresponding author: Barry R. Bloom, Harvard T. H. Chan School of Public Health, Boston, Massachusetts, United States; bbloom@hsph.harvard.edu.

who are ill and who seek care at a health facility. The premise is that, if patients with active disease are cured, mortality will disappear, prevalence of disease will decline, transmission will decline, and therefore incidence should decline. The reality in many countries is more complex, and overall the decline in incidence (only about 1.5 percent per year) has been unacceptably slow.

Chemotherapy for TB is one of the most cost-effective of all health interventions (McKee and Atun 2006). This evidence has been central to the global promotion of the WHO and Stop TB Partnership policy of directly observed therapy, short course (DOTS) strategy, the package of measures combining best practices in the diagnosis and care of patients with TB (UN General Assembly 2000). The DOTS strategy to control tuberculosis promotes standardized treatment, with supervision and patient support that may include, but is far broader than, direct observation of therapy (DOT), where a health care worker personally observes the patient taking the medication (WHO 2013a).

Thanks in part to these efforts and national and international investments, much progress has been made in TB control over the past several decades. Between 1990 and 2010, absolute global mortality from TB declined 18.7 percent, from 1.47 million to 1.20 million (Lozano and others 2012) and by 22 percent between 2000 and 2015 (WHO 2016a). By 2015, an estimated 49 million lives had been saved (WHO 2016a). The internationally agreed targets for TB, embraced in the United Nations (UN) Millennium Development Goals (MDGs), sought "to halt and reverse the expanding incidence of tuberculosis by 2015," and this target has been met to some extent in all six WHO regions and in most, but not all, of the world's 22 high-burden countries (WHO 2014c).

Despite progress, major gaps persist. Although the Sustainable Development Goals (SDGs) seek to end the tuberculosis epidemic altogether (WHO 2015a, 2015c), the decline in incidence has been disappointing. One of every three TB patients remains "unknown to the health system," many are undiagnosed and untreated, and case detection and treatment success rates remain too low in the high-burden countries. Ominously, rates of multidrug-resistant (MDR) TB—defined as resistance to the two major TB drugs, isoniazid and rifampicin—are rising globally (WHO 2011a) with the emergence of extensively drug-resistant (XDR) TB, resistant to many second-line drugs, as well as strains resistant to all current drugs (Dheda and others 2014; Udwadia and others 2012; Uplekar and others 2015). These are now primarily the result of transmission rather than inadequate treatment (Shah and others 2017).

Moreover, the TB problem has become more pressing because of co-infection with HIV/AIDS. While globally HIV/AIDS and TB co-infection represents only 11 percent of the total TB burden, in some areas of Sub-Saharan Africa with a high burden of TB, as many as three-quarters of TB patients are co-infected with HIV/AIDS. In those countries, efforts to control TB are overwhelmed by the rising number of TB cases occurring in parallel with the HIV/AIDS epidemic. And after decades of steady decline, the incidence of TB is also increasing in some high-income countries (HICs), mainly as the result of outbreaks in vulnerable groups (WHO 2015b).

If the ultimate goal of controlling an infectious disease is to interrupt transmission, turning the tide on TB will require early and accurate case detection, rapid commencement of and adherence to effective treatment that prevents transmission, and, where possible, preventive treatment of latent TB. It is universally understood that new strategies and more effective tools and interventions will be required to reach post-2015 targets (Bloom and Atun 2016; WHO 2015a). These interventions must be not only cost-effective, but also affordable and capable of having an impact on a very large scale.

TB control will need three new advances—development of new point-of-care diagnostics, more effective drug regimens to combat drug-susceptible and drug-resistant TB, and more effective vaccines. As argued in this chapter, these require new strategies and tools that include moving away from the traditional DOTS passive case finding and toward more active case finding in high-burden regions; service delivery that is targeted to the most vulnerable populations and integrated with other services, especially HIV/AIDS services; and care that is based at the primary health care and community levels. Specifically, in high-burden countries, many individuals with TB are asymptomatic, such that waiting for patients to become sick enough to seek care has not been sufficient to reduce transmission and incidence markedly (Bates and others 2012; Mao and others 2014; Willingham and others 2001; Wood and others 2007). A more active and aggressive approach is needed that tackles health system barriers to effective TB control.

The strategies for controlling TB recommended by the WHO have evolved significantly over time. In the early formulations, the central tenets of the global TB control strategy were clinical and programmatic in nature, focusing principally on the delivery of standardized drug regimens; the underlying assumption was that the problem could be solved largely by existing biomedical tools (Atun, McKee, and others 2005; Schouten and others 2011).

Yet, in many LMICs, health system weaknesses in governance, financing, health workforce, procurement and supply chain management, and information systems have impeded TB control (Elzinga, Raviglione, and Maher 2004; Marais and others 2010; Travis and others 2004) and not been adequately addressed by TB control efforts. The current global TB strategy, formulated as the End TB Strategy, is the most comprehensive ever, with three major pillars:

- Integrated, patient-centered care and prevention
- Social and political action to address determinants of disease
- Recognition of the urgent need for research to provide new tools (WHO 2015a).

Health systems are important and need to be strengthened. As with other health interventions, the success of tuberculosis treatment and control in a country is often determined by the strength of its health system (McKee and Atun 2006; WHO 2003). A health system can be defined in many ways, perhaps best as "all the activities whose primary purpose is to promote, restore, or maintain health" (WHO 2000, 5).

In a sense, the major risk factor for acquiring TB is breathing. Thus, people of all social and economic statuses are at risk. While TB disproportionately affects the poor, the narrative that TB is a disease only of the poor is misleading and counterproductive, if it leads either to further stigmatization of the disease or to the view that middle- and high-income countries need not worry about the disease. In the case of co-infection with HIV/AIDS, evidence suggests that HIV/AIDS is often more prevalent in better-off populations in Africa that suffer high rates of TB.

The analytical framework underlying this chapter defines key functions of the health system, ultimate goals, and contextual factors that affect the health system (figure 11.1). It builds on the WHO framework (WHO 2000) as well as health system frameworks developed by Frenk (1994), Hsiao and Heller (2007), and Roberts and others (2004), and national accounts (OECD, Eurostat, and WHO 2011). It also draws on earlier studies by Atun (2012); Atun and Coker (2008); Atun, Samyshkin, and others (2006); Samb and others (2009); and Swanson and others (2012).

Figure 11.1 Schematic Health Systems Framework

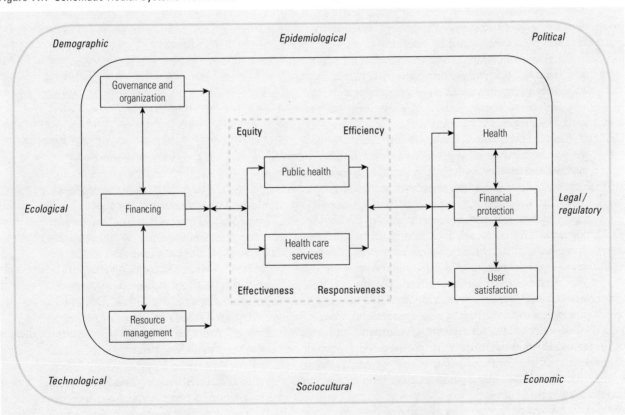

The four key health system functions represented in the framework are as follows:

- *Governance and organization.* The policy and regulatory environment; stewardship and regulatory functions of the ministry of health and its relation to other levels of the health system; and structural arrangements for insurers and purchasers, health care providers, and market regulators
- *Financing.* The way funds are collected, funds and risks are pooled, finances are allocated, and health care providers are remunerated
- *Resource management.* The way resources—physical, human, and intellectual—are generated and allocated, including their geographic and needs-based allocation
- *Service delivery.* Both population- and individual-level public health interventions and health care services provided in community, primary health care, hospitals, and other health institutions.

Each of these functions is influenced by the economic, demographic, legal, cultural, and political context.

As the framework suggests, health system goals include better health, financial protection, and user satisfaction. Personal health services and public health interventions should be organized to achieve an appropriate balance of equity (including reducing out-of-pocket [OOP] expenditures and impoverishment of individuals and families), efficiency, effectiveness (that is, the extent to which interventions are evidence based and safe), responsiveness, equity, and client satisfaction (as perceived by the users of services).

This chapter is organized as follows. First, we provide a detailed discussion of the global burden of disease and clinical context, followed by a review of approaches to diagnosis, treatment, and prevention. The aim throughout is to approach TB through a health system lens and, in the latter part of the chapter, to provide recommendations for improving delivery strategies and strengthening health systems, including care, supply chain, and information systems. Because the current tools for combating TB are seriously inadequate, we conclude with sections on critical research and development and economic analyses of new interventions for diagnosis, treatment, and vaccines. Throughout, emphasis is placed on data or modeling of the economic costs and benefits, where available, of current or possible future interventions to combat this disease.

The chapter recommends moving toward active case finding in high-burden countries; greater investments in health systems; community-based rather than hospital-based service delivery; and greater support for research on new tools—that is, developing better diagnostics, treatment regimens, and vaccines. Most of these approaches were included in earlier WHO policies, but were not emphasized. They are now part of the WHO's End TB Strategy, with which this report is fully consistent (WHO 2015a, 2015c).

HISTORICAL TRENDS, CURRENT BURDEN, AND GLOBAL RESPONSE

TB has been a major killer worldwide for centuries and has now exceeded HIV/AIDS and malaria as the world's largest cause of death from an infectious disease (Dye 2015; WHO 2016a).

Historical Trends

TB rates have been declining in North America and Western Europe since the early nineteenth century, prior to the introduction of chemotherapy in the 1950s. The decline may be partly due to the natural waning of the epidemic (Blower and others 1995), but the trend has been too prolonged for this to provide the whole explanation. Researchers have recently suggested that dramatic differences between cities experiencing marked declines prior to chemotherapy (for example, New York City in the United States; London in the United Kingdom) and cities where TB remained high (Cape Town in South Africa) may be explained by the quality and organization of the local health system (Hermans, Horsburgh, and Wood 2015). Other potential explanations for the 150-year decline have been the subject of debate and include the following:

1. Reduced opportunities for transmission per case, which may have occurred due to lower living density, better ventilation within homes, patient isolation within sanatoriums, and declining contacts among elderly cases (McFarlane 1989)
2. Reduced susceptibility of contacts, which may have been the result of improved nutrition and genetic pressures (Lipsitch and Sousa 2002; McKeown and Record 1962; Shetty and others 2006)
3. Reduced virulence of the pathogen, although there is little evidence to that effect.

While untreated TB has traditionally had a case fatality rate of 50 percent, there are differing opinions on the role of natural selection in resistance to pulmonary TB in humans prior to the availability of TB drugs

(Lipsitch and Sousa 2002). It is not possible to disentangle all of the factors that contributed to the decline of TB before the widespread introduction of chemotherapy or the reasons why progress has since stalled. What is clear is that the TB death rate in Western Europe fell 5 percent a year in the era before chemotherapy, with declines in the United States and Western Europe associated with active case finding, for example, X-ray screening.

By the 1990s, however, TB had emerged as a major global health issue, driven largely by an increase in the number of cases in the former Soviet Union and Sub-Saharan Africa. As the number of cases fell in other parts of the world, TB incidence per capita rose in these two regions.

In the Russian Federation and other former Soviet countries, TB incidence and deaths rose sharply between 1990 and 2000. Understanding precisely why is nearly as difficult as understanding the decline in Europe and North America. It is clear that there was a marked deterioration in case finding and cure rates in Russia, but this likely does not explain all of the increase (Shilova and Dye 2001). Other factors include enhanced transmission due to the mixing of prison and civilian populations; an increase in susceptibility to disease following infection, likely linked to alcoholism and stress; poor nutrition; emphasis on hospital-based treatment and extended hospitalization; poor service delivery; the spread of drug resistance; and, more recently, the rise of HIV/AIDS infection (Atun, Samyshkin, and others 2005; Toungoussova, Bjune, and Caugant 2006).

Current Burden

Global Progress

Although the overall burden of disease remains large, substantial progress has been made in TB control worldwide. Between 1995 and 2013, the TB case detection rate increased from 46 percent to 64 percent. In the same period, between 41 million and 56 million people were successfully treated, and by 2015 as many as 49 million lives were saved (Glaziou and others 2011; WHO 2015b, 2016a). TB prevalence worldwide fell 47 percent by 2015, and the TB-attributable mortality rate had declined 45 percent compared with a 1990 baseline.

Since the mid-2000s, the global incidence of TB has been declining, albeit slowly, along with the absolute number of new TB cases reported each year. However, incidence rates remain discouragingly high in high-burden countries in South-East Asia and Sub-Saharan Africa (figure 11.2).

Despite global progress, uncertainties remain in the burden and trends in TB. For example, while estimates of the WHO and of the Institute for Health Metrics and Evaluation (IHME) were similar on prevalence of TB in 2012, the trends differed: the WHO estimated a decline in cases, while the IHME estimated an increase in cases over the same interval.

The progress of individual countries, organized by major international TB targets and goals in 22 high-burden countries—that is, those defined by the WHO as the 22 countries accounting for approximately 80 percent of the world's TB cases in 2015—is shown in table 11.1 (WHO 2015b).

Figure 11.2 Estimated TB Incidence: Top-10 Countries, 2014

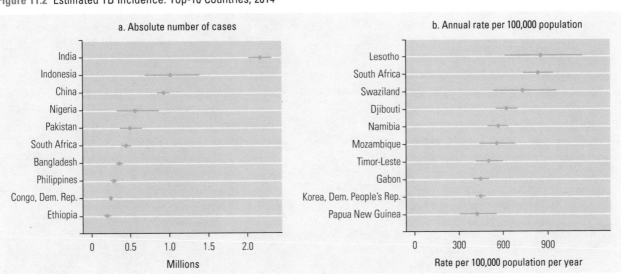

Source: WHO 2015b.

Note: TB = tuberculosis. The range shows the lower and upper bounds of the 95% uncertainty interval. The bullet indicates the best estimate.

Table 11.1 2015 Target Assessment: Global, WHO Regions, and 22 High-Burden Countries

Indicator		TB/HIV: 2015 Global Plan Targets			MDR-TB: 2015 Global Plan Targets	
		TB patients with known HIV status (%)	Notified HIV-positive TB patients started on ART (%)	People living with HIV newly enrolled in HIV care who were started on IPT	Estimated MDR-TB cases that were detected and notified (%)	Treatment success rate: confirmed MDR-TB cases, 2011 cohort (%)
Target		100%	100%	50%	100%	≥75%
Global						
Global		48	70		45	48
WHO region						
African (AFR)		76	69		74	47
Americas (AMR)		69	65		47	56
Eastern Mediterranean (EMR)		11	38		22	64
European (EUR)		59	54		61	46
South-East Asia (SEAR)		43	81		45	54
Western Pacific (WPR)		35	60		16	52
22 High-burden countries						
AFR	Congo, Dem. Rep	44	48		9	59
	Ethiopia	71	68		40	72
	Kenya	94	84		6	70
	Mozambique	91	72	17	19	31
	Nigeria	88	67	3.5	18	63
	South Africa	90	66	>100	>100	45
	Uganda	91	65		12	77
	Tanzania	83	73	0.4	10	75
	Zimbabwe	92	77	3.5	53	81
AMR	Brazil	65			39	56
EMR	Afghanistan	26		23	6	29
	Pakistan	2.8			20	70
EUR	Russian Federation				33	37
SEAR	Bangladesh	1.1	100	0	22	68
	India	63	88		57	50
	Indonesia	2.3	21		13	60
	Myanmar	12	74	19	22	71
	Thailand	83	59		12	
WPR	Cambodia	82	89	55	24	86
	China	39	67		8	50
	Philippines	2.1			47	41
	Vietnam	70	61		24	72

table continues next page

Table 11.1 2015 Target Assessment: Global, WHO Regions, and 22 High-Burden Countries (continued)

Indicator	TB/HIV: 2015 Global Plan Targets			MDR-TB: 2015 Global Plan Targets	
	TB patients with known HIV status (%)	Notified HIV-positive TB patients started on ART (%)	People living with HIV newly enrolled in HIV care who were started on IPT	Estimated MDR-TB cases that were detected and notified (%)	Treatment success rate: confirmed MDR-TB cases, 2011 cohort (%)
Target	100%	100%	50%	100%	≥75%
Classification					
	≥80% tested	≥80%	≥50%	≥80% detected and notified	≥75%
	50–79% tested	50–79%	25–49%	50–79% detected and notified	50–74%
	<50% tested	<50%	<25%	<50% detected and notified	<50%

Source: WHO 2015b.

Note: A blank cell indicates that no data are available. TB = tuberculosis; MDR TB = multidrug-resistant TB; HIV = human immunodeficiency virus; ART = antiretroviral treatment; IPT = isoniazid preventive therapy; WHO = World Health Organization.

Remaining Challenges

Despite significant progress, TB remains a formidable global health threat. The overall rate of decline in incidence, by any calculation, has been frustratingly slow (1.5 percent a year), and some countries and regions are still reporting rises in TB incidence, particularly in drug-resistant TB. Based on notification reports and surveys, there were an estimated 10.4 million new TB cases in 2015 (WHO 2016a). Assuming lifelong latent infection, about one-third of humanity could still be infected with Mtb (Dye and others 1999; Sudre, ten Dam, and Kochi 1992).

The estimation of TB incidence and prevalence remains imprecise, especially in high-burden countries where precision is most needed. Over the past decade, national surveys of the prevalence of tuberculosis disease have been undertaken in more than 20 countries, including 15 of the 22 highest-burden countries (WHO 2015b). These prevalence surveys provide vital data in high-burden settings. Great investment is needed in high-quality routine surveillance that builds on existing systems and produces robust data for assessment and future planning (Dye and others 2008; WHO 2012b). Since a quarter of TB patients are in India, the National Survey planned for 2017–18 will be very important.

Many factors drive the persistence and fatality of the disease. First, case detection has been insufficient: in 2014, only about 64 percent of people who developed TB were notified as newly diagnosed cases, leaving approximately 3 million to 4 million cases that either were not diagnosed or were diagnosed but not reported to national TB programs.

The emergence of highly drug-resistant tuberculosis, including MDR TB (resistance to at least isoniazid and rifampicin) and XDR TB (MDR plus resistance to at least one fluoroquinolone and one injectable antitubercular antibiotic), has proved a serious hurdle for effective control of tuberculosis in many settings. The most recent estimates of the burden of MDR TB suggest that approximately 480,000 new cases of MDR TB occur each year, of which only 20 percent are enrolled in treatment (WHO 2016a). Sufficiently strong surveillance and drug resistance laboratory testing are not yet adequate to establish whether MDR TB is rising or falling in most countries where MDR is of concern.

HIV/AIDS is another factor that challenges effective control of TB, especially in Southern African countries. Of the 10.4 million new cases of TB in 2014, 1.2 million occurred in HIV-positive individuals. Among the approximately 1.5 million deaths from TB in 2014, 400,000 were among individuals co-infected with HIV/AIDS (WHO 2015b). Globally, around half of patients diagnosed with TB were tested for HIV/AIDS, although that number has increased to 79 percent in the African region. Treating TB patients co-infected with HIV/AIDS with antiretroviral therapy (ART) rose to 77 percent globally, which is crucial, given that treating HIV-positive patients with ART reduces the risk of clinical TB by 64 percent.

Although dramatic improvements in TB control have been achieved over the last 25 years, the benefits have not been equally distributed among geographic regions. Falling mortality rates were often fueled by rapid economic development in Asian countries. Three WHO regions—the Americas, South-East Asia, and Western Pacific—reduced prevalence 50 percent by 2013, but the other three regions have not yet achieved that goal.

In 2014, the WHO Africa region had the highest incidence rates (about 280 cases per 100,000 population) and 28 percent of the estimated number of cases globally. Asia had 58 percent of total cases. China and India alone accounted for more than one in three (35 percent) of the world's new TB cases in 2013. Approximately 78 percent of total TB deaths and 73 percent of TB deaths among HIV-negative people occurred in the Africa and South-East Asia regions.

The spatial and temporal variation in TB incidence in Africa is strongly correlated with the prevalence of HIV/AIDS infection (Corbett and others 2003). Globally, an estimated 11 percent of all new adult TB cases were infected with HIV/AIDS in 2015. In the WHO Africa region, the percentage of incident TB cases with HIV/AIDS varied from 8 percent in Eritrea to 77 percent in Swaziland.

Many of the gains in TB control globally are stalling, with TB incidence no longer falling in some East Asian settings, notably Hong Kong SAR, China; Japan; the Republic of Korea; and Singapore. Part of the explanation could be that more cases are arising by reactivation from a previously infected aging human population (Vynnycky and others 2008; Wu and others 2010). Additionally, immigration from high-incidence countries is part of the reason why the decline of TB in North America and Western Europe has plateaued. Immigrants infected in their country of origin contribute, in varying degrees, to further transmission and outbreaks in the country where they have come to live or work (Verver and others 2005).

Global Response

Following its declaration in 1993 that tuberculosis was a global health emergency, the WHO launched the DOTS strategy in 1994 (WHO 1994). Prior to DOTS, there were at least five recommended regimens for treatment of TB, with varying effectiveness, serious adverse effects, and varying costs (Murray, Styblo, and Rouillon 1990). DOTS aimed to create a single common best-practice strategy that would be applicable to all countries and would include not just observing treatment but also securing political commitments as well as adequate and sustained financing:

- Ensure early case detection and diagnosis through quality-assured bacteriology
- Provide standardized treatment with supervision and patient support
- Ensure effective drug supply and management
- Monitor and evaluate performance and impact.

Emerging drug resistance compelled the WHO to introduce DOTS-plus in 1998, with two additional requirements: (1) the capacity to perform drug-sensitivity testing (DST) and (2) the ability to ensure access to second-line drugs (Stop TB Working Group on DOTS-Plus for MDR-TB 2003).

DOTS expanded further in 2014 to reflect six programmatic actions critical to an effective global TB control strategy (box 11.1). Thus, the history of TB response reflects attempts to tackle ever more fundamental causes of TB by addressing health system drivers of the epidemic.

Major organizational initiatives have sought to intensify the fight against TB: the TB Alliance in 2000; the Green Light Committee at the WHO in 2000; the Stop TB Initiative in 2001; the Global Fund to Fight AIDS, Tuberculosis, and Malaria (Global Fund), which was created as a major funder of country programs in 2002; UNITAID in 2006; and the Stop TB Partnership in 2008, which was created to coordinate, together with the WHO, the many provider, advocacy, and donor groups engaged in fighting TB. The Stop TB Partnership has 1,200 partners in 100 countries. Further, the Global Laboratory Initiative was established in 2007 to strengthen laboratory capacity in LMICs.

Increased attention and initiatives have been coupled with significant increases in international and domestic funding for TB. Funding for TB prevention, diagnosis, and treatment reached US$6.6 billion in 2016, almost double the level in 2006 (WHO 2015b). Overall about 84 percent (US$5.5 billion) of reported TB funding was derived from domestic sources; nevertheless, low-income countries (LICs) have benefited from Global Fund financing, which accounts for about 67 percent of total TB funding for these countries. In 2016, most TB

Box 11.1

WHO DOTS Strategy, 2014

- Pursue high-quality DOTS expansion and enhancement
- Address TB and HIV/AIDS co-infection, MDR TB, and the needs of poor and vulnerable populations
- Contribute to health system strengthening based on primary health care
- Engage all care providers
- Empower people with TB and communities through partnership.

Source: WHO 2014b.

funding (US$ 4.9 billion) was spent on drug-susceptible TB, with MDR TB receiving about US$1.7 billion. The WHO estimates that the gap in funding to achieve the SDG for TB is on the order of US$2 billion per year (WHO 2015a, 2016a).

Evolving Targets

The initial DOTS targets aimed to achieve a global tuberculosis detection rate of 70 percent and a treatment success rate of 85 percent. In 2000, the UN Millennium Declaration (UN General Assembly 2000), which established the MDGs, set in motion worldwide concerted efforts to alleviate poverty and improve global health. Astonishingly, the MDG goals did not specifically mention tuberculosis, which was then causing more than 9 million new cases and 1.5 million deaths annually. However, MDG 6, which aimed to halt and begin to reverse HIV/AIDS, malaria, and "other infectious diseases," provided sufficient language for international targets to be established for TB control.

The Global Plan to Stop TB 2001–15 of the Stop TB Partnership established two targets in addition to the general goal in MDG 6, for a total of three targets often referred to in the TB literature:

- Halt and reverse the global growth in TB incidence
- Decrease TB prevalence 50 percent from 1990 baseline levels by 2015
- Decrease TB mortality 50 percent from 1990 baseline levels by 2015.

The current UN Sustainable Development Goals seek to reduce tuberculosis deaths 95 percent and reduce the TB incidence rate 90 percent by 2035, effectively eliminating the disease. These are ambitious goals, and experts have outlined milestones in five-year increments to track progress and hold governing bodies accountable. With evidence that transmission and treatment failures in many countries continue at high levels, other metrics, including case detection and treatment success rates, are important indicators of progress.

Dye and others (2013) modeled what would be required to eliminate TB as a public health problem (less than 1 case per 100,000 population) by 2015. A projection of the decline in incidence at current rates (around 1 percent annually) indicates that MDG goals would not be met for more than 50 years. An updated model requires that incidence decrease 10 percent in 2020 and 17 percent a year thereafter (figure 11.3).

Figure 11.3 Projected Acceleration in the Decline of Global Tuberculosis Incidence Rates to Target Levels, 2015–35

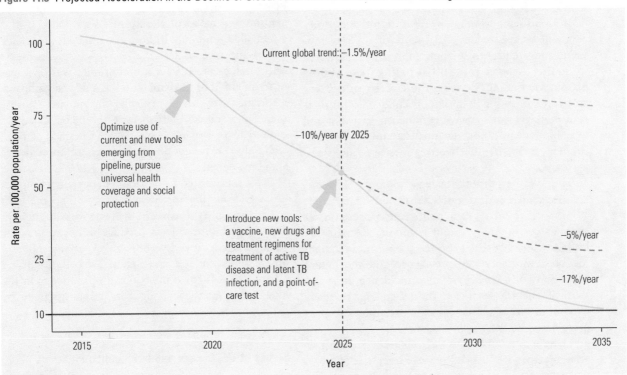

Source: WHO 2015c.
Note: TB = tuberculosis.

WHO End TB Strategy

Integrated, patient-centered care and prevention

- Early diagnosis of tuberculosis, including universal drug-susceptibility testing and systematic screening of contacts and high-risk groups
- Treatment of all people with tuberculosis, including drug-resistant tuberculosis, and patient support
- Collaborative tuberculosis and HIV/AIDS activities and management of comorbidities
- Preventive treatment of persons at high risk and vaccination against tuberculosis.

Bold policies and supportive systems

- Political commitment with adequate resources for tuberculosis care and prevention

- Engagement of communities, civil society organizations, and public and private care providers
- Universal health coverage policy and regulatory frameworks for case notification, vital registration, quality and rational use of medicines, and infection control
- Social protection, poverty alleviation, and actions on other determinants of tuberculosis.

Intensified research and innovation

- Discovery, development, and rapid uptake of new tools, interventions, and strategies
- Research to optimize implementation and impact and to promote innovations.

Source: WHO 2015a, 2015c.

However, such a "rate of decline has never been achieved on any geographical scale for any period of time and is not possible globally with the present suite of tools and systems for their delivery" (Dye 2013, 272–73).

It is difficult to conceive that significant progress will be realized by 2035 without the development and application of new tools and investment in health systems for TB, including reinstituting active case finding, devising more effective delivery strategies, investing in the supply chain and information management systems, conducting research and development into new diagnostics, and implementing new and more effective treatment regimens and vaccines.

The WHO's current strategic plan for TB control, the End TB Strategy (Uplekar and others 2015; WHO 2015c, 2016a) is a multifaceted program far more extensive than previous iterations. Recognizing both the successes of previous programs in reducing both mortality and prevalence and the failure of present programs to reduce incidence at a rate that will enable countries to meet the SDG targets by 2035, it proposes a broader and more ambitious program based on three pillars (box 11.2).

These are very ambitious and important goals that, to a large extent, will depend on investments in research and development of new tools and more effective use of the available tools.

INFECTION AND DISEASE IN INDIVIDUALS AND POPULATIONS

Tuberculosis is an infectious bacterial disease caused by *Mycobacterium tuberculosis*, which is transmitted by aerosols and most commonly affects the lungs. Mtb is essentially found only in humans, although the related pathogenic mycobacteria, *M. bovis*, causes disease in cattle and, before Pasteurization of milk, was the cause of scrofula, TB of the lymph nodes. A related pathogen, *M. leprae*, is the cause of leprosy in humans. Because there is no animal reservoir for Mtb, the pathogen has evolved to persist in people for long periods of time, with only a portion of people developing clinical disease with lung damage.

TB is transmitted from person to person via aerosol droplets from the throat and lungs of people with active respiratory disease. Individuals with pulmonary or laryngeal tuberculosis produce airborne droplets while coughing, sneezing, or simply speaking (Lin and others 2008; Loudon and Spohn 1969; Rodrigo and others 1997). Inhaled infectious droplets lodge in the lung alveoli and bacilli and are taken up there by macrophages.

Stages of TB Disease and Intervention Points

TB is best understood not as a single clinical entity but as a spectrum, which generally correlates with the immune responses. A high, but unknown, percentage of people infected with Mtb develop latent or persistent infection, but only about 10 percent develop disease in a lifetime (Chee and others 2005; Hanifa and others 2009). For immune-compromised individuals, the risk is about 8 percent a year (Selwyn and others 1989). A portion of highly exposed individuals likely to be infected with Mtb fail to develop tuberculin skin tests (TSTs) but remain healthy, suggesting that they are protected by yet-unknown immune mechanisms. Another unknown proportion of individuals with tubercle bacilli in sputum remain asymptomatic but it must be presumed capable of transmitting infection (Bates and others 2012; Mao and others 2014; Willingham and others 2001; Wood and others 2007).

Multiple possible points for interventions exist along the care continuum, including preventing infections, preventing establishment of latency, preventing transition from latent TB to active disease (chemoprophylaxis), and treating persons with active disease to achieve cure, thereby reducing morbidity, mortality, and transmission intensity (figure 11.4).

In most healthy people, infection with *M. tuberculosis* often causes no symptoms, since the person's immune system, through innate and acquired immunity, acts to kill or wall off the bacteria. Acquired cell-mediated immunity develops two to eight weeks after infection, and granulomas—that is, infiltrating macrophages and lymphocytes—wall off the infection and limit further replication and spread of the organism (Aziz, Ishaq, and Akhwand 1985), although this is only partially protective (Andrews and others 2012; Bates and others 2007; da Silva and others 2014; Lin, Ezzati, and Murray 2007; Slama and others 2007).

There is a widespread belief that infection does not confer significant subsequent immunity (Achkar and Jenny-Avital 2011; Barry and others 2009), which is used to explain why reinfection is not uncommon (Luzze and others 2013; Verver and others 2005). However, recent reanalysis of many studies reveals that latent TB infection does protect against active disease, almost certainly by engendering protective innate or acquired immune responses, but that this protection is only partial (Andrews and others 2012). Molecular fingerprinting techniques can be used to distinguish bacteria obtained during relapses of prior infection from reinfection with new strains. The original infecting strain can reemerge after apparent cure or ineffective treatment and reestablish active disease (relapse) (Khan, Minion, and others 2012; Luzze and others 2013). Reactivation rates vary from 1 percent to 30 percent a year in different populations. Whether latent bacilli remain viable for the full life span of all infected people

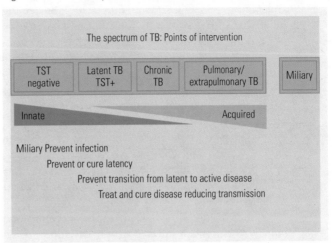

Figure 11.4 The TB Spectrum and Possible Points of Intervention

Note: TB = tuberculosis; TST = tuberculin skin test. Infection with *Mycobacterium tuberculosis* can lead to subclinical infection, which is cured by innate or acquired immune responses; latent infection that persists; chronic or asymptomatic TB in which tubercle bacilli are found in sputum of otherwise apparently healthy individuals; and active TB disease. In a small proportion of individuals, infection can lead directly to rapidly progressing disease, known as primary progressive TB. Miliary TB is widely disseminated, occurring primarily in children and severely immunodeficient individuals.

is unknown, but the risk of reactivation persists into old age (Stead and Dutt 1989).

The phenomenon of reactivation, often long after infection or after treatment, reflects the limitations of immune responses in assuring protection and indicates the challenge facing the development of effective vaccines that can provide long-term protection (Lin and others 2014; Lönnroth and others 2010; Selwyn and others 1989). Bacille Calmette-Guérin (BCG) is the only licensed vaccine available today and has been used for more than 90 years with a good safety record, except in immunodeficient children. However, its efficacy in preventing TB in adults has varied in different parts of the world, while consistently protecting children against the most severe forms of disease: disseminated miliary TB and TB meningitis (Mangtani and others 2014; Roy and others 2014). BCG vaccination is discussed further in the section on prevention.

Primary infection in some individuals leads to active TB (primary progressive tuberculosis) when the host immune response cannot effectively suppress the replication of bacilli. The symptoms of active TB of the lung are coughing, sometimes with blood in sputum; chest pains; weakness; weight loss; fever; and night sweats. Clinical tuberculosis is the sum of complex interactions between the pathogen and an individual's immune response that facilitate mycobacterial replication and cause illness, including wasting and granulomatous inflammation with tissue damage, for example, caseation, vasculitis, and fibrosis (Jagirdar and Zagzag 1996; O'Garra and others 2013; Shaler and others 2013). The most common clinical manifestation of TB is pulmonary disease, and, in the most infectious patients, bacilli are visible microscopically on stained sputum smears (50–70 percent of pulmonary cases) (Huang, Tchetgen, Becerra, Cohen, Galea, and others 2014; Huang, Tchetgen, Becerra, Cohen, Hughes, and others 2014). Extrapulmonary tuberculosis accounts for 10–30 percent of disease, but is more common among women and children (particularly lymphatic tuberculosis) and in people infected with HIV/AIDS (Chadha and others 2005; Lowell, Edwards, and Palmer 1969; MacIntyre and others 1997).

In the absence of other predisposing conditions, only 5–10 percent of infected people develop progressive primary disease within five years of infection (Chee and others 2005; Hanifa and others 2009; van Rie and others 2013). After five years, there is a much lower annual risk of developing TB by the reactivation of latent infection. However, the risk in HIV-positive individuals is on the order of 10 percent a year after infection (Selwyn and others 1989). The risk of progressing to active disease is relatively high in infancy, is lower in older children, increases quickly during adolescence (earlier in girls), and then increases more slowly throughout adulthood (da Silva and others 2014; Hanifa and others 2009; Isler and others 2013; Lienhardt and others 2003). The lifetime risk of developing TB following infection clearly depends on the prevailing transmission rate, but is generally estimated to be about 10 percent.

Latent TB, which exists in an unknown percentage of people infected with *M. tuberculosis*, has significant impact on the epidemiology and population dynamics of tuberculosis. It represents a huge reservoir of potential disease and further transmission. Concomitantly, long-term latent infection appears to provide partial protection against developing disease (Andrews and others 2012).

Following Mtb infection, whether the infection remains latent or develops into active disease is thought to depend largely on the host's ability to generate protective innate and cell-mediated immunity. There is at present little evidence that serum antibodies provide protection, although recent studies of serum from TST-negative highly exposed individuals indicate they may have antibodies capable of enabling macrophages to kill some bacilli in vitro (Lu and others 2016). Human T-cells are highly heterogeneous. From animal studies, both CD4 cells and cytotoxic CD8 T-cells are important for protection against Mtb infection. CD4+ cells are functionally heterogeneous. In the simplest

case, two antagonistic subclasses of CD4+—Th1 and Th2—have been described, each with its own set of cytokine mediators. Th1 responses, characterized by production of interferon gamma (IFN-γ), are associated with protection, while Th2 responses, characterized predominantly by Th2 cytokines (for example, IL-4, IL-10), are associated with antibody, inflammatory responses and tissue damage. A unique subset of human Th1 cells has recently been described that appears strongly to correlate with protection against mycobacterial disease. These Th1* cells constitute a unique subset of human CD4+ T-cells expressing the chemokine receptors—CCR6, CCR4, and the RORγ nuclear transcription factor, which exclusively appears to produce IFN-γ to mycobacteria (Sallusto 2016).

The importance of TB among infectious diseases is attributable to the high case fatality rate among untreated or improperly treated cases. About two-thirds of untreated smear-positive TB cases will die within five to eight years; most will die within the first two years (Huang, Tchetgen, Becerra, Cohen, Hughes, and others 2014; Libshitz and others 1997). As illustrated in figure 11.4, the rest will remain latent, chronically ill, or asymptomatic, or will self-cure. The case fatality rate for untreated microscopy smear-negative cases is lower, but still on the order of 10–15 percent (Chadha and others 2005; Khan, Minion, and others 2012; Libshitz and others 1997). Even among smear-positive patients receiving TB drugs, the case fatality rate can exceed 10 percent if adherence is low or if rates of HIV/AIDS infection and drug resistance are high.

M. tuberculosis Strains

There is striking evidence that the major strains of *M. tuberculosis* co-evolved with the major migrations of humans from Africa to Asia, Europe, and the Americas (Gagneux 2012). Many strains of Mtb can be revealed by molecular analyses, and the diversity is thought to exacerbate drug resistance and to affect the effectiveness of interventions to control the disease. While early targeted genetic analyses suggested only minimal within-species diversity of *M. tuberculosis* (Keane and others 2001; Yokoyama and others 2004), genomic studies have revealed much more variation (Alhajri and others 2011). Subsequent examination has provided increasing understanding of Mtb strains and how they spread globally (Talat and others 2010). Other investigations aim to discover whether differences between or within (according to Cegielski, Arab, and Cornoni-Huntley 2012) strains modify the ability of the pathogen to infect hosts or are associated with differences in the natural history of disease (Alhajri and others 2011; Wilkinson and others 2000). The number and scope of such studies is still limited, but a recent study has associated differences in Mtb strains with the probability of transmission of disease among household exposures in Brazil (Lopez and others 2003).

Evidence is accumulating that strain lineages vary in strength and mechanism of host-immune stimulation after infection (Baker and others 2012), within-host competitive ability (Boelaert and others 2007), rates of acquiring mutations (Bellamy and others 1998; Ford and others 2013) and drug resistance (Borrell and Gagneux 2011), and the specific mutations acquired (Fenner and others 2012), each of which may affect the within-host course of infection, disease, and response to therapy (Gagneux 2012). In general, the fitness of pathogens diminishes as mutations accumulate. A variety of evidence indicates that MDR TB strains are heterogeneous in their transmissibility in animal models and human populations (Grandjean and others 2015; Lee, Radmonski, and others 2015). It is likely that compromised transmissibility can change if compensatory mutations arise that reestablish fitness. A particular concern is the enhanced transmissibility of the Beijing strain with antibiotic resistance (Ford and others 2013; Hanekom and others 2007). Mathematical modeling similarly indicates that strain diversity may affect the emergence of drug resistance (Basu and Galvani 2008) and interventions (Cohen and others 2008; Colijn and others 2009), but improved projections will require additional data, especially from whole-genome sequencing and long-term monitoring of strain types within human populations.

TB and HIV/AIDS Co-Infection

The extent to which HIV/AIDS is fueling TB transmission (in addition to provoking reactivation) remains poorly understood. One analysis suggested that 1–2 percent of all transmission events were from HIV-positive, smear-positive TB cases in 2000 (Corbett and others 2003). The co-infection of TB and HIV/AIDS is geographically heterogeneously distributed. In countries in Eastern Europe and Southern Africa, as many as 75 percent of all TB patients are HIV-positive; in others, such as China and India, only a small fraction of TB cases are HIV-positive (Dye 2015).

The fraction of TB infections attributable to persons co-infected with HIV/AIDS depends on the prevalence of HIV/AIDS as well as on the infectiousness of HIV/AIDS-associated Mtb compared with that of TB cases not affected by HIV/AIDS. This fraction is influenced by biological factors (for example, the probability of smear-positive pulmonary disease) and how rapidly

individuals are diagnosed and receive effective treatment. The duration of HIV/AIDS-associated TB appears to be shorter than the duration of HIV-negative TB (Corbett and others 2004) or about the same (Wood and others 2007), depending on the setting.

Clearly, HIV/AIDS infection exerts a multifaceted suppression of the innate and acquired T-cell responses. In a sense, TB is often a sentinel for HIV/AIDS infection in high HIV/AIDS-endemic areas. Even prior to significant CD4+ T-cell depletion, individuals with latent TB can progress to active disease. Not only does HIV/AIDS infection suppress immune responses to Mtb, but the stimulation of T-cells by antigens of Mtb may contribute to T-cell activation, leading to the increased production of HIV/AIDS and acceleration of the disease process.

Clinically, the prevalence of extrapulmonary TB and disseminated TB are both increased in HIV-positive patients. Low CD4 cell counts are associated with an increased frequency of extrapulmonary TB, positive mycobacterial blood cultures, and atypical chest radiographic findings, reflecting an inability of the impaired immune response to contain infection. The rise in TB incidence attributable to HIV/AIDS appears to have peaked in most countries, as HIV/AIDS incidence has declined (Dye 2015).

Effect of TB on the Distribution of Other Diseases

TB affects the presence and nature of other diseases, possibly conferring protective effects. Microbial infections have the potential to influence the balance between CD4+ T-cell functional subsets by stimulating innate immune responses and by altering cytokine profiles, with positive or negative consequences for health (Sallusto 2016). Mtb infection may also protect against asthma, possibly by shifting the innate and acquired Th2 response to a Th1 subset that reduces the inflammatory response. One study of Japanese children found that strong tuberculin responses following BCG immunization were associated with less asthma, rhinoconjunctivitis, and eczema in later childhood (Shirakawa and others 1997). A study of South African children found an inverse association between *M. tuberculosis* infection and atopic rhinitis (Obihara and others 2005). Comparisons among countries have found that asthma tends to be more common where TB is less common (Shirtcliffe, Weatherall, and Beasley 2002; von Mutius and others 2000).

Interactions between other infections have also been investigated. Vigorous Th2 responses are seen in protective immune reactions to helminth infections, and helminths can shift the balance of immune responses to enhance allergic responses and thus compromise

Th1 immune responses to BCG and *M. tuberculosis* (Hopkin 2000). Conversely, a mycobacterial-based vaccine could potentially be constructed to prevent allergic responses and reduce asthma. Mtb infection may protect against leprosy, as does BCG (Karonga Prevention Trial Group 1996), and natural TB transmission may have contributed to the decline of leprosy in Europe (Lietman, Porco, and Blower 1997).

There is no information at present on whether the human microbiome affects responses to mycobacteria, but this is an area of research worthy of investigation. While the synergistic and antagonistic interactions between bacterial, viral, and parasitic infections are complex and unresolved, these examples raise the general likelihood that mycobacteria influence, and are influenced by, the presence of other infections.

Risk Factors for TB

Risk factors influence the probability of infection, disease, or outcome and operate on many scales (physiological, genetic, environmental, and behavioral). Once an individual has been exposed to a person with infectious pulmonary TB, his or her risk of developing subclinical TB infection depends on factors that influence either the ability of the person infected to transmit the disease or the susceptibility of the person exposed to infection and disease. Infected persons who are acid-fast bacillus smear- or culture-positive (Riley and Moodie 1974; Ross and Willison 1971; Tornee and others 2005), who have cavitary disease (destructive lesions in the lung where the bacilli multiply to high levels; Rodrigo and others 1997) or frequent cough (Loudon and Spohn 1969), or who have delayed treatment (Aziz, Ishaq, and Akhwand 1985; Lin and others 2008) are major transmitters of TB infection.

Risk factors relevant to the exposed host most often reflect the social and environmental determinants of heavy exposure and include living in densely populated spaces (Chadha and others 2005; Lowell, Edwards, and Palmer 1969; MacIntyre and others 1997), being incarcerated (Chadha and others 2005; Chee and others 2005), and working in occupations such as health care that involve frequent social or direct contact with TB patients (Hanifa and others 2009; Isler and others 2013; van Rie and others 2013). Most studies suggest that, among similarly exposed contacts, the risk of TB infection does not vary much by host attributes. However, some recent studies report that genetic loci are associated with differential risk of infection among household contacts exposed to an infectious case (da Silva and others 2014; Lienhardt and others 2003), while evidence indicates that smoking increases the

risk of TB (Bates and others 2007; Lin, Ezzati, and Murray 2007; Slama and others 2007).

In contrast to infection, disease progression is known to be highly dependent on host risk factors, the most important of which include HIV/AIDS co-infection (Selwyn and others 1989), low body mass index (Lönnroth and others 2010), exposure to tobacco (WHO 2015d) and biomass fuels (indoor air pollution; Bates and others 2007; Lin, Ezzati, and Murray 2007; Lin and others 2014; Slama and others 2007), diabetes mellitus (Jeon and Murray 2008), and heavy alcohol use (Lönnroth and others 2008; Rehm and others 2009; WHO 2014a). Host-specific risk factors also affect TB outcomes, including the risks of failing therapy, relapsing after treatment, and dying a TB-related death. In addition to HIV/AIDS, smoking and diabetes are recognized biological risk factors for poor treatment outcomes (Kim and others 2014), and some studies have implicated other comorbidities such as iron overload (Yokoyama and others 2004), renal dysfunction (Keane and others 2001), and hematological malignancies (Keane and others 2001).

Abundant evidence indicates that undernutrition is associated with TB in LMICs. In national surveys in India, the population-attributable risk of TB in undernourished adults and adolescents was two-fold or greater and greatest in rural areas (Bhargava and others 2014).

Table 11.2 lists the risk factors for TB progression and summarizes the relative risks for selected determinants for which meta-analyses have been conducted. Although HIV/AIDS is a much stronger risk factor for disease progression than other exposures, the relatively frequent occurrence of other determinants means that they explain a higher proportion of global TB cases than does HIV/AIDS. Table 11.3 estimates the most common

Table 11.2 Key Risk Factors for Tuberculosis from Meta-Analyses of Randomized Controlled Trials

Key risk factor	Odds ratio
Cigarette smoking	2.01–2.66
Indoor air pollution	1.4
Low body mass index	2.45[a]
Alcohol use (daily or alcohol use disorder)	2.94
Diabetes mellitus	3.11

Source: International Institute for Population Sciences and Macro International 2007.
Note: Human immunodeficiency virus/acquired immune deficiency syndrome (HIV/AIDS) does not appear in the table because once it was clear that HIV/AIDS was a major risk factor for TB, it became unethical to do a prospective study that did not offer HIV-positive patients isoniazid.
a. Odds of tuberculosis for body mass index of 18.5 compared to 25.

Table 11.3 Attributable Fraction of Key Risk Factors for Tuberculosis Disease Progression in India, by Socioeconomic Strata

Key risk factor	Population-Attributable Fraction (%)		
	Lowest socioeconomic stratum	Middle socioeconomic stratum	Highest socioeconomic stratum
Cigarette smoking	16	10	6
Indoor air pollution	29	25	6
Low body mass index	34	27	20
Alcohol use, daily	4	2	1
HIV/AIDS seroprevalence	9	10	6

Source: Oxlade and Murray 2012.
Note: HIV/AIDS = human immunodeficiency virus/acquired immune deficiency syndrome.

Table 11.4 Global Prevalence, Relative Risk, and Attributable Fraction for Incident Tuberculosis

Key risk factor	Global prevalence	Relative risk	Attributable fraction (%)	References
HIV/AIDS	0.008	8.3	5.5	WHO 2009a
Undernourishment	0.11	2.1	10.7	Lönnroth and others 2010
Diabetes mellitus	0.085	3.0	14.5	Jeon and Murray 2008
Heavy alcohol use	0.075	2.9	12.5	Lönnroth and others 2008
Cigarette smoking	0.21	2.6	25.1	Lin, Ezzati, and Murray 2007; Slama and others 2007
Indoor air pollution	0.41	1.5	17.0	Lin, Ezzati, and Murray 2007

Note: Relative risk estimates the magnitude of an association between exposure and disease on the basis of the incidence of disease in the exposed group relative to the unexposed group. Attributable risk is the absolute difference in incidence between an exposed and unexposed group that quantifies the risk of disease in the exposed group attributable to the exposure by removing the risk that would have occurred due to other causes.

attributable risk factors in different economic strata in India using data from the Indian National Family Health Survey (International Institute for Population Sciences and Macro International 2007). These data show that multiple risk factors often converge in individuals living in poverty, further amplifying their risk of disease.

HIV/AIDS is associated with only about 11 percent of TB patients worldwide. Other risk factors, such as diabetes mellitus and smoking, occur more widely. The population-attributable fraction is the proportional reduction in population disease or mortality that would occur if exposure to a risk factor were reduced to an alternative ideal exposure scenario, for example, no smoking. A global estimate of population-attributable factors for TB is given in table 11.4. It is not possible to estimate accurately the number of people with each of the risk factors because the data on background risk are uncertain and risks overlap. Nevertheless, the greater numbers of smokers and rapidly expanding number of people with diabetes mellitus allow us to infer that the proportion of all cases due to malnutrition and diabetes is five times higher and the proportion due to smoking is eight times greater than the proportion due to HIV/AIDS.

Risk factors also vary by socioeconomic status, as illustrated for India. While infection with Mtb is a risk for people of any economic stratum, the data from India indicate that some known risk factors for TB are greatest in the lowest socioeconomic group, a finding likely to be true for most populations.

Other less common comorbidities also modify the risk of disease. Persons are more likely to progress to active tuberculosis if they suffer from silicosis (Corbett and others 2000; Snider 1978), kidney disease (Mitwalli 1991), or solid (Libshitz and others 1997) and hematological (Khan and others 2005) malignancies; have undergone gastrectomy or ileojejunal bypass surgery (Choi and others 2015; Kim and others 2014; Yokoyama and others 2004); or have received the tumor necrosis factor alpha (TNF-α) inhibitor infliximab for the treatment of rheumatoid arthritis (Keane and others 2001). While these exposures are rare, some dramatically increase the risk of TB; older forms of weight-loss surgery, for example, can profoundly increase risk. To date, although several case reports document TB among patients undergoing gastric bypass, no systematic epidemiologic studies have been conducted on this risk factor (Alhajri and others 2011).

In addition to low body mass index, several micronutrient deficiencies have been associated with TB progression. In vitro studies suggest a role for vitamin D in host susceptibility to disease and, in one clinical study conducted in Pakistan, 25-hydroxy-vitamin D—25(OH)D—levels less than 9 nanograms per milliliter increased the risk of progression to active disease fivefold (Talat and others 2010). Vitamin A deficiency was found to be associated with a 2.8 increased risk of TB in the United States, although this finding was not statistically significant (Cegielski, Arab, and Cornoni-Huntley 2012), and reciprocal seasonal variation in vitamin D levels in South Africa correlate with TB notifications (Martineau and others 2011).

Nutritional factors may also interact with genetic polymorphisms to increase TB risk. Polymorphisms in the 25(OH)D receptor have been associated with TB risk, and several studies have demonstrated a gene-environment interaction between 25(OH)D levels and 25(OH)D receptor mutations (Wilkinson and others 2000); there is considerable evidence that 25(OH)D3 is essential for human macrophages to kill Mtb in vitro (Fabri and others 2011; Liu and others 2007). Vitamin D is produced in the skin by exposure to ultraviolet light, and seasonal variation in vitamin D has been correlated with the number of TB cases (Wilkinson and others 2000). This finding and the role of the skin pigment melanin to absorb ultraviolet light may explain the increased susceptibility of dark-skinned individuals to TB infection and more severe disease (Martineau and others 2011; Modlin and Bloom 2013). But correlation does not imply causation, and there is a critical need for well-designed clinical trials to ascertain the importance of these factors.

Much recent work has focused on identifying the genetic determinants of TB progression (Abel and others 2014). Twin studies strongly support the hypothesis that genetic factors play a role in TB susceptibility, and multiple loci have been implicated through candidate gene studies (Snider 1978). Some of these are rare variants that lead to alterations in the interferon-γ pathway required to develop acquired immunity to mycobacteria. Multiple defects in this pathway result in Mendelian susceptibility to mycobacterial diseases, which predisposes individuals not only to disseminated infections with nontuberculous mycobacteria, but also to tuberculosis (Bustamante and others 2014; Mitwalli 1991). Other studies have implicated candidate genes that affect innate immune responses (Png and others 2012). Several genome-wide association studies have also been reported, as reviewed in Naranbhai (2016). Some have identified alleles, which occur in "gene-free"

regions of the human genome, but these have not been consistently validated in separate populations. A locus on chromosome 11 has been associated with susceptibility in multiple populations (Chimusa and others 2014; Thye and others 2012). Of particular interest is a locus on chromosome 5 that encodes a component of interleukin 12 (IL-12) required for differentiating T-cells, which appears to confer resistance in highly susceptible HIV-positive populations in East Africa and for which there is evidence of positive selection (Sobota and others 2016).

TB DIAGNOSIS AND SCREENING

In simplest terms, the DOTS strategy for TB control has been to test individuals who seek care at a health facility for clinical symptoms of TB and to provide appropriate drug treatment for a period of 6–24 months. With timely diagnosis and correct treatment, almost all people with drug-sensitive TB can be cured, and even a short duration of treatment reduces the bacillary load and likelihood of transmission. Nevertheless, worldwide, the TB case detection rate remains low: in 2012, about 66 percent (5.7 million) of the estimated 10.4 million people who developed TB were newly diagnosed cases, with an estimated 3 million to 4 million cases remaining undiagnosed or unknown to health systems. Case detection in children is of particular concern: an estimated 1 million children developed tuberculosis in 2010, with about 32,000 children contracting multidrug-resistant TB disease (Seddon and others 2015).

In most countries, the most common diagnostic test is microscopic scanning of acid-fast stained bacilli in sputum smears—a technique dating to the 1880s. It is convenient but insensitive, diagnosing only about half of all TB cases in adults (Frieden 2004) and fewer in children (Detjen and others 2015) and HIV-positive individuals (Harries 1997). Diagnostic certainty is obtained when the organism is demonstrated in a laboratory after clinical evaluation of symptoms (usually cough) compatible with tuberculosis. In the absence of diagnostic laboratory tests, clinicians need to review clinical information and decide whether to initiate treatment for tuberculosis, weighing the risks of leaving possible TB untreated against adverse drug reactions and the social and financial costs of committing to months of therapy (WHO 2007). Often treatment, appropriate or not, is instituted before it is clear whether the patient has TB and whether the infection is drug-susceptible or drug-resistant.

Diagnosis of MDR and XDR TB

Diagnosis and treatment of MDR TB, in particular, has largely faltered worldwide. Only 30 of 107 countries are treating 75 percent or more of patients with MDR TB, with countries experiencing high levels of loss to follow-up (WHO 2013a). Of the estimated 450,000 people who developed MDR TB in 2012, only 94,000 (20.9 percent) were detected, and just 77,000 were started on second-line treatment. MDR and XDR TB also represent a threat to health care personnel and health infrastructure. Unknown numbers of nurses and physicians have acquired MDR and XDR TB, and in 2014, there were an estimated 210,000 deaths from MDR TB (WHO 2015b).

The diagnosis of drug-resistant TB and its treatment are complex, requiring laboratory capability for drug-sensitivity testing and between 9 and 20 months of daily administration of drugs that are both more toxic and less efficacious than the drugs used to treat drug-sensitive TB (Nathanson and others 2010). Inadequate human resources, poor access to laboratory services, and low capacity to do drug-susceptibility testing and analysis partly account for low case detection for MDR TB (Shin and others 2008). Health system approaches that favor hospital-based management of MDR TB frequently have limited access to service delivery, and scale-up of new diagnostic tools and treatment regimens is often weak in health systems where MDR TB dominates (Keshavjee and Farmer 2010; Nardell and Dharmadhikari 2010).

Several economies—including Estonia; Hong Kong SAR, China; Latvia; and Singapore—that have strengthened their health systems by improving access to diagnosis and primary care treatment have halted the rise in MDR TB incidence (Cohen and others 2014; Cuevas and others 2011; Dye 2009). Strong laboratory capacity, which has enabled rapid and definitive determination of drug sensitivity, strong supply chain management systems, and successful scale-up of effective treatment regimens have contributed to this success (Gandhi and others 2010). In this context, it is technically difficult for countries to diagnose patterns of drug resistance. For this reason, the WHO created the TB Supranational Reference Laboratory Network of 24 quality-control laboratories, which are located in every continent and able to carry out sophisticated testing for drug resistance (WHO 2015a).

Recent Advances in TB Diagnostics

Tuberculosis diagnostics have advanced steadily over the past decade (see box 11.3). As a result, between 2007 and 2012, the WHO issued 10 new policy statements on TB diagnosis covering an array of approaches (Lawn 2015).

Box 11.3

New Strategies for TB Diagnosis

- Use of light-emitting diode (LED) microscopy as an alternative to conventional Ziehl-Neelsen light microscopy, which has been the mainstay of TB diagnosis for decades (Cuevas and others 2011)
- Use of nucleic acid amplification tests (NAATs) for diagnosis of active TB, including manual technologies such as loop-mediated isothermal amplification as well as automated technologies such as Xpert MTB/RIF (Pai, Kalantri, and Dheda 2006)
- Use of nucleic acid amplification technology approaches for rapid screening for drug resistance, for example, based on line probe assays (Pai, Kalantri, and Dheda 2006)

- Use of liquid culture systems as a more rapid and sensitive alternative to conventional solid culture (Palacios and others 1999).

Other avenues for developing new TB diagnostics hold promise:

- Urine-based diagnostics for detecting *M. tuberculosis* antigen, for example, assays to detect lipoarabinomannan, especially in HIV-positive patients (Green and others 2009; Nakiyingi and others 2014)
- Immunochromatographic tests for rapid confirmation of Mtb in culture (Hasegawa and others 2002)
- Exhaled air mass spectrometry for volatiles and chemical analysis (Phillips and others 2007).

Among the new diagnostic options that have emerged in recent years, the Xpert MTB/RIF test has received the most attention. Xpert MTB/RIF is an automated deoxyribonucleic acid (DNA) amplification test that provides rapid and sensitive detection of TB and rifampicin resistance. It uses a cartridge-based system that integrates sample processing and real-time polymerase chain reactions, accommodates use by relatively unskilled health care workers, and provides results in less than two hours. The system is expensive, costing about US$17,000 per unit, and the tests, currently subsidized, cost about US$10. The ability to diagnose TB and identify MDR TB from sputum in less than two hours is a major step forward in linking diagnosis to rapid initiation of treatment. However, Xpert MTB/RIF is currently not a technology for point-of-care diagnosis. In December 2010, the WHO recommended that the device be used for initial diagnosis in patients suspected of having MDR TB or HIV/AIDS-associated TB disease. Subsequently, some countries, including China, India, and South Africa, have purchased Xpert equipment at reduced prices and taken advantage of volume pricing to purchase test cartridges.

The Xpert system is a significant advance in accelerating the diagnosis of TB, particularly MDR TB, and will likely be a valuable new tool for major hospital and TB diagnostic laboratories, despite being dependent on a sophisticated and expensive device and relatively expensive costs for each sample tested. However, a multicenter trial in four African countries failed to demonstrate lower TB-related morbidity (Theron and others 2014). A new device model being developed, the GeneXpert Omni, which is portable and battery operated, has the potential to become a point-of-care diagnostic test in many more sites and is to be released later in 2017.

Since shortening the time between diagnosis and initiation of appropriate treatment is a major factor in reducing transmission, technologies that allow diagnosis and drug-sensitivity testing at the point of care are ideal. Some innovative research is under way to achieve that goal, but point-of-care testing remains a formidable challenge. Considering the sheer number of patients queued in busy outpatient departments, it is unlikely that cough screening and sputum testing can be effectively implemented in many of the highest-risk ambulatory settings—or in all resource-limited settings. Even the DNA amplification methods lack the sensitivity to detect many patients with early disease. Potentially infectious TB cases will be missed, delays in diagnosis will occur, and patients with XDR TB will likely not respond promptly to current therapy. Traditional methods of control will be necessary for the foreseeable future (WHO 2009a).

A recently developed molecular approach examining gene expression of peripheral blood cells rather than sputum has the potential to identify the subset of healthy individuals with latent TB who are likely to progress to active disease (Zak and others 2016). Rather than detecting components of the pathogen, this novel method measures gene expression signatures in peripheral white blood cells that are elevated in healthy individuals with latent infection prior to their progression to active TB. In a panel of 16 gene probes in three separate cohorts in different countries, it was possible to predict persons who progressed to active disease six months to one year before any symptoms could be detected clinically. At the one-year point prior to diagnosis, the specificity of the test was around 61 percent; in HIV-positive individuals, it was significantly higher, at around 80 percent. The molecular exploration of host responses offers new possibilities for diagnosing infection and defining the gene signatures of persons who do not progress to active disease, potentially enabling understanding of the genes required for resistance to disease. In a similar approach, gene expression in the whole blood of patients with either latent tuberculosis or other diseases versus patients with active tuberculosis was compared using a validated multicohort analytical framework. The diagnostic capacity of a three-gene set was found to be 88–90 percent in active and latent TB in samples from children and adults in 10 countries (Sweeney and others 2016). Such molecular host signatures could potentially serve as biomarkers for defining determinants of protection against infection or disease in future studies and vaccine trials.

TB TREATMENT

Treatment aims to cure the disease process, rapidly stop transmission, and prevent relapse (WHO 2006). Current treatment of tuberculosis requires multiple antibiotics, guided by predicted or demonstrated antibiotic susceptibility and taken for many months. Context-specific treatment guidelines are usually developed by local health authorities with guidelines and oversight from the WHO. Clinical trials in the twentieth century established current first-line drug regimens (Fox, Ellard, and Mitchison 1999; Mitchison 2004). Treatment success rates of 85 percent or more for new drug-sensitive cases are regularly reported to the WHO from a wide variety of clinical settings (WHO 2012a, 2015b).

Treatment effectiveness has been eroded, however, by the evolution and transmission of multidrug-resistant tuberculosis. Treatment for MDR TB, which is defined as resistance to isoniazid and rifampicin (the two most effective TB drugs) is longer and requires more expensive and more toxic drugs. For most patients with MDR TB, the current regimens recommended by the WHO last 18–24 months, and treatment success rates are much lower, around 60 percent. The WHO now conditionally recommends using seven drugs to reduce the time of treatment to nine months for uncomplicated pulmonary disease (WHO 2016b). New drug combinations, for example, including bedaquiline or delaminid, which are thought to act on new molecular targets, are being introduced, but an ideal combination is likely several years away (Villemagne and others 2012; Zumla, Nahid, and Cole 2013).

Patients who are effectively treated for tuberculosis usually show clinical response within 8–12 weeks, both subjectively (reduced cough, fatigue, fevers, and sweats; increased appetite) and objectively (sputum smear or culture conversion from positive to negative; weight gain) (WHO 2010). Failure to respond to treatment is typically due to poor drug quality, underdosing or malabsorption, nonadherence, drug resistance (which may broaden while on treatment), paradoxical reactions or immune reconstitution inflammatory syndrome (IRIS), adverse drug effects, or another disease process (bronchiectasis, malignancy, pneumoconiosis, autoimmune disease, or organ failure).

One of the embarrassing deficits in the field of TB control is the ambiguous definition of "cure." In the twenty-first century, it should be shocking that accurate biomarkers for treatment response, or in fact cure, are essentially nonexistent, as is the ability to predict relapses after treatment (Walzl and others 2008). Within clinical trials, cure is defined as no relapse after one year after completing therapy. In LMICs the general criterion of cure for individual patients is two negative sputum smears a month apart (WHO 2014b). Yet sputum smears are not sufficiently sensitive or precise to be certain that there is true sterilization of the infection. Bacterial culture, though more sensitive, is also more time-consuming and less frequently used in resource-poor countries (Phillips and others 2016). There are no microbiological or molecular biomarkers to establish whether an individual's infection has been sterilized by treatment. Recurrence can be due either to reactivation of a previously treated strain or to reinfection with a new strain. Reinfection in previously treated patients may be as common as relapse and can be distinguished from relapse by comparing mycobacterial DNA sequences from both the original isolate and the recurrence (Marx and others 2014).

Treatment Regimens

Effective tuberculosis treatment needs to overcome the organism's ability to persist in diverse microenvironments under extreme conditions, including immunological attack, prolonged antibiotic exposure, and nutrient and oxygen depletion (Islam, Richards, and Ojha 2012; Shaler and others 2013). Standardized treatment regimens and fixed-dose combination medications simplify good clinical care in resource-limited settings. Table 11.5 presents current treatment regimens, with an intensive phase followed by a continuation phase (Chakraborty and others 2013; Donald and McIlleron 2009; Shi and others 2011; WHO 2010, 2013b, 2016a, 2016b).

First-Line Treatment of Drug-Susceptible TB
Rifampicin and isoniazid are the most potent drugs for susceptible TB and are taken throughout the course of first-line treatment (Donald and McIlleron 2009; WHO 2010). Pyrazinamide synergistically reinforces the sterilizing activity of rifampicin and, when added to the first two months of treatment, reduces the duration of treatment to six months (Fox, Ellard, and Mitchison 1999; Hong Kong Chest Service and British Medical Research Council 1979). Ethambutol is added to the regimen for two months to reduce on-treatment development of drug resistance (WHO 2010) and is continued for the full duration of therapy in settings with high background prevalence of isoniazid resistance. As effective as standard treatment has been, resistance to isoniazid, rifampicin, and pyrazinamine is increasing in many countries, indicating that new regimens will need to be increasingly incorporated into TB treatment.

Second-Line Treatment of MDR TB
The treatment of drug-resistant TB is evolving, and recommendations are changing rapidly. Four factors make it difficult to arrive at clear, generalizable recommendations. First, individual strains vary in their susceptibility, and customized regimens might be more appropriate, when possible. Second, testing susceptibility to pyrazinamide and second- and third-line agents is neither widely available nor consistently reliable. Third, many agents have limited availability due to their cost or limited production. Finally, few comparative studies are available to provide data on which to make optimal treatment decisions.

While drug-resistant disease is curable, the cure rate in several studies is lower than for drug-sensitive disease. In some studies of MDR TB, only 54 to 70 percent of patients achieve treatment completion or cure (Ahuja and others 2012; Bassili and others 2013;

Table 11.5 Tuberculosis Treatment Regimens Currently Recommended by the WHO

Type of case and phase	Length of regimen (months)	Drug used
New tuberculosis case		
Intensive phase	2	Rifampicin, isoniazid, pyrazinamide, ethambutol
Continuation phase	4	Rifampicin, isoniazid (low risk of isoniazid resistance) or rifampicin, isoniazid, ethambutol (high risk[a] of isoniazid resistance)
Previously treated tuberculosis case (relapse or default)[b]		
Intensive phase	2	Rifampicin, isoniazid, pyrazinamide, ethambutol, streptomycin
Continuation phase	1	Rifampicin, isoniazid, pyrazinamide, ethambutol
	5	Rifampicin, isoniazid, ethambutol
Previously treated tuberculosis case (treatment failure)[c]		
Intensive phase	8	MDR TB regimen (see below)
Continuation phase	12	MDR TB regimen (see below)
MDR TB cases		
2010 guideline	20	Kanamycin (or amikacin), moxifloxacin[d] (ethionamide, cycloserine (or terizidone), pyrazinamide
Intensive phase	8	Bedaquiline or delamanid, where sensitivity following the initial regimen cannot be assured (up to six months)
Continuation phase	12	Moxifloxacin,[d] ethionamide, cycloserine, pyrazinamide
2016 short regimen (conditional recommendation)		
Intensive phase	4–6	Kanamycin, moxifloxacin,[d] prothionamide, clofazimine, pyrazinamide, high-dose isoniazid, ethambutol
Continuation phase	5	Moxifloxacin,[d] clofazimine, ethambutol, and pyrazinamide

Note: MDR TB = multidrug-resistant tuberculosis defined as resistance to isoniazid and rifampicin; WHO = World Health Organization.

a. Using local epidemiological data.

b. Low risk of MDR TB using local epidemiological data. The WHO recommends treatment guided by drug-susceptibility testing, especially rapid molecular tests, and suggests that standard first-line treatment be used if there is no evidence of drug resistance to isoniazid and rifampicin.

c. Defined as smear positive after five months of first-line treatment, relapse or default after second or subsequent course of treatment, or active tuberculosis after contact with an MDR TB case.

d. Or high-dose levofloxacin or gatifloxacin.

James and others 2011; Loveday and others 2012; Nathanson and others 2010). Treatment requires new drugs, with regimens containing anywhere from three to seven drugs that have not been previously employed (Mitnick and others 2008). In general, these second- and third-line agents are less potent and must be administered for a more extended period of time, ranging from 9 to 24 months. They are also more difficult to administer, as most regimens contain agents such as kanamycin and amikacin that must be administered by injection. These drugs are far more toxic than first-line agents, causing a range of drug-specific side effects. Nevertheless, it has been possible to achieve MDR TB cure rates of 60–80 percent irrespective of HIV/AIDS status in settings with severe resource constraints and patients with advanced disease (Meressa and others 2015; WHO 2016a).

Key strategies that have contributed to successful treatment include intensive management of adverse effects, nutritional supplementation, adherence interventions, and collaboration between the public health service and nongovernmental organizations (NGOs). These approaches should be routinely incorporated into programs wherever possible.

Generally, MDR TB has substantial human, economic, and social consequences (Rouzier and others 2010). The cost of treating MDR TB using conventional regimens ranges from US$2,500 to US$10,000, compared with US$100–US$1,000 for drug-susceptible TB cases (Floyd and others 2013), placing substantial costs on high-burden countries. For example, in South Africa, although MDR TB and XDR TB represent less than 3 percent of all TB cases detected, they consume an estimated 35 percent of the national health budget allocated to tuberculosis control (Pooran and others 2013). In some countries, the costs to treat MDR TB are estimated to exceed the total budget for TB control.

In May 2016, the WHO issued a conditional recommendation on use of the shorter MDR TB regimen, which would shorten the duration of treatment (to 9–12 months), increase adherence and retention in care, and lower costs (about US$1,000 in drug costs per patient) (WHO 2016a). Routine analysis of mutations conferring resistance to isoniazid may further inform the choice of MDR TB treatment: isolates with mutations in the promoter region of the *inhA* gene are susceptible to high-dose isoniazid but resistant to ethionamide, while those with *katG* mutations are resistant to high-dose isoniazid but sensitive to ethionamide (WHO 2016a).

Ongoing clinical studies are beginning to form the evidential basis for the WHO guidelines given in table 11.5, and are discussed in more detail in the section titled "Research and Development." In this rapidly changing area, encouraging data suggest that higher cure rates are possible, perhaps with shorter courses using newer agents (see the review by Zumla, Nahid, and Cole 2013). Bedaquiline and delamanid, two newly approved drugs, both lead to more rapid clearance of organisms and higher cure rates for MDR TB when administered with an optimized regimen. Similarly, the oxazolidinone antibiotic linezolid, which is used largely to treat Gram-positive infections, accelerates clearance and increases cure. Clofazimine, a riminophenazine dye used to treat leprosy, is now recommended for the shortened MDR TB regimen. These new treatments may cause significant side effects. Clofazamine may cause skin discoloration. For unclear reasons, bedaquiline therapy has been associated with a higher death rate, while linezolid produces a range of dose-limiting toxicities, including neuropathy and myelosuppression.

Treatment in Specific Situations

Regimens for treating tuberculosis in children are identical to those for adults. Correct dosing by weight is essential, and the most appropriate formulation of combination medications receives ongoing advocacy (WHO 2013c).

Tuberculosis in pregnancy can be treated with isoniazid, rifampicin, pyrazinamide, and ethambutol. Streptomycin, amikacin, and kanamycin may cause fetal ototoxicity and should not be used if possible (Donald 2016). The safety of other drugs used to treat MDR TB has not been well studied in pregnancy.

Treatment should be individualized, with expert review. Contraceptive advice during MDR TB treatment is essential.

Glucocorticoids may limit the inflammatory damage associated with tuberculosis (Critchley and others 2013). Evidence supports the use of glucocorticoids for tuberculous meningitis (Prasad and Singh 2008). Additionally, surgery may be necessary to improve the chance of cure by removing localized disease (Marrone and others 2013) and to decompress vital structures that are compromised by the tuberculous cavities.

A particularly devastating form of TB, tuberculous meningitis, has a rapid onset and is frequently fatal. Current treatments are less effective for TB meningitis, and higher doses of drugs may be needed to reach therapeutic levels in the central nervous system (Donald 2016).

Drug Toxicities and Interactions

Prompt detection and effective management of adverse drug effects is essential to the integrity of a treatment program. TB antibiotics, like other medications, may interfere with drug metabolism and excretion. Rifampicin potently induces expression of hepatic cytochrome P450 enzymes (McIlleron and others 2007), substantially reducing levels of several clinically important drugs including HIV/AIDS protease inhibitors, warfarin, phenytoin, carbamazepine, and estrogen-containing contraceptives. Antiretroviral drugs nevirapine and efavirenz interact with rifampicin; however, only the nevirapine interaction is clinically significant, and current recommendations are to use efavirenz with rifampicin. The newer drugs, bedaquiline and delamanid, which in small studies seem to be effective against MDR- or XDR-TB, increase the QT interval with a risk of arythmia, and linezolid has serious effects on bone marrow and neurologic function. Clinically significant interactions should be checked regularly online.[1]

Antiretroviral Therapy

In 2014, there were 10.4 million new cases of TB, of which 1.2 million (11 percent) were among people living with HIV/AIDS. Over the past 30 years, antiretroviral therapy for HIV/AIDS infection has improved to the point where effective therapy is widely available in LMICs, with strikingly improved mortality in patients co-infected with HIV/AIDS and tuberculosis (Khan, Minion, and others 2012).

Early initiation of ART reduces mortality risk in HIV-positive patients co-infected with tuberculosis and is therefore recommended, irrespective of CD4 count

(WHO 2013a). To reduce mortality risk, it should be commenced within two weeks of TB treatment.[2] The goal of ART is to achieve long-term viral load suppression assessed with regular viral load measurements. Cotrimoxazole prophylaxis for *Pneumocystis* pneumonia, toxoplasmosis, bacterial sepsis, and malaria reduces mortality in patients co-infected with TB and HIV/AIDS and should be given until the CD4 count recovers to above 200 cells per microliter after at least six months of ART.

One significant adverse effect of combined treatment is the development of IRIS, which is characterized by persisting or recurring fevers and a worsening of the focal tuberculous process (in profoundly immune-suppressed patients with CD4 count below 50 cells per microliter) starting combination ART shortly after commencing tuberculosis treatment (Meintjes and others 2008; Meintjes and others 2010). IRIS can usually be controlled with steroids and nonsteroid anti-inflammatory agents.

Antidiabetic Treatment

Diabetes is a significant risk factor for tuberculosis but has received less attention than HIV/AIDS in LMICs. This will likely change given the increasing life expectancy and prevalence of obesity and type 2 diabetes globally. All patients with tuberculosis should be screened for diabetes (Faurholt-Jepsen and others 2012; WHO 2011a). Diabetic patients should have their glucose control assessed regularly while on TB treatment as part of integrated clinical care, and treatment should be optimized with oral antidiabetic agents and insulins.

Surgery

With treatment outcomes for multidrug-resistant tuberculosis patients achieving only about 50 percent success, surgery, once a major tool in the pre-antibiotic era, has reemerged as an adjuvant therapeutic strategy. A systematic review and meta-analysis to assess the evidence for the effect of surgery as an adjunct to chemotherapy found that there was little substantial data on which to base recommendations, but there appeared to be some enhancement of successful outcomes from surgery on adults treated for MDR TB (Harris and others 2016).

Palliative Care

Tuberculosis remains a leading cause of death in LMICs. Suffering and the process of dying are important clinical consequences of advanced tuberculosis that should be detected and communicated by an experienced clinician who can initiate effective palliative treatment (Connor

and others 2012; Smart 2010). Terminally ill patients may decide to improve their quality of life by discontinuing tuberculosis treatment. Physical discomfort, psychological distress, and unresolved end-of-life social issues can all potentially be addressed by trained community health workers (CHWs) once the need has been identified. These structures need ongoing local support and advocacy (Harding and others 2012).

The Cascade of Care and Completion of Treatment

The DOTS strategy to control tuberculosis promotes standardized treatment, with supervision and patient support, which may include direct observation of therapy, where a health care worker personally observes the patient taking the medication (WHO 2013b). The scientific evidence on the effectiveness of DOT compared to self-administered therapy is mixed. Despite the galvanizing impact of the DOTS strategy in mobilizing support and treatment activities, a systematic comparison of the effectiveness of DOT relative to self-medication in 11 random control trials failed to establish its unique effectiveness in ensuring either compliance or cure (Karumbi and Garner 2015).

DOTS has been associated with reduced prevalence of drug resistance in the United States (Moonan and others 2011; Pasipanodya and Gumbo 2013); other HICs; and many LMICs, such as Cambodia, China, and Ethiopia (WHO 2014b, 2015b). However, in highly endemic countries, especially those burdened with HIV/AIDS, even where adequate diagnosis and effective treatment are provided, the strategy has not dropped incidence or transmission as much as needed. As discussed in the section on research and development, additional strategies will be needed where the forces of infection, environment, and HIV/AIDS are driving the infection rate, despite effective treatment of incident cases (Middelkoop and others 2015).

Some countries have experimented with involving community members to make treatment supervision more acceptable to individual patients (Datiko and Lindtjørn 2009), but the operational issues are substantial, and a meta-analysis after DOTS implementation that included community members in China found that 52 percent of patients still took self-administered therapy (Hou and others 2012). Nonadherent patients need to be identified early and offered practical interventions to assist their return into care (Toczek and others 2013; Yin and others 2012), including hospitalization for supervised treatment and physical rehabilitation. Clinic staff who know the patient and community are in the best position to decide which patients need the intense adherence support implicit in DOTS.

It is important to emphasize that early case detection, whether by passive or active case finding, is a necessary but not sufficient condition for effective control of TB. A recent analysis of the cascade of care of TB in India reveals the challenges of ensuring treatment completion (Subbaraman and others 2016). In this important study of about 2 million cases of conventional TB evaluated through the Revised National Tuberculosis Control Program, the authors created a framework and followed the cascade of care from the number of prevalent cases to those reaching TB diagnostic centers, those diagnosed with TB, those registered for treatment, those who completed treatment, and finally those with recurrence-free survival at one year. The results indicated for conventional TB that 45 percent completed treatment and 39 percent were disease free after one year. Of patients diagnosed with MDR TB, only 14 percent completed treatment and 11 percent remained disease free at one year. These striking results clearly indicate the critical need for support of treatment to enable greater treatment completion in India and most LMICs.

TB PREVENTION

There are three obvious strategies for preventing TB: vaccination, infection control, and chemoprophylaxis or isoniazid preventive therapy (IPT). Arguably, the most useful but perhaps least appreciated preventive intervention is simply the early diagnosis and rapid initiation of effective treatment of TB cases, thus reducing the infectious burden and reducing transmission. TB is unusual among infectious diseases, in that appropriate (and effective) treatment of the individual patient may be the most effective public health intervention to protect the population.

Vaccination: Natural and Acquired Immunity

BCG Vaccine
The most widely used vaccine in the world is BCG, which is given to about 100 million children annually. Isolated in 1908, following attenuation through 431 passages of a virulent *M. bovis* isolated from a human TB case, BCG was found to be protective to some extent in multiple animal models of TB. In its first human trial in 1921, it was found to protect a child heavily exposed in a household at high risk.

BCG has several advantages: it can be given at birth or at any time after birth; a single inoculation produces long-lasting skin test positivity to tuberculin; it is relatively stable; it produces a scar useful for epidemiological

surveillance of access to immunization; and it is inexpensive.

Considerable evidence indicates that giving BCG to young children is effective at preventing tuberculous meningitis and disseminated (miliary) TB (Mangtani and others 2014; Rodrigues, Diwan, and Wheeler 1993). Random control trials and case control studies have shown consistently high protective efficacy of BCG against serious childhood forms of disease (73 percent), meningitis, and miliary TB (77 percent). The most complete analysis of the effect of BCG vaccine suggests that giving BCG to children born in 2002 prevented about 29,000 cases of childhood meningitis and 11,500 cases of miliary TB during the first five years of life or one case of meningitis for every 3,400 vaccinated children and one case of miliary TB for every 9,300 vaccinated children (Trunz, Fine, and Dye 2006). A recent report indicates that deferring BCG immunization to six weeks after birth generates stronger and longer-lasting specific Th1 cellular immune responses (Kagina and others 2009; Lutwama and others 2014). In some countries, children were repeatedly vaccinated over time, and there is some evidence from Taiwan, China, that multiple vaccinations may increase protection (Chan and others 2013). A worrisome drawback, however, is the incidence of disseminated BCG infection in HIV-positive children (Hesseling and others 2007).

Successful vaccines ideally prevent both infection and disease among persons exposed to the pathogen. While it is generally believed that BCG protects against disease rather than infection, recent findings, using Interferon-Gamma Release Assays (IGRAs) that can distinguish Mtb infection from BCG vaccination, suggest that BCG may protect to varying degrees against infection as well (Eisenhut and others 2009; Mangtani and others 2014; Soysal and others 2005).

The cost-effectiveness of BCG was estimated in 2006 to be between US$40 and US$170 per disability-adjusted life year (DALY), US$8,000 and US$11,000 per life saved, or US$5,000 and US$8,000 per case averted (Dye 2006), making it a very cost-effective intervention.

Despite positive evidence regarding the impact of BCG on children, BCG remains the most controversial of all currently used vaccines, because its protective efficacy has varied widely in different parts of the world, from 77 percent protection in adolescents in the United Kingdom (Sutherland and Springett 1987) to 0 percent protection in all age groups in South India (Bloom 1994; Mangtani and others 2014). Because young children represent only a minor contributor to TB transmission, BCG immunization of infants has only a relatively small impact on transmission within populations (Knight and others 2014). This finding is borne out by outcomes in parts of Europe and North America that did not use BCG, where TB declined at rates that were not measurably different from those in regions that used the vaccine (Styblo 1991). In a recent analysis using South African data, Dye (2013) found that BCG vaccination would reduce TB in HIV-negative individuals by about 17 percent, to which would be added the value of preventing transmission to HIV-positive individuals. He estimated that revaccination with BCG would be highly cost-effective at all combinations of cost (US$1–US$10 per child) and efficacy (10–80 percent).

BCG immunization has also been shown to have extremely variable protective efficacy against adult TB in randomized trials and observational studies (Bloom and Fine 1994; Fine 1995; Mangtani and others 2014). Explanations for the variation remain unclear. Suggestions include the fact that BCG lacks more than 100 genes of Mtb, including some putative protective antigens; the genetic make-up of different human populations; the variable persistence of different BCG strains or preparations; and the interference by atypical mycobacteria in the environment. It was shown many years ago that guinea pigs immunized with different species of environmental atypical mycobacteria showed different degrees of protection against Mtb. Some, such as *M. kansasii*, were as effective as BCG in animals (Palmer and Long 1966). It is often forgotten that *M. microti*, a murine mycobacterium, was as effective as BCG in the British Medical Research Council human vaccine trials (Bloom and Fine 1994; Hart and Sutherland 1977). This suggests that, if exposure to environmental mycobacteria in a population provides some degree of protection, the effects of BCG observed in that population will be comparably less than in a naïve population. This could explain the large differences in BCG efficacy in populations living in different geographic locations (Weir and others 2006), where children in tropical latitudes show less protection (Mangtani and others 2014). For example, in the South India trial area, two-thirds of the individuals were positive to an *M. avium* purified protein derivative skin test by age 9 years and 97 percent were positive by ages 15–19 years (Tuberculosis Prevention Trial 1979). Understanding the degree of environmental exposure to nontuberculous mycobacteria will be important in planning and evaluating any new vaccines against TB.

A Rationale for Vaccines: Latent Infection Can Prevent Reinfection

It is widely believed that a protective vaccine is unlikely to be developed against TB because natural infection with Mtb is ineffective at preventing reinfection. However,

there is a remarkable amount of epidemiologic evidence that, in fact, Mtb latent infection does indeed provide significant protection against reinfection by engendering protective immune responses that likely persist (reviewed by Andrews and others 2012). Early experiments of Heimbeck (1938) in Norwegian nurses and Sutherland, Svandova, and Radhakrishna (1982) found that, among healthy young individuals, being TST-positive provided up to 80 percent protection against reinfection (ranging from 45 to 81 percent in multiple studies) compared to being TST-negative. In a more recent study from South Africa where it was possible to measure infections in the apparently uninfected group and to observe cases of tuberculosis directly, the estimated immunological protection conferred by latent TB infection was 79 percent (Andrews and others 2012). These results encourage the view that new vaccines with better efficacy than BCG could provide relatively high levels of protection, if the protective immune responses generated are sustained over time, as is the case of latent TB.

Innate Immune Responses

The body's immune response is critical in protecting against infection and disease, through both innate and acquired immunity. This is perhaps best exemplified by the fact that, although only 10 percent of persons infected with TB develop disease in their lifetime, immune-compromised individuals have a risk of almost 10 percent *per year* (Selwyn and others 1989). Immunodeficient individuals, such as persons infected with HIV/AIDS (Gandhi and others 2006) or receiving anti-TNF immunotherapy for autoimmune diseases (Wolfe and others 2004), have a markedly increased incidence of TB. In immune-compromised HIV-positive patients in KwaZulu-Natal, the mean time from diagnosis to death from XDR or drug-resistant TB was an astonishing 16 days (Gandhi and others 2006). And the increased prevalence of drug-resistant TB in immune-compromised individuals is consistent with the view that the effectiveness of antibiotics depends to some extent on the antimicrobial immune response. It is intriguing that a population of healthy contacts exists in high-burden countries, who almost certainly have been exposed repeatedly to infection yet remain TST-negative, IGRA-negative, and apparently healthy. This suggests that mechanisms of innate immunity may have the ability to kill the relatively small numbers of infecting tubercle bacilli early after respiratory infection even before they can grow to numbers able to sensitize and expand T-cells able to respond to TB antigens. These mechanisms are currently not understood, and greater research is needed.

Preventive Therapy

There are two approaches to preventive therapy. For HIV-positive individuals at high risk for many opportunistic infections, cotrimoxazole is recommended routinely, and in high-burden countries between 50 and 87 percent of HIV-positive patients are receiving this preventive therapy (WHO 2015b).

The major approach to prevent development of TB in persons at high risk, particularly household contacts and HIV-positive individuals, is to screen them with a TST and, ideally, to offer persons found to be HIV-positive chemoprophylaxis, most commonly IPT, for a latent infection (Rangaka and others 2015). In perhaps the most dramatic studies, a community-based trial of IPT among BCG-unvaccinated Alaska Eskimos, a community with a high risk of infection, produced a 60 percent decline in TB incidence that lasted more than two decades in treated households (Comstock, Baum, and Snider 1979). Overall in an analysis of randomized controlled trials, preventive therapy has clear benefits. In 2011, the WHO began recommending that HIV-positive individuals free of symptoms suggestive of tuberculosis receive treatment with IPT for at least six months (WHO 2011a). The risk of clinically active TB disease is reduced 60 percent in immunocompetent, HIV-negative individuals (Smieja and others 2000) and 32–62 percent in HIV-positive adults who are treated with preventive therapy lasting 3 to 12 months (Akolo and others 2010). Since these guidelines came into force, the number of HIV-positive people receiving IPT has increased sharply, rising to approximately 933,000 in 2014 (WHO 2015b). The high risk of TB among persons co-infected with *M. tuberculosis* and HIV/AIDS motivates those encouraging wider use of preventive therapy, especially in Africa (Stop TB Partnership 2011), but questions have been raised about the methods of screening to ensure that the persons most likely to benefit receive this treatment (Lawn and others 2012) and that the persons with subclinical TB are not inadvertently treated with isoniazid monotherapy that could lead to resistance. Studies among child contacts of active cases have demonstrated that giving isoniazid daily for 12 months provides 30–60 percent protection against active TB (Ayieko and others 2014). Recent work suggests that isoniazid can be continued for longer than six months in HIV-positive adults with minimal adverse effects and longer protection (den Boon and others 2016).

At a population level, a randomized trial in high-incidence urban communities in Brazil found that TB incidence was 15 percent lower in intervention than in nonintervention communities after five years (Cavalcante and others 2010). Yet IPT is not widely used. Of the highest-burden countries, only Brazil and South Africa have policies to scale up the use of IPT. Even with the resources available in the United States, the implementation of contact tracing and IPT has fallen short of recommendations (Lee and others 2006). In trials of IPT in high-burden countries, protection of TST-positive adults infected with HIV/AIDS averaged about 60 percent, but the effects were lost soon after the IPT treatment ended, and there was little or no impact on mortality (Churchyard and others 2012; Samandari and others 2011). By contrast, IPT was shown to reduce both TB incidence and mortality among HIV-positive children (Zar and others 2007). A randomized controlled trial, the Temprano study, compared early versus later treatment with ART and early versus later treatment with IPT and various combinations in 2,050 HIV-positive individuals with high CD4+ counts in Côte d'Ivoire. The results showed that six months of IPT resulted in a 44 percent lower risk of severe HIV/AIDS-related illness and a 35 percent lower risk of death from any cause than the risks with deferred initiation of ART and no IPT and that the combination reduced TB by 73 percent (Temprano ARNS Study Group 2015). Use of IPT for six months reduced the incidence of TB in Brazil not only for the duration of treatment but over a seven-year follow-up (Golub and others 2015). The strong inference from this work is that the combination of early initiation of both ART and IPT in HIV-positive individuals, now adopted by the WHO, should become the norm in HIV/AIDS and TB control.

Real challenges are associated with the use of IPT: active disease must be excluded, where practical by radiography, before isoniazid is taken alone, and adherence to six or more months of daily treatment tends to be poor among healthy people. Even in the United States, fewer than 50 percent of individuals who initiated IPT completed six months of treatment (Hirsch-Moverman and others 2015). Adverse effects include a risk of hepatitis, especially in persons co-infected with HIV/AIDS (Ayles and Muyoyeta 2006), if IPT is administered for long periods of time. In the United States, adverse effects are on the order of 1 percent but rise to 4 percent if IPT is given with rifapentine (Getahun and others 2015). A recent cluster randomized trial of mass screening and IPT was carried out for tuberculosis control among gold miners in multiple mines in Thibela in South Africa, a community known to be at high risk for TB. Miners were given IPT for 9 months, and the effect on prevention of disease was followed for 12 months. Despite the positive effect of isoniazid in preventing tuberculosis during the period of treatment, IPT had no significant sustained impact on TB control in South African gold mines (Churchyard and others 2014). Most discouraging, the results of a systematic review and meta-analysis of the cascade of care in latent TB indicated that completion of preventive treatment was only 19 percent (Alsdurf and others 2016).

It remains unclear, other than in the case of HIV-positive individuals and child household contacts, how feasible and cost-effective IPT scale-up would be in high-burden countries. It has been a challenge for health systems in LMICs, which are finding it difficult to provide treatment for diagnosed TB patients and to maintain IPT for healthy contacts. A recent approach to shortening preventive therapy derives from studies of a combination of long-acting rifapentine plus isoniazid, which reduced the time of treatment from nine to three months and was better tolerated, if more expensive (Sterling and others 2011).

The critical question of the best preventive therapy with which to combat MDR TB remains unsettled. The significant adverse effects of MDR TB regimens are a serious trade-off against prevention of the 10 percent of cases likely to result from preventive treatment, and no optimal regimen using newer drugs has been established (Moore 2016). The alternative is registering all such contacts, monitoring them carefully, and instituting treatment at the earliest sign of disease.

It may not be altogether fanciful to imagine, with advances in research, that more effective drug regimens for latent infection could have a profound effect on reducing the global burden of TB. It is unknown what proportion of the one-third of people on the planet exhibiting positive TST retain viable tubercle bacilli capable of reactivating and transmitting disease. But, if a practical drug regimen could sterilize the infection in all of these individuals, this enormous reservoir of the pathogen could be eliminated in a short period of time. Rather than passively detecting patients with disease, screening populations for persons who were infected as determined by tuberculin positivity and applying the hoped-for effective mycobactericidal regimen, the great burden of latent TB could conceivably be reduced or eliminated. This approach should be considered in future research.

Impact of Effective Treatment on Transmission

Of the interventions available to control transmission, it has long been taught that effective treatment ranks highest. Treatment can be applied only to known or suspected cases, and, to be effective, requires knowledge of drug resistance. It has traditionally been thought that, for drug-susceptible TB, at least two weeks of effective

treatment are required to reduce the risk of transmission substantially, regardless of sputum smear status (Rouillon, Perdrizet, and Parrot 1976). For drug-resistant TB, however, the two-week rule appeared to have failed as a policy during the outbreaks in New York City and Miami in the 1980s and 1990s, when patients with unsuspected drug resistance on conventional four-drug therapy transmitted their infection after isolation ended (Coronado and others 1993). Therefore, current guidelines generally recommend isolating MDR TB patients until smear or culture conversion.

The rate at which treatment renders tuberculosis cases noninfectious was recently reexamined, employing the classic model of transmission from humans to guinea pigs, wherein TB transmission was established by passing exhaust air from the ward past a panel of guinea pigs highly susceptible to TB (Dharmadhikari and others 2014). The study suggested that, like drug-susceptible TB, MDR TB transmission also responds rapidly to effective treatment, well before sputum smear or culture conversion (Dharmadhikari and others 2014). In a series of five exposure studies where mostly smear-positive, coughing patients with confirmed MDR TB were admitted and promptly started on therapy, transmission to guinea pigs appears to have occurred predominantly from patients with unsuspected XDR TB who were not responsive to effective treatment.

Infection Control of TB Transmission in Congregate Settings

Transmission and reinfection, especially of drug-resistant strains, is a key driver of the global TB epidemic (Wood, Lawn, Caldwell, and others 2011; Wood, Lawn, Johnstone-Robertson, and others 2011). The benefit of isoniazid prophylaxis in high-risk HIV-positive populations, for example, has been rapidly reversed by ongoing transmission and reinfection soon after isoniazid is stopped (Samandari and others 2011). Likewise, the challenge in high-transmission settings is to provide greater protection against reinfection than is currently provided by BCG immunization at birth as well as subsequent natural exposure to Mtb and environmental mycobacteria (Tameris and others 2013).

Transmission control was not specifically mentioned in the original Global Plan to Stop TB 2006–15, but the mostly hospital-based outbreak of XDR TB in 2006 dramatically called attention to the problem (Gandhi and others 2006). Since then, control efforts have centered on health care facilities, although it is widely understood that transmission also occurs in homes, schools, churches, shelters, refugee camps, and correctional facilities, among other congregate settings (WHO 2009b).

Still, because they specifically bring together infectious and vulnerable persons, health care facilities dominate the list of environments that amplify transmission at the population level.

Hospitals as Epicenters of Transmission

One key epicenter of transmission is hospitals where TB patients reside. Because hospital exposure is better documented than many other congregate interactions, there is a likely bias toward indicting hospitals, but it is also likely that hospital transmission is underestimated, for example, by not counting infecting strains for which DNA fingerprints are not available.

The significant reduction of the TB epidemic in New York City from 3,800 cases in the 1980s to 577 in 2015 indicates that multifaceted efforts are needed in large urban multicultural environments with large numbers of visitors, migrants, and homeless people and increasing rates of HIV/AIDS.[3] Clearly DOT was helpful in ensuring compliance in a portion of TB patients, but perhaps more significant was the major effort to institute infection control in hospitals, prisons, shelters, and congregate housing facilities (Frieden and others 1995).

Using network analysis, Gandhi and others (2013) concluded that most strain-specific XDR TB transmission in KwaZulu-Natal occurred in hospitals due to prolonged stay, congregate settings, and delayed recognition of drug resistance. Transmission patterns are similar as far away as Tomsk Oblast, Siberia. A retrospective study of the causes of drug resistance in the Tomsk Oblast showed a greater than sixfold higher risk among treatment-adherent patients hospitalized for drug-susceptible TB than among patients not hospitalized (Gelmanova and others 2007). Anyone familiar with treatment practices common to Eastern Europe will understand why this might occur. Although Tomsk predominantly uses ambulatory treatment for new TB cases, hospitalized patients are admitted to poorly ventilated, multibed rooms, tightly sealed against the cold. Drug susceptibility is normally only tested when patients fail to respond to first-line treatment, usually following months of ineffective treatment. Drug susceptibility testing by conventional methods requires additional months. During this prolonged period of ineffective treatment, there is ample opportunity for transmission and reinfection. This scenario is not unique to Tomsk, as delays in drug-susceptibility testing occur in most TB programs where laboratory services are inadequate. Treatment failure is the usual indication for drug-susceptibility testing, and molecular methods are only slowly reducing the time required for results on first-line and, much less often, second-line drugs. However, despite hospital transmission, ambulatory treatment is highly effective, and Tomsk is among the few high-burden places in the world where MDR TB rates may be declining (WHO 2010).

Principles of TB Transmission Control

Since the 1985–92 resurgence of TB in the United States and several European settings, where institutional transmission played an important role, a three-tiered hierarchical approach has been adopted, based on a paradigm used in industry: administrative controls, engineering (or environmental) controls, and personal protection (respirators). Administrative controls entail the rapid diagnosis of symptomatic, potentially infectious cases and drug resistance and the prompt initiation of effective therapy. This has recently been promoted under the acronym, FAST (Find cases Actively by cough surveillance, Separate temporarily, and Treat effectively), as a way to communicate the key components and facilitate adoption. Environmental controls have focused on natural and mechanical ventilation and on the evolving technology of sustainable ultraviolet germicidal (UVGI) air disinfection. Personal respiratory protection is the last tier of protection, assuming incomplete protection from administrative and engineering controls. Ironically, although the last tier of protection, respirators are often the only protection available to health care workers, cannot be worn continuously, and are unlikely to be worn when treating a patient with unsuspected TB.

Measures of the Efficacy of TB Transmission Control

Measuring the efficacy of transmission control interventions has been elusive. Among process indicators are questions regarding whether windows are open or respirators are available, although these factors may be tied too loosely to exposure to be useful. However, to the extent that undiagnosed TB patients and undiagnosed drug resistance are key exposure factors, process indicators tied to unprotected exposure time can be measured and reported. Institutions can document, for example, the percentage of admissions that are screened for cough and had sputum sent to a lab; the turnaround time from submission until results are obtained; and the time from admission until the onset of effective treatment based on drug-sensitivity testing. Such measures should become routine in hospitals with access to rapid diagnostic tests.

Few studies have been conducted not only of the efficacy of TB infection control methods, but also of their cost. Apart from the great difficulty of measuring the efficacy of interventions to prevent transmission, isolating the costs of infection control activities can be challenging, as many infection control interventions are integral to hospital functions more generally. Assuming the presence of unsuspected, untreated patients in the hospital, ventilation is a key intervention, and natural ventilation ranks high among recommendations in suitable climates. The added cost of designing and constructing a naturally ventilated patient waiting area is difficult to separate from the routine capital costs of hospitals. Some insights can be gleaned from unpublished data from a high-risk setting in Vladimir, Russia, a training center of excellence in TB control (box 11.4).

Cost-Effective Air Disinfection

Natural ventilation alone does not provide adequate ventilation for airborne infection control in many settings. However, mechanical ventilation systems are often prohibitively expensive and often fail due to lack of maintenance. Room air cleaners (with filters, UVGI, or both) are often sold to hospital administrators as a simple, inexpensive fix, but they rarely move enough air to achieve the 12 or more equivalent air changes per hour recommended to control airborne infections. Reentrapment and recirculation of the same air through the device (short-circuiting) also lead to low rates of effective clean air delivery.

As noted in the Vladimir study, upper-room germicidal UVGI (with room air-mixing fans) is among the most effective and least expensive ways to achieve high-volume air disinfection. Hospital studies have shown 70–80 percent efficacy. But like mechanical ventilation and room air cleaners, caution is required. Although they are under development, international standards and guidelines for safe and effective application and maintenance are not widely available. No agency currently regulates this small industry, and few experts are qualified to plan installations. Still, as back-up technology for natural ventilation, they are a logical choice. Low-velocity ceiling fans are recommended to assure essential room air mixing. With the development of LED (light-emitting diode) UVGI, the prospect of solar-powered systems with battery back-up may make upper-room germicidal UVGI more sustainable in the near future.

Masks and Respirators

Assuming incomplete efficacy of both source control and engineering or environmental control strategies, the last-tier intervention is respiratory protection—that is, use of a device designed to exclude infectious droplet nuclei from inhaled air.

Masks and respirators are easily confused. Surgical masks are designed to protect the environment by blocking the aerosolization of some portion of exhaled respiratory droplets and droplet nuclei, but they do not adequately protect the wearer and have a limited role in TB transmission control when worn short-term by patients. MDR TB patients wearing masks were 53 percent less likely to infect guinea pigs breathing exhaust air from the ward (Dharmadhikari and others 2012). Recently, using the same transmission model in South Africa, Mphaphlele and others (2015) tested the efficacy of several control interventions in preventing transmission from patients in hospital rooms to guinea pigs. The study confirmed the previous report and showed 70–80 percent efficacy of upper-room UVGI air disinfection.

Box 11.4

Real Costs of Infection Control in Vladimir Oblast TB Dispensary, Russia

Costs for high-level infection control are difficult to obtain. The TB Dispensary, with assistance from the Centers for Disease Control and Prevention, has over the past decade painstakingly introduced and studied the impact of a variety of conventional and novel TB infection control interventions in Vladimir Oblast, an area with high rates of TB and drug resistance. For the entire Vladimir region (population 1.5 million), accurate estimates of annual cost are US$350 for health care worker training; US$12,000 for ventilation system maintenance; US$10,000 for respirators; US$300 for respirator fit testing; and US$3,000 for health care worker screening. For the multistory hospital, with floor area of 17,000 cubic meters, the capital cost of a new, high-capacity ventilation system with negative-pressure isolation rooms was US$345,000, and the cost of maintenance was US$4,425 per year. Of three ventilation systems studied, the upper-room UVGI system was the least expensive intervention, at US$14 per equivalent-room air change, more than nine times more cost-effective than expensive mechanical systems per equivalent-room air change.

In contrast, respirators are designed to protect the wearer. Properly fitted, certified N-95 (or equivalent) respirators can be 85–90 percent protective. However, as an intervention, respiratory protection often fails either because the face seal leaks due to improper fit or adjustment or, more important, because the masks are not worn consistently. The cost of respirator programs is easily assessed, but their effectiveness is not.

Lessons for Household Transmission

Since TB is transmitted largely by aerosol droplets, transmission is affected by the built household environment. One study from South Africa found evidence that transmission of infection was greater, as determined by DNA fingerprinting of the strains, in modern-built brick housing with windows than in older shacks (Wood and others 2010). The reason may be that residents in modern housing kept windows closed in an effort to maintain cleanliness, whereas shacks simply had more ventilation. Another study measured the effects of increasing natural ventilation in traditional housing and demonstrated that natural ventilation was facilitated by opening doors and windows and extrapolated that such a change could potentially reduce the risk of household transmission by 80 percent (Lygizos and others 2013).

TURNING THE TIDE AGAINST TB

Despite the progress made in TB control over the past two decades, serious gaps persist. Although TB can be treated and cured, it is still one of the deadliest infectious diseases in the world today.

Three key elements are needed to achieve effective TB control and to meet the Sustainable Development Goals: (1) early and accurate diagnosis and drug-sensitivity testing, (2) patient access to and completion of effective treatment, and (3) prevention of progression from latent infection to disease. Obviously, these categories are not distinct; each affects and is related to the others, and all face both technical and system challenges. Without greater effectiveness of these key elements, it will not be possible to bend the curve and dramatically reduce transmission and incidence rates in all countries. Turning the tide against TB therefore requires investing in new technologies—diagnostics, treatment regimens, and vaccines—and tackling the system and strategic challenges that influence the degree to which technological advances reach the people who need them and translate into better heath.

Earlier Diagnosis: Toward Active Case Finding

Limitations of Passive Case Finding

Even with modern technology, effective case detection in resource-poor communities with weak health systems has been difficult to introduce (Kranzer and others 2010; Kranzer and others 2013). The principal paradigm for diagnosing cases of TB is passive case finding, which depends on the TB-infected individual seeking medical care. But passive case finding faces many challenges. TB is most prevalent in marginalized communities that are less visible to conventional health systems. Patients are typically poor, from disadvantaged groups, prone to other diseases such as HIV/AIDS and diabetes that increase their vulnerability to TB, and often migrants. Even when symptoms are present, in many countries, up to a third of TB patients either fail to seek treatment or do so from traditional healers before seeking medical treatment, leading to more severe illness, delayed treatment, and increased transmission (Brouwer and others 1998; Sreeramareddy and others 2014).

TB control is premised fundamentally on the assumption that, if active TB cases are identified and treated, transmission will be diminished and ultimately interrupted. The issue of unsuspected cases is, however, a serious problem that has received very little attention. Traditional guidelines tend to focus on known or suspected cases with classic symptoms and active disease. However, some forms of TB, such as asymptomatic and chronic tuberculosis, do not present with clinical symptoms for months or years and can transmit infection over extended periods of time.

Evidence strongly indicates that the problem of unsuspected or asymptomatic cases of TB and unsuspected cases of drug resistance is significant, contributing to the one-third of TB patients being "unknown to the health system." These patients are capable of transmitting disease but not ill enough to seek care or to be detected by passive case finding. In a teaching hospital in Lusaka, Zambia, for example, 900 newly admitted patients (70.6 percent HIV-positive) who were able to produce sputum without induction were screened. Testing by fluorescent microscopy and automated liquid culture detected TB in 22 percent of patients, of which 13.4 percent were unsuspected (Bates and others 2012). This number included 18 MDR TB cases, 5 of which were unsuspected. In the same hospital, 94 patients with cough, who were admitted primarily for obstetric or gynecological indications (73.4 percent HIV-positive), had sputum processed in the same way; in addition, Xpert MTB/RIF was used for rapid diagnosis (Friedich and others 2013). TB was diagnosed in 28 percent of the

94 sputum specimens, of which the Xpert device detected 80.8 percent compared to 50 percent by standard smear microscopy. Results of this kind are not new: similar results were reported more than a decade ago in a low-HIV/AIDS setting in Lima, Peru, where 250 of 349 consecutive new admissions to a female general medical ward were screened for TB by sputum smear, culture, and radiographs. Of these, 16 percent had culture-proven TB, one-third of which were unsuspected, including 6 unsuspected MDR cases (Willingham and others 2001).

The DOTS strategy in high-burden countries, even when implemented more effectively, will simply not be sufficient to overcome the challenge of unsuspected cases or drug resistance. In a groundbreaking population-based active case finding survey of HIV/AIDS and TB in Sub-Saharan Africa, where the population has a 23 percent prevalence of HIV/AIDS infection, Wood and others (2007) found that, despite a highly effective DOTS TB control program with high rates of compliance, 63 percent of adult cases with pulmonary TB were not known to the health system. Among HIV-negative individuals, passive case finding identified 67 percent of prevalent smear-positive cases, the target recognized for adequate DOTS implementation. But among individuals with HIV/AIDS infection, passive case finding identified only 33 percent of those with smear-positive TB.

Similar findings were obtained in a large survey of 47,000 individuals in Cambodia, in which 12 percent of individuals were examined clinically and sputa were tested by smear and by culture. Only one-third of TB cases were detected by sputum smears. Importantly, 44 percent of the sputum-positive cases and 23 percent of the smear-negative culture-positive cases exhibited none of the signs of clinical tuberculosis (Mao and others 2014). A surprising demographic finding was that people over age 50 years accounted for more than half of all detected infections, a trend evident in other Asian countries.

Clearly, in many parts of the world where the burden of TB is low and control programs have been effective, the need for active case finding is not great, and cost-effectiveness would argue against recommending it. However, in high-burden communities, passive case finding fails to detect early and asymptomatic cases, leaving a third of TB patients not known to the health system.

Active Case Finding: What Does the Evidence Show?

Active case finding—mass screening and surveillance—almost certainly contributed to the rapid decline of TB in European countries and the Americas (5–8 percent a year) following World War II—that is, prior to the introduction of antibiotics (Dye 2015; Golub and others 2005). In 1974, the WHO recommended discontinuing active case finding with radiography, since it was no longer necessary or cost-effective in populations with low prevalence of TB and good access to high-quality health care, particularly in HICs. The WHO reiterated this policy in 2014, again finding that it would not be cost-effective, and recommended that indiscriminate mass screening be avoided (WHO 2013c). However, it did recommend systematic screening for active TB in geographically defined subpopulations with extremely high levels of undetected TB (1 percent prevalence or higher). Regrettably, this WHO recommendation has not been sufficiently emphasized to stimulate countries and donors to initiate and support active case finding in high-burden countries or to have an impact on transmission in those countries.

One strategy for active case finding has been to use X-radiography, particularly mobile X-ray units, to detect lung lesions with computer-assisted detection in people who are relatively asymptomatic (Melendez and others 2016; Philipsen and others 2015). This strategy is able to detect many more patients with infection than is possible through passive case finding, screening for coughs, or self-reporting. In South Africa, for example, the only period in which incidence of TB cases declined occurred between 1950 and 1975, when X-ray surveillance captured about 10 percent of the population annually (R. Wood, personal communication). While in Europe and North America TB control programs dramatically reduced the annual risk of infection in successive cohorts (Cauthen, Pio, and ten Dam 2002), such a decline has not occurred in countries with high prevalence of TB and HIV/AIDS (Kritzinger and others 2009).

In recent studies in Kenya, abnormal chest radiography had high sensitivity (94 percent) and reasonable specificity (73 percent) for detecting tuberculosis (van't Hoog and others 2012). Radiography represents a potentially valuable population-based screen to determine which individuals should have their sputum tested by culture or by an Xpert device for definitive diagnosis. With rapid technical developments, computerized reading of X-radiograms could allow high-throughput screening of larger numbers of individuals in a cost-effective way (see box 11.5). This is particularly true when combined with clinical symptoms, where it was found that a sensitivity of 95 percent and negative predictive value of 98 percent could be achieved. (Melendez and others 2016).

Active Case Finding in Targeted Regions

In many LMICs, patients with TB often seek care from one or more traditional providers before seeking

Undetected Cases in Hospitals: The Case of FAST

TB infection control needs to focus on prompt screening of admitted patients with chronic cough. This concept has been formulated into a transmission control strategy called FAST (Find cases Actively by cough surveillance, Separate temporarily, and Treat effectively).

Several pilot FAST projects have begun around the world, including in Bangladesh and Russia. In a TB hospital in Veronesh, Russia, of almost 1,000 patients hospitalized with suspected pulmonary TB, 93.5 percent were tested by Xpert MTB/RIF within two days of admission. Of these, 407 were positive, and 161 were rifampin-resistant, of whom 159 received MDR TB treatment within three working days of receiving the result. Under normal operating conditions, treatment failure would have been

identified months after admission, and drug-susceptibility testing would have taken several more months, during which time, other patients and staff would have been exposed. FAST, in other words, was a dramatic improvement from the status quo.

Similar results are being obtained in a pilot study at the National Institute of Diseases of the Chest Hospital (NIDCH), a 680-bed facility in Dhaka, Bangladesh. Because respiratory symptoms are common in patients admitted to NIDCH, a decision was made to conduct universal sputum sampling. Of the TB cases identified, 13 percent were unsuspected and an additional 1.3 percent were infected with MDR TB. Diagnoses were available within one to two days of collection, and treatment was initiated within one day of a confirmed diagnosis.

---

medically appropriate care (Satyanarayana and others 2011). Even symptomatic surveillance for classic signs of TB—cough, fever, and weight loss—fails to detect a substantial number of cases, especially in persons who are HIV-positive (Corbett and others 2010).

In cluster randomized trials in Brazil, intensified case finding had a significant impact on reducing TB (Cavalcante and others 2010). The WHO commissioned several studies on the effectiveness and acceptability of active case finding or systematic screening of active TB (WHO 2013d). The studies reported that active case finding was highly acceptable to populations in Sub-Saharan Africa.

In a recent review of undiagnosed TB that would not be found by passive case finding, Yuen and others (2015) found that it is precisely in high-risk populations, as well as in persons infected with HIV/AIDS, where intensive case finding and early initiation of treatment or preventive therapy would likely have the greatest impact for the fewest resources.

In another study in South Africa (Shapiro and others 2012), a group of 2,800 individuals in households with a detected TB index case were enrolled to determine community prevalence of undetected TB and HIV/AIDS. Field teams screened participants for TB symptoms, collected sputum specimens for smear microscopy and culture, and provided HIV/AIDS

counseling and testing. They found that 6,075 per 100,000 of the household contacts were sputum-positive compared with 477 residents of random households without an index case. This finding demonstrated the value of screening contacts of index cases in a high-burden area and cautioned against random screening of total populations. Of the 169 previously unidentified cases with TB detected by culture, only 6 percent were found to be sputum-positive, and only 11 percent were symptomatic; the remaining 89 percent would not have been diagnosed with passive case finding.

However, the evidence is mixed. In a large, complex community randomized trial, the Zamstar study (Ayles and others 2013), 64,000 individuals in Zambia and the Western Cape, South Africa, were surveyed for TB symptoms, sputa were taken for identifying individuals with disease, and one arm employed enhanced household active case finding with counseling. Clearly, screening households with index cases revealed a greater number of TB cases. The adjusted ratio for prevalence and the adjusted ratio for incidence did not differ significantly for the enhanced case finding versus usual practice or for the household versus nonhousehold groups. The study identified no evidence that enhanced case finding had an effect on the burden of tuberculosis at the community level. However, despite not reaching statistical significance, the findings suggested that the household intervention did reduce the burden of tuberculosis in these communities.

A meta-analysis of controlled studies found that screening increased the number of cases found in the short term and tended to find cases earlier and with less severe disease (Kranzer and others 2013). Treatment outcomes among people identified through screening were similar to outcomes among people identified through passive case finding. Once again, this analysis confirmed that, in many settings, more than half of the prevalent TB cases remain undiagnosed.

A recent transmission modeling study of TB in South Africa suggested that the current DOTS approach of passive case finding is unlikely to permit the country to reach the WHO targets for 2050. The model predicts that interventions such as active case finding, with early initiation of treatment and reduction of pretreatment loss to follow-up, could have a large impact (Knight and others 2015). Thus, defining the high-burden target populations where active case finding is likely to be most effective is an important analysis to be undertaken.

Although most official data on TB incidence and prevalence are estimated for entire countries, a recent innovative epidemiological approach asked whether high-burden regions within countries—TB hot spots—might lend themselves to targeted control efforts. Such hot spots have been identified in a few countries, such as Moldova, and it will be of interest to learn whether targeted control efforts can improve their effectiveness at lower cost than the usual countrywide programs (Dowdy and others 2012; Jenkins and others 2013; Manjourides and others 2012; Zelner and others 2016). These population experiments for TB control need to be supported and evaluated.

We therefore recommend identifying countries and high-risk populations that are not responding effectively to the standard DOTS strategy and designing targeted active case finding interventions that could have a greater impact on earlier case detection and successful treatment.

Initiating active case finding interventions in high-burden countries will clearly require external financial assistance. Nevertheless, given the limitations of current tools and increasing threat of MDR TB, active case finding may be the best strategy for reducing incidence and prevalence in the long run in high-burden areas. And although active case finding is more expensive than passive case finding, added costs will be more than offset by the diagnostic and treatment costs averted—that is, TB transmitted in the hospital and in the community by unsuspected cases, especially MDR TB cases. The questions of how much screening, in what

places, and at what cost need to be answered if we are to avert each additional case of drug-susceptible or MDR TB. If interrupting transmission and reducing incidence more rapidly is the goal, the evidence suggests that active case finding targeted to high-burden areas can make a difference.

Community-Based, Integrated Delivery of TB Care

Service delivery—from screening and diagnosing patients to administering treatment and monitoring progress—is a key challenge in TB control, as with other health care services (Farmer 2013; Kim, Farmer, and Porter 2013).

Dominance (and Costs) of Hospital-Based Care

The costs of health service delivery are the largest cost of tuberculosis control. While the mean costs of diagnostics and tests do not vary significantly across income groups, the costs of drugs and hospitalization do (Laurence, Griffiths, and Vassall 2015), particularly the costs of treatment (WHO 2013b, 2014b, 2016a). For example, the costs per patient of drug-sensitive TB treatment were US$14,659 in HICs, US$840 in upper-middle-income countries, US$273 in lower-middle-income countries, and US$258 in LICs, with strong positive correlation with income (Laurence, Griffiths, and Vassall 2015). However, the mean costs of treating drug-susceptible TB were highly variable in countries at the same income level (Floyd and others 2013; Laurence, Griffiths, and Vassall 2015).

Hospitalization accounts for an average of 74 percent of all drug-susceptible TB costs (although this varies widely between individual studies) and 64 percent of all MDR TB costs. Conversely, mean costs of outpatient treatment were 12 times less than hospitalization costs, accounting for 6 percent of total costs. In one study, in the LMIC group, India consistently had the lowest costs for hospitalization and Ukraine had the highest costs for hospitalization and outpatient care (Laurence, Griffiths, and Vassall 2015). In Ukraine, high hospitalization costs, where patients also incurred costs, led to treatment default (Vassall and others 2009). In 2013, in countries with a high burden of TB and MDR TB (excluding China and Russia), almost 38 percent of funding (US$919 million) was allocated to hospital inpatient and hospital outpatient care of drug-susceptible TB (WHO 2013b). In addition, in 2013 Russia spent US$1.6 billion on TB control, most of which went toward hospital-based TB care (Atun, Samyshkin, and others 2006). However, funding allocated to neglected high-transmission areas, such as prisons, remains woefully low (Lee and others 2012).

Efficient and effective delivery of health services for TB is critical for improving TB outcomes globally. Yet, the delivery of TB services is inefficient and ineffective due to the high reliance on hospital services and the vertical delivery of DOTS (Atun, Samyshkin, and others 2006; Atun, Weil, and others 2010; Samb and others 2009). For example, from 2008 to 2010 in most of the world's 22 high-burden countries, the average cost of treating a patient with drug-susceptible TB was US$100–US$500. However, the average costs varied from US$100 to US$10,000 when Russia (a hospital-based service delivery model) was included (Floyd and others 2013).

In 2014, in most of the 22 high-burden countries for drug-susceptible TB, the WHO estimated that the share of hospital inpatient and outpatient costs ranged from 30 to 60 percent, with durations of stay ranging from 5 to 56 days (WHO 2014b). In the 22 high-burden TB countries, the costs of hospital inpatient and outpatient care for managing drug-susceptible TB as a proportion of the national TB program budget were 1–10 percent in the Democratic Republic of Congo, Ethiopia, Tanzania, Thailand, and Uganda; 11–20 percent in Bangladesh, Kenya, Myanmar, and Pakistan; and in excess of 40 percent in India (46 percent), Mozambique (51.8 percent), and Vietnam (74.2 percent) (WHO 2013b). While the WHO report did not have data for China and Russia, earlier studies suggested that, in Russia, where drug-susceptible TB is treated predominantly in hospitals, patients are kept under observation long after treatment completion; as a result, hospital inpatient costs account for around 60 percent of the total costs of treatment (Atun, Samyshkin, and others 2006). It is difficult to understand why China has shifted most TB care from outpatient to hospital-based care.

In South Africa, which has the second-highest number of confirmed cases of MDR TB (WHO 2011b) and the highest number of confirmed cases of XDR TB, MDR TB accounts for only 3.5 percent of the TB disease burden, but absorbs almost half of the US$218 million national TB program budget (WHO 2011c). Patients with MDR TB are hospitalized from the initiation of treatment until culture conversion, and the cost per patient of treating MDR TB was US$17,164, more than 40 times the cost of treating drug-susceptible TB (Schnippel and others 2013), which was estimated to be US$314–US$392 for community-based treatment (Sinanovic and others 2003). Around 95 percent of these costs were hospitalization costs (Schnippel and others 2013). More recent studies in South Africa have put the cost of inpatient treatment of MDR TB at US$6,772 (compared with treatment of drug-susceptible TB at US$256), with estimates suggesting that 45 percent of total costs are hospitalization costs (Pooran and others 2013).

The cost situation in South Africa is similar to that observed in countries where drug-susceptible and MDR TB are treated as inpatient care, such as Estonia (US$10,880) and Russia (Tomsk region, US$14,657). These high costs contrast with the lower costs recorded in countries where MDR TB is managed in outpatient clinics and at home—for example, Peru (US$2,423) and the Philippines (US$3,613). In Estonia and Russia, hospital costs accounted for 43 and 52 percent, respectively, of the total cost of treating an MDR TB patient (Fitzpatrick and Floyd 2012). Estimates suggest that the global average cost per patient of treating MDR TB is US$13,259 (5th–95th percentiles US$2,797–US$42,040) using an outpatient model and US$34,599 (5th–95th percentiles US$6,959–US$109,154) using an inpatient model (Fitzpatrick and Floyd 2012).

High hospital costs crowd out funding for cost-effective interventions, such as those aimed at addressing the social determinants of health, as well as new diagnostics and medicines that could be delivered in the community or in primary care settings.

Worldwide, there is substantial variation in the cost of treating patients using DOTS. Among the 22 high-burden countries, the cost per successfully treated patient varies from less than US$100 to more than US$10,000 for a standardized treatment. Even in countries with similar per capita income levels, the cost per successfully treated patient varies 50-fold (Floyd and others 2013). According to recent cost-effectiveness studies, the cost of treating one MDR TB case ranges from nearly US$15,000 in a hospital-based program in Tomsk, Siberia, to US$2,400 in a community-based program in Lima, Peru (Fitzpatrick and Floyd 2012).

The failure to prioritize MDR TB adequately or to achieve adequate cure rates is a major problem exemplified by the situation in two large countries. In India, the MDR TB cure rate is about 11 percent (Subbaraman and others 2016). In China, only about 5 percent of MDR patients are being treated, and the policy is formulated entirely around hospital-based treatment, with high relapse rates after discharge (Zhao and others 2012).

Efficiency and Effectiveness of Community-Based TB Treatment

A great deal of evidence points to the effectiveness of transitioning hospital-based TB care to primary health care settings (Edginton 1999) and to community-based models (Ayles and others 2013; Binagwaho 2013; Cavalcante and others 2007; Cavalcante and others 2010; Corbett and others 2010; Islam and others 2002; Shapiro and others 2012), even for management of MDR TB (Fitzpatrick and Floyd 2012; Furin and others 2011; Heller and others 2010; Luyirika and others 2012;

Mitnick and others 2003; Mukherjee and others 2002; Nathanson and others 2006; Seung and others 2009; Smart 2010). In addition to clinical effectiveness and improved outcomes, community-based models appear to be more acceptable to patients (Horter and others 2014).

A recent community-based model for providing TB treatment was developed in Bangladesh by BRAC, the world's largest NGO (Islam and others 2002; Islam and others 2011). Individuals diagnosed with tuberculosis are given free treatment but asked to provide a small bond, equivalent to about US$3.25, to assure that they will complete treatment. Upon successful completion of treatment, the funds are returned. The treatment cost per patient was US$312 in 2010. For patients unable to afford the bond, the community acts as underwriter, which establishes a social incentive to complete treatment. Program cure rates are up to 92 percent, which is comparable to a government-run program, yet the costs of the community-based program are half those of a public program (Islam and others 2002).

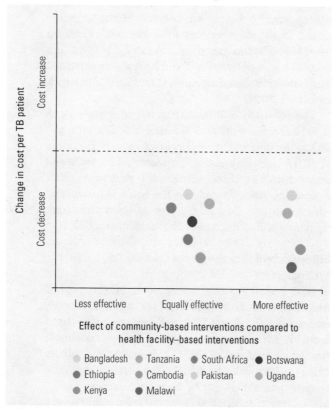

Figure 11.5 Cost-Effectiveness of Community-Based Interventions Compared to Health Facility–Based Interventions for Tuberculosis Treatment in Select Countries

Note: TB = tuberculosis.

Several countries transitioning from hospital-based services to primary health care or community settings have improved quality and outcomes of TB care—for example, Haiti (Farmer and others 1991), Latvia (Leimane and Leimans 2006), Moldova (Soltan and others 2008), Romania (Marica and others 2009), and Zambia (Miti and others 2003). Ethiopia has introduced the use of health extension workers to scale up access to primary health care services, including TB services, with improved compliance and treatment outcomes (Bilal and others 2011; Datiko and Lindtjørn 2009, 2010), and employed village outreach programs in rural settings (Shargie, Mørkve, and Lindtjørn 2006). Similarly, India has engaged urban community volunteers to supervise DOTS (Singh and others 2004). South Africa and Tanzania have used CHWs to expand access to TB services (Sinanovic and others 2015; Wandwalo and others 2004), and Rwanda has achieved effective community-based treatment (Binagwaho and others 2014). In addition to community-based care, a public-private mix with NGOs has been used in India, South Africa, and beyond to expand access to TB services and improve outcomes (Lal and others 2011; Pantoja, Floyd, and others 2009; Sinanovic and Kumaranayake 2006; Wells, Uplekar, and Pai 2015).

In the case of drug-susceptible TB, early indications are that outpatient treatment in the community is not poorer than hospitalized care (Bassili and others 2013; Loveday and others 2012). Although current guidelines recommend isolating MDR TB patients until smear or culture conversion, community-based treatment of drug-resistant TB is growing in acceptance due to its cost-effectiveness and a shortage of long-term hospital beds—for example, in South Africa (Brust and others 2012).

The benefits of transitioning facility-based services to community-based care are substantial. In six studies, where outcomes between community-based and health facility–based TB care were similar, the costs of community-based care were 33 to 70 percent lower (figure 11.5). In the four countries where the treatment outcomes in community-based TB care and health facility-based TB care were better, costs were 32 to 77 percent lower.

Community-based DOTS in Tanzania reduced costs 35 percent: from US$203 per patient treated at a health center to US$128 per patient treated in the community, with almost identical treatment outcomes. This program reduced costs by lowering the number of visits to the clinic (Wandwalo, Robberstad, and Morkve 2005). In Malawi and Kenya, moving to a community-based model reduced costs even more: 67 and 77 percent, respectively (Floyd and others 2003; Nganda and others 2003) (table 11.6).

Table 11.6 Costs and Effectiveness Comparing Community-Based Tuberculosis Care to Health Facility–Based Tuberculosis Care

Study	Study country	Community cost (2012 US$)	Health facility cost (2012 US$)	% difference in cost per patient	Effectiveness of community-based care vs. health facility–based care
Islam and others 2002	Bangladesh	172.80	259.20	33	Similar
Wandwalo, Robberstad, and Morkve 2005	Tanzania	216.10	331.90	35	Similar
Dick and Henchie 1998	South Africa	1,296.10	2,073.10	37	Similar
Moalosi and others 2003	Botswana	5,135.90	8,543.40	40	Similar
Datiko and Lindtjørn 2010	Ethiopia	138.00	332.70	59	Similar
Pichenda and others 2012	Cambodia	639.30	2,131.10	70	Similar
Khan, Khowaja, and others 2012	Pakistan	320.83	471.16	32	Higher
Okello and others 2003	Uganda	796.52	1,405.63	43	Higher
Nganda and others 2003	Kenya	752.65	2,250.51	67	Higher
Floyd and others 2003	Malawi	1,040.94	4,477.99	77	Higher

Human Resource Challenges to Community-Based Care

Despite the evidence, many countries have not transitioned to community-based models of service delivery for TB. Barriers to adoption of innovative models of care delivery are often related to health system governance, organization, and financing, in particular (external and domestic) financing flows that reinforce vertical programing; provider payment systems that allocate large proportions of the budget to structures and inputs (hospitals and hospital activities), rather than health outcomes; and a health workforce that lacks suitable skills (in particular, trained CHWs who underpin community-based service delivery). A general reluctance to adopt innovations may also impinge the move to community-based models, including public-private partnerships, which in several countries have helped to improve outcomes while lowering costs (Atun, de Jongh, and others 2010; Atun, Lazarus, and others 2010; Atun, McKee, and others 2005; Atun and others 2012; Howitt and others 2012; Khan, Khowaja, and others 2012).

Both active case finding and community-based TB delivery models require a competent, motivated health workforce, both at health facilities and in communities. Following patient diagnosis, treatment must be adhered to, and factors that drive patient adherence to medication are complex and relate both to patients' willingness and ability to seek health care and their experiences within the health system (Munro and others 2007; Podewils and others 2013). Clinic staff with limited resources need to provide accurate information to their patients and make it easy for patients to access and take good-quality treatment consistently until cured.

Inadequate human resource capacity remains an important health system barrier for TB control (Figueroa-Munoz and others 2005; Harries and others 2005), especially for MDR TB, which requires longer and more complex interventions than drug-susceptible TB (Keshavjee and Farmer 2010). Several factors, such as weak planning, absolute shortage of health staff, limited training, inadequate skills, lack of incentives to motivate and retain staff, and inappropriate distribution of the available health workforce, have contributed to the human resource crisis confronting global efforts to contain TB (Awofeso, Schelokova, and Dalhatu 2008; Buchan and Dal Poz 2002; Caminero 2003).

While community-based TB treatment certainly requires initial investments, including training, supervision, and management of CHWs, the initial investment is generally offset in the long run by savings accrued from community-based treatment rather than hospital care (Wandwalo, Robberstad, and Morkve 2005).

Private Sector Challenges

Some high-burden countries, such as India, have health care systems in which private sector rather than public sector care predominates. In India, about 75 percent of health care is provided by the private sector, most often based on OOP payments (Pai, Daftary, and Satyanarayana 2016). A high proportion of providers in many countries are not medically trained, and appropriate care is often not provided (Udwadia, Pinto, and Uplekar 2010). Patients with TB often seek care initially from private providers and may consult three to five providers before receiving a correct diagnosis of TB, which delays the average time to initiate treatment to 60–66 days (Satyanarayana and others 2011; Sreeramareddy and others 2014).

In studies using surrogate patients presenting to physicians with cardinal TB symptoms, correct diagnosis by physicians may be as low as a third (Das and others 2015), and surveying physicians for how they would treat a new patient diagnosed with TB revealed that no more than a third recommended the WHO standard treatment protocol. In this context, private practitioners often do not register TB patients in the health system; without notifications, it is difficult for state and national TB programs to conduct planning and to improve control of TB. Such countries need to improve the communication between private providers and the health system. Innovative approaches in India and Pakistan have included the creation of public-private mixes using interface organizations and information technology to improve treatment of TB (Khan, Minion, and others 2012; Wells, Uplekar, and Pai 2015).

From Vertical to Targeted, Integrated Delivery
Another challenge for TB service delivery is the dominance of vertically organized and financed TB programs, supported by external institutions (Katz and others 2010), which circumvent and fail to strengthen weak health systems in LMICs in an effort to deliver accessible and quality TB services (Atun, Weil, and others 2010; Car and others 2012; Coker, Atun, and McKee 2004; Coker and others 2005; Samb and others 2009; Shigayeva and others 2010; Wood and others 2010).

Integrated service delivery has been shown to be beneficial. By 2008, TB services were being delivered at the primary health care level in 20 of the 22 high-burden countries and 83 percent of 173 countries reported making progress in TB control (WHO 2013b). However, these services were not effectively integrated with other disease control programs as part of comprehensive primary health care. In Cambodia, hospital-based DOTS care was the norm until stronger primary health care enabled the introduction of integrated community-based TB services. Similarly, the National Rural Health Mission in India has expanded integrated service delivery, including rapid scale-up of child health, TB, and combined TB and HIV/AIDS services. Thailand extended access to primary health care–based TB services as part of universal health coverage.

In Vietnam, tuberculosis control services, which were historically operated through a vertical network, are now embedded in general health services (Atun, Weil, and others 2010). Integration between care delivery domains—for example, civilian and prison health care (Shin and others 2006)—has also been shown to improve patient outcomes.

Vertical delivery of TB services is especially inefficient in the context of concurrent tuberculosis and HIV/AIDS epidemics (Drobniewski and others 2004). As noted, the burden of TB and HIV/AIDS co-infection is substantial, most acutely in Sub-Saharan Africa, and there is a demonstrable need to integrate TB and HIV/AIDS services (Corbett and others 2006; Creswell and others 2011; DeLuca, Chaisson, and Martinson 2009; Perumal, Padayatchi, and Stiefvater 2009; Sylla and others 2007). Emerging evidence indicates the benefits of integrating TB control with HIV/AIDS control (Gandhi and others 2009; Gasana and others 2008; Harris and others 2008; Huerga and others 2010; Jack and others 2004; Legido-Quigley and others 2013; Miti and others 2003; Pevzner and others 2011; Phiri and others 2011; Uwinkindi and others 2014; Uyei and others 2011; Walton and others 2004; Zachariah and others 2003) and other targeted programs (Howard and El-Sadr 2010; Zwarenstein and others 2011) in the primary health care setting. Integration improves outcomes—for example, through concurrent screening or through provision of cotrimoxazole during routine TB care or isoniazid during routine HIV/AIDS care and at voluntary counseling and testing centers (Uyei and others 2011).

Treatment for both tuberculosis and HIV/AIDS should be integrated at the clinic as a standardized package of care, with adherence support and HIV/AIDS drug-resistance testing. It is essential that all HIV-positive individuals be tested for TB. In 2004, the WHO introduced integrated activities to improve prevention, diagnosis, and treatment of TB in people living with HIV/AIDS (box 11.6), but the achievements have been mixed. Creating positive synergies through effective integration of TB control with HIV/AIDS and other targeted programs has been arduous (Ansa and others 2012; Atun and Cooker 2008; Atun, Lazarus, and others 2010; Marais and others 2010; Okot-Chono and others 2009; Uwimana, Hausler, and Zarowsky 2012; Uwimana and Jackson 2013). Integration must be site- and service-specific.

While integrating diagnostic and laboratory services makes great sense, integrating patients with undiagnosed TB in health care clinics and hospitals without the benefit of proper infection control measures poses serious risks to persons with HIV/AIDS. Moreover,

WHO-Recommended Collaborative TB and HIV/AIDS Activities

In 2004, the WHO recommended a set of collaborative activities to improve prevention, diagnosis, and treatment of TB in people living with HIV/AIDS (WHO 2004). These recommendations were updated in 2010 and 2011 (WHO 2012b). Collaborative activities include the following:

1. Establish and strengthen coordination mechanisms for delivering integrated TB and HIV/AIDS services.
2. Test TB patients for HIV/AIDS.

3. Provide ART and cotrimoxazole preventive therapy to TB patients living with HIV/AIDS.
4. Provide HIV/AIDS prevention services for TB patients.
5. Intensify TB case finding among people living with HIV/AIDS.
6. Offer isoniazid preventive treatment to people living with HIV/AIDS who do not have active TB.
7. Control the spread of TB infection in health care and congregate settings.
8. Use Xpert MTB/RIF as the primary test for diagnosing TB in people living with HIV/AIDS who have signs and symptoms of TB.

an anticipated consequence of integrating HIV/AIDS and TB care is the exposure of immune-compromised HIV-positive patients to undiagnosed TB, making it essential to control infection and separate patients.

Effective TB control will require health systems to interact with sectors that address the social determinants of health. However, it has been argued that the programmatic and biomedical focus fostered by DOTS may have, in some instances, hindered multisectoral collaboration and effective coverage of vulnerable communities (Ayles and others 2009; den Boon and others 2007; Gler, Podewils, and others 2012; van't Hoog and others 2011; Wood and others 2007); geographically concentrated groups (de Vries and others 2014); groups at risk, such as women, children, and adolescents (Ettehad and others 2012; Isaakidis and others 2013; Marais and others 2010; Moyo and others 2014; Sheriff and others 2010); and disenfranchised populations (Corbett and others 2009), for example, persons imprisoned in penitentiary facilities (O'Grady, Hoelscher, and others 2011; O'Grady, Maeurer, and others 2011).

Stronger Supply Chains

A robust and well-functioning supply chain is a complex but essential component of any country's health system. An uninterrupted supply of high-quality drugs is imperative to treat TB effectively and to prevent transmission of the disease or its escalation to drug-resistant strains. Weak systems of supply chain management, with inadequate

demand forecasting, ineffective drug procurement, long procurement cycles, poor-quality drugs, and delays in the delivery of diagnostics and medicines, have led to treatment interruptions, exacerbating drug-susceptible and MDR TB epidemics (Mathew and others 2006; van der Werf and others 2012; Victor and others 2007). The lack of availability or poor quality of TB drugs in public clinics run by national TB programs or in private facilities leads to patients missing doses, creating increased risks for relapse and the emergence of drug-resistant forms of the disease.

Stock-outs of TB medicines have many causes. While some stock-outs are related to poor planning, distribution bottlenecks, and poor demand visibility, there are global shortages for some drugs. The problem of global shortages affects many antimicrobials, especially generic injectable agents. Very often, given the small number of manufacturers, when one manufacturer experiences problems related to quality or manufacturing, global shortages can arise.

Global Supply Chain

The global supply chain of TB medicines, from the manufacturer to the patient, can be divided into two distinct segments: the upstream supply chain (global supply chain) and the in-country supply chain (figure 11.6). The global, or upstream, segment consists of the processes related to global demand forecasting, procurement, and financing. The in-country segment includes the quantification of needs by national TB programs,

Figure 11.6 A Simplified Supply Chain from Manufacturer to Patient

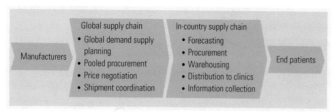

Source: Yadav 2010.

procurement by ministries of health, warehousing, distribution, and information collection about patients regarding treatment and future needs.

The upstream supply chain for TB medicines is fraught with market shortcomings. All commonly used TB drugs are off-patent, holding little interest for large pharmaceutical companies. As a consequence, there are few producers for most drugs. In particular, timely provision of life-saving second-line medicines for MDR TB has been woefully inadequate, with estimates suggesting that less than 0.5 percent of the MDR TB cases in 2002–09 were treated with drugs of known quality (Keshavjee and Farmer 2012). Stock-outs of TB medicines are frequent in LICs, and shortages exist even in HICs, where standard isoniazid has not been available for more than a year.

Apart from the lack of manufacturer interest in these low-demand, limited-profit-potential medicines, the lack of procurement coordination across low- and high-demand countries further fragments the small market. Lack of proper quantification at the country level translates into a lack of robust global forecasts for TB medicines. The upstream supply chain for the donor-funded portion of the TB market currently operates through a pooled procurement mechanism operated by the Global Drug Facility. The Global Drug Facility attempts to coordinate the orders from multiple countries, especially lower-demand countries. For MDR TB medicines, it also runs a strategic rotating stockpile to reduce stock-outs and volatility in orders to the manufacturer. However, the global supply chain is far from optimal and requires significant strengthening of its technical capacity to manage a small market with highly uncertain demand and a fragile supply base (Institute of Medicine 2013).

It is important to examine how the global supply chain for TB medicines has evolved over time. The Green Light Committee was developed in the 2000s to approve programs that deliver MDR TB treatment and provide access to low-cost second-line drugs. However, the Green Light Committee approved a small number of MDR TB treatments, creating long delays in receiving approvals

and drugs, limited demand for second-line drugs, and constrained supply, with few producers providing medicines that met stringent regulatory approval.

In a typical healthy pharmaceutical supply chain, some upstream steps such as active pharmaceutical ingredient (API) manufacturing, formulation, and packaging are carried out before the buyer places an order. These forecast-driven steps lead to the finished product or the API manufacturer holding some inventory, which reduces the time required to fulfill a confirmed order.

In the TB medicines supply chain, however, many of these processes are order driven as opposed to forecast driven. Manufacturers hold little, if any, finished product inventory and little, if any, API inventory. All steps in the upstream supply chain start only after a confirmed order is placed. And the order stream from the pooled purchaser is lumpy, meaning that it occurs in large quantities at certain times of the year. These problems lead to suboptimal holding of inventory, poor planning of batch size, subscale manufacturing of the finished product, higher costs, and excessively long lead times. These issues constrain national TB programs, which are unable to plan much in advance due to uncertain financing and delayed disbursement and thus face further delays in receiving supplies after they place an order. Together, these factors contribute to stock-outs of TB medicines at the national level.

Possible mechanisms to address these problems include the creation of an accurate global demand forecast system, the development of supply-contracting structures that provide limited-volume guarantees to manufacturers, and a buffer inventory or stockpile to smooth demand. Their applicability and cost-effectiveness depend on careful analysis of the nature of demand uncertainty, supply lead times, and ability of global program staff to operate these mechanisms.

Some of these mechanisms are now starting to be used by the Global Drug Facility (Arinaminpathy and others 2015), but they require adequate technical resourcing. Also, while Global Drug Facility purchasing may lead to greater coordination and pooling of orders from many LICs, a significant portion of the TB burden is in middle-income countries, which do not procure through the Global Drug Facility. Overcoming the excessive fragmentation in the global TB drug market, especially for low-demand drugs for MDR TB, requires not only robust technical solutions but also strong political will.

In-Country Supply Chains
In HICs, while the nature of health care provision and financing varies considerably, medicines are distributed primarily by private sector agencies. In LICs, and in many

of the TB-endemic countries, in particular, medicines are distributed to health facilities primarily through a central medical store, regional or district stores, or a transport fleet owned by the government or a central medical store. Global donor–funded or national government–funded TB drugs also flow primarily through this government-run distribution system (figure 11.7).

A multitiered distribution structure wherein TB medicines are stored at multiple levels (national, regional, district) before reaching TB clinics is common in most countries. The distribution system maps directly to the administrative structure of the health system, for ease of administration and governance, as opposed to technical or operational imperatives (Yadav 2010).

Successfully managing a multitiered distribution system for TB medicines is an information-intensive operation. Data on stock levels at each stage, past consumption, and future requisitioning need to flow through different levels of the system. Such data are recorded on store ledgers, stock control cards, and requisition forms at the district and health facility levels but rarely get reported to higher levels of the distribution system. The lack of consumption data prohibits better overall supply planning. There is a critical need for a simple and robust logistics management information system to record and report these data systematically.

Staff need to be well trained to forecast need and place orders, yet staff at health facilities often have inadequate capacity to estimate the quantity of medicines needed, resulting in under- or over-ordering. One solution is to deploy trained staff from district or regional delivery teams to visit health facilities, check the stock they have used, help them to estimate how much is needed for the next period, and replenish that quantity

Figure 11.7 Flow of Medicines through the Public, Private, and NGO Sector in Low- and Middle-Income Countries

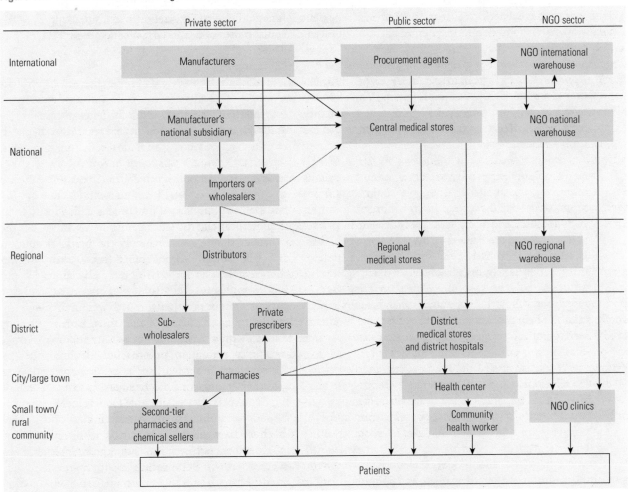

Source: Yadav, Tata, and Babaley 2011.
Note: NGO = nongovernmental organization.

from the supply they carry with them. Zimbabwe has implemented such a system, called Delivery Team Top Up (Yadav, Tata, and Babaley 2011). In a large-scale randomized pilot study in Zambia, relatively simple changes to the information and product flow system significantly improved the availability of essential drugs (Vledder and others 2015). HIV/AIDS medicine programs in multiple countries have also experimented with different variants of the distribution, requisitioning, and information flow model. Such innovation has been lacking for the distribution of TB medicines.

With the recent explosion of inexpensive information technology such as mobile phones, new options have become available for collecting and using information about clinic-level consumption. However, technology will not fix all of the problems in the distribution system.

Apart from lack of information, another crucial cause of poor supply chain performance relates to the lack of incentives (Yadav, Stapleton, and Van Wassenhove 2013): public sector supply chains often lack the ability to reward good performance or to remove incompetent workers. Better mechanisms are needed to align incentives and motivate the supply chain workforce (Spisak and others 2016), but greater accountability in the distribution system for TB drugs requires richer information about stock and consumption data. These models have not yet been leveraged to their fullest, but they have the potential to be the backbone of planning in the supply system.

Having a healthy and robust supply chain for TB medicines in the private sector is as important as improving the publicly run supply chain. Significant proportions of TB patients in high-burden countries such as China and India seek TB treatment in private clinics or obtain medicines in private pharmacies (Wells, Uplekar, and Pai 2015); in some countries, public-private models rely on the availability and quality of drugs in the private sector. While countries such as Brazil and China have created social insurance programs to help patients to cover the cost of private sector services, in most countries patients themselves pay out of pocket for private sector treatment for TB.

TB medicines in the private sector are distributed through a network of importers, wholesalers, sub-wholesalers, pharmacies, and drug stores. Compared to private sector pharmaceutical supply chains in HICs, private sector supply chains in most TB-endemic countries are excessively fragmented, with myriad small wholesalers and distributors; intermediaries between the manufacturer and the patient; and poor information technology and communication systems, which result in poor coordination across the distribution channel.

Fragmentation of the supply chain makes it difficult to achieve scale economies and to improve or verify quality, especially given the severe resource constraints of regulatory authorities.

In some countries where medicine wholesaling is highly fragmented, consolidation of wholesaling and distribution in the supply chain is being driven by policy measures such as better enforcement of distribution practices and stricter reporting requirements. For instance, when a nationwide Good Supply Practice enforcement campaign was launched in China in 2004, the number of pharmaceutical wholesalers dropped from 16,000 to 7,445 (Yadav 2015).

Better Information Management and New Technologies

The lack of reliable and timely information impedes the organization of TB control and effective discharge by ministries of health of their stewardship function. In 2009, only 4 of the 22 high-burden countries had well-functioning vital registration systems that appropriately coded causes of death (Glaziou and others 2011).

Challenges

As both an infectious and chronic disease, TB presents a range of challenges for collecting and managing information. First, there is the challenge of case finding and surveillance. Once patients are identified, diagnosis requires sputum smear and, ideally, culture and drug-sensitivity testing, a challenge in low-income settings where good laboratory facilities are rare. Sputum smears can be collected in small clinics, but culture and DST is a specialized process. New diagnostic techniques, particularly GeneXpert, have improved the situation significantly, avoiding the need for sputum smear or culture in initial diagnostic work-up in sites that have the machines. However, many clinics have to send samples to other sites with machines, and any patient found positive for Mtb requires follow-up testing to assess their response to treatment. Patients found resistant to rifampicin require follow-up drug-sensitivity testing to permit individualized therapy (Lessem and others 2015). It is therefore critical to capture lab data from all locations and sources, including GeneXpert. Newer, portable models in development (GeneXpert Omni) with potential for point-of-care diagnosis have the ability to transfer results in real time by short message service or through the Internet. Even in countries with sophisticated health care systems, like South Africa, there are enormous problems getting the data on a sputum sample to the appropriate clinic, physician, and patient.

Once patients have been diagnosed successfully, they need to be tracked in a longitudinal record that captures data on demographics, clinical condition, current and previous medication, lab results, complications, and treatment response and outcomes. For first-line TB treatment with DOTS, the record is typically a paper register in the clinic. This usually supplements other registers, including primary care visits and maternal health. While well-designed paper registers can be effective, they are typically challenging for busy staff to keep up to date and accurate and lead to much duplication of data. This problem becomes much more severe with large numbers of patients and mobile populations. Drug-resistant TB is a particular challenge due to the complexity of recording treatment and clinical data and the long treatment times.

E-health systems are playing an increasingly important role in the management of TB and are especially important for drug-resistant TB in LMICs. Labrique and others (2013) describe 12 key functions of m-health (and e-health tools more generally). All of these are relevant to TB care:

1. Client education and behavior change communication (short message service reminders to take medication or attend appointments)
2. Sensors and point-of-care diagnostics (attachments for microscopy)
3. Registries and vital events tracking (community case finding and registration)
4. Data collection and reporting (research data collection; Fraser and others 2012)
5. Electronic health (medical) records
6. Electronic decision support (information, protocols, algorithms, checklists)
7. Provider-to-provider communication (telemedicine consultations)
8. Provider work planning and scheduling (to help community health workers to manage their patients)
9. Provider training and education (Web-based resources and video on mobile phone memory cards)
10. Human resource management (tracking activities, patient contacts, and location of community health workers)
11. Supply chain management
12. Financial transactions and incentives.

New Technologies to Improve TB Information Management

Several recent e-health applications have addressed case finding. An m-health application was developed to assist nonclinical CHWs to screen patients in general medical clinics in Karachi, Pakistan (Theron and others 2015).

Staff used the built-in interactive questionnaire to identify symptoms and signs of TB in patients who were coughing for two weeks or more. In the intervention area overall, notification of TB cases to the national TB program increased from 1,569 to 3,140 cases between 2010 and 2011. Increasingly, CHWs in rural communities in LMICs are using m-health applications to find unknown patients with TB and other diseases (Were and others 2009).

Some groups have developed Web-based electronic medical record (EMR) systems for managing drug-resistant TB (Fraser and others 2013). EMRs were one of the first e-health applications for managing TB. Partners In Health developed and deployed a Web-based medical record for managing MDR TB in Peru in 2001, with tools to allow clinicians to view trends in lab data and changes in medications as well as to create reports for the national TB program and funders (Fraser and others 2002). The system was also used to collect core data for subsequent research studies after additional data collection and cleaning. Image data of chest X-rays captured with a digital camera were included for most patients, and psychiatric records were added later. The system was extensively evaluated to determine its performance and potential impact on quality of data and delivery of care (Fraser and others 2006).

From 2000 onward, Peru scaled up the individualized treatment of drug-resistant TB, including upgrading laboratory facilities at local, district, and national levels. Two e-health systems were implemented as part of Peru's system. The first was an early m-health application to assist staff in collecting smear and culture data from 98 small clinics in northern Lima. The system reduced the median processing time for cultures from 23 days to 8 days and for smears from 25 days to 12 days and significantly reduced the number of errors. The intervention reduced the number of work-hours necessary to process results by 70 percent and was preferred by all users.

Blaya and others (2007) evaluated a Web-based laboratory management and reporting system, eChasqui, also in Lima, in a large random control trial of 1,671 patients in 44 clinics, 12 of which were randomized to receive initial access to the system. Error rates (mainly missing results) fell 87 percent for cultures and 82 percent for DSTs. Delays for cultures were reduced from a median of 8 days to 5 days and for DSTs from a median of 17 days to 11 days. In addition, the time to culture conversion fell 20 percent (Blaya and others 2014). Results similar to those seen here in TB patients have been replicated for other diseases, particularly HIV/AIDS (Amoroso and others 2010; Siedner and others 2015).

Several EMR systems have been developed to assist in the management of MDR TB, including eTB manager, initially developed in Brazil and now deployed in many countries (Fraser and others 2013).

In 2008, a new EMR system was developed for MDR TB care based on the open-source EMR system OpenMRS platform (Mamlin and others 2006). The OpenMRS-TB system provided similar functionality to Peru's EMR, but was embedded in a general-purpose EMR platform that was also used to support a range of clinical care, including HIV/AIDS, primary care, maternal health, and oncology. It has been deployed in Haiti, Indonesia, Pakistan, and several African countries. A version of OpenMRS-TB was created and deployed in Peru for a large epidemiological study of MDR TB (Fraser and others 2012). A new version of OpenMRS-TB is currently under development for clinical and research purposes in a collaboration between Partners In Health, Médecins Sans Frontières, and ThoughtWorks. OpenMRS has been developed as open-source software and also supports open standards for the coding of medical data. OpenMRS is now used to support the care of patients in more than 40 LMICs (Mohammed-Rajput and others 2011; Seebregts and others 2009), with versions to support the management of HIV/AIDS, maternal-child health, and, more recently, heart disease and primary care.

The design of OpenMRS offers some advantages for the development of research data management tools. Due to the focus on safe collection, storage, and management of clinical data, it includes auditing of data changes in the main database tables. This feature allows tracking of the history of changes in data items linked to the login of the user. OpenMRS is designed around a flexible data dictionary, called the concept dictionary, which allows new data items to be added without changing the underlying structure of the database. The dictionary simplifies the translation and maintenance of items in additional languages like Spanish and has led to the development of a core dictionary mapped to coding standards such as ICD-10 and SNOMED-CT and shared by most users of the system. A major advantage of OpenMRS from a developer's perspective is its modular software architecture, which allows software modules, either from the OpenMRS module library or newly developed modules, to be plugged into the main system, adding functions without changing the core system.

Telemedicine to Support Health Workers

While clinics can generally manage the DOTS protocols for treating drug-sensitive TB, management of drug-resistant TB can be complex, especially for patients with second-line resistance, including XDR TB. Expertise in managing such patients is limited, which is one of the reasons why only a minority of patients receive fully effective treatment. Telemedicine is a potential strategy to support clinicians with limited knowledge of these complex treatment protocols. This can be as simple as an e-mail question to a specialist for advice on a specific patient's drug regimen and resistance or a video conference with both clinicians and the patient. Many projects use "store and forward telemedicine" typically involving e-mailing text and attached images (Della Mea 1999). Studies have shown that even modest-specification digital cameras can capture images of chest X-rays good enough for diagnosis and management of TB (Szot and others 2004).

Telemedicine approaches often work well in small-scale projects but are difficult to scale up. Individual e-mails are not suitable for large numbers of referrals due to the difficulty of ensuring that all of the correct information is recorded accurately in the referral and the resulting assessment is recorded in the patients' notes. A more effective approach is to share data in a secure, Web-based EMR system like Peru's EMR, OpenMRS-TB, or eTB manager (Fraser and others 2013), giving the remote specialist access to the individual patient's record. The remote specialist can see the full range of clinical data, lab results, and often imaging and record an assessment directly in the clinical record. Another challenge with scale-up is that clinical expertise is limited and cannot be "spread too thin." A more effective and scalable strategy can be to use telemedicine as part of training initiatives (Geissbuhler and others 2003), along with better clinical guidelines and decision support for local staff.

SMS Reminders to Improve Adherence

With the importance of achieving good adherence for managing TB and preventing the emergence of drug resistance, there is great interest in tools and strategies to improve adherence. DOT is the best-established approach, but questions have been raised about its scalability and cost. With mobile phones widely available in LMICs, m-health may provide tools to support treatment adherence. Most work has focused on improving adherence to ART with text messages or interactive voice prompts, with evidence of improvements in adherence in some random control trials (Lester and others 2010; Pop-Eleches and others 2011), but also some negative results (Cameroon, India).

Analysis of these studies suggests that messages customized to each patient and the ability of patients to communicate with actual staff (not just automated prompts) improve adherence. To date, these tools have not matched the adherence rates of effective DOT, and there is evidence of messaging fatigue among patients.

Further work is under way to design interventions based on established psychological models of behavior change accompanied by rigorous evaluation.

Information Technology to Manage Supply Chains

An additional challenge for managing drug-resistant TB has been establishing effective medication supply chains, and information systems are increasingly important for forecasting requirements, tracking medication shipments, and managing inventory at clinics.

Lack of supply of second-line TB medications is a key factor in poor scale-up of treatment. While first-line drugs are low cost and generally widely available, second-line drugs are mostly used for drug-resistant TB and often manufactured to order. Orders have to be placed months in advance to ensure continuity of care, and accurate forecasting is essential. Information systems can assist in multiple steps in this process, including forecasting, ordering, tracking shipments, and managing inventory.

In Peru, the EMR was used to forecast medication requirements for treating drug-resistant TB. Combining data on the number of patients enrolled, their length of time in treatment, recruitment rate, and current regimens resulted in error rates of 3 percent or less for more than 1,000 patients in both 2003 and 2004 (Fraser and others 2013). A related study looked at forecasting medication for 68 patients in the same cohort and compared that to the usual manual methods. In one study, Peru's EMR predicted 99 percent of one year's needed supply of medicines, while more manual methods predicted 149 percent (Fraser and others 2013).

New tools are becoming available for managing shipments and inventory in LMICs.[4] One information system for drug-resistant TB, eTB Manager, includes inventory management for each clinic linked to requirements forecasting (Fraser and others 2013). These tools are now available for general use in drug forecasting. M-health tools are also being used to track inventory in local clinics in East Africa using text messages (SMS for Life) and have been shown to reduce stock-outs dramatically for antimalarial drugs (Barrington and others 2010). They are also being used for TB medication. Other systems have been developed to detect counterfeit medication in countries like Nigeria by allowing patients to text a unique code printed on the medication container to a free number.[5]

As noted, the OpenMRS-TB EMR platform supports the management of a wide range of diseases and primary care. Its use of open standards for storing and exchanging data supports interoperability with other e-health systems, allowing systems with a range of functionality to be linked together—for example, EMR systems, laboratory information systems, pharmacy systems, m-health applications, and national reporting systems, such as the District Health Information System (DHIS 2).

Such e-health architecture approaches are being deployed in several LMICs, including Bangladesh, India, Kenya, the Philippines, and Rwanda. Many countries have now adopted the DHIS 2 to collect, manage, and report on health data at the district and national levels. The system can take direct feeds of data from systems such as OpenMRS and some m-health applications, improving the accuracy and timeliness of data. Embedding the specialized data collection and analysis tools for TB care in broader e-health systems has large benefits, such as facilitating case finding through primary care visits and lab data, identifying potential risk factors like diabetes, maintaining a complete and accurate list of medications, and providing effective decision support based on the sharing of all key data.

Further evaluation is needed on the performance of e-health systems in LMICs as well as the clinical impact on TB management. In addition, there are only limited data at present on the costs of deploying such systems and maintaining good performance and usage levels in the long term (Blaya, Fraser, and Holt 2010). There is, however, some evidence that effective EMR and laboratory information systems can save money in LMICs by reducing errors and waste and speeding patient management (Driessen and others 2013). It is also very likely to be more cost-effective to embed TB management tools in existing e-health systems than to run parallel systems.

RESEARCH AND DEVELOPMENT

In addition to requiring new care delivery and health system strategies, turning the tide against TB will likely require technological advances that could accelerate cure, reduce transmission and incidence, and prevent disease. Despite the effectiveness of standard drug regimens for drug-sensitive TB, resistance is increasing, compliance with long treatment times is problematic, and new drugs and regimens are needed.

Current TB therapy has many advantages: the standard drugs are remarkably safe, with little toxicity even in vulnerable populations such as pregnant women and children; a complete course is highly effective against drug-sensitive disease; and the drugs themselves are affordable in the poorest parts of the world. Despite these advantages, first-line drugs are ineffective against multidrug-resistant strains. And rifampin, perhaps the most effective agent in the current first-line therapy, has pharmacologic interactions with many other drugs, most notably HIV/AIDS protease inhibitors taken by many co-infected individuals.

The most important limitation of the current regimen is the extended time required for effective therapy. "Short course" chemotherapy is anything but short; failing to complete six months of treatment leads to significant rates of relapse. Because patients feel better in a matter of weeks, they often have little motivation to continue taking their medications. In addition, the extended course means that a substantial investment is needed to ensure a continuous drug supply. These requirements add substantially to the cost of what otherwise would be an inexpensive undertaking. This, together with the training and logistics necessary to ensure adequate DOTS implementation, has led to remarkably poor results and continued treatment failure, leading to millions of deaths each year. Thus, the challenge is to develop not just new drugs, but ideally new drug regimens effective in treating drug-sensitive and drug-resistant TB and shortening the time of treatment.

Better drugs and regimens could have a substantial impact. To be most useful, they would have the following attributes:

- Rapid activity, shortening the course of therapy required for cure
- Safety, allowing use in a wide range of patients without requiring substantial prescreening
- Easy administration, preferably oral, so that health professionals are not required
- Limited interactions with other drugs, particularly antiretroviral drugs
- Limited cost, making them affordable in the poorest parts of the world.

There are two general paths to achieving these goals: optimizing the use of currently available medications and developing completely new drugs. Phase III clinical trials are expensive and will always be rare. It will likely be impossible to test each new drug serially.

Given the enormous cost of developing new drugs (the average cost of developing a new drug to licensure is on the order of US$1 billion or more), the former is the most attractive path to making rapid changes to recommended therapy.

Optimizing the Use of Current Medications

Is it possible to reconfigure the current drug regimen to produce better efficacy against a broader range of organisms? The evidence so far is mixed. Animal studies and human pharmacokinetic observations have suggested some modifications of TB drug therapy that might produce better results. For example, many

patients who receive rifampin at recommended doses have low serum levels. Increasing the dosage of rifampin or using a different rifamycin might enhance the clearance of infection. Several studies are looking at altered dosing regimens for rifampin or substitution of the long-acting drug rifapentine. As measured by a surrogate endpoint—culture conversion at two months—rifapentine is no better than rifampin. In multiple short-term controlled trials that included fluoroquinolones to shorten therapy, the failure rate of cures at two to four months was unacceptably high. None of those shortened regimens was effective enough to offer substantial advantages in treatment (Gillespie and others 2014; Jindani and others 2014; Merle and others 2014).

The fluoroquinolone trials were phase III studies designed to permit U.S. Federal Drug Administration (FDA) approval for these regimens, if successful. Performing such a trial is an enormous undertaking. The current treatment regimen is highly successful in some patients, with a less than 5 percent relapse rate in most settings. Showing improved efficacy requires an enormous number of patients, which is why the fluoroquinolone study was designed to show noninferiority, a criterion that does not require the same level of evidence. Nevertheless, these studies require thousands of patients to provide confidence in the results and investments in infrastructure in the low-income settings where the trials are conducted, making them extremely expensive and logistically challenging.

To mitigate the costs associated with such trials, some studies are experimenting with alternative trial designs. For example, one study investigated the efficacy of the oxazolidinone linezolid. Instead of recruiting patients with drug-sensitive disease, these investigators studied patients with MDR TB, a group where success rates are historically lower (Gler, Skripconoka, and others 2012; Lee, Song, and others 2015). They compared regimens that had been individually designed for each patient with the same regimen plus linezolid. This study showed a faster rate of clearance of bacteria and a lower relapse rate in the linezolid-treated patients, suggesting that this drug has properties that might allow a shorter regimen, at least in this setting. However, linezolid treatment was associated with very high levels of toxicity, far higher than could be tolerated by patients with drug-sensitive disease. Still, this class of compounds shows promise. In another study, delamanid (OPC-67683), a nitro-dihydro-imidazooxazole derivative, was found to accelerate sputum clearance of Mtb by 45 percent in two months, somewhat better than standard treatment (30 percent). These studies suggest that the priority given to shortening treatment time to sputum conversion may be compromising the need to assure cure and prevent treatment failure and relapse.

Finding New Treatments

Producing novel agents is in some ways superior to optimizing the use of current drugs. The length of therapy cannot be shortened with current drugs. And because antibiotic resistance arises from mutations rather than acquisition of broad determinants of resistance, virtually all bacteria, including MDR TB strains, should be sensitive to completely new classes of antibiotics. These advantages must be balanced, however, against the substantial costs involved in developing new drugs. Preclinical development costs tens of millions of dollars, while completing all of the clinical studies necessary for drug approval can run into the hundreds of millions. And there are substantial risks along the way: only a small minority of compounds that enter clinical trials are approved; many more fail to make it into clinics.

Nonetheless, new drug development for TB already has achieved some notable successes (Hoagland and others 2016). Two new drugs have recently received approval for human use for MDR TB under certain conditions. Both bedaquiline and delamanid have been approved in Europe; bedaquiline also has received FDA approval. These agents have interesting and novel mechanisms of action. Bedaquiline, a diarylquinoline, inhibits bacterial adenosine triphosphate synthesis by directly blocking the adenosine triphosphate synthase complex. Delamanid, a nitroimidazole, is converted by bacterial enzymes to its active form, which may liberate toxic nitric oxide in the process. As predicted for drugs with new molecular mechanisms, there is little cross-resistance to existing antibiotics (although altered activity of an efflux pump might decrease the efficacy of both clofazimine and bedaquiline). It is not clear how these agents will be used. In rather small clinical trials, bedaquiline was effective, but patients who received the drug had higher death rates, largely after treatment was completed, for unknown reasons (Cox and Laessig 2014; Diacon and others 2014; Gupta and others 2015). Until more is known, bedaquiline use will likely be restricted to persons with drug-resistant TB (WHO 2013e). Less is known about delamanid and its optimal use at this point.

The path to obtaining approval for bedaquiline and delamanid is both interesting and illustrative. Both were tested in patients with MDR disease in much the way that linezolid was used, adding them to optimized therapies. Patients treated with the new drugs cleared infection significantly more rapidly and had lower rates of relapse when treatment was stopped. The small numbers in these trials provided the basis for "conditional" approval

of both drugs for use in MDR infections. However, final approval and an expanded indication for drug-sensitive disease will require larger phase III trials.

Several new regimens are currently undergoing testing in clinical trials. Like the fluoroquinolone trials, many of these target drug-sensitive TB with the aim of shortening the duration of therapy without compromising the rate of cure. As of this writing, trials are planned, enrolling participants, or under way that will test whether treatment can be shortened to as little as two months using a variety of regimens. Of these, a phase III trial testing pretomanid/moxifloxacin/pyrazinamide (PaMZ) was the farthest along. However, the trial was put on hold due to unexpected toxicity, and its future is uncertain.

In addition to drugs that either have already been approved or are in late clinical trials, several preclinical compounds are undergoing development. These include both new members of existing classes, such as oxazolidinones that might have less toxicity than linezolid, and completely new classes of compounds. Compounds with novel mechanisms of action are particularly attractive. Not only are they generally active against drug-resistant disease, but they may exploit pathways that could clear disease more rapidly.

However, two issues have arisen with these new compounds. First, many compounds with antibacterial activity seem to target a very limited number of bacterial processes. These often induce cross-resistant mutations. Therefore, there is far less diversity than desired. Second, and perhaps more concerning, much remains unknown about the fundamental biology of infection. A principal goal of new drug development is to shorten the course of therapy. However, there are no in vitro correlates that confidently predict that an early-stage compound will result in more effective therapy. This presents a considerable obstacle to the drug development process. And differences in the effectiveness of drugs between laboratory studies and patients question whether in vitro and animal models adequately predict the most effective compounds.

Do standard markers of rapid clearance in clinical trials correlate with ultimate treatment success? It is likely that some drugs used in TB act more slowly and might not be seen to be effective in early bacterial clearance studies and, conversely, that some drugs act rapidly but do not sustain their effects and control infection over the longer term. Without biomarkers for the state of viability and magnitude of the TB bacillus in the host, answering these questions will likely require large trials (Wallis and Nacy 2013).

Even in the best of circumstances, serial testing of individual drugs in large trials is unlikely ever to be affordable. Moreover, these drugs will never be used alone; instead, they will always be used in combination with other drugs. And these combinations might be more (or, conceivably, less) efficacious than would be predicted for individual drugs. Indeed, experiments in animal models suggest that some drugs can act synergistically to effect much more rapid cure. This has led to the model of testing regimens rather than individual drugs. In this model, which has been advanced by the TB Alliance, new drugs would be tested and approved in combinations. While the characteristics of individual drugs might never be determined (and, in this model, would not necessarily be approved as individual agents), this strategy would provide a much more rapid and practical path to drug approval, albeit at the risk of missing information about individual agents.

Because of the cost of developing new drugs and regimens and the fact that the populations in greatest need are in LMICs, an enormous challenge remains: how can countries afford new more effective regimens, and how can the international community contribute to making them available to the populations that need them? Pharmaceutical companies have few private sector incentives to invest in TB drug development or, more generally, in antibiotic development at present, and some sort of public-private mechanisms will need to be developed.

Developing New Vaccines

In the past two decades, there has been a renewed effort to develop vaccines against TB that would provide greater protection than BCG. There are at least three strategies for contributing to TB control where vaccines are being tested in clinical trials. One strategy is to determine whether vaccines can prevent infection with TB (prevention-of-infection trial), in which IGRAs are used to detect infection by Mtb. A second is to test whether vaccines can prevent recurrence of TB or MDR TB after treatment (prevention-of-recurrence trial) or possibly be used therapeutically with chemotherapy to accelerate cure. Finally, the ultimate goal is large-scale immunization for prevention of disease (POD). About 40 vaccine candidates are at various stages of preclinical testing, and 15 vaccine candidates are currently in clinical trials (Jiménez-Levi 2012).

Among the candidates in the pipeline (Evans and others 2013) are (1) recombinant vaccine candidates expressing Mtb antigens in BCG, adenovirus, cytomegalovirus (CMV), or other vectors; (2) genetically attenuated whole-cell Mtb strains, lacking either virulence determinants or ability to replicate; (3) and a variety of subunit protein antigen candidates with adjuvants that would be used as boosters in children or adolescents primed with BCG. All of these vaccines are being tested

in preclinical studies in experimental animals, and some are being tested in nonhuman primates.

The scientific basis for development of any effective vaccine includes (1) significant understanding of immunological mechanisms of protection against infection or disease; (2) molecular correlates of mechanisms that would diminish the need for large, multiyear efficacy trials; (3) definition of Mtb antigens that engender those protective mechanisms; (4) means of delivering those antigens that generate or prime for protective rather than pathogenic responses; and (5) animal models that are more predictive of protection in humans than current models appear to be. None of these criteria has been met for any TB vaccine candidate at present.

Several special considerations are necessary in vaccine testing. Since vaccines, in contrast to most drugs, are given to healthy children or adults, their safety must be the foremost concern. In addition, they need to be tested in places with a high TB burden that have laboratories capable of analyzing the immune correlates of protection; they cannot compromise the ability to test for infection with Mtb in IGRAs; and the preexposure to environmental mycobacteria in places where they are tested cannot compromise detection of protection.

From animal studies and human Mendelian genetic studies, it appears that both CD4+ and CD8+ T-cells and IFN-γ, TNF-α, and other cytokines are *necessary* to protect against disease (Modlin and Bloom 2013; O'Garra and others 2013). The challenge is to learn what responses are *sufficient* for protection. It is unclear how faithful small animal models of TB will be to the human response to vaccine candidates. There is hope that nonhuman primates may be the most predictive model of human protection. Human vaccine trials showing at least partial protection may be the only way to establish those conditions. The first new candidate, MVA85A, expressing a major Mtb antigen, 85A, in modified vaccinia Ankara vector, was tested in more than 3,000 South Africa infants in a well-executed phase IIb trial (Tameris and others 2013). The candidate, which was reported to induce IFN-γ and engender some protection in four animal species, failed to protect children against either infection or disease.

BCG is known to induce Th1 T-cells and a number of cytokines—for example, IFN-γ, TNF-α, IL-12—that, in animal models and in human Mendelian genetic deficiency studies, appear to be *necessary* for protection against TB. However, the immunological factors that are *sufficient* to engender protection are not yet understood (Modlin and Bloom 2013). It is very unlikely that large-scale trials of new vaccines, such as the South India trial, which followed 360,000 people for 15 years and failed to show protection in any age group, will soon be undertaken for new candidate vaccines. Thus, there is an urgent scientific need to develop molecular "correlates of protection" that can be measured in small numbers of recipients, that will predict which new vaccine candidates are likely to protect against infection and disease, and that will identify which individuals are likely to remain susceptible or relapse after treatment. In the absence of molecular markers of protection—for example, either involved in protecting against infection or preventing latent TB from progressing to active disease—serious consideration will have to be given to the development of a safe, attenuated, but live genetically engineered Mtb challenge. This development could be as valuable to TB vaccine development as live challenges have been in malaria and enteric vaccines.

Modeling the impact of possible new TB vaccines has been enormously valuable. It has shown that, because children contribute little to transmission, giving a more effective vaccine than BCG only to infants and children would have little effect on the epidemic (Knight and others 2014). Modeling suggests that, in high-endemic countries, vaccinating adolescents, who were the recipient population found to be highly protected (about 80 percent) in the original trials of BCG and M. microti in the United Kingdom (Hart and Sutherland 1977; Sutherland and Springett 1987), would be more effective than vaccinating infants. Immunizing or boosting adolescents just before they enter the age of highest risk would likely have the greatest impact on the disease burden.

Because of the need to immunize large numbers of people in a general population to obtain enough statistical power to establish vaccine efficacy, the approach of the field is to test smaller numbers of individuals in high-burden countries to learn about immunological parameters that may correlate with protection. For example, an experimental trial with a small targeted population could ascertain whether immunization could prevent reinfection and relapse (at the end of treatment). Targeting vaccines to a group of treated patients would shorten the time to learn whether there was an effect on relapse and reduce the costs and time required for disease prevention trials in large populations. It is remarkable how little research has been devoted to combining chemotherapy and immunotherapy in TB.

Understanding the Immune Mechanisms Necessary and Sufficient for Protection

Current thinking is that a single vaccine given at birth is unlikely to provide sufficient protection to prevent disease in adults, who have the highest risk of developing disease. Because the duration and costs of vaccine efficacy

trials are great, several strategies are being developed to gain insights into the critical immune mechanisms necessary for protection in humans. Testing vaccine candidates in TST-negative individuals and evaluating their ability to prevent infection as measured by IGRAs could be accomplished in a shorter time than disease prevention trials. As discussed, vaccinating patients at the completion of drug treatment to prevent relapses or reinfection in high-burden areas could provide information in as little as one to two years. In all such trials, it will be essential to study multiple molecular and immunological markers to develop correlates of protection. Finally, the most promising candidates need to be tested in small groups of volunteers to understand which of the different mechanisms each candidate engenders, which are likely to correlate with protection, and which can be used as biomarkers for protection. Here innovative trial designs, such as matched-pair randomized trials, could provide power and information with much fewer volunteers (King and others 2009).

Relevant are the older studies indicating that latent TB seems to engender persisting immune responses that afford significant protection from disease (Andrews and others 2012), when compared with the risks of reinfection of TB patients who have been cured (Middelkoop and others 2015). This raises the concern that, if chemotherapy kills most of the Mtb organisms, the susceptibility of people successfully cured of TB will revert back to that of naïve individuals. This suggests that the immunologic value of latency may lie in the persistence of the pathogen and microbial antigens. Thus, the duration of protective immune responses engendered by new vaccines may be critical to protecting against reinfection and relapse. These findings reinforce the approach of vaccinating or revaccinating individuals who have been "cured" by treatment to test whether vaccination will reduce the incidence of relapse or reinfection.

Since BCG is the most widely used vaccine in the world, particularly in high-burden TB countries, the most likely vaccine strategy will be priming with BCG or another whole-cell candidate in early childhood and boosting with a live attenuated TB vaccine, a vaccine with Mtb antigens expressed in a viral vector (such as an adenovirus or CMV), or a subunit vaccine containing multiple epitopes plus an adjuvant. Particularly exciting are new vaccine platforms that offer the possibility of generating long-enduring immune responses to Mtb antigens, including recombinant BCG vaccines designed to engender both CD4 and CD8 T-cells (Kaufmann and others 2014), attenuated TB vaccine (Spertini and others 2015), attenuated recombinant CMV vectors (Hansen and others 2013), and mRNA (messenger ribonucleic acid) vaccines (Chahal and others 2016; Petsch and others 2012). Clearly, vaccine trials comparing multiple candidate vaccines in phases II and III are enormously expensive and time-consuming (on the order of US$50 million per trial over a period of three to five years). This is why there is an urgent need to define molecular or immunological correlates of protection that would enable the up-selection of the most promising candidates from small-scale human studies.

An alternative being pursued is developing a safe, genetically engineered Mtb live challenge strain that could persist long enough to enable rapid assessment of the effectiveness of a vaccine to induce killing of the challenge strain, but totally lacking the potential to cause disease. With phase I human studies in a small number of individuals, the ability of a vaccine candidate to kill the challenge strain would support conducting a small number of phase II and phase III clinical trials to test the efficacy of a particularly effective vaccine candidate against TB infection and disease. Historically, all vaccines have been iterative processes with continuous learning and improvements. The development of biomarkers of protection that would enable identification of the most promising candidates for large clinical trials would profoundly accelerate TB vaccine development.

Effective new vaccines are essential for TB control, yet their development, testing, and regulatory approval require many years and considerable investment. The slow decline in TB incidence globally, especially in high-burden countries, even as mortality and prevalence are declining, compels us to recognize the serious possibility that tuberculosis may not be controlled without a protective vaccine.

FINANCING FOR TB PROGRAMS

The WHO estimates that funding for prevention, diagnosis, and treatment of TB reached US$6.6 billion, of which US$5.3 billion was for diagnosis and treatment of drug-susceptible TB and US$1.8 billion was for MDR TB (WHO 2014b). Of those funds, 84 percent derives from domestic sources, which vary across countries (WHO 2016a).

In 2014, development assistance allocated US$1.4 billion to TB (IHME 2015), a drop of 9 percent from 2013, two-thirds of which came from the Global Fund. The WHO estimates the shortfall in funds necessary to expand TB programs at about US$2.0 billion (WHO 2016a). The Global Fund is the single largest funder of TB assistance globally committing about 55 percent of its funds to HIV/AIDS, 27 percent to malaria, and 18 percent to TB (IHME 2015). Yet financing from the Global Fund represents about 50 percent of all current development assistance for health devoted to TB. The United States does not have a separate entity for funding TB as it does for HIV/AIDS and malaria, instead channeling half of its US$500 million in TB assistance through the Global Fund; the remainder is channeled bilaterally. In 2014, the Bill & Melinda Gates Foundation provided about 12.6 percent of all development assistance for health dedicated to TB. Other government donors were the United Kingdom (7.7 percent), France (7.0 percent) Germany (5.1 percent), Japan (3.4 percent), Canada (4.7 percent), and Australia (2.2 percent) (IHME 2015). Of these funds, about 78 percent were provided through the Global Fund.

The WHO estimates that the level of funding required to enable a comprehensive approach to controlling TB would be on the order of US$8.8 billion, two-thirds of which would be for diagnosis and treatment of drug-susceptible TB and 20 percent for drug-resistant TB (WHO 2016a). This figure does not include the costs of research needed to develop new drugs, vaccines, and diagnostics, which the WHO estimates would require an additional US$2.0 billion.

Given the magnitude of the TB epidemic, the emergence of MDR and XDR TB, and the need to strengthen health systems for TB, a greater level of funding will be required to extend current efforts and enable the new approaches recommended here to reduce incidence and transmission of the disease dramatically (figures 11.8 and 11.9). A summary of the latest 2015 recommendations of the Copenhagen Consensus Center, a consortium of international economists, suggested that additional investment in TB would represent a good buy (*Economist* 2015). For every US$1 invested, the return was estimated to be US$43. Were US$2 billion invested to cover the shortfall, the potential economic savings could

Figure 11.8 Funding for Tuberculosis Prevention, Diagnosis, and Treatment, by Intervention Area, 2006–14

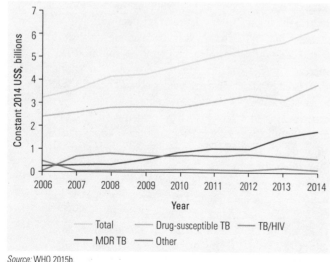

Source: WHO 2015b.
Note: TB = tuberculosis; HIV = human immunodeficiency virus; MDR = multidrug-resistant.

be on the order of US$300 billion (Lundgrun 2015). But despite increases in domestic and international financing, the WHO estimates the current funding gap to be US$2.0 billion for extending current measures and an additional US$1.3 billion for research and new technologies. That leaves a funding gap of US$2.7 billion per year to assure a full response to the TB epidemic.

ECONOMIC ANALYSES AND COST-EFFECTIVENESS

As the pipeline for new TB diagnostic technologies continues to expand, health and economic evaluations are needed to inform decisions about the most promising options to pursue in different settings and patient populations. Economic evaluation of new diagnostic approaches can seem deceptively simple, but several factors should be considered if these evaluations are to provide credible and useful guidance for policy. These factors pertain both to quantifying potential impact and to estimating costs.

First, it is important to consider the pathway(s) by which new diagnostics are expected to lead to improved health outcomes. For instance, aspirations for new point-of-care diagnostics point to the benefits of returning rapid test results, which can reduce loss to follow-up by eliminating the need for a return visit. Quicker diagnosis may increase the rate of initiating treatment, improve patient outcomes, and reduce transmission by decreasing the period of infectiousness. However, imperfections in implementation may cause real-world application to fall short of the maximum theoretical potential.

Moreover, evaluating the impact and cost-effectiveness of a new approach requires comparing the new approach to the status quo that it will displace. For example, a comparative evaluation of a new diagnostic approach should specify (1) where the diagnostic will be used (for example, only in central facilities such as district hospitals or also in peripheral health centers); (2) the sequence of tests and associated responses that will guide decision making in different types of individuals or be based on particular population-level factors (for example, in individuals with HIV/AIDS or a history of treatment or in a setting with a particular population-level HIV/AIDS prevalence); and (3) the current diagnostic approach in these settings that constitutes the status quo comparator (that is, the extent to which bacterial culture or drug-sensitivity testing is currently being used).

It is also crucial to estimate the costs associated with scale-up and implementation, which are often significantly greater than the costs of the commodities per se or even the costs including other health care services that are consumed at the patient level (for example, the opportunity costs of provider time). At the simplest

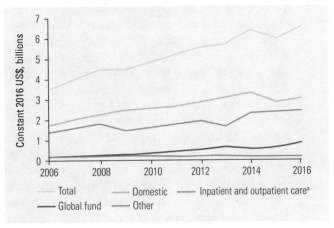

Figure 11.9 Funding for Tuberculosis Prevention, Diagnosis, and Treatment by Funding Source, 2006–16

Total — Domestic — Inpatient and outpatient care[a]
Global fund — Other

Source: WHO 2016a.
a. 91 percent of funding for inpatient and outpatient care is accounted for by middle- and high-income countries; such countries do not typically receive international donor funding for inpatient and outpatient care services. Data are estimates based on country-reported utilization.

level, scaling up new technologies often involves economies (or costs) of scale that relate to the shape of the average cost function in relation to the quantity, which reflects different mixtures of fixed and variable costs at different scales. At a more complex level, achieving population coverage requires paying attention to health system capacity, reflecting constraints not only on the budget but also on infrastructure and human and other resources. The validity of cost-effectiveness estimates depends on quantifying the costs of delivering an intervention or strategy in a way that is consistent with the benefits ascribed to that intervention or strategy. Many published studies fail to meet this requirement.

With regard to diagnostic approaches, important questions should be addressed regarding patient pathways to care, how a new diagnostic technology or strategy will alter the pathways, and where delays or loss to follow-up may occur, particularly as these might attenuate the expected benefits of a diagnostic. In HIV/AIDS, considerable attention has recently been given to the so-called "cascade of care," and similar considerations are highly salient to tuberculosis control interventions, including those relating to diagnosis (Subbaraman and others 2016).

Cost-Effectiveness of Using Xpert MTB/RIF

Xpert MTB/RIF represents a significant technological advance in accelerating diagnosis of TB and MDR disease in many settings. However, it has significant limitations. Several studies have examined the cost-effectiveness of Xpert MTB/RIF in different LMICs. A cost-effectiveness study published in 2011 by Vassall and colleagues (2011) and focusing on India, South Africa, and Uganda estimated that Xpert devices used in combination with smear would have an incremental cost-effectiveness ratio of between US$41 and US$110 compared to conventional use of smear plus clinical diagnosis. A 2012 modeling study (Abimbola and others 2012) estimated cost-effectiveness of Xpert at the regional level in Sub-Saharan Africa and found that Xpert would reduce mortality and lower overall costs. Another 2012 study focusing on screening with Xpert prior to initiating ART in HIV/AIDS patients (Andrews and others 2012) found much less favorable results, indicating that using Xpert would cost US$5,100 per year of life saved compared to the next most attractive strategy, which involved smear and culture. A third study from 2012 (Menzies and others 2012) examined the cost-effectiveness of Xpert in five Southern African countries and found a cost-effectiveness ratio of around US$1,000 per DALY averted. Other studies have shown smaller-than-projected benefits of Xpert.

Widely divergent results reflect the many challenges of evaluating new diagnostic technologies and point to several areas for further investigation, including the extent to which frequent empirical treatment would reduce the potential benefit of Xpert technology measured against a counterfactual of diagnosis based strictly on the results from smear microscopy. As dramatic scale-up of Xpert has been pursued in South Africa and other settings, other implementation challenges have come to light, including the high overall budgetary impact of seeking high coverage of Xpert, the feasibility of deploying Xpert at the point of care, inability to link Xpert findings to health information systems, and limits on the potential benefit of faster diagnosis arising from the failure to translate diagnostic improvements into faster initiation of treatment (Lawn 2015).

New technologies that can be used at the point of care are needed, and portable devices (for example, GeneXpert Omni) are under development that can be used as a point-of-care diagnostic test. Nevertheless, expanding their capacity for drug-sensitivity testing against the multiple drugs used in secondary and tertiary drug regimens remains a daunting challenge.

Cost-Effectiveness of Developing New Drugs and Regimens

The public health case for investing in new TB drugs is clear (Zumla, Nahid, and Cole 2013), but the substantial cost of drug development remains a significant obstacle to progress. Even if the efficiency of new drug development can be improved, new TB drug development is likely to remain a challenging investment decision for many years to come.

The cost-effectiveness and affordability of first-line regimens for TB treatment have been long established (World Bank 1993), and attention has focused on exploring the most cost-effective way to deliver treatment. For countries providing TB treatment through hospitals, studies have demonstrated the relative cost-effectiveness of ambulatory treatment (Floyd, Wilkinson, and Gilks 1997; Vassall and others 2002; Vassall and others 2009). Economic analysis in other settings has focused on delivering care through community structures (Floyd and others 2003; Moalosi and others 2003; Nganda and others 2003) and ensuring effective cooperation with the private sector (Floyd, Arora, and others 2006; Pantoja, Floyd, and others 2009; Pantoja, Lönnroth, and others 2009). Although these studies demonstrate feasible and cost-effective approaches to delivering TB treatment, the high costs of delivering relatively long antibiotic therapies in poorly resourced health systems is a concern, as are the high default rates in some settings (Kruk, Schwalbe, and Aguiar 2008). These concerns are heightened by evidence of the substantial economic and poverty impact of TB treatment on patients (and households), with numerous studies finding that the multiple health service visits required can have a severe impact on the economic welfare of TB patients (Barter and others 2012).

The current approach to the treatment of MDR TB presents a particular challenge from an economic perspective. Several studies (Floyd and others 2012; Resch and others 2006; Suarez and others 2002; Tupasi and others 2006) have suggested that the treatment of MDR TB is cost-effective. A recent systematic review found that the cost per DALY averted was lower than gross domestic product per capita in all 14 of the WHO subregions considered (Fitzpatrick and Floyd 2012). However, the absolute price of second-line drug regimens, even for LICs, can run into the thousands of dollars, with a three- or fourfold burden on total costs of the health system. For example, in South Africa, treating MDR TB costs more than half of the total national budget for TB control (Schnippel and others 2013), with hospitalized treatment costing more than US$15,000 per person treated (Pooran and others 2013; Schnippel and others 2013). However, these costs may be substantially reduced given the efforts to decentralize MDR TB treatment and care. Also potentially cost-effective, the cost of drug-susceptibility testing required to confirm a diagnosis of MDR TB treatment can also be substantial (Acuna-Villaorduna and others 2008; Floyd and others 2012), and, as highlighted in previous sections, culture-based DST provides a substantial practical challenge in settings with limited laboratory capacity. Additionally, the economic burden of MDR TB on households may be substantially higher than the costs of first-line treatment and is likely to be catastrophic (Ramma and others 2015; survey of MDR TB patient costs in South Africa, unpublished data).

In light of these challenges, increasing attention is being placed on developing low-cost models of MDR TB diagnosis and treatment for scale-up—for example, new ambulatory models of care (Sinanovic and others 2015; Weiss and others 2014). In short, although the current approaches to the treatment of both drug-susceptible TB and MDR TB are widely accepted to be cost-effective, the relatively high cost of treatment for both patients and health systems, the cost of DST, the high levels of default, and the limited effectiveness of MDR TB treatment in low- and middle-income health systems make a strong economic and public health case for investing in new TB drugs.

In recent years, substantial investments have been made in clinical trials of new TB drugs and regimens (Hoagland and others 2016; Zumla, Nahid, and Cole 2013). Candidate drugs affect treatment efficacy or effectiveness and cost through different pathways, but the broad aim has been to improve one or more of the following three dimensions:

- Shorten the duration of treatment; trialed examples for first-line regimens include four-month moxifloxacin-based regimens (Gillespie and others 2014; Jindani and others 2014) and the Bangladesh regimen and bedaquiline-based regimens for MDR TB (Diacon, Donald, and others 2012).
- Increase the efficacy of treatment, particularly for MDR TB; trialed examples include delamanid (Gler, Skripconoka, and others 2012) and bedaquiline (Diacon, Donald, and others 2012).
- Develop regimens that are effective in both drug-susceptible and MDR TB. This will require new drugs for which drug resistance does not currently exist in most populations.

In order to justify and support investment, various economic and modeling efforts have explored the potential gains from improving these dimensions of TB treatment in terms of cost-effectiveness, direct effect on treatment success, broader impact on transmission, and patient and provider costs. In recent years, academic interest in both the investment in new drugs and these analyses has increased. At the time of writing, considerable work is ongoing, with much new work expected on the horizon.

Shortening Treatment Regimens to Reduce Incidence

To date, modeling analyses of TB treatment have focused on the population-level health gains from investing in shortening treatment regimens. For example, examining first-line treatment, both Salomon and others (2006) and Abu-Raddad and others (2009) used a transmission model calibrated to the South-East Asia region and found a substantial impact on incidence due to the introduction of shortened regimens. Salomon and others (2006) found that a noninferior two-month first-line regimen would prevent around 13–21 percent of all new TB cases and 19–25 percent of TB deaths, depending on assumptions made regarding the scale-up of current regimens over an 18-year period. The study suggested that, if the cost savings generated by treatment shortening were invested in TB case detection, two- or threefold reductions in incidence might be possible. Abu-Raddad and others (2009) found that a four-month regimen with efficacy similar to that of the standard of care would achieve up to a 10 percent reduction in incidence over 35 years and a two-month regimen with increased efficacy would achieve a 23 percent reduction in incidence over the same period of time. A more recent effort by Fofana and others (2014) suggested a more modest, but still positive, impact, estimating a 3 percent reduction in incidence from a four-month regimen and a 7 percent reduction from a two-month regimen over a 10-year period.

The analysis of the economic gains from treatment shortening has relied primarily on decision analytic models of patient cohorts. A study by Owens, Fofana, and Dowdy (2013) examined a hypothetical noninferior first-line regimen and explored trade-offs between drug price, treatment duration, and health system treatment costs for a cohort of new TB patients. This study found that a novel regimen with a four-month duration costing US$1 per day would at worst be highly cost-effective and at best be cost saving, depending on the current level of treatment costs.

Ongoing work using an individual-based cohort model is exploring these trade-offs in specific country settings, using primary cost data from Bangladesh, Brazil, South Africa, and Tanzania (Zwerling and others 2016). This study found that, at the cost of US$1 per day, a four-month noninferior first-line TB drug regimen would be cost saving in South Africa (reducing costs about 10 percent) and in Brazil (reducing costs 20 percent), highly cost-effective in Tanzania (saving about US$120 per DALY averted), but not cost-effective in Bangladesh. Even if new first-line drugs cost up to US$10 and US$58 in South Africa and Brazil, respectively, using threshold analysis, Trajman and others (2016) found that the new TB regimen would be a cost-effective option compared to the standard regimen. This threshold price is US$0.97 in Bangladesh and US$1.13 in Tanzania (Zwerling and others 2016). In all settings, the impact on health would be modest and dependent on current default rates;

settings with higher health system and TB treatment delivery costs would have the highest gain. Unfortunately, the initial first-line regimens with potential regimen-shortening effects coming out of trials in 2014 (moxifloxacin-based regimens) failed to achieve adequate levels of cure, so these gains, at the time of writing, remain hypothetical.

Zwerling and others (2016) also drew attention to the importance of patient costs, with the largest savings achieved through reductions in the economic burden of TB treatment on households. Patient cost savings ranged from US$175 (South Africa) to US$45 (Bangladesh), depending on the setting.

Improving Therapeutic Efficacy in Patients with MDR TB

Compared to drug-resistant TB treatment regimens, much less research has been conducted on the potential cost-effectiveness and impact of new MDR TB regimens. In the last few years, two new MDR TB drugs (bedaquiline and delamanid) have come up for regulatory authority and programmatic approval by the WHO. As part of the process, an exploratory cost-effectiveness analysis was conducted using a decision analytic model of a cohort of new MDR TB cases (Vassall 2013). These analyses found both drugs to be potentially cost-effective, given their impact on efficacy. However, uncertainty around bedaquiline's impact on mortality and, in the case of delamanid, the lack of randomization used when assessing long-term outcomes, combined with the potential cardiotoxic effects, have raised concerns. The DALYs averted varied by setting, with countries already having good outcomes benefiting less. However, increased efficacy, even without treatment shortening, also reduced costs in some cases, as the need for MDR TB retreatment and management of chronic cases was reduced. The results were less certain for LICs; because the potential benefits of increased efficiency for transmission were not included, no definitive conclusion could be reached for these settings.

In the case of bedaquiline, the impact on cost-effectiveness of a shortened MDR TB regimen was also examined, given that the trial results suggested that time to sustained sputum conversion may be reduced (Vassall 2013). Examining a reduction in treatment of two months, the cost-effectiveness analysis found cost savings at current drug prices. However, the extent of cost savings depended on the duration of hospitalization during treatment. The benefits in terms of DALYS averted were less clear due to the trade-off between the reduction in default and cure rates. Further trials, with an integrated economic analysis, are ongoing that test the use of bedaquiline as part of a nine-month MDR TB regimen, the STREAM (Standardized Treatment

Regimen of Anti-Tuberculosis Drugs for Patients with Multi-Drug-Resistant Tuberculosis) Trial (Nunn and others 2014). In 2016, the WHO recommended the new shortened regimen, which offers the promise of both lower drug prices and lower health system costs, while being as effective as longer-course treatments (WHO 2016b). Economic analyses are ongoing.

Developing New Drugs for Treating Drug-Susceptible and MDR TB as First-Line Therapies

For the drugs discussed here, most of the work to date has explored the economic and health benefits of reducing the length of treatment and improving efficacy. However, new drugs or regimens that hold promise for treating both drug-susceptible and rifampicin-resistant TB also may have significant benefits. One example is PaMZ (Diacon and others 2010; Diacon, Dawson, and others 2012), a trial currently on hold. This new treatment regimen was assumed to have a dual benefit: a shortened first-line treatment for drug-susceptible patients (four months) with an efficacy noninferior to the current standard treatment and a shortened second-line treatment for patients with rifampicin-resistant TB (six months) with an efficacy noninferior to first-line treatment for drug-susceptible TB patients. In this case, introduction of the new regimen could result in substantial cost savings (at least 35 percent reduction) from a societal perspective. The mean cost per presumptive TB patient was reduced by US$23 (28 percent) for health service treatment-related costs and US$42 (42 percent) for patient treatment-related costs in South Africa. When the introduction of PaMZ in a cohort of only rifampicin-resistant patients was modeled, both the reduction in costs and the gain in effect were greater. The clinical safety and effectiveness of this new regimen remains to be determined, but the economic modeling can be applied to any new regimen effective for treating both drug-resistant and drug-susceptible TB.

This model can be extended to explore the gains from a drug with the following optimal characteristics in all dimensions:

1. Short duration (two weeks maximum shortening)
2. High efficacy (95 percent cure rate for drug-susceptible TB, 85 percent for rifampicin-resistant TB)
3. Ability to treat all forms of TB (that is, with no circulating resistance and no need for initial DST)
4. Drug price set at US$5 per day.

Using the same model, Zwerling and others (2016) found that such a drug would be cost saving in a setting such as South Africa. Even with a comparatively high daily cost compared to current treatment, these authors estimated a potential reduction of 51 percent of total TB diagnostic and treatment costs when modeling a cohort of 10,000 presumptive TB patients from a societal perspective. This is primarily a gain on the patient side, including a reduction in the direct costs of treatment and a more rapid return to full productivity. In this high-HIV/AIDS-prevalence setting, there is a slight increase in ART-related costs (from the health service perspective) of 4 percent and an increase in DALYs averted of 6.5 percent, primarily from a reduction in defaults and an increase in cure rates for persons with MDR TB.

In summary, while much of the evidence on the potential economic and health benefits of investment in new TB drugs is based on models, emerging findings suggest that reducing the duration, improving the efficacy, and expanding the range of use of TB regimens may have the potential for substantial economic and public health gains in most settings (table 11.7). In a field with no new drugs for the last half century up until the past five years, the biomedical and drug development challenges cannot be underestimated, but new drugs are now being trialed, and much work refining and validating these nascent predictions is expected to emerge in the coming years.

Costs to Patients of TB Treatment

For diagnosis and many months of treatment for TB, out-of-pocket costs can be catastrophic for patients and their families. Data on patient costs in LMICs are limited and incomplete. In a systematic analysis of 11 publications on patient costs in eight countries in Africa, Ukwaja and others (2012) estimated that mean patient prediagnostic costs varied between US$36 and US$196, corresponding to 10.4 and 35.0 percent of their annual income, respectively. Average patient treatment costs ranged between US$3 and US$662, corresponding to 0.2–30.0 percent of their annual income. Prediagnostic household costs accounted for 13–18.8 percent of patients' annual household income, while total household treatment costs ranged between US$26 and US$662, accounting for 2.9–9.3 percent of annual household income. Consequently, 18 percent to 61 percent of patients received financial assistance from outside their household to cope with the cost of TB care. Patient costs in South Africa for diagnosis and treatment of MDR TB were even more expensive: only 3 percent of patients were still employed, and disability grants were the primary source of income for 44 percent of patients

Table 11.7 Population Impact, Patient Impact, Cost, and Cost-Effectiveness of New Tuberculosis Drugs

Study and goal	Regimen	Setting	Time horizon	Impact (reduction)	Cost	Cost-effectiveness
Shortening treatment duration						
Salomon and others 2006	First-line, 2 month	South-East Asia	2012–30: 18 years	13–21% incidence; 19–25% mortality	—	—
Abu-Raddad and others 2009	First-line, 4 month, noninferior to standard	South-East Asia	2015–50: 35 years	10% incidence	—	—
	First-line, 2 month, 90% efficacy in drug-resistant cases			23% incidence		
	First-line, 10 days, 90% efficacy in drug-resistant cases			27% incidence		
Fofana and others 2014	First-line, 4 month, noninferior to standard	Global, nonspecific	10 years	1.9% incidence; 3.5% mortality	—	—
	First-line, 2 month, noninferior to standard			4.3% incidence; 7.5% mortality		
	First-line, 2 weeks, noninferior to standard			6.7% incidence; 13.1% mortality		

table continues next page

Table 11.7 Population Impact, Patient Impact, Cost, and Cost-Effectiveness of New Tuberculosis Drugs (continued)

Study and goal	Regimen	Setting	Time horizon	Impact (reduction)	Cost	Cost-effectiveness
Owens, Fofana, and Dowdy 2013	First-line, 4 month, noninferior to standard, US$1 per day	Global, nonspecific	Cohort lifetime	7.9 DALYs averted (100 cohort)	Health service cost: cost saving to US$5,900 (2012)	Highly cost-effective to cost saving, depending on current treatment costs
	First-line, 2 month, noninferior to standard, US$5 per day			14.6 DALYs averted (100 cohort)	Health service cost: cost saving to US$20,200 (2012)	Cost saving
Trajman and others 2016	First-line, 4 month, noninferior to standard, US$1 per day	South Africa	Cohort lifetime	Equivalent effect	10% societal cost reduction	Cost saving
		Brazil			20% societal cost reduction	Cost saving
		Bangladesh			3.5% cost increase	Not cost-effective (ICER: 997)
		Tanzania			Cost neutral	Cost-effective (ICER: 120)

Increasing efficacy for MDR TB treatment

Study and goal	Regimen	Setting	Time horizon	Impact (reduction)	Cost	Cost-effectiveness
Vassall 2013	Bedaquiline	China, Estonia, Nepal, Russian Federation, Peru, Philippines	Cohort lifetime	Varied by setting from 0.94 to 5.27 incremental DALYs, depending on current treatment success	Varied by setting from US$823 to US$2,930, depending on ability to reduce retreatment costs	Varied from US$202 to US$2,042 per DALY averted; likely to be cost-effective in all settings except low income, but ICER highly uncertain, depending on assumptions regarding trial results
Vassall 2013	Delamanid	China, Estonia, Nepal, Russian Federation, Peru, the Philippines	Cohort lifetime	Varied by setting from 0.94 to 1.65 incremental DALYs depending on current treatment success	Varied by setting from US$757 to US$2,548	Varied from US$501 to US$1,654 per DALY averted; likely to be cost-effective in all settings except low income, but ICER highly uncertain, depending on assumptions regarding trial results

Developing regimens that are effective in both drug-susceptible and MDR TB

Study and goal	Regimen	Setting	Time horizon	Impact (reduction)	Cost	Cost-effectiveness
Gomez and others 2016	First- (4 month) and second-line (6 month), PaMZ, noninferior to standard for first-line and equivalent to first-line treatment of drug-sensitive TB for MDR patients, less than US$1 per day	South Africa	Cohort lifetime	Equivalent effect estimated, presumptive TB cohort	35% societal cost reduction	Cost saving
				16% increase in DALYs averted, MDR cohort	60% societal cost reduction	Cost saving

Future developments

Study and goal	Regimen	Setting	Time horizon	Impact (reduction)	Cost	Cost-effectiveness
Gomez and others 2016	Optimal: first- and second-line, 2 weeks, high efficacy, US$5 per day, no extra DST	South Africa	Cohort lifetime	6.5% increase in DALYs averted	51% societal cost reduction; 58.1% patient costs reduction; 56.5% treatment costs reduction; no change in diagnosis costs	Cost saving

Note: DALY = disability-adjusted life year; ICER = incremental cost-effectiveness ratio; MDR = multidrug resistant; TB = tuberculosis; PaMZ = pretomanid/moxifloxacin/pyrazinamide; DST = drug-sensitivity testing; — = not available.

(Ramma and others 2015). Many of the patients reported having no source of income before (56 percent) and during (47 percent) treatment. These costs were likely catastrophic for many patients.

Modeling the Impact of New Vaccines

The last decade has seen a significant increase in the level of investment in TB vaccine development: more than 14 TB vaccine candidates have been tested in 50 human trials, with funding of more than US$600 million (Jiménez-Levi 2012). Despite the significant costs of vaccine development (Brennan and Thole 2012), the complex task of selecting vaccine candidates must now occur. Therefore, there is an effort to determine globally acceptable criteria for differentiating and subsequently maintaining the most promising candidates in the vaccine pipeline (Brennan and Thole 2012).

Mathematical modeling can be used to differentiate candidates on the basis of the potential impact that different vaccine characteristics targeted at different population groups may have on the future TB burden. For example, modeling the impact of vaccines targeted at uninfected infants in South-East Asia has suggested that a novel vaccine introduced in 2015 could avert more than 40 percent of the TB burden by 2050 (Abu-Raddad and others 2009) and that, to have the most rapid impact on TB burden, such a vaccine would need to be efficacious in both uninfected and latently infected individuals (Dye and Williams 2008). Linking such work to the economics of TB vaccines has shown that different TB vaccine profiles can also be cost-effective (BIO Ventures for Global Health 2006; Ditkowsky and Schwartzman 2014; Tseng and others 2011). However, uncertainty remains about how various vaccine characteristics (efficacy, duration of protection) and targeting strategies (age, HIV/AIDS status) may combine to maximize impact in countries with the largest TB burden.

The underlying economics of TB vaccines are also unclear. For example, depending on the vaccine profile, the likely price of both vaccine delivery and dose remains uncertain. TB vaccines for infants could be incorporated into the standard infant vaccination program (DTP3 [diphtheria-tetanus-pertussis]), and cost estimates are straightforward to generate. However, the economics of targeting adolescents and older populations are largely unknown, and only recently are these populations being considered as a new platform for other vaccines, such as human papillomavirus (Sinanovic and others 2009) or measles booster. In the future, with these and other potential vaccines (for example, measles, human papillomavirus, or a future HIV/AIDS vaccine) for adolescents and adults, the targeting of adolescents via schools is likely to become

increasingly common, and thus the costs may decrease. Due to the pervasiveness of Mtb infection in high-burden settings, TB vaccines targeted at adults may be used in mass campaigns to prevent disease. There are few precedents for such campaigns, and the levels of coverage that could be achievable are open to debate. Similarly, the lack of acceptability of frequent mass campaigns could limit the potential impact of a TB vaccine for adults. Finally, it is possible that vaccines could be targeted to patients being treated with TB or MDR TB either to accelerate treatment times or to prevent recurrence after drug treatment.

Knight and others (2014) have explored a wide range of vaccine profiles to understand what type of vaccine profile, targeted at what age group, would have the biggest impact on TB incidence in LMICs (Knight and others 2014). Vaccine profiles were defined by both efficacy and duration of protection, with a range from 40 to 80 percent and from five years to lifetime, respectively. The vaccine was assumed to be introduced in 2024. A comparison was then made between targeting infants and targeting adolescents or adults in mass campaigns. A new TB vaccine would likely be used as a booster to BCG, due to the broad use of BCG and its efficacy in infants. The vaccine was assumed to prevent active disease in both uninfected and latently infected individuals, with 40 percent less efficacy in persons with HIV/AIDS. Vaccine "take" was modeled with an exact duration of protection. Each country was modeled separately, with calibration methods used to capture both uncertainty in natural history parameters and the data on TB burden (WHO 2013b). Vaccine coverage was taken from similar mass campaigns in each country, such as for rubella, and were timed to occur with a frequency of every 10 years or the duration of protection (whichever was shorter) from 2024 onward. Cost-effectiveness was defined as cost per DALY averted compared against gross national income per capita from a health sector perspective, with tiered vaccine pricing by income group.

By estimating the burden of TB in all LMICs for which data were available, the model was able to predict that a vaccine targeted at adolescents or adults would have a far greater impact on TB burden before 2050 than one targeted at infants (figure 11.10) (Knight and others 2014). This is due to the differential burden of disease between these two age groups, with infants suffering from greater levels of extrapulmonary TB and therefore contributing less to transmission (Styblo 1991). This conclusion remained valid over the 2024–50 period, even when considering lifetime duration of protection.

Knight and others (2014) reported that vaccines targeted at adolescents or adults with 10-year durations of protection and 60 percent efficacy could be cost-effective in LICs at US$149 (95 percent range cost saving of US$387) per DALY averted at a cost of US$1 per dose.

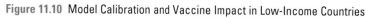

Figure 11.10 Model Calibration and Vaccine Impact in Low-Income Countries

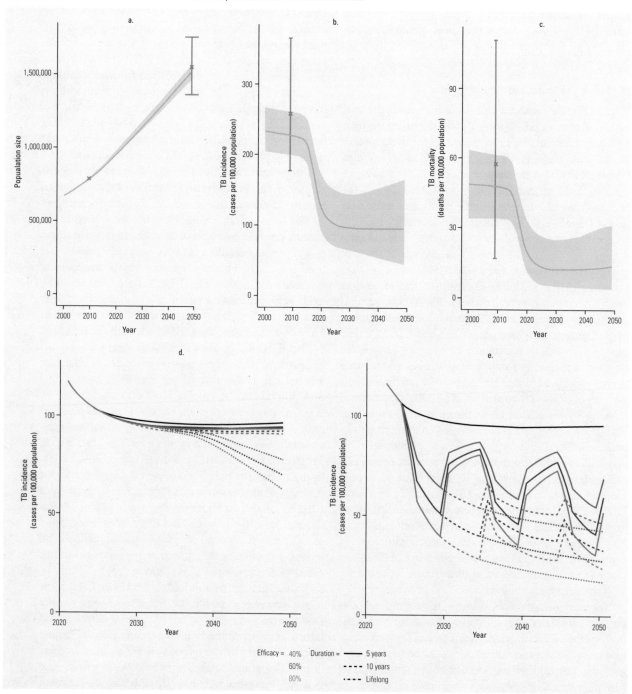

Note: Model calibration (panels a–c) and vaccine impact (panels d–e) in low-income countries. Panels a–c show median (solid dark blue line) and 95% range (blue cloud) of model fits to data. (Panel a) Human population size (per 1,000) in low-income countries, 2000–50. (Panel b) Tuberculosis (TB) incidence: cases per 100,000 population per year, 2000–50 (Panel c) TB mortality: deaths per 100,000 population per year, 2000–50. (Panels d–e) TB incidence (cases per 100,000 population per year), 2000–50, with median model output (black line) and vaccine profile impact: characteristics of efficacy (color) and duration of protection (line type) for vaccines targeted at infants (panel d) or at adolescent or adults (panel e). A vaccine targeted at infants (panel d) has a smaller impact on TB disease incidence than one targeted at adolescents or adults (panel e). The "waves" within the adolescent or adult incidence figure (panel e) are due to the impact of mass campaigns.

The same profile targeted at infants would avert only 0.89 (0.42–1.58) million TB cases while averting 17 (11–24) million TB cases in adolescents or adults and would not be considered cost-effective at US$1,692 (US$634–US$4,603) per DALY averted. In threshold analysis, the price per dose at which the vaccine profile would be cost-effective was determined. For example, a vaccine with 10-year duration of protection and 60 percent efficacy targeted at adolescents or adults could be priced at up to US$20 in upper-middle-income countries and still be considered cost-effective. This reflects the large number of cases that could be averted by targeting the age group in which most cases of disease occur and in which most sources of transmission are found. Vaccines with short duration (five years) and low efficacy (40 percent) were also found to be cost-effective if targeted at adolescents and adults.

A recent review pointed out that funding for TB vaccine development significantly lacks the same support provided to other vaccine development efforts (Manjelievskaia and others 2016). For example, funding to develop an Ebola vaccine ramped up quickly following the 2013–14 epidemic in Guinea, Liberia, and Sierra Leone, an outbreak that killed approximately 11,310 persons. The global response to the outbreak was enormous; the U.S. government alone appropriated more than US$5.4 billion for the Ebola emergency response in 2015, of which a large portion was directed to research, including developing Ebola vaccines. In comparison, funding to develop a TB vaccine received only US$85 million to US$90 million in 2015 (based on prior years' funding numbers), despite an estimated 29,000 people dying of TB per week (based on 2014 mortality estimates) and little sign of meaningful diminution in the global spread of Mtb and the continuing spread of MDR and XDR TB (Frick, Henry, and Lessem 2016; TAG 2016).

In conclusion, vaccines have an enormous potential to reduce the incidence and prevalence of TB if they are targeted at adolescents or adults, suggesting that increased investments in candidate vaccines targeting this group are warranted. Vaccines are also likely to be highly cost-effective, even if only having relatively modest clinical effectiveness. Given the age-dependent period of risk, special consideration should be given to developing candidate vaccines providing long-term protection.

EXTENDED COST-EFFECTIVENESS ANALYSIS OF UNIVERSAL PUBLIC FINANCING OF TB TREATMENT

Tuberculosis causes approximately 28 million active infections and 480,000 deaths in India annually (WHO 2016a). The disease burden is concentrated largely within the poorer parts of the population: TB has a four times greater incidence among persons in lower socio-economic groups, and incidence is greater in rural than urban areas (Muniyandi and others 2007). Private health expenditures also constitute a large majority of India's total health expenditures, and most TB patients consult private practitioners for their first visit, resulting in substantial OOP spending on TB (Satyanarayana and others 2011; Uplekar and others 1998; Uplekar, Pathania, and Raviglione 2001). In India, as in many countries, OOP medical costs are a leading cause of impoverishment. Kruk, Goldmann, and Galeo (2009) and Sengupta and Nundy (2005) found, for example, that about 40 percent of Indian households borrowed money or sold assets to pay for health care. In light of such findings, the government is increasingly assuming responsibility for financing TB treatment (Jha and Laxminarayan 2009).

Universal public finance (UPF) is when government finances an intervention irrespective of who is receiving it. For any given health intervention, UPF entails consequences in multiple domains. First, UPF increases intervention uptake. Second, it eliminates the need for private expenditures. Finally, it provides financial risk protection (insurance) by covering catastrophic expenditures that would otherwise throw households into poverty. This section reports on these three consequences of UPF using extended cost-effectiveness analysis (ECEA) findings on DOTs expansion in India (Verguet, Laxminarayan, and Jamison 2015).

Because of the importance of OOP costs, international agencies have supported the use of health sector policies to attenuate health-related financial risks (WHO 1999, 2010; World Bank 1993). Despite the attention paid to its significant potential as part of broader social insurance, UPF in practice covers few interventions in most LMICs, with little consensus on what to cover in highly resource-constrained environments. In India, UPF has typically financed condition-specific programs (for example, against leprosy, HIV/AIDS, and cataract blindness) or, more recently, secondary and tertiary care insurance such as the Rashtriya Swasthya Bima Yojana and the Arogyasri (in Andhra Pradesh) programs. These insurance programs are thought to provide significant financial protection since they defray the high OOP costs associated with hospitalizations.

Currently, about 70 percent of TB cases receive DOTS; only about half of these services are obtained for free in the public sector. People do not always obtain TB treatment at the public hospital level for various reasons, including transportation cost and waiting time. Most lower-income people prefer to see a private physician after working hours than to take a day off work without pay to visit a public hospital (Kumar and Kumar 1997).

Table 11.8 Public Finance of Tuberculosis Treatment to 90 Percent Coverage in India, by Income Quintile
per million population

Outcome	Total	Income Quintile				
		I	II	III	IV	V
TB deaths averted	80	40	25	12	3	0
Private expenditures crowded out[a]	29	6	6	7	6	4
Insurance value[a]	9	5	2	1	1	0

Note: TB = tuberculosis.
a. Figures expressed in 2011 US$, thousands.

Table 11.9 Borrowing to Finance Tuberculosis Treatment in India, by Income Quintile
per million population

Outcome	Total	Income Quintile				
		I	II	III	IV	V
TB deaths averted	29	13	10	5	1	0
Private expenditures crowded out[a]	−25	−12	−8	−4	−1	0
Insurance value[a]	0	0	0	0	0	0

Note: TB = tuberculosis.
a. Figures expressed in 2011 US$, thousands.

Yet, privately purchased TB treatment is often ineffective because private doctors do not necessarily provide the standard regimen with proven efficiency (Satyanarayana and others 2011; Udwadia, Pinto, and Uplekar 2010; Uplekar and Shepard 1991). A potential virtue of UPF is to eliminate low-quality treatment in the private sector, enabling the uptake of higher-quality treatment and increasing technical efficiency. However, this requires a well-managed public sector program, something widely achieved only in parts of India.

We estimated the results of expanding DOTS through UPF to cover 90 percent for an Indian population of 1 million (table 11.8). The total number of lives saved would be about 80 per 1 million per year, and the health benefits would be concentrated among the bottom two income quintiles (80 percent), as TB has a higher incidence among these socioeconomic groups. The total number of private expenditures averted by the program would be about US$30,000 per 1 million population per year, and the bottom two quintiles would benefit from about 40 percent of the private expenditures averted. The total financial protection provided for this population sample (measured as a money-metric value of insurance) would be about US$10,000, 80 percent of which would accrue to the bottom two quintiles. The total (incremental) treatment costs incurred by UPF for the sample would be about US$65,000.

This analysis illustrates how UPF can be used to improve financial protection and technical efficiency by eliminating the purchase of lower-quality treatments. It is only a limited take on greater possibilities. For example, a detailed assessment could provide more comprehensive estimates of TB costs (for example, households' transportation costs, earnings, and productivity impacts). The focus here is on the OOP cost of treatment and excludes the cost of earnings reduced by the disease. For example, the number of working days lost due to TB can range from 30 to 90 in South India (Muniyandi and others 2006; Muniyandi and others 2008). Indirect costs from lost earnings can be substantial (Ananthakrishnan and others 2012), which would—in the absence of other forms of social insurance—increase the insurance benefits provided by UPF.

A limitation of focusing on the financial cost of treatment is that individuals do not get care for other reasons as well, including lack of information about TB and its treatment. Primary health centers in India may be difficult to reach due to poor travel conditions (Muniyandi and others 2006), be overcrowded, and not respect the dignity of patients. Health services may not always be available, even after informational and financial barriers have been removed: increasing coverage may thus not be feasible, and the extent of subsequent health gains from UPF may be significantly reduced in the absence of supply-side intervention. If demand for TB treatment for any of these reasons does not match disease incidence, the level of coverage achievable will be constrained.

Yet, using ECEA, Verguet, Laxminarayan, and Jamison (2015) demonstrated that the potential benefits of UPF for health and financial risk protection would accrue primarily to the poor. Reductions in OOP expenditures would also benefit the poor because UPF crowds out private financing of the inferior treatments frequently purchased by persons with income constraints. Lowering the costs of borrowing for the poor could potentially achieve some of the health gains of UPF, but at the cost of leaving the poor more deeply in debt (table 11.9).

SUMMARY AND RECOMMENDATIONS

While much progress has been made over the past several decades, particularly in reducing mortality, TB remains a major infectious disease, whose severity is exacerbated by the growing problem of multidrug-resistant TB, extensively drug-resistant TB, and co-infection with HIV/AIDS. Progress in TB control requires early and accurate case detection, rapid commencement of and adherence to effective treatment, and prevention of transmission.

The great challenge is to reduce transmission by identifying and treating patients with TB who are asymptomatic, unaware of their status, or unable to gain access to treatment.

This chapter offers four overarching recommendations: (1) strengthen the current WHO End TB Strategy to emphasize active case finding in targeted high-burden countries; (2) strengthen health systems in those countries, particularly emphasizing community-based care; (3) strengthen information systems; and (4) invest far more in research to develop the tools necessary to control TB. Fundamentally, it is necessary to revise the current global TB control strategies in most high-burden countries and to make significant new investments in health systems and research.

Rethinking and Revising the DOTS Strategy

Since the WHO designated tuberculosis as a global emergency in 1993, the DOTS strategy has been the mainstay of TB control worldwide. It is based on the premise that patients with TB will be sufficiently ill to seek care from the health system and, if appropriately treated, be cured and that transmission will be reduced. Since 1994, the DOTS strategy has significantly improved the diagnosis and treatment of individuals identified with tuberculosis in all countries and reduced mortality. The prevalence and treatment of drug-susceptible TB is a "best buy" at US$100–US$500 per case cured. Treatment of MDR TB remains limited and more expensive. Yet the decline of TB incidence globally, particularly in the 22 highest-burden countries, has lagged the declines in HIV/AIDS and malaria and is far below the MDG targets set by the Stop TB Partnership to reduce TB incidence, prevalence, and mortality by 50 percent compared with a baseline of 1990. With TB exceeding HIV/AIDS and malaria as the largest cause of death from any single infectious disease and drug resistance increasing, it is critical to reconsider how to control the epidemic more effectively.

DOTS has the great advantage of being a single, unifying global strategy that, in principle, can be applied to all patients in all countries. Yet, while effective in countries with strong health systems, DOTS is failing to bend the incidence curve rapidly, especially in LICs with high TB burdens and weak health systems. Management of TB has been particularly challenging in LMICs with high incidence and prevalence of co-infection with HIV/AIDS, which makes treatment more difficult and relapse or reinfection more common. Of particular concern is the limited impact of DOTS on the effective control of MDR TB, which requires complex diagnostic testing and is enormously expensive (US$5,000–US$10,000 per case cured) and only partially effective. TB, especially MDR TB, represents a serious threat to health personnel in high-burden countries. Even with high patient treatment compliance, in these contexts, DOTS as commonly implemented is not reducing the transmission and incidence of disease sufficiently rapidly. As this chapter discusses, substantial numbers of individuals with TB have tubercle bacilli in their sputa and yet are asymptomatic and not likely to report to a health facility and thus be detected by passive case finding.

In this context, the WHO has revised and promulgated the End TB Strategy, which emphasizes patient-centered care, treatment for all patients with drug-susceptible and drug-resistant TB, increased community engagement, and, for the first time, an explicit focus on research. Consistent with the End TB Strategy (WHO 2015a), this chapter suggests that a stratified approach with improved targeting in high-burden countries will be necessary in these contexts. Such a diversified and better-targeted strategy, should seek to accomplish the following:

1. Identify high-transmission countries and hot spots within countries where targeted efforts can be more effective and cost-effective.
2. Increase the capacity for surveillance.
3. Strengthen early TB detection and diagnosis by active case finding in certain countries and populations.
4. Provide rapid diagnosis and enable more rapid initiation and better maintenance of treatment for both drug-susceptible and multidrug-resistant TB.
5. Expand preventive therapy of the contacts of TB patients, children, and HIV-positive individuals.
6. Combine these strategies with an approach rooted in community-based delivery of TB services and support, wherever possible.
7. Improve the drug supply chain to improve access to TB treatments that have very small markets, and improve information technology to enable more effective control.
8. Significantly increase resources for research on developing new diagnostic technologies, development and testing of new drug regimens, and new vaccines to prevent TB.

All of these recommendations, while at some variance with previous DOTS protocols, are fully consistent with the new WHO End TB strategic goals (WHO 2015a). The new Stop TB Partnership's Zero TB Initiative seeks to apply these recommendations to demonstrate in a small number of high-burden cities that a comprehensive program of active case finding, effective treatment, and prevention in households can be effective in limiting transmission and reducing the incidence of TB (Stop TB Partnership 2016).

Expanding Active Case Finding

In high-burden, low-income countries, particularly those with a high incidence and prevalence of TB and HIV/AIDS co-infection, earlier and more comprehensive case finding and treatment are required. Passive case finding and screening of populations for classic symptoms clearly fail to detect a major proportion of existing TB cases, which are asymptomatic or unknown to the health system—representing up to one-third or 3 million cases—leading to continued transmission of TB infection. In low-burden countries where DOTS is effective in reducing incidence, prevalence, and mortality, the current approach should be expanded, and investments in active case finding are not likely to be cost-effective. But, in high-burden countries, targeted introduction of active case finding with modern rapid and point-of-care diagnostic tests and mobile X-radiography for screening populations could significantly improve early diagnosis and early institution of treatment and dramatically reduce transmission. As this chapter discusses, TB treatment regimens are lengthy and not without drug-related adverse events, which, in weak health systems, create challenges to maintaining consistent adherence to recommended drugs (Schaaf and others 2009; Verma and others 2004). Health systems that can provide patient support, including mechanisms to incentivize treatment completion, can bolster the effectiveness of active case finding.

Strengthening Health Systems

With drug-resistant TB now a global crisis, early diagnosis and effective treatment, either through improved access to bacterial culture and drug-sensitivity testing (Dowdy and others 2008; Uys and others 2009) or through rapid molecular diagnostics (Lin and others 2012), are essential to reduce the burden of drug-resistant TB in high-prevalence settings. Modeling studies suggest that these interventions could be highly cost-effective, because they provide not only potentially life-saving care but also prevent further spread of drug-resistant disease (Menzies and others 2012). Modeling studies also suggest that infection-control interventions can be very cost-effective (Basu and others 2007), especially when aimed at health care workers and the patients responsible for most transmission (Andersson 2006; Woolhouse and others 1997).

Although some new diagnostics and care delivery models have emerged, the uptake of new tools and innovations for TB control has been suboptimal in weak health systems (Cobelens and others 2012). New tools such as the Xpert MTB/RIF assay enable rapid and effective diagnosis of TB and MDR TB (Boehme and others 2010; Boehme and others 2011; Chang and others 2012), do not require highly skilled health workers (Rachow and others 2011), and have been demonstrated to be cost-effective (Vassall and others 2011). However, their rapid introduction has been hindered by weak health systems, specifically weak supply chain management systems, weak information systems linking diagnostic data to the site of treatment, and the need to address false-positive indications of rifampicin resistance (Dowdy and others 2011; Kirwan, Cárdenas, and Gilman 2012; Lawn and others 2011; Scott and others 2011; Trébucq and others 2011).

Increased numbers of better trained and motivated health workers at multiple levels, better information systems, and functioning logistics and supply chains are critical if TB is to be effectively controlled. TB transmission can be prevented through investments in infection control in clinics and hospitals; preventive therapy for household and HIV-positive contacts; better-designed housing for low-income populations; and better nutrition for at-risk populations. Efforts like these require technical and financial support, not only in TB programs per se, but also in complementary activities that support the delivery of TB services. Without improving health systems, extending the scope and targeting of TB programs, and providing additional technical and financial support, it is questionable how significantly and rapidly high-burden countries can improve TB control.

Expanding Community-Based Care

While in many countries, TB treatment has traditionally been hospital-based, in an increasing number of settings community-based treatment has been shown to be as clinically effective and significantly more cost-effective, even when compared with clinic-based management of TB. Efforts should be undertaken to transition health systems from hospital-based to community-based care in countries where doing so is feasible. Community-based care and treatment are effective and may offset some of the increases in financing required for active case finding. It will be important, in countries with large private health care providers, to develop public-private partnerships to engage the private sector in offering the best possible diagnostic and treatment protocols. Strengthening health systems to support more effective community-based TB care—including investing in community-based health workers, information systems, and supply chains—can have significant impact, not only on TB, but also on other infectious and chronic diseases, including HIV/AIDS and noncommunicable diseases such as diabetes and cardiovascular disease, which similarly require long-term or continuous treatment.

Strengthening Research and Development

The current tools for combatting TB are woefully inadequate, yet funding for TB research lags that for HIV/AIDS and malaria. Reducing the burden of TB and MDR TB will require greater funding for more intensive research into new approaches to point-of-care diagnosis, shorter and more effective treatment regimens for both TB and MDR TB, and better service delivery. But the current drug pipeline is thin. There is an urgent need for new drugs and regimens that will be cost-effective and affordable. Of particular urgency is the need to develop new multidrug regimens that shorten the duration of treatment, increase the number of cures of drug-susceptible TB, and, ideally, increase the number of cures of both drug-susceptible *and* drug-resistant TB. A small number of new drugs appear promising in this regard, but require further clinical evaluation. New regimens capable of effectively treating both drug-susceptible and drug-resistant TB would reduce the need for expensive drug-sensitivity testing and could be highly cost-effective. Several molecular tools are being developed that could allow prediction of risk for patients with latent infection to progress to active disease and, possibly, of when treated cases are truly cured. This approach could enable preventive treatment of individuals at high risk of progression to disease. The same molecular tools may be able to identify host gene signatures that would identify protective immune responses that could become biomarkers for predicting the efficacy of new vaccines.

Developing more effective vaccines to prevent TB infection, disease, relapse, or reinfection will be essential, since even a modestly successful vaccine would be highly cost-effective. BCG remains the most widely used vaccine in the world; while its ability to prevent severe childhood consequences of TB is cost-effective, its impact on preventing disease in adults is questionable at best. Preventing infection and disease is the major goal of vaccine research, and, given the challenges to case detection, drug resistance, and cure, it remains uncertain whether TB can be eliminated as a global public health problem without an effective preventive vaccine.

Drug, device, and vaccine companies are essential to developing the new tools required for TB, but they have few incentives to invest in a disease that occurs primarily in resource-poor countries where the returns on investments in long-term development and trials will be few, if any. Public-private collaborations could make a major difference to developing new technologies for TB.

The Bottom Line

TB remains the largest cause of death from an infectious disease, and, in contrast to HIV/AIDS and malaria, the incidence is not declining at a rate required to bring this epidemic under control. This chapter urges that the traditional strategy to control TB most commonly implemented in many countries, which has been successful in low-burden countries of the Americas and Europe, needs to evolve into a more stratified and targeted approach in order to meet the needs of high-burden populations where it has not been effective in controlling transmission and reducing incidence of TB. The WHO's End TB Strategy now emphasizes differences in the epidemic in different countries and the need for research to develop new tools (WHO 2015a, 2015c). The recommendations of this chapter are fully consistent with the WHO's End TB Strategy.

This chapter argues that new investments are needed to make health systems more responsive and effective by providing greater access to improved technologies for rapid diagnosis and to drug-sensitivity testing. It advocates for introducing new modalities, such as active case finding and community-based care in high-burden settings. Finally, it emphasizes the urgent need for greater investments in research to develop new tools for diagnosis, drug regimens for treatment, and vaccines for prevention. Such investments will be costly—and more funding will be required to extend current efforts and enable the new approaches recommended here—but ultimately highly cost-effective for both individuals and countries. Only with new thinking and new approaches will it be possible to transform TB control to a level that can achieve the ultimate goal of eliminating TB as a global public health problem. To reduce significantly the largest cause of death from infectious disease in the world and to improve the lives of people who suffer from it, greater financial investments will be necessary and indeed justified.

NOTES

World Bank Income Classifications as of July 2014 are as follows, based on estimates of gross national income (GNI) per capita for 2013:

- Low-income countries (LICs) = US$1,045 or less
- Middle-income countries (MICs) are subdivided:
  (a) lower-middle-income = US$1,046 to US$4,125
  (b) upper-middle-income (UMICs) = US$4,126 to US$12,745
- High-income countries (HICs) = US$12,746 or more.

1. For example, http://reference.medscape.com/drug-interactionchecker or http://www.hiv-druginteractions.org.
2. For the WHO recommendations, see http://www.who.int/hiv/topics/tb/art_hivpatients/en.
3. Described at http://www1.nyc.gov/assets/doh/downloads/pdf/tb/tb2015.pdf.

4. For example, OpenBoxes (https://openboxes.com) and OpenLMIS (https://www.villagereach.org).

5. Sproxil (https://www.sproxil.com).

REFERENCES

Abel L, J. El-Baghdadi, A. A. Bousfiha, J. L. Casanova, and E. Schurr. 2014. "Human Genetics of Tuberculosis: A Long and Winding Road." *Archive of Philosophical Transitions of the Royal Society of London* 12: 369 (1645): 20130428.

Abimbola, T. O., B. J. Marston, A. A. Date, J. M. Blandford, N. Sangrujee, and others. 2012. "Cost-Effectiveness of Tuberculosis Diagnostic Strategies to Reduce Early Mortality among Persons with Advanced HIV Infection Initiating Antiretroviral Therapy." *Journal of Acquired Immune Deficiency Syndromes* 60 (1): e1–7.

Abu-Raddad, L. J., L. Sabatelli, J. T. Achterberg, J. D. Sugimoto, I. M. Longini Jr., and others. 2009. "Epidemiological Benefits of More-Effective Tuberculosis Vaccines, Drugs, and Diagnostics." *Proceedings of the National Academy of Sciences* 106 (33): 13980–85.

Achkar, J. M., and E. R. Jenny-Avital. 2011. "Incipient and Subclinical Tuberculosis: Defining Early Disease States in the Context of Host Immune Response." *Journal of Infectious Diseases* 204 (Suppl 4): S1179–86.

Acuna-Villaorduna, C., A. Vassall, G. Henostroza, C. Seas, H. Guerra, and others. 2008. "Cost-Effectiveness Analysis of Introduction of Rapid, Alternative Methods to Identify Multidrug-Resistant Tuberculosis in Middle-Income Countries." *Clinical Infectious Diseases* 47 (4): 487–95.

Ahuja, S. D., D. Ashkin, M. Avendano, R. Banerjee, M. Bauer, and others. 2012. "Multidrug Resistant Pulmonary Tuberculosis Treatment Regimens and Patient Outcomes: An Individual Patient Data Meta-Analysis of 9,153 Patients." *PLoS Medicine* 9 (8): e1001300.

Akolo, C., I. Adetifa, S. Shepperd, and J. Volmink. 2010. "Treatment of Latent Tuberculosis Infection in HIV Infected Persons." *Cochrane Database of Systematic Reviews* 20: CD000171.

Alhajri, K., N. Alzerwi, K. Alsaleh, H. Bin Yousef, and M. Alzaben. 2011. "Disseminated (Miliary) Abdominal Tuberculosis after Laparoscopic Gastric Bypass Surgery." *BMJ Case Reports* 2011 (May 12): bcr1220103591.

Alsdurf, H., P. C. Hill, A. Matteelli, H. Getahun, and D. Menzies. 2016. "The Cascade of Care in Diagnosis and Treatment of Latent Tuberculosis Infection: A Systematic Review and Meta-Analysis." *The Lancet Infectious Diseases* 16: 1269–78.

Amoroso, C., B Akimana, B. Wise, and H. S. F. Fraser. 2010. "Using Electronic Medical Records for HIV Care in Rural Rwanda." *Studies Health Technology and Informatics* 160 (Pt. 1): 337–41.

Ananthakrishnan, R., M. Muniyandi, A. Jeyaraj, G. Palani, and B. W. C. Sathiyasekaran. 2012. "Expenditure Pattern for TB Treatment among Patients Registered in an Urban Government DOTS Program in Chennai City, South India." *Tuberculosis Research and Treatment* 2012: 747924.

Andersson, D. I. 2006. "The Biological Cost of Mutational Antibiotic Resistance: Any Practical Conclusions?" *Current Opinion in Microbiology* 9 (5): 461–65.

Andrews, J. R., F. Noubary, R. P. Walensky, R. Cerda, E. Losina, and others. 2012. "Risk of Progression to Active Tuberculosis Following Reinfection with *Mycobacterium tuberculosis*." *Clinical Infectious Diseases* 54 (6): 784–91.

Ansa, G. A., J. D. Walley, K. Siddiqi, and X. Wei. 2012. "Assessing the Impact of TB/HIV Services Integration on TB Treatment Outcomes and Their Relevance in TB/HIV Monitoring in Ghana." *Infectious Diseases of Poverty* 1 (December 24): 13.

Arinaminpathy, N., T. Cordier-Lassalle, K. Lunte, and C. Dye. 2015. "The Global Drug Facility as an Intervention in the Market for Tuberculosis Drugs." *Bulletin of the World Health Organization* 93 (4): 237–48A.

Atun, R. 2012. "Health Systems, Systems Thinking and Innovation." *Health Policy and Planning* 27 (Suppl 4): iv4–8.

Atun, R., and R. Coker. 2008. "Health Systems and Communicable Disease Control: Emerging Evidence and Lessons from Central and Eastern Europe." In *Health Systems and the Challenge of Communicable Diseases: Experiences from Europe and Latin America*, edited by R. Coker, R. Atun, and M. McKee, 193–208. Maidenhead, U.K.: Open University Press.

Atun, R., T. de Jongh, F. Secci, K. Ohiri, and O. Adeyi. 2010. "Integration of Targeted Health Interventions into Health Systems: A Conceptual Framework for Analysis." *Health Policy and Planning* 25 (2): 104–11.

Atun, R., F. M. Knaul, Y. Akachi, and J. Frenk. 2012. "Innovative Financing for Health: What Is Truly Innovative?" *The Lancet* 380 (9858): 2044–49.

Atun, R., J. V. Lazarus, W. Van Damme, and R. Coker. 2010. "Interactions between Critical Health System Functions and HIV/AIDS, Tuberculosis, and Malaria Programmes." *Health Policy and Planning* 25 (Suppl 1): 11–13.

Atun, R., M. McKee, F. Drobniewski, and R. Coker. 2005. "Analysis of How the Health Systems Context Shapes Responses to the Control of Human Immunodeficiency Virus: Case-Studies from the Russian Federation." *Bulletin of the World Health Organization* 83 (10): 730–38.

Atun, R., N. Menabde, K. Saluvere, M. Jesse, and J. Habicht. 2006. "Introducing a Complex Health Innovation— Primary Health Care Reforms in Estonia (Multimethods Evaluation)." *Health Policy* 79 (1): 79–91.

Atun, R., Y. Samyshkin, F. Drobniewski, Y. Balabanova, I. Fedorin, and others. 2006. "Costs and Outcomes of Tuberculosis Control in the Russian Federation: Retrospective Cohort Analysis." *Health Policy and Planning* 21 (5): 353–64.

Atun, R., Y. Samyshkin, F. Drobniewski, N. M. Skuratova, G. Gusarova, and others. 2005. "Barriers to Sustainable Tuberculosis Control in the Russian Federation Health System." *Bulletin of the World Health Organization* 83 (3): 217–23.

Atun, R., D. E. Weil, M. Tan Eang, and D. Mwakyusa. 2010. "Health-System Strengthening and Tuberculosis Control." *The Lancet* 375 (9732): 2169–78.

Awofeso, N., I. Schelokova, and A. Dalhatu. 2008. "Training of Front-line Health Workers for Tuberculosis Control:

Lessons from Nigeria and Kyrgyzstan." *Human Resources for Health* 6 (20): 1–9.

Ayieko, J., L. Abuogi, B. Simchowitz, E. A. Bukusi, A. H. Smith, and others. 2014. "Efficacy of Isoniazid Prophylactic Therapy in Prevention of Tuberculosis in Children: A Meta-Analysis." *BMC Infectious Diseases* 14: 91.

Ayles, H., and M. Muyoyeta. 2006. "Isoniazid to Prevent First and Recurrent Episodes of TB." *Tropical Doctor* 36 (2): 83–86.

Ayles, H., M. Muyoyeta, E. Du Toit, A. Schaap, S. Floyd, and others. 2013. "Effect of Household and Community Interventions on the Burden of Tuberculosis in Southern Africa: The ZAMSTAR Community-Randomised Trial." *The Lancet* 382 (9899): 1183–94.

Ayles, H., A. Schaap, A. Nota, C. Sismanidis, R. Tembwe, and others. 2009. "Prevalence of Tuberculosis, HIV, and Respiratory Symptoms in Two Zambian Communities: Implications for Tuberculosis Control in the Era of HIV." *PLoS One* 4 (5): e5602.

Aziz, A., M. Ishaq, and R. Akhwand. 1985. "Infection Risk of Sputum Positive Tuberculosis Patients to Their Family Contacts with and without Chemotherapy." *Journal of Pakistan Medical Association* 35 (8): 249–52.

Baker, M. A., D. Wilson, K. Wallengren, A. Sandgren, O. Iartchouk, and others. 2012. "Polymorphisms in the Gene That Encodes the Iron Transport Protein Ferroportin 1 Influence Susceptibility to Tuberculosis." *Journal of Infectious Diseases* 205 (7): 1043–47.

Barrington, J., O. Wereko-Brobby, P. Ward, W. Mwafongo, and S. Kungulwe. 2010. "SMS for Life: A Pilot Project to Improve Anti-Malarial Drug Supply Management in Rural Tanzania Using Standard Technology." *Malaria Journal* 9 (298): 1–9.

Barry, C. E., H. I. Boshoff, V. Dartois, T. Dick, S. Ehrt, and others. 2009. "The Spectrum of Latent Tuberculosis: Rethinking the Biology and Intervention Strategies." *Nature Reviews Microbiology* 7 (12): 845–55.

Barter, D. M., S. O. Agboola, M. B. Murray, and T. Bärnighausen. 2012. "Tuberculosis and Poverty: The Contribution of Patient Costs in Sub-Saharan Africa—A Systematic Review." *BMC Public Health* 12 (November 14): 980.

Bassili, A., C. Fitzpatrick, E. Qadeer, R. Fatima, K. Floyd, and others. 2013. "A Systematic Review of the Effectiveness of Hospital- and Ambulatory-Based Management of Multidrug-Resistant Tuberculosis." *American Journal of Tropical Medicine and Hygiene* 89 (2): 271–80.

Basu, S., J. R. Andrews, E. M. Poolman, N. R. Gandhi, N. S. Shah, and others. 2007. "Prevention of Nosocomial Transmission of Extensively Drug-Resistant Tuberculosis in Rural South African District Hospitals: An Epidemiological Modelling Study." *The Lancet* 370 (9597): 1500–07.

Basu, S., and A. P. Galvani. 2008. "The Transmission and Control of XDR TB in South Africa: An Operations Research and Mathematical Modelling Approach." *Epidemiology and Infection* 136 (12): 1585–98.

Bates, M., J. O'Grady, P. Mwaba, L. Chilukutu, J. Mzyece, and others. 2012. "Evaluation of the Burden of Unsuspected Pulmonary Tuberculosis and Co-Morbidity with Non-Communicable Diseases in Sputum Producing Adult Inpatients." *PLoS One* 7 (7): e40774.

Bates, M. N., A. Khalakdina, M. Pai, L. Chang, F. Lessa, and K. R. Smith. 2007. "Risk of Tuberculosis from Exposure to Tobacco Smoke: A Systematic Review and Meta-Analysis." *Archives of Internal Medicine* 167 (4): 335–42.

Bellamy, R., C. Ruwende, T. Corrah, K. P. McAdam, H. C. Whittle, and others. 1998. "Variations in the NRAMP1 Gene and Susceptibility to Tuberculosis in West Africans." *New England Journal of Medicine* 338 (10): 640–44.

Bhargava, A., A. Benedetti, O. Oxlade, M. Pai, and D. Menzies. 2014. "Undernutrition and the Incidence of Tuberculosis in India: National and Subnational Estimates of the Population-Attributable Fraction Related to Undernutrition." *National Medical Journal of India* 27 (3): 128–33.

Bilal, N. K., C. H. Herbst, F. Zhao, A. Soucat, and C. Lemiere. 2011. "Health Extension Workers in Ethiopia: Improved Access and Coverage for the Rural Poor." In *Yes Africa Can: Success Stories from a Dynamic Continent*, edited by P. Chuhan-Pole and M. Angwafo, 433–43. Washington, DC: World Bank.

Binagwaho, A. 2013. "Resistant TB: Use the Tools Available." *Nature* 494 (7436): 176.

Binagwaho, A., P. E. Farmer, S. Nsanzimana, C. Karema, M. Gasana, and others. 2014. "Rwanda 20 Years on: Investing in Life." *The Lancet* 384 (9940): 371–75.

BIO Ventures for Global Health. 2006. "Tuberculosis Vaccines: The Case for Investment." Washington, DC: BIO Ventures for Global Health. http://www.bvgh.org/Portals/0/Reports/2006_10_tb _vaccines,_the_case_for_investment.pdf.

Blaya, J. A., H. S. F. Fraser, and B. Holt. 2010. "E-Health Technologies Show Promise in Developing Countries." *Health Affairs* 29 (2): 244–51.

Blaya, J. A., S. S. Shin, M. Yagui, C. Contreras, P. Cegielski, and others. 2014. "Reducing Communication Delays and Improving Quality of Care with a Tuberculosis Laboratory Information System in Resource Poor Environments: A Cluster Randomized Controlled Trial." *PLoS One* 9 (4): e90110.

Blaya, J. A., S. S. Shin, M. Yagui, G. Yale, C. Z. Suarez, and others. 2007. "A Web-Based Laboratory Information System to Improve Quality of Care of Tuberculosis Patients in Peru: Functional Requirements, Implementation and Usage Statistics." *BMC Medical Informatics and Decision Making* 7: 33.

Bloom, B. R. 1994. *Tuberculosis: Pathogenesis, Protection, and Control*. Washington, DC: ASM Press.

Bloom, B. R., and R. Atun. 2016. "Rethinking Global Control of Tuberculosis." *Science Translational Medicine* 8 (329): 329.

Bloom, B. R., and P. E. M. Fine. 1994. "The BCG Experience: Implications for Future Vaccines against Tuberculosis." In *Tuberculosis: Pathogenesis, Protection, and Control*, edited by B. R. Bloom, 531–57. Washington, DC: ASM Press.

Blower, S. M., A. R. Mclean, T. C. Porco, P. M. Small, P. C. Hopewell, and others. 1995. "The Intrinsic Transmission Dynamics of Tuberculosis Epidemics." *Nature Medicine* 1 (8): 815–21.

Boehme, C. C., P. Nabeta, D. Hillemann, M. P. Nicol, S. Shenai, others. 2010. "Rapid Molecular Detection of Tuberculosis and Rifampin Resistance." *New England Journal of Medicine* 363 (11): 1005–15.

Boehme, C. C., M. P. Nicol, P. Nabeta, J. S. Michael, E. Gotuzzo, and others. 2011. "Feasibility, Diagnostic Accuracy, and

Effectiveness of Decentralised Use of the Xpert MTB/RIF Test for Diagnosis of Tuberculosis and Multidrug Resistance: A Multicentre Implementation Study." *The Lancet* 377 (9776): 1495–505.

Boelaert, J. R., S. J. Vandecasteele, R. Appelberg, and V. R. Gordeuk. 2007. "The Effect of the Host's Iron Status on Tuberculosis." *Journal of Infectious Diseases* 195 (12): 1745–53.

Borrell, S., and S. Gagneux. 2011. "Strain Diversity, Epistasis, and the Evolution of Drug Resistance in *Mycobacterium tuberculosis*." *Clinical Microbiology and Infection* 17 (6): 815–20.

Brennan, M. J., and J. Thole. 2012. "Tuberculosis Vaccines: A Strategic Blueprint for the Next Decade." *Tuberculosis* 92 (Suppl 1): S6–13.

Brouwer, J. A., M. J. Boeree, P. Kager, C. M. Varkevisser, and A. D. Harries. 1998. "Traditional Healers and Pulmonary Tuberculosis in Malawi." *International Journal of Tuberculosis and Lung Disease* 2 (3): 231–34.

Brust, J. C., N. S. Shah, M. Scott, K. Chaiyachati, M. Lygizos, and others. 2012. "Integrated, Home-Based Treatment for MDR-TB and HIV in Rural South Africa: An Alternate Model of Care." *International Journal of Tuberculosis and Lung Disease* 16 (8): 998–1004.

Buchan, J., and M. R. Dal Poz. 2002. "Skill Mix in the Health Care Workforce: Reviewing the Evidence." *Bulletin of the World Health Organization* 80 (7): 575–80.

Bustamante, J., S. Boisson-Dupuis, L. Abel, and J. L. Casanova. 2014. "Mendelian Susceptibility to Mycobacterial Disease: Genetic, Immunological, and Clinical Features of Inborn Errors of IFN-γ Immunity." *Seminars in Immunology* 26 (6): 454–70.

Caminero, J. 2003. "Is the DOTS Strategy Sufficient to Achieve Tuberculosis Control in Low- and Middle-Income Countries? 1. Need for Interventions in Universities and Medical Schools [Unresolved Issues]." *International Journal of Tuberculosis and Lung Disease* 7 (6): 509–15.

Car, J., T. Paljärvi, M. Car, A. Kazeem, A. Majeed, and others. 2012. "Negative Health System Effects of Global Fund's Investments in AIDS, Tuberculosis. and Malaria from 2002 to 2009: Systematic Review." *Journal of the Royal Society of Medicine Short Reports* 3 (10): 70.

Cauthen, G. M., A. Pio, and H. G. ten Dam. 2002. "Annual Risk of Tuberculosis Infection." *Bulletin of the World Health Organization* 80 (6): 503–11.

Cavalcante, S., B. Durovni, G. L. Barnes, F. B. A. Souza, R. F. Silva, and others. 2010. "Community-Randomized Trial of Enhanced DOTS for Tuberculosis Control in Rio de Janeiro, Brazil." *International Journal of Tuberculosis and Lung Disease* 14 (2): 203.

Cavalcante, S., E. Soares, A. G. F. Pacheco, R. E. Chaisson, B. Durovni, and others. 2007. "Community DOT for Tuberculosis in a Brazilian Favela: Comparison with a Clinic Model." *International Journal of Tuberculosis and Lung Disease* 11 (5): 544–49.

Cegielski, J. P., L. Arab, and J. Cornoni-Huntley. 2012. "Nutritional Risk Factors for Tuberculosis among Adults in the United States, 1971–1992." *American Journal of Epidemiology* 176 (5): 409–22.

Chadha, V., P. Kumar, P. S. Jagannatha, P. S. Vaidyanathan, and K. P. Unnikrishnan. 2005. "Average Annual Risk of Tuberculous Infection in India." *International Journal of Tuberculosis and Lung Disease* 9 (1): 116–18.

Chahal, J. S., O. F. Khan, C. L. Cooper, J. S. McPartlan, J. K. Tsosie, and others. 2016. "Dendrimer-RNA Nanoparticles Generate Protective Immunity against Lethal Ebola, H1N1 Influenza, and *Toxoplasma gondii* Challenges with a Single Dose." *Proceedings of the National Academy of Sciences* 113 (29): E4133–42.

Chakraborty, S., T. Gruber, C. E. Barry, H. I. Boshoff, and K. Y. Rhee. 2013. "Para-Aminosalicylic Acid Acts as an Alternative Substrate of Folate Metabolism in *Mycobacterium tuberculosis*." *Science* 339 (6115): 88–91.

Chan, P. C., C. H. Yang, L. Y. Chang, K. F. Wang, Y. C. Kuo, and others. 2013. "Lower Prevalence of Tuberculosis Infection in BCG Vaccinees: A Cross-Sectional Study in Adult Prison Inmates." *Thorax* 68 (3): 263–68.

Chang, K., W. Lu, J. Wang, K. Zhang, S. Jia, and others. 2012. "Rapid and Effective Diagnosis of Tuberculosis and Rifampicin Resistance with Xpert MTB/RIF Assay: A Meta-Analysis." *Journal of Infection* 64 (6): 580–88.

Chee, C., M. Teleman, I. C. Boudville, and Y. T. Wang. 2005. "Contact Screening and Latent TB Infection Treatment in Singapore Correctional Facilities." *International Journal of Tuberculosis and Lung Disease* 9 (11): 1248–52.

Chimusa, E. R., N. Zaitlen, M. Daya, M. Moller, P. D. van Helden, and others. 2014. "Genome-Wide Association Study of Ancestry-Specific TB Risk in the South African Coloured Population." *Human Molecular Genetics* 23 (3): 796–809.

Choi, I. J., Y. W. Kim, H. S. Lee, K. W. Ryu, H. M. Yoon, and others. 2015. "Risk Factors for TB in Patients with Early Gastric Cancer: Is Gastrectomy a Significant Risk Factor for TB?" *Chest* 148 (3): 774–83.

Churchyard, G., K. Fielding, J. Lewis, L. Coetzee, E. Corbett, and others. 2012. "Community-Wide Isoniazid Preventive Therapy Does Not Improve TB Control among Gold Miners: the Thibela TB Study, South Africa." Paper presented at the 19th Conference on Retroviruses and Opportunistic Infections, Seattle, March 5–8.

———. 2014. "A Trial of Mass Isoniazid Preventive Therapy for Tuberculosis Control." *New England Journal of Medicine* 370 (17): 301–10.

Cobelens, F., S. van Kampen, E. Ochodo, R. Atun, and C. Lienhardt. 2012. "Research on Implementation of Interventions in Tuberculosis Control in Low- and Middle-Income Countries: A Systematic Review." *PLoS Medicine* 9 (12): e1001358.

Cohen, T., C. Colijn, A. Wright, M. Zignol, A. Pym, and others. 2008. "Challenges in Estimating the Total Burden of Drug-Resistant Tuberculosis." *American Journal of Respiratory and Critical Care Medicine* 177 (12): 1302–06.

Cohen, T., H. E. Jenkins, C. Lu, M. McLaughlin, K. Floyd, and others. 2014. "On the Spread and Control of MDR-TB Epidemics: An Examination of Trends in Anti-Tuberculosis Drug Resistance Surveillance Data." *Drug Resistance Updates* 17 (4–6): 105–23.

Coker, R., R. A. Atun, and M. McKee. 2004. "Health-Care System Frailties and Public Health Control of Communicable Disease on the European Union's New Eastern Border." *The Lancet* 363 (9418): 1389–92.

Coker, R., B. Dimitrova, F. Drobniewski, Y. Samyshkin, J. Pomerleau, and others. 2005. "Health System Frailties in Tuberculosis Service Provision in Russia: An Analysis through the Lens of Formal Nutritional Support." *Public Health* 119 (9): 837–43.

Colijn, C., A. Brandes, J. Zucker, D. S. Lun, B. Weiner, and others. 2009. "Interpreting Expression Data with Metabolic Flux Models: Predicting *Mycobacterium tuberculosis* Mycolic Acid Production." *PLoS Computational Biology* 5 (8): e1000489.

Comstock, G. W., C. Baum, and D. E. Snider Jr. 1979. "Isoniazid Prophylaxis among Alaskan Eskimos: A Final Report of the Bethel Isoniazid Studies." *American Review of Respiratory Disease* 119 (5): 827–30.

Connor, S., K. Foley, R. Harding, and E. Jaramillo. 2012. "Declaration on Palliative Care and MDR/XDR-TB." *International Journal of Tuberculosis and Lung Disease* 16 (6): 712–13.

Corbett, E. L., T. Bandason, Y. B. Cheung, B. Makamure, E. Dauya, and others. 2009. "Prevalent Infectious Tuberculosis in Harare, Zimbabwe: Burden, Risk Factors and Implications for Control." *International Journal of Tuberculosis and Lung Disease* 13 (10): 1231.

Corbett, E. L., T. Bandason, T. Duong, E. Dauya, B. Makamure, and others. 2010. "Comparison of Two Active Case-Finding Strategies for Community-Based Diagnosis of Symptomatic Smear-Positive Tuberculosis and Control of Infectious Tuberculosis in Harare, Zimbabwe (DETECTB): A Cluster-Randomised Trial." *The Lancet* 376 (9748): 1244–53.

Corbett, E. L., S. Charalambous, V. M. Moloi, K. Fielding, A. D. Grant, and others. 2004. "Human Immunodeficiency Virus and the Prevalence of Undiagnosed Tuberculosis in African Gold Miners." *American Journal of Respiratory and Critical Care Medicine* 170 (6): 673–79.

Corbett, E. L., G. J. Churchyard, T. C. Clayton, B. G. Williams, D. Mulder, and others. 2000. "HIV Infection and Silicosis: The Impact of Two Potent Risk Factors on the Incidence of Mycobacterial Disease in South African Miners." *AIDS* 14 (17): 2759–68.

Corbett, E. L., B. Marston, G. J. Churchyard, and K. M. De Cock. 2006. "Tuberculosis in Sub-Saharan Africa: Opportunities, Challenges, and Change in the Era of Antiretroviral Treatment." *The Lancet* 367 (9514): 926–37.

Corbett, E. L., C. J. Watt, N. Walker, D. Maher, B. G. Williams, and others. 2003. "The Growing Burden of Tuberculosis: Global Trends and Interactions with the HIV Epidemic." *Archives of Internal Medicine* 163 (9): 1009–21.

Coronado, V. G., C. M. Beck-Sague, M. D. Hutton, B. J. Davis, P. Nicholas, and others. 1993. "Transmission of Multidrug-Resistant *Mycobacterium tuberculosis* among Persons with Human Immunodeficiency Virus Infection in an Urban Hospital: Epidemiologic and Restriction Fragment Length Polymorphism Analysis." *Journal of Infectious Diseases* 168 (4): 1052–55.

Cox, E., and K. Laessig. 2014. "FDA Approval of Bedaquiline—the Benefit-Risk Balance for Drug-Resistant Tuberculosis." *New England Journal of Medicine* 371 (8): 689–91.

Creswell, J., M. Raviglione, S. Ottmani, G. B. Migliori, M. W. Uplekar, and others. 2011. "Tuberculosis and Noncommunicable Diseases: Neglected Links and Missed Opportunities." *European Respiratory Journal* 37 (5): 1269–82.

Critchley, J. A., F. Young, L. Orton, and P. Garner. 2013. "Corticosteroids for Prevention of Mortality in People with Tuberculosis: A Systematic Review and Meta-Analysis." *The Lancet Infectious Diseases* 13 (3): 223–37.

Cuevas, L. E., N. Al-Sonboli, L. Lawson, M. A. Yassin, I. Arbide, and others. 2011. "LED Fluorescence Microscopy for the Diagnosis of Pulmonary Tuberculosis: A Multi-Country Cross-Sectional Evaluation." *PLoS Medicine* 8(7): e1001057.

Das, J., A. Kwan, B. Daniels, S. Satyanarayana, R. Subbaraman, and others. 2015. "Use of Standardised Patients to Assess Quality of Tuberculosis Care: A Pilot, Cross-Sectional Study." *The Lancet Infectious Diseases* 15 (11): 1305–13.

da Silva, R. C., L. Segat, H. L. da Cruz, H. C. Schindler, L. M. Montenegro, and others. 2014. "Association of CD209 and CD209L Polymorphisms with Tuberculosis Infection in a Northeastern Brazilian Population." *Molecular Biology Reports* 41 (8): 5449–57.

Datiko, D. G., and B. Lindtjørn. 2009. "Health Extension Workers Improve Tuberculosis Case Detection and Treatment Success in Southern Ethiopia: A Community Randomized Trial." *PLoS One* 4(5): e5443.

———. 2010. "Cost and Cost-Effectiveness of Smear Positive Tuberculosis Treatment by Health Extension Workers in Southern Ethiopia: A Community Randomized Trial." *PLoS One* 5 (2): e9158.

Della Mea, V. 1999. "Internet Electronic Mail: A Tool for Low-Cost Telemedicine." *Journal of Telemedicine and Telecare* 5 (2): 84–89.

DeLuca, A., R. E. Chaisson, and N. A. Martinson. 2009. "Intensified Case Finding for Tuberculosis in Prevention of Mother to Child Transmission Programs; a Simple and Potentially Vital Addition for Maternal and Child Health." *Journal of Acquired Immune Deficiency Syndromes* 50 (2): 196–99.

den Boon, S., A. Matteelli, N. Ford, and H. Getahun. 2016. "Continuous Isoniazid for the Treatment of Latent Tuberculosis Infection in People Living with HIV." *AIDS* 30 (5): 797–801.

den Boon, S., S. W. P. van Lill, M. W. Borgdorff, D. A. Enarson, S. Verver, and others. 2007. "High Prevalence of Tuberculosis in Previously Treated Patients, Cape Town, South Africa." *Emerging Infectious Diseases* 13 (8): 1189.

Detjen, A. K., A. R. DiNardo, J. Leyden, K. R. Steingart, D. Menzies, and others. 2015. "Xpert MTB/RIF Assay for the Diagnosis of Pulmonary Tuberculosis in Children: A Systematic Review and Meta-Analysis." *The Lancet Respiratory Medicine* 3 (6): 451–61.

de Vries, G., R. Aldridge, J. A. Cayla, W. H. Haas, A. Sandgren, and others. 2014. "Epidemiology of Tuberculosis in Big Cities of the European Union and European Economic Area Countries." *Eurosurveillance* 19 (9): pii=20726.

Dharmadhikari, A. S., M. Mphahlele, A. Stoltz, K. Venter, R. Mathebula, and others. 2012. "Surgical Face Masks Worn by Patients with Multidrug-Resistant Tuberculosis: Impact on Infectivity of Air on a Hospital Ward." *American Journal of Respiratory and Critical Care Medicine* 185 (10): 1104–19.

Dharmadhikari, A. S., M. Mphahlele, K. Venter, A. Stoltz, R. Mathebula, and others. 2014. "Rapid Impact of Effective Treatment on Transmission of Multidrug-Resistant Tuberculosis." *International Journal of Tuberculosis and Lung Disease* 18 (9): 1019–25.

Dheda, K., T. Gumbo, N. R. Gandhi, M. Murray, G. Theron, and others. 2014. "Global Control of Tuberculosis: From Extensively Drug-Resistant to Untreatable Tuberculosis." *The Lancet Respiratory Medicine* 2 (4): 321–38.

Diacon, A. H., R. Dawson, M. Hanekom, K. Narunsky, S. J. Maritz, and others. 2010. "Early Bactericidal Activity and Pharmacokinetics of PA-824 in Smear-Positive Tuberculosis Patients." *Antimicrobial Agents and Chemotheraphy* 54 (8): 3402–07.

Diacon, A. H., R. Dawson, F. von Groote-Bidlingmaier, G. Symons, A. Venter, and others. 2012. "14-Day Bactericidal Activity of PA-824, Bedaquiline, Pyrazinamide, and Moxifloxacin Combinations: A Randomised Trial." *The Lancet* 380 (9846): 986–93.

Diacon, A. H., P. R. Donald, A. Pym, M. Grobusch, R. F. Patientia, and others. 2012. "Randomized Pilot Trial of Eight Weeks of Bedaquiline (TMC207) Treatment for Multidrug-Resistant Tuberculosis: Long-Term Outcome, Tolerability, and Effect on Emergence of Drug Resistance." *Antimicrobial Agents and Chemotheraphy* 56 (6): 3271–76.

Diacon, A. H., A. Pym, M. P. Grobusch, J. M. de los Rios, E. Gotuzzo, and others. 2014. "Multidrug-Resistant Tuberculosis and Culture Conversion with Bedaquiline." *New England Journal of Medicine* 371 (8): 723–32.

Dick, J., and S. Henchie. 1998. "A Cost Analysis of the Tuberculosis Control Programme in Elsies River, Cape Town." *South African Medical Journal* 88 (Suppl 3): 380–83.

Ditkowsky, J. B., and K. Schwartzman. 2014. "Potential Cost-Effectiveness of a New Infant Tuberculosis Vaccine in South Africa—Implications for Clinical Trials: A Decision Analysis." *PLoS One* 9 (1): e83526.

Donald, P. R. 2016. "Chemotherapy for Tuberculous Meningitis." *New England Journal of Medicine* 374 (2): 179–81.

Donald, P. R., and H. McIlleron. 2009. "Antituberculosis Drugs." In *Tuberculosis: A Comprehensive Clinical Reference*, edited by H. S. Schaaf and A. Zumla. Philadelphia: Saunders Elsevier.

Dowdy, D. W., A. Cattamanchi, K. R. Steingart, and M. Pai. 2011. "Is Scale-Up Worth It? Challenges in Economic Analysis of Diagnostic Tests for Tuberculosis." *PLoS Medicine* 8 (7): e1001063.

Dowdy, D. W., R. E. Chaisson, G. Maartens, E. L. Corbett, and S. E. Dorman. 2008. "Impact of Enhanced Tuberculosis Diagnosis in South Africa: A Mathematical Model of Expanded Culture and Drug Susceptibility Testing." *Proceedings of the National Academy of Sciences* 105 (32): 11293–98.

Dowdy, D. W., J. E. Golub, R. E. Chaisson, and V. Saraceni. 2012. "Heterogeneity in Tuberculosis Transmission and the Role of Geographic Hotspots in Propagating Epidemics." *Proceedings of the National Academy of Sciences* 109 (24): 9557–62.

Driessen, J., M. Cioffi, N. Alide, Z. Landis-Lewis, G. Gamadzi, and others 2013. "Modeling Return on Investment for EMR System in Lilongwe, Malawi." *Journal of American Medical Informatics Association* 20 (4): 743–48.

Drobniewski, F. A., R. Atun, I. Fedorin, A. Bikov, R. Coker, and others. 2004. "The 'Bear Trap': The Colliding Epidemics of Tuberculosis and HIV in Russia." *International Journal of STD and AIDS* 15 (10): 641–46.

Dye, C. 2009. "Doomsday Postponed? Preventing and Reversing Epidemics of Drug-Resistant Tuberculosis." *Nature Reviews Microbiology* 7 (1): 81–87.

———. 2013. "Making Wider Use of the World's Most Widely Used Vaccine: Bacille Calmette–Guérin Revaccination Reconsidered." *Journal of the Royal Society Interface* 10 (87): 20130365.

———. 2015. *The Population Biology of Tuberculosis.* Princeton, NJ: Princeton University Press.

Dye, C., A. Bassili, A. L. Bierrenbach, J. F. Broekmans, V. K. Chadha, and others. 2008. "Measuring Tuberculosis Burden, Trends, and the Impact of Control Programmes." *The Lancet Infectious Diseases* 8 (4): 233–43.

Dye, C., and K. Floyd. 2006. "Tuberculosis." In *Disease Control Priorities in Developing Countries* (second edition), edited by D. T. Jamison, J. G. Breman, A. R. Measham, G. Alleyne, M. Claeson, D. B. Evans, P. Jha, A. Mills, and P. Musgrove. Washington, DC: World Bank and Oxford University Press.

Dye, C., P. Glaziou, K. Floyd, and M. Raviglione. 2013. "Prospects for Tuberculosis Elimination." *Annual Review of Public Health* 34 (December 14): 271–86.

Dye, C., S. Scheele, P. Dolin, V. Pathania, and M. C. Raviglione. 1999. "Global Burden of Tuberculosis: Estimated Incidence, Prevalence, and Mortality by Country." *Journal of the American Medical Association.* 282 (7): 677–86.

Dye, C., and B. G. Williams. 2008. "Eliminating Human Tuberculosis in the Twenty-First Century." *Journal of the Royal Society Interface* 5 (23): 653–62.

Economist. 2015. "The Economist Special Online Supplement." *Economist,* Copenhagen Consensus. http://www.copenhagen consensus.com/post-2015-consensus/economist.

Edginton, M. 1999. "Tuberculosis Patient Care Decentralised to District Clinics with Community-Based Directly Observed Treatment in a Rural District of South Africa." *International Journal of Tuberculosis and Lung Disease* 3 (5): 445–50.

Eisenhut, M., S. Paranjothy, I. Abubakar, S. Bracebridge, M. Lilley, and others. 2009. "BCG Vaccination Reduces Risk of Infection with *Mycobacterium tuberculosis* as Detected by Gamma Interferon Release Assay." *Vaccine* 27 (44): 6116–20.

Elzinga, G., M. C. Raviglione, and D. Maher. 2004. "Scale Up: Meeting Targets in Global Tuberculosis Control." *The Lancet* 363 (9411): 814–19.

Ettehad, D., H. S. Schaaf, J. A. Seddon, G. S. Cooke, and N. Ford. 2012. "Treatment Outcomes for Children with Multidrug-Resistant Tuberculosis: A Systematic Review and Meta-Analysis." *The Lancet Infectious Diseases* 12 (6): 449–56.

Evans, T. G., M. J. Brennan, L. Barker, and J. Thole. 2013. "Preventive Vaccines for Tuberculosis." *Vaccine* 31 (Suppl 2): B223–26.

Fabri, M., S. Stenger, D.-M. Shin, J.-M. Yuk, P. T. Liu, and others. 2011. "Vitamin D Is Required for IFN-γ–Mediated Antimicrobial Activity of Human Macrophages." *Science Translational Medicine* 3 (104): 104.

Farmer, P. 2013. "Chronic Infectious Disease and the Future of Health Care Delivery." *New England Journal of Medicine* 369 (25): 2424–36.

Farmer, P., S. Robin, S. L. Ramilus, and J. Y. Kim. 1991. "Tuberculosis, Poverty, and 'Compliance': Lessons from Rural Haiti." *Seminars in Respiratory Infections* 6 (4): 254–60.

Faurholt-Jepsen, D., N. Range, G. PrayGod, K. Jeremiah, M. Faurholt-Jepsen, and others. 2012. "The Role of Anthropometric and Other Predictors for Diabetes among Urban Tanzanians with Tuberculosis." *International Journal of Tuberculosis and Lung Disease* 16 (12): 1680–85.

Fenner, L., M. Egger, T. Bodmer, E. Altpeter, M. Zwahlen, and others. 2012. "Effect of Mutation and Genetic Background on Drug Resistance in *Mycobacterium tuberculosis.*" *Antimicrobial Agents and Chemotherapy* 56 (6): 3047–53.

Figueroa-Munoz, J., K. Palmer, M. R. Dal Poz, L. Blanc, K. Bergström, and others. 2005. "The Health Workforce Crisis in TB Control: A Report from High-Burden Countries." *Human Resources for Health* 3 (1): 2.

Fine, P. E. 1995. "Variation in Protection by BCG: Implications of and for Heterologous Immunity." *The Lancet* 346 (8986): 1339–45.

Fitzpatrick, M. C., and K. Floyd. 2012. "A Systematic Review of the Cost and Cost Effectiveness of Treatment for Multidrug-Resistant Tuberculosis." *Pharmacoeconomics* 30 (1): 63–80.

Floyd, K., V. K. Arora, K. J. Murthy, K. Lonnroth, N. Singla, and others. 2006. "DOTS for Tuberculosis Control: Evidence from India." *Bulletin of the World Health Organization* 84: 437–45.

Floyd, K., C. Fitzpatrick, A. Pantoja, and M. Raviglione. 2013. "Domestic and Donor Financing for Tuberculosis Care and Control in Low-Income and Middle-Income Countries: An Analysis of Trends, 2002–11, and Requirements to Meet 2015 Targets." *The Lancet Global Health* 1 (2): e105–15.

Floyd, K., R. Hutubessy, K. Kliiman, R. Centis, N. Khurieva, and others. 2012. "Cost and Cost-Effectiveness of Multidrug-Resistant Tuberculosis Treatment in Estonia and Russia." *European Respiratory Journal* 40 (1): 133–42.

Floyd, K., J. Skeva, T. Nyirenda, F. Gausi, and F. Salaniponi. 2003. "Cost and Cost-Effectiveness of Increased Community and Primary Care Facility Involvement in Tuberculosis Care in Lilongwe District, Malawi." *International Journal of Tuberculosis and Lung Disease* 7 (Suppl 1): S29–37.

Floyd, K., D. Wilkinson, and C. Gilks. 1997. "Comparison of Cost Effectiveness of Directly Observed Treatment (DOT) and Conventionally Delivered Treatment for Tuberculosis: Experience from Rural South Africa." *BMJ* 315 (7120): 1407–11.

Fofana, M. O., G. M. Knight, G. B. Gomez, R. G. White, and D. W. Dowdy. 2014. "Population-Level Impact of Shorter-Course Regimens for Tuberculosis: A Model-Based Analysis." *PLoS One* 9 (5): e96389.

Ford, C. B., R. R. Shah, M. K. Maeda, S. Gagneux, M. B. Murray, and others. 2013. "*Mycobacterium tuberculosis* Mutation Rate Estimates from Different Lineages Predict Substantial Differences in the Emergence of Drug-Resistant Tuberculosis." *Nature Genetics* 45 (7): 784–90.

Fox, W., G. A. Ellard, and D. A. Mitchison. 1999. "Studies on the Treatment of Tuberculosis Undertaken by the British Medical Research Council Tuberculosis Units, 1946–1986, with Relevant Subsequent Publications." *International Journal of Tuberculosis and Lung Disease* 3 (10, Suppl 2): S231–79.

Fraser, H. S., J. Blaya, S. S. Choi, C. Bonilla, and D. Jazayeri. 2006. "Evaluating the Impact and Costs of Deploying an Electronic Medical Record System to Support TB Treatment in Peru." *AMIA Annual Symposium Proceedings* 2006: 265–68.

Fraser, H. S., A. Habib, M. Goodrich, D. Thomas, J. A. Blaya, and others. 2013. "E-Health Systems for Management of MDR-TB in Resource-Poor Environments: A Decade of Experience and Recommendations for Future Work." In *MedInfo*, vol. 192, 627–31. Amsterdam: IOS Press E Books.

Fraser, H. S., D. Jazayeri, C. D. Mitnick, J. S. Mukherjee, and J. Bayona. 2002. "Informatics Tools to Monitor Progress and Outcomes of Patients with Drug Resistant Tuberculosis in Perú." *AMIA Annual Symposium Proceedings* 2002: 270–74.

Fraser, H. S., D. Thomas, J. Tomaylla, N. Garcia, L. Lecca, and others. 2012. "Adaptation of a Web-Based, Open Source Electronic Medical Record System Platform to Support a Large Study of Tuberculosis Epidemiology." *BMC Medical Informatics and Decision Making* 12 (1): 125.

Frenk, J. 1994. "Dimensions of Health System Reform." *Health Policy* 27 (1): 19–34.

Frick, M., I. Henry, and E. Lessem. 2016. "Falling Short of the Rights to Health and Scientific Progress: Inadequate TB Drug Research and Access." *Health and Human Rights* 18 (1): 9–24.

Frieden, T. R., ed. 2004. *Toman's Tuberculosis: Case Detection, Treatment, and Monitoring.* Geneva: World Health Organization.

Frieden, T. R., P. I. Fujiwara, R. M. Washko, and M. A. Hamburg. 1995. "Tuberculosis in New York City—Turning the Tide." *New England Journal of Medicine* 333 (4): 229–33.

Friedich, S. O., A. Rachow, E. Saathoff, K. Singth, C. D. Mangu, and others. 2013. "Assessment of the Sensitivity and Specificity of Xpert MTB/RIF Assay as an Early Sputum Biomarker of Response to Tuberculosis Treatment." *The Lancet Respiratory Medicine* 1 (6): 432–70.

Furin, J., J. Bayona, M. Becerra, P. Farmer, A. Golubkov, and others. 2011. "Programmatic Management of Multidrug-Resistant Tuberculosis: Models from Three Countries." *International Journal of Tuberculosis and Lung Disease* 15 (10): 1294–300.

Gagneux, S. 2012. "Host–Pathogen Coevolution in Human Tuberculosis." *Philosophical Transactions of the Royal Society B: Biological Sciences* 367 (1590): 850–59.

Gandhi, N. R., A. P. Moll, U. Lalloo, R. Pawinski, K. Zeller, and others. 2009. "Successful Integration of Tuberculosis and HIV Treatment in Rural South Africa: The Sizonq'oba

Study." *Journal of Acquired Immune Deficiency Syndromes* 50 (1): 37–43.

Gandhi, N. R., A. Moll, A. W. Sturm, R. Pawinski, T. Govender, and others. 2006. "Extensively Drug-Resistant Tuberculosis as a Cause of Death in Patients Co-Infected with Tuberculosis and HIV in a Rural Area of South Africa." *The Lancet* 368 (9547): 1575–80.

Gandhi, N. R., P. Nunn, K. Dheda, H. S. Schaff, M. Zignol, and others. 2010. "Multidrug-Resistant and Extensively Drug-Resistant Tuberculosis: A Threat to Global Control of Tuberculosis." *The Lancet* 375 (9728): 1830–43.

Gandhi, N. R., D. Weissman, P. Moonley, M. Ramathal, I. Elson, and others. 2013. "Nosocomial Transmission of Extensively Drug-Resistant Tuberculosis in a Rural Hospital in South Africa." *Journal of Infectious Diseases* 207 (1): 9–17.

Gasana, M., G. Vandebriel, G. Kabanda, S. J. Tsiouris, J. Justman, and others. 2008. "Integrating Tuberculosis and HIV Care in Rural Rwanda." *International Journal of Tuberculosis and Lung Disease* 12 (Suppl 1): S39–43.

Geissbuhler, A., O. Ly, C. Lovis, and J.-F. L'Haire. 2003. "Telemedicine in Western Africa: Lessons Learned from a Pilot Project in Mali, Perspectives and Recommendations." In *Annual Symposium Proceedings*, vol. 2003, 249. Bethesda, MD: American Medical Informatics Association.

Gelmanova, I. Y., S. Keshavjee, V. T. Goluchikova, V. I. Berzina, A. K. Strelis, and others. 2007. "Barriers to Successful Tuberculosis Treatment in Tomsk, Russian Federation: Non-Adherence, Default, and the Acquisition of Multidrug Resistance." *Bulletin of the World Health Organization* 85 (9): 649–732.

Getahun, H., A. Matteelli, R. E. Chaisson, and M. Raviglione. 2015. "Latent *Mycobacterium tuberculosis* Infection." *New England Journal of Medicine* 372 (May 28): 2127–35.

Gillespie, S. H., A. M. Crook, T. D. McHugh, C. M. Mendel, S. K. Meredith, and others. 2014. "Four-Month Moxifloxacin-Based Regimens for Drug-Sensitive Tuberculosis." *New England Journal of Medicine* 371 (17): 1577–87.

Glaziou, P., K. Floyd, E. L. Korenromp, C. Sismanidis, A. Bierrenbach, and others. 2011. "Lives Saved by Tuberculosis Control and Prospects for Achieving the 2015 Global Target for Reducing Tuberculosis Mortality." *Bulletin of the World Health Organization* 89 (8): 573–82.

Gler, M., L. Podewils, N. Munez, M. Galipot, M. I. D. Quelapio, and others. 2012. "Impact of Patient and Program Factors on Default during Treatment of Multidrug-Resistant Tuberculosis." *International Journal of Tuberculosis and Lung Disease* 16 (7): 955–60.

Gler, M. T., V. Skripconoka, E. Sanchez-Garavito, H. Xiao, J. L. Cabrera-Rivero, and others. 2012. "Delamanid for Multidrug-Resistant Pulmonary Tuberculosis." *New England Journal of Medicine* 366 (23): 2151–60.

Golub, J. E., S. Cohn, V. Saraceni, S. C. Cavalcante, A. G. Pacheco, and others. 2015. "Long-Term Protection from Isoniazid Preventive Therapy for Tuberculosis in HIV-Infected Patients in a Medium-Burden Tuberculosis Setting: The TB/HIV in Rio (THRio) Study." *Clinical Infectious Diseases* 60 (4): 639–45.

Golub, J. E., C. I. Mohan, G. W. Comstock, and R. E. Chaisson. 2005. "Active Case Finding of Tuberculosis: Historical Perspective and Future Prospects." *International Journal of Tuberculosis and Lung Disease* 9 (11): 1183–203.

Gomez, G. B., D. W. Dowdy, M. L Bastos, A. Zwerling, S. Sweeney, and others. 2016. "Cost and Cost-Effectiveness of Tuberculosis Treatment Shortening: A Model-based Analysis." *BMC Infectious Diseases*. 16 (1): 726.

Grandjean, L., R. H. Gilman, L. Martin, E. Soto, and others. 2015. "Transmission of Multidrug-Resistant and Drug Susceptible Tuberculosis within Households: A Prospective Cohort Study." *PLoS Medicine* 12 (6): e1001843.

Green, C., J. F. Huggett, E. Talbot, P. Mwaba, K. Reither, and A. Zumla. 2009. "Rapid Diagnosis of Tuberculosis through the Detection of Mycobacterial DNA in Urine by Nucleic Acid Amplification Methods." *The Lancet Infectious Diseases* 9 (8) 505–11.

Gupta, R., M. Gao, A. Cirule, H. Xiao, L. Geiter, and others. 2015. "Delamanid for Extensively Drug-Resistant Tuberculosis." *New England Journal of Medicine* 373 (3): 291–92.

Hanekom, M., G. D. van der Spuy, E. Streicher, S. L. Ndabambi, C. R. McEvoy, and others. 2007. "A Recently Evolved Sublineage of the *Mycobacterium tuberculosis* Beijing Strain Family Is Associated with an Increased Ability to Spread and Cause Disease." *Journal of Clinical Microbiology* 45 (5): 1483–90.

Hanifa, Y., A. Grant, J. Lewis, E. L. Corbett, K. Fielding, and others. 2009. "Prevalence of Latent Tuberculosis Infection among Gold Miners in South Africa." *International Journal of Tuberculosis and Lung Disease* 13 (1): 39–46.

Hansen, S. G., M. Piatak Jr., A. B. Ventura, C. M. Hughes, R. M. Gilbride, and others. 2013. "Immune Clearance of Highly Pathogenic SIV Infection." *Nature* 502 (7469): 100–04.

Harding, R., K. M. Foley, S. R. Connor, and E. Jaramillo. 2012. "Palliative and End-of-Life Care in the Global Response to Multidrug-Resistant Tuberculosis." *The Lancet Infectious Diseases* 12 (8): 643–6.

Harries, A. D. 1997. "Tuberculosis in Africa: Clinical Presentation and Management." *Pharmacology and Therapeutics* 73 (1): 1–50.

Harries, A. D., R. Zachariah, K. Bergström, L. Blanc, F. M. Salaniponi, and others. 2005. "Human Resources for Control of Tuberculosis and HIV-Associated Tuberculosis [Unresolved Issues]." *International Journal of Tuberculosis and Lung Disease* 9 (2): 128–37.

Harris, J. B., S. M. Hatwiinda, K. M. Randels, B. H. Chi, N. G. Kancheya, and others. 2008. "Early Lessons from the Integration of Tuberculosis and HIV Services in Primary Care Centers in Lusaka, Zambia." *International Journal of Tuberculosis and Lung Disease* 12 (7): 773–79.

Harris, R. C., M. S. Khan, L. J. Martin, V. Allen, D. A. Moore, and others. 2016. "The Effect of Surgery on the Outcome of Treatment for Multidrug-Resistant Tuberculosis: A Systematic Review and Meta-Analysis." *BMC Infectious Diseases* 16: 262.

Hart, P. A., and I. Sutherland. 1977. "BCG and Vole Bacillus Vaccines in the Prevention of Tuberculosis in Adolescence and Early Adult Life." *BMJ* 2 (6082): 293.

Hasegawa, N, T. Miura, K. Ishii, K. Yamaguchi, T. H. Lindner, and others. 2002. "New Simple and Rapid Test for Culture Confirmation of *Mycobacterium tuberculosis* Complex: A Multicenter Study." *Journal of Clinical Microbiology* 40 (3): 908–12.

Heimbeck, J. 1938. "Incidence of Tuberculosis in Young Adult Women with Special Reference to Employment." *British Journal of Tuberculosis* 32 (3): 154–66.

Heller, T., R. Lessells, C. G. Wallrauch, T. Bärnighausen, C. S. Cooke, and others. 2010. "Community-Based Treatment for Multidrug-Resistant Tuberculosis in Rural KwaZulu-Natal, South Africa." *International Journal of Tuberculosis and Lung Disease* 14 (4): 420–26.

Hermans, S., C. R. Horsburgh Jr., and R. Wood. 2015. "A Century of Tuberculosis Epidemiology in the Northern and Southern Hemisphere: The Differential Impact of Control Interventions." *PLoS One* 10 (8): e0135179.

Hesseling, A. C., B. J. Marais, R. P. Gie, H. S. Schaaf, P. E. Fine, and others. 2007. "The Risk of Disseminated Bacille Calmette-Guerin (BCG) Disease in HIV-Infected Children." *Vaccine* 25 (1): 14–18.

Hirsch-Moverman, Y., R. Shrestha-Kuwahara, J. Bethel, H. M. Blumberg, T. K. Venkatappa, and others. 2015. "Latent Tuberculous Infection in the United States and Canada: Who Completes Treatment and Why?" *International Journal of Tuberculosis and Lung Disease* 19 (1): 31–38.

Hoagland, D. T., J. Liu, R. B. Lee, and R. E. Lee. 2016. "New Agents for the Treatment of Drug-Resistant *Mycobacterium tuberculosis*." *Advanced Drug Delivery Reviews* 102: 55–72.

Hong Kong Chest Service and British Medical Research Council. 1979. "Controlled Trial of 6-Month and 8-Month Regimens in the Treatment of Pulmonary Tuberculosis: The Results up to 24 Months." *Tubercle* 60 (4): 201–10.

Hopkin, J. 2000. "Atopy, Asthma, and the Mycobacteria." *Thorax* 55 (6): 443–45.

Horter, S., B. Stringer, L. Reynolds, M. Shoaib, S. Kasozi, and others. 2014. "'Home Is Where the Patient Is': A Qualitative Analysis of a Patient-Centred Model of Care for Multi-Drug Resistant Tuberculosis." *BMC Health Services Research* 14 (1): 1–8.

Hou, W. L., F. Song, N. X. Zhang, X. X. Dong, S. Y. Cao, and others. 2012. "Implementation and Community Involvement in DOTS Strategy: A Systematic Review of Studies in China." *International Journal of Tuberculosis and Lung Disease* 16 (11): 1433–40.

Howard, A. A., and W. M. El-Sadr. 2010. "Integration of Tuberculosis and HIV Services in Sub-Saharan Africa: Lessons Learned." *Clinical Infectious Diseases* 50 (Suppl 3): S238–44.

Howitt, P., A. Darzi, G. Z. Yang, H. Ashrafian, and R. Atun. 2012. "Technologies for Global Health." *The Lancet* 380 (9840): 507–35.

Hsiao, W. C., and P. S. Heller. 2007. "What Should Macroeconomists Know about Health Care Policy?" Working Paper WP/07/13, International Monetary Fund, Washington, DC.

Huang, C.-C., E. T. Tchetgen, M. C. Becerra, T. Cohen, J. Galea, and others. 2014. "Cigarette Smoking among Tuberculosis Patients Increases Risk of Transmission to Child Contacts." *International Journal of Tuberculosis and Lung Disease* 18 (11): 1285–91.

Huang, C.-C., E. T. Tchetgen, M. C. Becerra, T. Cohen, K. C. Hughes, and others. 2014. "The Effect of HIV-Related Immunosuppression on the Risk of Tuberculosis Transmission to Household Contacts." *Clinical Infectious Diseases* 58 (6): 765–74.

Huerga, H., H. Spillane, W. Guerrero, A. Odongo, and F. Varaine. 2010. "Impact of Introducing Human Immunodeficiency Virus Testing, Treatment and Care in a Tuberculosis Clinic in Rural Kenya." *International Journal of Tuberculosis and Lung Disease* 14 (5): 611–15.

IHME (Institute for Health Metrics and Evaluation). 2015. "Financing Global Health 2014. Shifts in Funding as the MDG Era Closes." IHME, Seattle.

Institute of Medicine. 2013. *Developing and Strengthening the Global Supply Chain for Second-Line Drugs for Multidrug-Resistant Tuberculosis: Workshop Summary*. Washington, DC: National Academies Press.

International Institute for Population Sciences and Macro International. 2007. *National Family Health Survey (NFHS-3), 2005–2006*. Mumbai: International Institute for Population Sciences.

Isaakidis, P., R. Paryani, K. Samsuddin, H. Mansoor, M. Manglani, and others. 2013. "Poor Outcomes in a Cohort of HIV-Infected Adolescents Undergoing Treatment for Multidrug-Resistant Tuberculosis in Mumbai, India." *PLoS One* 8 (7): e68869.

Islam, A., M. A. May, F. Ahmed, R. A. Cash, and J. Ahmed. 2011. *Making Tuberculosis History: Community-Based Solutions for Millions*. Dhaka: University Press Limited.

Islam, M. D., S. Wakai, N. Ishikawa, A. M. R. Chowdhury, and J. P. Vaughan. 2002. "Cost-Effectiveness of Community Health Workers in Tuberculosis Control in Bangladesh." *Bulletin of the World Health Organization* 80 (6): 445–50.

Islam, M. S., J. P. Richards, and A. K. Ojha. 2012. "Targeting Drug Tolerance in Mycobacteria: A Perspective from Mycobacterial Biofilms." *Expert Review of Anti-Infective Therapy* 10 (9): 1055–66.

Isler, M., P. Rivest, J. Mason, and P. Brassard. 2013. "Screening Employees of Services for Homeless Individuals in Montréal for Tuberculosis Infection." *Journal of Infection and Public Health* 6 (3): 209–15.

Jack, C., U. Lalloo, Q. A. Karim, S. A. Karim, W. El-Sadr, and others. 2004. "A Pilot Study of Once-Daily Antiretroviral Therapy Integrated with Tuberculosis Directly Observed Therapy in a Resource-Limited Setting." *Journal of Acquired Immune Deficiency Syndromes* 36 (4): 929–34.

Jagirdar, J., and D. Zagzag. 1996. "Pathology and Insights into Pathogenesis of Tuberculosis." In *Tuberculosis*, edited by W. N. Rom and S. Garay, 467–91. Boston: Little, Brown.

James, P., R. Gupta, D. J. Christopher, B. Thankagunam, and B. Veeraraghavan. 2011. "MDR- and XDR-TB among

Suspected Drug-Resistant TB Patients in a Tertiary Care Hospital in India." *Clinical Respiratory Journal* 5 (1): e19–25.

Jenkins, H. E., V. Plesca, A. Ciobanu, V. Crudu, I. Galusca, and others. 2013. "Assessing Spatial Heterogeneity of Multidrug-Resistant Tuberculosis in a High-Burden Country." *European Respiratory Journal* 42 (5): 1291–301.

Jeon, C. Y., and M. B. Murray. 2008. "Diabetes Mellitus Increases the Risk of Active Tuberculosis: A Systematic Review of 13 Observational Studies." *PLoS Medicine* 5 (7): e152.

Jha, P., and R. Laxminarayan. 2009. "Choosing Health in India: An Entitlement for All Indians." University of Toronto and Resources for the Future, New Delhi.

Jiménez-Levi, E. 2012. *Tuberculosis Research and Development: 2012 Report on Tuberculosis Research Funding Trends, 2005–2011.* New York: Treatment Action Group.

Jindani, A., T. S. Harrison, A. J. Nunn, P. P. Phillips, G. J. Churchyard, and others. 2014. "High-Dose Rifapentine with Moxifloxacin for Pulmonary Tuberculosis." *New England Journal of Medicine* 371 (October 23): 1599–608.

Kagina, B. M., B. Abel, M. Bowmaker, T. J. Scriba, S. Gelderbloem, and others. 2009. "Delaying BCG Vaccination from Birth to 10 Weeks of Age May Result in an Enhanced Memory CD4 T Cell Response." *Vaccine* 27 (40): 5488–95.

Karonga Prevention Trial Group. 1996. "Randomised Controlled Trial of Single BCG, Repeated BCG, or Combined BCG and Killed *Mycobacterium leprae* Vaccine for Prevention of Leprosy and Tuberculosis in Malawi." *The Lancet* 348 (9019): 17–24.

Karumbi, J., and P. Garner. 2015. "Directly Observed Therapy for Treating Tuberculosis." *Cochrane Database of Systematic Reviews* 5: CD003343.

Katz, I., M. Aziz, M. Olszak-Olszewski, R. Komatsu, D. Low-Beer, and others. 2010. "Factors Influencing Performance of Global Fund-Supported Tuberculosis Grants." *International Journal of Tuberculosis and Lung Disease* 14 (9): 1097–103.

Kaufmann, S. H. E., M. F. Cotton, B. Eisele, M. Gengenbacher, L. Grode, and others. 2014. "The BCG Replacement Vaccine VPM1002: From Drawing Board to Clinical Trial." *Expert Review of Vaccines* 13 (5): 619–30.

Keane, J., S. Gershon, R. P. Wise, E. Mirabile-Levens, J. Kasznica, and others. 2001. "Tuberculosis Associated with Infliximab, A Tumor Necrosis Factor A–Neutralizing Agent." *New England Journal of Medicine* 345 (15): 1098–104.

Keshavjee, S., and P. E. Farmer. 2010. "Picking Up the Pace: Scale-Up of MDR Tuberculosis Treatment Programs." *New England Journal of Medicine* 363 (19): 1781–84.

———. 2012. "Tuberculosis, Drug Resistance, and the History of Modern Medicine." *New England Journal of Medicine* 367 (10): 931–36.

Keshavjee, S., and K. Seung. 2008. "Stemming the Tide of Multidrug-Resistant Tuberculosis: Major Barriers to Addressing the Growing Epidemic." Institute of Medicine report, Institute of Medicine, Washington, DC. https://www.ncbi.nlm.nih.gov/books/NBK45010.

Khan, A. J., S. Khowaja, F. S. Khan, F. Qazi, I. Lotia, and others. 2012. "Engaging the Private Sector to Increase Tuberculosis Case Detection: An Impact Evaluation Study." *The Lancet Infectious Diseases* 12 (8): 608–16.

Khan, B., P. Ahmed, K. Ullah, C. A. Hussain, I. Hussain, and S. Raza. 2005. "Frequency of Tuberculosis in Haematological Malignancies and Stem Cell Transplant Recipients." *Journal of the College of Physicians and Surgeons–Pakistan* 15 (1): 30–3.

Khan, F. A., J. Minion, A. Al-Motiri, A. Benedetti, A. D. Harries, and others. 2012. "An Updated Systematic Review and Meta-Analysis on the Treatment of Active Tuberculosis in Patients with HIV Infection." *Clinical Infectious Diseases* 55 (8): 1154–63.

Kim, C. H., K. H. Im, S. S. Yoo, S. Y. Lee, S. I. Cha, and others. 2014. "Comparison of the Incidence between Tuberculosis and Nontuberculous Mycobacterial Disease after Gastrectomy." *Infection* 42 (4): 697–704.

Kim, J. Y., P. Farmer, and M. E. Porter. 2013. "Redefining Global Health-Care Delivery." *The Lancet* 382 (9897): 1060–69.

King, G., E. Gakidou, K. Imai, J. Lakin, R. T. Moore, and others. 2009. "Public Policy for the Poor? A Randomised Assessment of the Mexican Universal Health Insurance Programme." *The Lancet* 373 (9673): 1447–54.

Kirwan, D. E., M. K. Cárdenas, and R. Gilman. 2012. "Rapid Implementation of New TB Diagnostic Tests: Is it Too Soon for a Global Roll-Out of Xpert MTB/RIF?" *American Journal of Tropical Medicine and Hygiene* 87 (2): 197–201.

Knight, G. M., P. J. Dodd, A. D. Grant, K. L. Fielding, G. J. Churchyard, and others. 2015. "Tuberculosis Prevention in South Africa." *PLoS One* 10 (4): e0122514.

Knight, G. M., U. K. Griffiths, T. Sumner, Y. V. Laurence, A. Gheorghe, and others. 2014. "Impact and Cost-Effectiveness of New Tuberculosis Vaccines in Low- and Middle-Income Countries." *Proceedings of the National Academy of Sciences* 111 (43): 15520–25.

Kranzer, K., H. Afnan-Holmes, K. Tomlin, J. E. Golub, A. E. Shapiro, and others. 2013. "The Benefits to Communities and Individuals of Screening for Active Tuberculosis Disease: A Systematic Review." *International Journal of Tuberculosis and Lung Disease* 17 (4): 432–46.

Kranzer, K., R. M. Houben, J. R. Glynn, L. G. Bekker, R. Wood, and others. 2010. "Yield of HIV-Associated Tuberculosis During Intensified Case Finding in Resource-Limited Settings: A Systematic Review and Meta-Analysis." *The Lancet Infectious Diseases* 10 (2): 93–102.

Kritzinger, F. E., S. den Boon, S. Verver, D. A. Enarson, C. J. Lombard and others. 2009. "No Decrease in Annual Risk of Tuberculosis Infection in Endemic Area in Cape Town, South Africa." *Tropical Medicine and International Health* 14 (2): 136–42.

Kruk, M. E., E. Goldmann, and S. Galeo. 2009. "Borrowing and Selling to Pay for Health Care in Low- and Middle-Income Countries." *Health Affairs* 28 (4): 1056–66.

Kruk, M. E., N. R. Schwalbe, and C. A. Aguiar. 2008. "Timing of Default from Tuberculosis Treatment: A Systematic Review." *Tropical Medicine and International Health* 13 (5): 703–12.

Kumar, M., and S. Kumar. 1997. "Tuberculosis Control in India: Role of Private Doctors." *The Lancet* 350 (9087): 1329–30.

Labrique, A. B., L. Vasudevan, E. Kochi, R. Fabricant, and G. Mehl. 2013. "mHealth Innovations as Health System Strengthening Tools: 12 Common Applications and a Visual Framework." *Global Health: Science and Practice* 1 (2): 160–71.

Lal, S., M. W. Uplekar, I. Katz, K. Lonnroth, R. Komatsu, and others. 2011. "Global Fund Financing of Public-Private Mix Approaches for Delivery of Tuberculosis Care." *Tropical Medicine and International Health* 16 (6): 685–92.

Laurence, Y. V., U. K. Griffiths, and A. Vassall. 2015. "Costs to Health Services and the Patient of Treating Tuberculosis: A Systematic Literature Review." *PharmacoEconomics* 33 (9): 1–17.

Lawn, S. D. 2015. "Advances in Diagnostic Assays for Tuberculosis." *Cold Spring Harbor Perspectives in Medicine* 5 (12): pii=a017806.

Lawn, S. D., S. V. Brooks, K. Kranzer, M. P. Nicol, A. Whitelaw, and others. 2011. "Screening for HIV-Associated Tuberculosis and Rifampicin Resistance before Antiretroviral Therapy Using the Xpert MTB/RIF Assay: A Prospective Study." *PLoS Medicine* 8 (7): e1001067.

Lawn, S. D., A. D. Kerkhoff, M. Vogt, and R. Wood. 2012. "Diagnostic Accuracy of a Low-Cost, Urine Antigen, Point-of-Care Screening Assay for HIV-Associated Pulmonary Tuberculosis before Antiretroviral Therapy: A Descriptive Study." *The Lancet Infectious Diseases* 12 (3): 201–09.

Lee, D., S. S. Lal, R. Komatsu, A. Zumla, and R. Atun. 2012. "Global Fund Financing of Tuberculosis Services Delivery in Prisons." *Journal of Infectious Diseases* 205 (Suppl 2): S274–83.

Lee, D. K., Y.-S. Cho, S. H. Hong, W. H. Chung, and Y. C. Ahn. 2006. "Inflammatory Pseudotumor Involving the Skull Base: Response to Steroid and Radiation Therapy." *Otolaryngology—Head and Neck Surgery* 135 (1): 144–48.

Lee, M., T. Song, Y. Kim, I. Jeong, S. N Cho, and C. E. Barry. 2015. "Linezolid for XDR-TB—Final Study Outcomes." *New England Journal of Medicine* 373 (3): 290–91. http://www.nejm.org/doi/full/10.1056/NEJMc1500286#t=article.

Lee, R. S., N. Radmonski, J. F. Proulx, I. Levade, B. J. Shapiro and others. 2015. "Population Genomics of *Mycobacterium tuberculosis* in the Inuit." *Proceedings of the National Academy of Sciences* 112 (44): 13609–14.

Legido-Quigley, H., C. M. Montgomery, P. Khan, R. Atun, A. Fakoya, and others. 2013. "Integrating Tuberculosis and HIV Services in Low- and Middle-Income Countries: A Systematic Review." *Tropical Medicine and International Health* 18 (2): 199–211.

Leimane, V., and J. Leimans. 2006. "Tuberculosis Control in Latvia: Integrated DOTS." *Eurosurveillance* 11 (3): 29–33.

Lessem, E., H. Cox, C. Daniels, J. Furin, L. McKenna, and others. 2015. "Access to New Medications for the Treatment of Drug-Resistant Tuberculosis: Patient, Provider and Community Perspectives." *International Journal of Infectious Diseases* 32: 56–60.

Lester, R. T., P. Ritvo, E. J. Mills, A. Kariri, S. Karanja, and others. 2010. "Effects of a Mobile Phone Short Message Service on Antiretroviral Treatment Adherence in Kenya (WelTel Kenya1): A Randomised Trial." *The Lancet* 376 (9755): 1838–45.

Libshitz, H. I., H. K. Pannu, L. S. Elting, and C. D. Cooksley. 1997. "Tuberculosis in Cancer Patients: An Update." *Journal of Thoracic Imaging* 12 (1): 41–46.

Lienhardt, C., K. Fielding, J. Sillah, A. Tunkara, S. Donkor, and others. 2003. "Risk Factors for Tuberculosis Infection in Sub-Saharan Africa: A Contact Study in the Gambia." *American Journal of Respiratory and Critical Care Medicine* 168 (4): 448–55.

Lietman, T., T. Porco, and S. Blower. 1997. "Leprosy and Tuberculosis: The Epidemiological Consequences of Cross-Immunity." *American Journal of Public Health* 87 (12): 1923–27.

Lin, H.-H., D. Dowdy, C. Dye, M. Murray, and T. Cohen. 2012. "The Impact of New Tuberculosis Diagnostics on Transmission: Why Context Matters." *Bulletin of the World Health Organization* 90 (10): 739–47.

Lin, H.-H., M. Ezzati, and M. Murray. 2007. "Tobacco Smoke, Indoor Air Pollution, and Tuberculosis: A Systematic Review and Meta-Analysis." *PLoS Medicine* 4 (1): e20.

Lin, H.-H., C. Suk, H. L. Lo, R. Y. Huang, D. A. Enarson, and others. 2014. "Indoor Air Pollution from Solid Fuel and Tuberculosis: A Systematic Review and Meta-Analysis." *International Journal of Tuberculosis and Lung Disease* 18 (5): 613–21.

Lin, X., V. Chongsuvivatwong, L. Lin, A. Geater, and R. Lijuan. 2008. "Dose–Response Relationship between Treatment Delay of Smear-Positive Tuberculosis Patients and Intra-Household Transmission: A Cross-Sectional Study." *Transactions of the Royal Society of Tropical Medicine and Hygiene* 102 (8): 797–804.

Lipsitch, M., and A. O. Sousa. 2002. "Historical Intensity of Natural Selection for Resistance to Tuberculosis." *Genetics* 161 (4): 1599–607.

Liu, P. T., S. Stenger, D. H. Tang, and R. L. Modlin. 2007. "Cutting Edge: Vitamin D-Mediated Human Antimicrobial Activity against *Mycobacterium tuberculosis* Is Dependent on the Induction of Cathelicidin." *Journal of Immunology* 179 (4): 2060–63.

Lönnroth, K., B. G. Williams, P. Cegielski, and C. Dye. 2010. "A Consistent Log-Linear Relationship between Tuberculosis Incidence and Body Mass Index." *International Journal of Epidemiology* 39 (1): 149–55.

Lönnroth, K., B. G. Williams, S. Stadlin, E. Jaramillo, and C. Dye. 2008. "Alcohol Use as a Risk Factor for Tuberculosis–A Systematic Review." *BMC Public Health* 8 (1): 289.

Lopez, B., D. Aguilar, H. Orozco, M. Burger, C. Espitia, and others. 2003. "A Marked Difference in Pathogenesis and Immune Response Induced by Different *Mycobacterium tuberculosis* Genotypes." *Clinical and Experimental Immunology* 133 (1): 30–37.

Loudon, R. G. and S. K. Spohn. 1969. "Cough Frequency and Infectivity in Patients with Pulmonary Tuberculosis." *American Review of Respiratory Disease* 99 (1): 109–11.

Loveday, M., K. Wallengren, A. Voce, B. Margot, T. Reddy, and others 2012. "Comparing Early Treatment Outcomes of MDR-TB in a Decentralised Setting with a Centralised Setting in KwaZulu-Natal, South Africa." *International Journal of Tuberculosis and Lung Disease* 16 (2): 209–15.

Lowell, A. M., L. B. Edwards, and C. E. Palmer. 1969. "Tuberculosis Morbidity and Mortality and Its Control." In *Tuberculosis,* edited by A. M. Lowell, L. B. Edwards, and C. E. Palmer, 129–66. Cambridge, MA: Harvard University Press.

Lozano, R., M. Naghavi, K. Foreman, S. Lim, K. Shibuya, and others. 2012. "Global and Regional Mortality from 235 Causes of Death for 20 Age Groups in 1990 and 2010: A Systematic Analysis for the Global Burden of Disease Study 2010." *The Lancet* 380 (9859): 2095–128.

Lu, L. L., A. W. Chung, T. R. Rosebrock, M. Ghebremichael, W. H. Yu, and others. 2016. "A Functional Role for Antibodies in Tuberculosis." *Cell* 167 (2): 433–43.

Lundgrun, B. 2015. "Ebola Kills Far Fewer Than AIDS, TB, and Malaria. What Should We Prioritise?" *The Guardian,* January 19.

Lutwama, F., B. M. Kagina, A. Waiswa, N. Mansoor, S. Kirimunda, and others. 2014. "Distinct T-Cell Responses When BCG Vaccination Is Delayed from Birth to 6 Weeks of Age in Ugandan Infants." *Journal of Infectious Diseases* 209 (6): 887–97.

Luyirika, E., H. Nsobya, R. Batamwita, P. Businge, W. Musoke, and others. 2012. "A Home-Based Approach to Managing Multi-Drug Resistant Tuberculosis in Uganda: A Case Report." *AIDS Research and Therapy* 9 (1): 12.

Luzze, H., D. F. Johnson, K. Dickman, H. Mayanja-Kizza, A. Okwera, and others. 2013. "Relapse More Common Than Reinfection in Recurrent Tuberculosis 1–2 Years Post Treatment in Urban Uganda." *International Journal of Tuberculosis and Lung Disease* 17 (3): 361–67.

Lygizos, M., S. V. Shenoi, R. P. Brooks, A. Bhushan, J. C. M. Brust, and others. 2013. "Natural Ventilation Reduces High TB Transmission Risk in Traditional Homes in Rural KwaZulu-Natal, South Africa." *BMC Infectious Diseases* 13 (July 1): 300.

MacIntyre, C. R., N. Kendig, L. Kummer, S. Birago, and N. M. Graham. 1997. "Impact of Tuberculosis Control Measures and Crowding on the Incidence of Tuberculous Infection in Maryland Prisons." *Clinical Infectious Diseases* 24 (6): 1060–67.

Mamlin, B. W., P. G. Biondich, B. A. Wolfe, H. S. F. Fraser, D. Jazayeri, and others. 2006. "Cooking Up an Open Source EMR for Developing Countries: OpenMRS, a Recipe for Successful Collaboration." *AMIA Annual Symposium Proceedings* 2006: 529–53.

Mangtani, P., I. Abubakar, C. A. Ariti, and J. A. C. Sterne. 2014. "Protection by BCG Vaccine Against Tuberculosis: A Systematic Review of Randomized Controlled Trials." *Clinical Infectious Diseases* 58 (4): 470–80.

Manjelievskaia, J., D. Erck, S. Piracha, and L. Schrager. 2016. "Drug-Resistant TB: Deadly, Costly, and in Need of a Vaccine." *Transactions of the Royal Society of Tropical Medicine and Hygiene* 110 (3): 186–91.

Manjourides, J., H. H. Lin, S. Shin, C. Jeffery, C. Contreras, and others. 2012. "Identifying Multidrug Resistant Tuberculosis Transmission Hotspots Using Routinely Collected Data." *Tuberculosis* 92 (3): 273–79.

Mao, T. E., K. Okada, N. Yamada, S. Peou, M. Ota, and others. 2014. "Cross-Sectional Studies of Tuberculosis Prevalence in Cambodia between 2002 and 2011." *Bulletin of the World Health Organization* 92 (8): 573–81.

Marais, B. J., M. C. Raviglione, P. R. Donald, A. D. Harries, A. L. Kritski, and others. 2010. "Scale-Up of Services and Research Priorities for Diagnosis, Management, and Control of Tuberculosis: A Call to Action." *The Lancet* 375 (9732): 2179–91.

Marica, C., C. Didilescu, N. Galie, D. Chiotan, J. P. Zellweger, and others. 2009. "Reversing the Tuberculosis Upwards Trend: A Success Story in Romania." *European Respiratory Journal* 33 (1): 168–70.

Marrone, M. T., V. V Venkataramanan, M. Goodman, A. C. Hill, J. A. Jereb, and others. 2013. "Surgical Interventions for Drug-Resistant Tuberculosis: A Systematic Review and Meta-Analysis." *International Journal of Tuberculosis and Lung Disease* 17 (1): 6–16.

Martineau, A. R., S. Nhamoyebonde, T. Oni, M. X. Rangaka, S. Marais, and others. 2011. "Reciprocal Seasonal Variation in Vitamin D Status and Tuberculosis Notifications in Cape Town, South Africa." *Proceedings of the National Academy of Sciences* 108 (47): 19013–17.

Marx, F. M., R. Dunbar, D. A. Enarson, B. G. Williams, R. M. Warren, and others. 2014. "The Temporal Dynamics of Relapse and Reinfection Tuberculosis after Successful Treatment: A Retrospective Cohort Study." *Clinical Infectious Diseases* 58 (12): 1676–83.

Mathew, T. A., T. N. Ovsyanikova, S. S. Shin, I. Y. Gelmanova, D. A. Balbuena, and others. 2006. "Causes of Death during Tuberculosis Treatment in Tomsk Oblast, Russia." *International Journal of Tuberculosis and Lung Disease* 10 (8): 857–63.

McFarlane, N. 1989. "Hospitals, Housing, and Tuberculosis in Glasgow, 1911–51." *Social History of Medicine* 2 (1): 59–85.

McIlleron, H., G. Meintjes, W. J. Burman, and G. Maartens. 2007. "Complications of Antiretroviral Therapy in Patients with Tuberculosis: Drug Interactions, Toxicity, and Immune Reconstitution Inflammatory Syndrome." *Journal of Infectious Diseases* 196 (Suppl 1): S63–75.

McKee, M., and R. Atun. 2006. "Beyond Borders: Public-Health Surveillance." *The Lancet* 367 (9518): 1224–26.

McKeown, T., and R. Record. 1962. "Reasons for the Decline of Mortality in England and Wales during the Nineteenth Century." *Population Studies* 16 (2): 94–122.

Meintjes, G., S. D. Lawn, F. Scano, G. Maartens, M. A. French, and others. 2008. "Tuberculosis-Associated Immune Reconstitution Inflammatory Syndrome: Case Definitions for Use in Resource-Limited Settings." *The Lancet Infectious Diseases* 8 (8): 516–23.

Meintjes, G., R. J. Wilkinson, C. Morroni, D. J. Pepper, K. Rebe, and others. 2010. "Randomized Placebo-Controlled Trial of Prednisone for Paradoxical TB-Associated Immune Reconstitution Inflammatory Syndrome." *AIDS* 24 (15): 2381.

Melendez, J., C. I. Sánchez, R. H. Philipsen, P. Maduskar, R. Dawson, and others. 2016. "An Automated Tuberculosis

Screening Strategy Combining X-Ray-Based Computer-Aided Detection and Clinical Information." *Scientific Reports* 6: 25265. doi:10.1038/srep25265.

Menzies, N. A., T. Cohen, H.-H. Lin, M. Murray, and J. A. Saloman. 2012. "Population Health Impact and Cost-Effectiveness of Tuberculosis Diagnosis with Xpert MTB/RIF: A Dynamic Simulation and Economic Evaluation." *PLoS Medicine* 9 (11): e1001347.

Meressa, D., R. M. Hurtado, J. R. Andrews, E. Diro, K. Abato, and others. 2015. "Achieving High Treatment Success for Multidrug-Resistant TB in Africa: Initiation and Scale-Up of MDR TB Care in Ethiopia: An Observational Cohort Study." *Thorax* 70 (12): 1181–88.

Merle, C. S., K. Fielding, O. B. Sow, M. Gninafon, M. B. Lo, and others. 2014. "A Four-Month Gatifloxacin-Containing Regimen for Treating Tuberculosis." *New England Journal of Medicine* 371 (17): 1588–98.

Middelkoop, K., B. Mathema, L. Myer, E. Shashkina, A. Whitelaw, and others. 2015. "Transmission of Tuberculosis in a South African Community with a High Prevalence of HIV Infection." *Journal of Infectious Diseases* 211 (1): 53–61.

Mitchison, D. A. 2004. "Antimicrobial Therapy of Tuberculosis: Justification for Currently Recommended Treatment Regimens." *Seminars in Respiratory and Critical Care Medicine* 24 (3): 307–15.

Miti, S., V. Mfungwe, P. Reijer, and D. Maher. 2003. "Integration of Tuberculosis Treatment in a Community-Based Home Care Programme for Persons Living with HIV/AIDS in Ndola, Zambia." *International Journal of Tuberculosis and Lung Disease* 7 (9, Suppl 1): S92–98.

Mitnick, C. D., J. Bayona, E. Palacios, S. Shin, J. Furin, and others. 2003. "Community-Based Therapy for Multidrug-Resistant Tuberculosis in Lima, Peru." *New England Journal of Medicine* 348 (2): 119–28.

Mitnick, C. D., S. S. Shin, K. J. Seung, M. L. Rich, S. S. Atwood, and others. 2008. "Extensively Drug-Resistant Tuberculosis: A Comprehensive Treatment Approach." *New England Journal of Medicine* 359 (6): 563–74.

Mitwalli, A. 1991. "Tuberculosis in Patients on Maintenance Dialysis." *American Journal of Kidney Diseases* 18 (5): 579–82.

Moalosi, G., K. Floyd, J. Phatshwane, T. Moeti, N. Binkin, and T. Kenyon. 2003. "Cost-Effectiveness of Home-Based Care versus Hospital Care for Chronically Ill Tuberculosis Patients, Francistown, Botswana." *International Journal of Tuberculosis and Lung Disease* 7 (Suppl 1): S80–85.

Modlin, R. L., and B. R. Bloom. 2013. "TB or Not TB: That Is No Longer the Question." *Science Translational Medicine* 5 (213): 213–16

Mohammed-Rajput, N. A., D. C. Smith, B. Mamlin, P. Biondich, and B. N. Doebbeling. 2011. "OpenMRS, a Global Medical Records System Collaborative: Factors Influencing Successful Implementation." *AMIA Annual Symposium Proceedings* 2011 (October 22): 960–68.

Moonan, P. K., T. N. Quitugua, J. M. Pogoda, G. Woo, G. Drewyer, and others. 2011. "Does Directly Observed Therapy (DOT) Reduce Drug Resistant Tuberculosis?" *BMC Public Health* 11 (1): 19.

Moore, D. A. J. 2016. "What Can We Offer to 3 Million MDRTB Household Contacts in 2016?" *BMC Medicine* 14: 64.

Moyo, S., J. J. Furin, J. Hughes, J. Daniels, L. Snyman, and others. 2014. "Outcomes in Adolescents Undergoing Treatment for Drug-Resistant Tuberculosis in Cape Town, South Africa, 2008–2013." *Archives of Pediatric Infectious Diseases* 3 (3): e17934.

Mphaphlele, M., A. S. Dharmadhikari, P. A. Jensen, S. N. Rudnick, T. H. van Reenen, and others. 2015. "Institutional Tuberculosis Transmission Controlled Trial of Upper Room Ultraviolet Air Disinfection: A Basis for New Dosing Guidelines." *American Journal of Respiratory and Critical Care Medicine* 192 (4): 477–84.

Mukherjee, J. S., S. Shin, J. Furin, M. L. Rich, F. Léandre, and others. 2002. "New Challenges in the Clinical Management of Drug-Resistant Tuberculosis." *Infectious Diseases in Clinical Practice* 11 (6): 329–39.

Muniyandi, M., R. Rajeswari, R. Balasubramanian, and P. R. Narayanan. 2008. "A Comparison of Costs to Patients with Tuberculosis Treated in a DOTS Programme with Those in a Non-DOTS Programme in South India." *Journal of Health Management* 10 (1): 9–24.

Muniyandi, M., R. Ramachandran, R. Balasubramanian, and P. R. Narayanan. 2006. "Socio-Economic Dimensions of Tuberculosis Control: Review of Studies over Two Decades from Tuberculosis Research Center." *Journal of Communicable Diseases* 38 (3): 204.

Muniyandi, M., R. Ramachandran, P. G. Gopi, V. Chandrasekaran, R. Subramani, and others. 2007. "The Prevalence of Tuberculosis in Different Economic Strata: A Community Survey from South India [Short Communication]." *International Journal of Tuberculosis and Lung Disease* 11 (9): 1042–45.

Munro, S. A., S. A. Lewin, H. J. Smith, M. E. Engel, A. Fretheim, and others. 2007. "Patient Adherence to Tuberculosis Treatment: A Systematic Review of Qualitative Research." *PLoS Medicine* 4 (7): e238.

Murray, C. J., K. Styblo, and A. Rouillon. 1990. "Tuberculosis in Developing Countries: Burden, Intervention and Cost. *Bulletin of the International Union Against Tuberculosis and Lung Disease* 65 (December 8): 6–24.

Nakiyingi, L., V. M. Moodley, Y. C. Manabe, M. P. Nicol, M. Holshouse, and others. 2014. "Diagnostic Accuracy of a Rapid Urine Lipoarabinomannan Test for Tuberculosis in HIV-Infected Adults." *Journal of Acquired Immune Deficiency Syndromes* 66 (3): 270–79.

Naranbhai, V. 2016. "The Role of Host Genetics (and Genomics) in Tuberculosis." *Microbiology Spectrum* 4 (5). doi: 10.1128/microbiolspec.TBTB2-0011-2016.

Nardell, E., and A. Dharmadhikari. 2010. "Turning off the Spigot: Reducing Drug-Resistant Tuberculosis Transmission in Resource-Limited Settings." *International Journal of Tuberculosis and Lung Disease* 14 (10): 1233.

Nathanson, E., C. Lambregts-van Weezenbeek, M. Rich, R. Gupta, J. Bayona, and others. 2006. "Multidrug-Resistant Tuberculosis Management in Resource-Limited Settings." *Emerging Infectious Diseases* 12 (9): 1389.

Nathanson, E., P. Nunn, M. W. Uplekar, K. Floyd, E. Jaramillo, and others. 2010. "MDR Tuberculosis: Critical Steps for

Prevention and Control." *New England Journal of Medicine* 363 (11): 1050–58.

Nganda, B., J. Wang'ombe, K. Floyd, and J. Kangangi. 2003. "Cost and Cost-Effectiveness of Increased Community and Primary Care Facility Involvement in Tuberculosis Care in Machakos District, Kenya." *International Journal of Tuberculosis and Lung Disease* 7 (9, Suppl 1): S14–20.

Nunn, A. J., I. D. Rusen, A. Van Deun, G. Torrea, P. P. Phillips, and others. 2014. "Evaluation of a Standardized Treatment Regimen of Anti-Tuberculosis Drugs for Patients with Multi-Drug-Resistant Tuberculosis (STREAM): Study Protocol for a Randomized Controlled Trial." *Trials* 15 (September 9): 353.

Obihara, C. C., N. Beyers, R. P. Gie, P. C. Potter, B. J. Marais, and others. 2005. "Inverse Association between *Mycobacterium tuberculosis* Infection and Atopic Rhinitis in Children." *Allergy* 60 (9): 1121–25.

OECD (Organisation for Economic Co-operation and Development), Eurostat, WHO (World Health Organization). 2011. *A System of Health Accounts.* Paris: OECD Publishing. http://www.who.int/health-accounts/methodology/sha2011.pdf.

O'Garra, A., P. S. Redford, F. W. McNab, C. I. Bloom, R. J. Wilkinson, and others. 2013. "The Immune Response in Tuberculosis." *Annual Review of Immunology* 31 (March): 475–527.

O'Grady, J., M. Hoelscher, R. Atun, M. Bates, P. Mwaba, and others. 2011. "Tuberculosis in Prisons in Sub-Saharan Africa: The Need for Improved Health Services, Surveillance, and Control." *Tuberculosis* 91 (2): 173–78.

O'Grady, J., M. Maeurer, R. Atun, I. Abubakar, P. Mwaba, and others. 2011. "Tuberculosis in Prisons: Anatomy of Global Neglect." *European Respiratory Journal* 38 (4): 752–54.

Okello, D., K. Floyd, F. Adatu, R. Odeke, and G. Gargioni. 2003. "Cost and Cost-Effectiveness of Community-Based Care for Tuberculosis Patients in Rural Uganda." *The International Journal of Tuberculosis and Lung Disease* 7 (9, Suppl 1): S72–79.

Okot-Chono, R., F. Mugisha, F. Adatu, E. Madraa, R. Dlodlo, and others. 2009. "Health System Barriers Affecting the Implementation of Collaborative TB-HIV Services in Uganda." *International Journal of Tuberculosis and Lung Disease* 13 (8): 955–61.

Owens, J. P., M. O. Fofana, and D. W. Dowdy. 2013. "Cost-Effectiveness of Novel First-Line Treatment Regimens for Tuberculosis." *International Journal of Tuberculosis and Lung Disease* 17 (May): 590–96.

Oxlade, O., and M. Murray. 2012. "Tuberculosis and Poverty: Why Are the Poor at Greater Risk in India?" *PLoS One* 7 (11): e47533.

Pai, M., A. Daftary, and S. Satyanarayana. 2016. "TB Control: Challenges and Opportunities for India." *Transactions of the Royal Society of Tropical Medicine and Hygiene* 110 (3): 158–60.

Pai, M., S. Kalantri, and K. Dheda. 2006. "New Tools and Emerging Technologies for the Diagnosis of Tuberculosis: Part II. Active Tuberculosis and Drug Resistance." *Expert Review of Molecular Diagnostics* 6 (3): 423–32.

Palacios, J. J., J. Ferro, N. Ruiz Palma, J. M. García, H. Villar, and others. 1999. "Fully Automated Liquid Culture System Compared with Löwenstein-Jensen Solid Medium for Rapid Recovery of Mycobacteria from Clinical Samples." *European Journal of Clinical Microbiology and Infectious Diseases* 18 (4): 265–73.

Palmer, C., and M. W. Long 1966. "Effects of Infection with Atypical Mycobacteria on BCG Vaccination and Tuberculosis." *American Review of Respiratory Disease* 94 (4): 553–68.

Pantoja, A., K. Floyd, K. P. Unnikrishnan, R. Jitendra, M. R. Padma, and others. 2009. "Economic Evaluation of Public-Private Mix for Tuberculosis Care and Control, India. Part I. Socio-Economic Profile and Costs among Tuberculosis Patients." *International Journal of Tuberculosis and Lung Disease* 13 (6): 698–704.

Pantoja, A., K. Lönnroth, S. S. Lal, L. S. Chauhan, M. W. Uplekar, and others. 2009. "Economic Evaluation of Public-Private Mix for Tuberculosis Care and Control, India. Part II. Cost and Cost-Effectiveness." *International Journal of Tuberculosis and Lung Disease* 13 (6): 705–12.

Pasipanodya, J. G., and T. Gumbo. 2013. "A Meta-Analysis of Self-Administered versus Directly Observed Therapy Effect on Microbiologic Failure, Relapse, and Acquired Drug Resistance in Tuberculosis Patients." *Clinical Infectious Diseases* 57 (1): 21–31.

Perumal, R., N. Padayatchi, and E. Stiefvater. 2009. "The Whole Is Greater Than the Sum of the Parts: Recognising Missed Opportunities for an Optimal Response to the Rapidly Maturing TB-HIV Co-Epidemic in South Africa." *BMC Public Health* 9 (1): 243.

Petsch, B., M. Schnee, A. B. Vogel, E. Lange, B. Hoffmann, and others. 2012. "Protective Efficacy of in vitro Synthesized, Specific mRNA Vaccines against Influenza A Virus Infection." *Nature Biotechnology* 30 (12): 1210–16.

Pevzner, E. S., G. Vandebriel, D. W. Lowrance, M. Gasana, and A. Finlay. 2011. "Evaluation of the Rapid Scale-Up of Collaborative TB/HIV Activities in TB Facilities in Rwanda, 2005–2009." *BMC Public Health* 11 (1): 550.

Philipsen, R. H., C. I. Sánchez, P. Maduskar, J. Melendez, L. Peters-Bax, and others. 2015. "Automated Chest-Radiography as a Triage for Xpert Testing in Resource-Constrained Settings: A Prospective Study of Diagnostic Accuracy and Costs." *Scientific Reports* 5:12215. doi: 10.1038/srep12215.

Phillips, M., R. N. Cataneo, R. Condos, G. A. Ring Erickson, J. Greenberg, and others. 2007. "Volatile Biomarkers of Pulmonary Tuberculosis in the Breath." *Tuberculosis* 87 (1): 44–52.

Phillips, P. P., C. M. Mendel, D. A. Burger, A. M. Crook, A. J. Nunn, and others. 2016. "Limited Role of Culture Conversion for Decision-Making in Individual Patient Care and for Advancing Novel Regimens to Confirmatory Clinical Trials." *BMC Medicine* 14 (February 4): 19.

Phiri, S., P. Khan, A. D. Grant, D. Gareta, H. Tweya, and others. 2011. "Integrated Tuberculosis and HIV Care in a Resource-Limited Setting: Experience from the Martin

Preuss Centre, Malawi." *Tropical Medicine and International Health* 16 (11): 1397–403.

Pichenda, K., K. Nakamura, A. Morita, M. Kizuki, K. Seino, and T. Takano. 2012. "Non-Hospital DOT and Early Diagnosis of Tuberculosis Reduce Costs while Achieving Treatment Success." *International Journal of Tuberculosis and Lung Disease* 16 (6): 828–34.

Png, E., B. Alisjahbana, E. Sahiratmadja, S. Marzuki, R. Nelwan, and others. 2012. "A Genome Wide Association Study of Pulmonary Tuberculosis Susceptibility in Indonesians." *BMC Medical Genetics* 13 (January 13): 5.

Podewils, L. J., M. T. S. Gler, M. I. Quelapio, and M. P. Chen. 2013. "Patterns of Treatment Interruption among Patients with Multidrug-Resistant TB (MDR TB) and Association with Interim and Final Treatment Outcomes." *PLoS One* 8 (7): e70064.

Pooran, A., E. Pieterson, M. Davids, G. Theron, and K. Dheda. 2013. "What Is the Cost of Diagnosis and Management of Drug Resistant Tuberculosis in South Africa?" *PLoS One* 8 (1): e54587.

Pop-Eleches, C., H. Thirumurthy, J. P. Habyarimana, J. G. Zivin, M. P. Goldstein, and others. 2011. "Mobile Phone Technologies Improve Adherence to Antiretroviral Treatment in a Resource-Limited Setting: A Randomized Controlled Trial of Text Message Reminders." *AIDS* 25 (6): 825–34.

Prasad, K., and M. B. Singh. 2008. "Corticosteroids for Managing Tuberculous Meningitis." *Cochrane Database of Systematic Reviews* 23 (1): CD002244.

Rachow, A., A. Zumla, N. Heinrich, G. Rojas-Ponce, B. Mtafya, and others. 2011. "Rapid and Accurate Detection of *Mycobacterium tuberculosis* in Sputum Samples by Cepheid Xpert MTB/RIF Assay: A Clinical Validation Study." *PLoS One* 6 (6): e20458.

Ramma, L., H. Cox, L. Wilkinson, N. Foster, L. Cunnama, and others. 2015. "Patients' Costs Associated with Seeking and Accessing Treatment for Drug-Resistant Tuberculosis in South Africa." *International Journal of Tuberculosis and Lung Disease* 19 (12): 1513–19.

Rangaka, M. X., S. C. Cavalcane, B. J. Marais, S. Thim, N. A. Martinson, and others. 2015. "Controlling the Seedbeds of Tuberculosis: Diagnosis and Treatment of Tuberculosis Infection." *The Lancet* 386 (10010): 2344–53.

Rehm, J., A. V. Samokhvalov, M. G. Neuman, R. Room, C. Parry, and others. 2009. "The Association between Alcohol Use, Alcohol Use Disorders and Tuberculosis (TB). A Systematic Review." *BMC Public Health* 9 (1): 450.

Resch, S. C., J. A. Salomon, M. Murray, and M. C. Weinstein. 2006. "Cost-Effectiveness of Treating Multidrug-Resistant Tuberculosis." *PLoS Medicine* 3 (7): e241.

Riley, R., and A. Moodie. 1974. "Infectivity of Patients with Pulmonary Tuberculosis in Inner City Homes." *American Review of Respiratory Disease* 110 (6): 810–12.

Roberts, M., W. Hsiao, P. Berman, and M. Reich. 2004. *Getting Health Reform Right: A Guide to Improving Performance and Equity.* Oxford: Oxford University Press.

Rodrigo, T., J. A. Caylà, G. de Olalla P., H. Galdós-Tangüis, J. M. Jansà, and others. 1997. "Characteristics of Tuberculosis Patients Who Generate Secondary Cases." *International Journal of Tuberculosis and Lung Disease* 1 (4): 352–57.

Rodrigues, L. C., V. K. Diwan, and J. G. Wheeler. 1993. "Protective Effect of BCG against Tuberculous Meningitis and Miliary Tuberculosis: A Meta-Analysis." *International Journal of Epidemiology* 22 (6): 1154–58.

Ross, J. D., and J. C. Willison. 1971. "The Relationship between Tuberculin Reactions and the Later Development of Tuberculosis: An Investigation among Edinburgh School Children in 1960–1970." *Tubercle* 52 (4): 258–65.

Rouillon, A., S. Perdrizet, and R. Parrot. 1976. "Transmission of Tubercle Bacilli: The Effects of Chemotherapy." *Tubercle* 57 (4): 275–99.

Rouzier, V. A., O. Oxlade, R. Verduga, L. Gresely, and D. Menzies. 2010. "Patient and Family Costs Associated with Tuberculosis, Including Multidrug-Resistant Tuberculosis, in Ecuador." *The International Journal of Tuberculosis and Lung Disease* 14 (10): 1316–22.

Roy, A., M. Eisenhut, R. J. Harris, L. C. Rodrigues, S. Sridhar, and others. 2014. "Effect of BCG Vaccination Against *Mycobacterium tuberculosis* Infection in Children: Systematic Review and Meta-analysis." *BMJ* 349 (August 5): g4643.

Sallusto, F. 2016. "Heterogeneity of Human CD4(+) T Cells against Microbes." *Annual Review of Immunology* 34 (May 24): 317–34.

Salomon, J. A., J. Lloyd-Smith, W. M. Getz, S. Resch, M. S. Sánchez, and others. 2006. "Prospects for Advancing Tuberculosis Control Efforts through Novel Therapies." *PLoS Medicine* 3 (8): e273.

Samandari, T., T. B. Agizew, S. Nyirenda. Z. Tedla, T. Sibanda, and others. 2011. "6-Month Versus 36-Month Isoniazid Preventive Treatment for Tuberculosis in Adults with HIV Infection in Botswana: A Randomised, Double-Blind, Placebo-Controlled Trial." *The Lancet* 377 (9777): 1588–98.

Samb, B., T. Evans, M. Dybul, R. Atun, J.-P. Moatti, and others. 2009. "An Assessment of Interactions between Global Health Initiatives and Country Health Systems." *The Lancet* 373 (9681): 2137–69.

Satyanarayana, S., S. A. Nair, S. S. Chadha, R. Shivashankar, G. Sharma, and others. 2011. "From Where Are Tuberculosis Patients Accessing Treatment in India? Results from a Cross-Sectional Community Based Survey of 30 Districts." *PLoS One* 6 (9): e24160.

Schaaf, H. S., B. J. Marais, A. C. Hesseling, W. Brittle, and P. R. Ronald. 2009. "Surveillance of Antituberculosis Drug Resistance among Children from the Western Cape Province of South Africa—An Upward Trend." *American Journal of Public Health* 99 (8): 1486–90.

Schnippel, K., S. Rosen, K. Shearer, N. Martinson, L. Long, and others. 2013. "Costs of Inpatient Treatment for Multi-Drug-Resistant Tuberculosis in South Africa." *Tropical Medicine and International Health* 18 (1): 109–16.

Schouten, E. J., A. Jahn, D. Midiani, S. D. Makombe, A. Mnthambala, and others. 2011. "Prevention of Mother-to-Child Transmission of HIV and the Health-Related Millennium Development Goals: Time for a Public Health Approach." *The Lancet* 378 (9787): 282–84.

Scott, L. E., K. McCarthy, N. Gous, M. Nduna, A. Van Rie, and others. 2011. "Comparison of Xpert MTB/RIF with Other Nucleic Acid Technologies for Diagnosing Pulmonary Tuberculosis in a High HIV Prevalence Setting: A Prospective Study." *PLoS Medicine* 8 (7): e1001061.

Seddon, J. A., H. E. Jenkins, L. Liu, T. Cohen, R. E. Black, and others. 2015. "Counting Children with Tuberculosis: Why Numbers Matter." *International Journal of Tuberculosis and Lung Disease* 19 (Suppl 1): 9–16.

Seebregts, C. J., B. W. Mamlin, P. G. Biondich, H. S. F. Fraser, B. A. Wolfe, and others. 2009. "The OpenMRS Implementers Network." *International Journal Medical Informatics* 78 (11): 711–20.

Selwyn, P. A., D. Hartel, V. A. Lewis, E. E. Schoenbaum, S. H. Vermund, and others. 1989. "A Prospective Study of the Risk of Tuberculosis among Intravenous Drug Users with Human Immunodeficiency Virus Infection." *New England Journal of Medicine* 320 (9): 545–50.

Sengupta, A., and S. Nundy. 2005. "The Private Health Sector in India." *BMJ* 331 (7526): 1157–58.

Seung, K. J., D. B. Omatayo, S. Keshavjee, J. J. Furin, P. E. Farmer, and others. 2009. "Early Outcomes of MDR-TB Treatment in a High HIV-Prevalence Setting in South Africa." *PLoS One* 4 (9): e7186.

Shah, N. S., S. C. Auld, J. C. M. Brust, B. Mathema, N. Ismail, and others. 2017. "Transmission of Extensively Drug-Resistant Tuberculosis in South Africa." *New England Journal of Medicine* 376: 243–53.

Shaler, C. R., C. N. Horvath, M. Jeyanathan, and Z. Xing. 2013. "Within the Enemy's Camp: Contribution of the Granuloma to the Dissemination, Persistence and Transmission of *Mycobacterium tuberculosis*." *Frontiers in Immunology* 4 (February 14): 30.

Shapiro, A. E., E. Variava, M. H. Rakgokong, N. Moodley, B. Luke, and others. 2012. "Community-Based Targeted Case Finding for Tuberculosis and HIV in Household Contacts of Patients with Tuberculosis in South Africa." *American Journal of Respiratory and Critical Care Medicine* 185 (10): 1110–16.

Shargie, E. B., O. Mørkve, and B. Lindtjørn. 2006. "Tuberculosis Case-Finding through a Village Outreach Programme in a Rural Setting in Southern Ethiopia: Community Randomized Trial." *Bulletin of the World Health Organization* 84 (2): 112–19.

Sheriff, F. G., K. P. Manji, M. M. Chagani, R. M. Mpembeni, A. M. Jusabani, and others. 2010. "Latent Tuberculosis among Pregnant Mothers in a Resource Poor Setting in Northern Tanzania: A Cross-Sectional Study." *BMC Infectious Diseases* 10 (1): 52.

Shetty, N., M. Shemko, M. Vaz, and G. D'Souza. 2006. "An Epidemiological Evaluation of Risk Factors for Tuberculosis in South India: A Matched Case Control Study." *International Journal of Tuberculosis and Lung Disease* 10 (1): 80–86.

Shi, W., X. Zhang, X. Jiang, H. Yuan, J. S. Lee, and others. 2011. "Pyrazinamide Inhibits Trans-Translation in *Mycobacterium tuberculosis*." *Science* 333 (6049): 1630–32.

Shigayeva, A., R. Atun, M. McKee, and R. Coker. 2010. "Health Systems, Communicable Diseases and Integration." *Health Policy and Planning* 25 (Suppl 1): i4–20.

Shilova, M. V., and C. Dye. 2001. "The Resurgence of Tuberculosis in Russia." *Philosophical Transactions of the Royal Society of London B: Biological Sciences* 356 (1411): 1069–75.

Shin, S. S., A. D. Pasechnikov, I. Y. Gelmanova, G. G. Peremitin, A. K. Strelis, and others. 2006. "Treatment Outcomes in an Integrated Civilian and Prison MDR-TB Treatment Program in Russia." *The International Journal of Tuberculosis and Lung Disease* 10 (4): 402–8.

Shin, S. S., M. Yagui, L. Ascencios, G. Yale, C. Suarez, and others. 2008. "Scale-Up of Multidrug-Resistant Tuberculosis Laboratory Services, Peru." *Emerging Infectious Diseases* 14 (5): 701.

Shirakawa, T., T. Enomoto, S. Shimazu, and J. M. Hopkin. 1997. "The Inverse Association between Tuberculin Responses and Atopic Disorder." *Science* 275 (5296): 77–79.

Shirtcliffe, P., M. Weatherall, and R. Beasley. 2002. "An Inverse Correlation between Estimated Tuberculosis Notification Rates and Asthma Symptoms." *Respirology* 7 (2): 153–55.

Siedner, M. J., A. J. Lankowski, M. Kanyesigye, M. B. Bwana, J. E. Haberer, and others. 2015. "A Combination SMS and Transportation Reimbursement Intervention to Improve HIV Care Following Abnormal CD4 Test Results in Rural Uganda: A Prospective Observational Cohort Study." *BMC Medicine* 13 (1): 160.

Sinanovic, E., K. Floyd, L. Dudley, V. Azevedo, R. Grant, and others. 2003. "Cost and Cost-Effectiveness of Community-Based Care for Tuberculosis in Cape Town, South Africa." *International Journal of Tuberculosis and Lung Disease* 7 (9, Suppl 1): S56–62.

Sinanovic, E., and L. Kumaranayake. 2006. "Financing and Cost-Effectiveness Analysis of Public-Private Partnerships: Provision of Tuberculosis Treatment in South Africa." *Cost Effectiveness and Resource Allocation* 4: 11.

Sinanovic, E., J. Moodley, M. A. Barone, S. Mall., S. Cleary, and others. 2009. "The Potential Cost-Effectiveness of Adding a Human Papillomavirus Vaccine to the Cervical Cancer Screening Programme in South Africa." *Vaccine* 27 (44): 6196–202.

Sinanovic, E., L. Ramma, A. Vassall, V. Azevedo, L. Wilkinson, and others. 2015. "Impact of Reduced Hospitalisation on the Cost of Treatment for Drug-Resistant Tuberculosis in South Africa." *International Journal of Tuberculosis and Lung Disease* 19 (2): 172–78.

Singh, A., D. Parasher, D. S. Shekhavat, S. Sahu, D. Wares, and others. 2004. "Effectiveness of Urban Community Volunteers in Directly Observed Treatment of Tuberculosis Patients: A Field Report from Haryana, North India [Notes from the Field]." *International Journal of Tuberculosis and Lung Disease* 8 (6): 800–802.

Slama, K., C. Chiang, D. A. Enarson, K. Hassmiller, A. Fanning, and others. 2007. "Tobacco and Tuberculosis: A Qualitative Systematic Review and Meta-Analysis [Review Article]."

International Journal of Tuberculosis and Lung Disease 11 (10): 1049–61.

Smart, T. 2010. "Decentralised, Patient-Centered Models of Delivering Treatment and Palliative Care for People with M/XDR-TB." *HIV and AIDS Treatment in Practice* 166 (October 8): 2–10.

Smieja, M. J., C. A. Marchetti, D. J. Cook, and F. M. Smaill. 2000. "Isoniazid for Preventing Tuberculosis in Non-HIV Infected Persons." *Cochrane Database of Systematic Reviews* 2: CD001363.

Snider, D. Jr. 1978. "The Relationship between Tuberculosis and Silicosis." *American Review of Respiratory Disease* 118 (3): 455–60.

Sobota, R. S., C. M. Stein., N. Kodaman, L. B. Scheinfeldt, I. Maro, and others. 2016. "A Locus at 5q33.3 Confers Resistance to Tuberculosis in Highly Susceptible Individuals." *American Journal of Human Genetics* 98 (3): 514–24.

Soltan, V., A. K. Henry, V. Crudu, and I. Zatusevski. 2008. "Increasing Tuberculosis Case Detection: Lessons from the Republic of Moldova." *Bulletin of the World Health Organization* 86 (1): 71–76.

Soysal, A., K. A. Millington, M. Bakir, D. Dosanjh, Y. Aslan, and others. 2005. "Effect of BCG Vaccination on Risk of *Mycobacterium tuberculosis* Infection in Children with Household Tuberculosis Contact: A Prospective Community-Based Study." *The Lancet* 366 (9495): 1443–51.

Spertini, F., R. Audran, R. Chakour, O. Karoui, V. Steiner-Monard, and others. 2015. "Safety of Human Immunisation with a Live-Attenuated *Mycobacterium tuberculosis* Vaccine: A Randomised, Double-Blind, Controlled Phase I Trial." *The Lancet Respiratory Medicine* 3 (12): 953–62.

Spisak, C., L. Morgan, R. Eichler, J. Rosen, B. Serumaga, and others. 2016. "Results-Based Financing in Mozambique's Central Medical Store: A Review after 1 Year." *Global Health: Science and Practice* 4 (1): 2–13.

Sreeramareddy, C. T., Z. Z. Qin, S. Satyanarayana, R. Subbaraman, and M. Pai. 2014. "Delays in Diagnosis and Treatment of Pulmonary Tuberculosis in India: A Systematic Review." *International Journal of Tuberculosis and Lung Disease* 18 (3): 255–66.

Stead, W. W., and A. K. Dutt. 1989. "Tuberculosis in the Elderly." *Seminars in Respiratory Infections* 4: 189–97.

Sterling, T. R., M. E. Villarino, A. S. Borisov, N. Shang, F. Gordin, and others. 2011. "Three Months of Rifapentine and Isoniazid for Latent Tuberculosis Infection." *New England Journal of Medicine* 365: 2155–66.

Stop TB Partnership. 2011. "The Global Plan to Stop TB." World Health Organization, Geneva.

———. 2016. "The 'Zero TB Initiative' Sparks New Action to End TB." World Health Organization, Geneva, July 26. http://us3.campaign-archive2.com/?u=85207b84f0f2d8ddc9bd878de&id=6f3e04fcc9&e=abd33e01a4.

Stop TB Working Group on DOTS-Plus for MDR-TB. 2003. "A Prioritised Research Agenda for DOTS-Plus for Multidrug-Resistant Tuberculosis (MDR-TB)." *International Journal of Tuberculosis and Lung Disease* 7 (5): 410–14.

Styblo, K. 1991. *Epidemiology of Tuberculosis: Selected Papers.* The Hague: KNCV Tuberculosis Foundation.

Suarez, P. G., K. Floyd, J. Portocarrero, E. Alarcon, E. Rapiti, and others. 2002. "Feasibility and Cost-Effectiveness of Standardised Second-Line Drug Treatment for Chronic Tuberculosis Patients: A National Cohort Study in Peru." *The Lancet* 359 (9322): 1980–89.

Subbaraman, R., R. R. Nathavitharana, S. Satyanarayana, M. Pai, B. E. Thomas, and others. 2016. "The Tuberculosis Cascade of Care in India's Public Sector: A Systematic Review and Meta-Analysis." *PLoS Medicine* 13 (10): e1002149. doi:10.1371/journal.pmed.1002149.

Sudre, P., G. ten Dam, and A. Kochi. 1992. "Tuberculosis: A Global Overview of the Situation Today." *Bulletin of the World Health Organization* 70 (2): 149.

Sutherland, I., and V. Springett. 1987. "Effectiveness of BCG Vaccination in England and Wales in 1983." *Tubercle* 68 (2): 81–92.

Sutherland, I., E. Svandova, and S. Radhakrishna. 1982. "The Development of Clinical Tuberculosis Following Infection with Tubercle Bacilli: 1. A Theoretical Model for the Development of Clinical Tuberculosis Following Infection, Linking from Data on the Risk of Tuberculous Infection and the Incidence of Clinical Tuberculosis in the Netherlands." *Tubercle* 63 (4): 255–68.

Swanson, R. C., A. Cattaneo, E. Bradley, S. Chunharas, R. Atun, and others. 2012. "Rethinking Health Systems Strengthening: Key Systems Thinking Tools and Strategies for Transformational Change." *Health Policy and Planning* 27 (Suppl 4): iv54–64.

Sweeney, T. E., L. Braviak, C. M. Tato, and P. Khatri. 2016. "Genome-Wide Expression for Diagnosis of Pulmonary Tuberculosis: A Multicohort Analysis." *The Lancet Respiratory Medicine* 4 (3): 213–24.

Sylla, L., R. D. Bruce, A. Kamarulzaman, and F. L. Altice. 2007. "Integration and Co-Location of HIV/AIDS, Tuberculosis, and Drug Treatment Services." *International Journal of Drug Policy* 18 (4): 306–12.

Szot, A., F. Jacobson, S. Munn, D. Jazayeri, E. Nardell, and others. 2004. "Diagnostic Accuracy of Chest X-rays Acquired Using a Digital Camera for Low-Cost Teleradiology." *International Journal of Medicine* 73 (1): 65–73.

TAG (Treatment Action Group). 2016. *Report on Tuberculosis Research Funding Trends, 2005–2015: No Time to Lose.* New York: TAG. http://www.treatmentactiongroup.org/sites/default/files/TB_FUNDING_2016.

Talat, N., S. Perry, J. Parsonnet, G. Dawood, and R. Hussain. 2010. "Vitamin D Deficiency and Tuberculosis Progression." *Emerging Infectious Diseases* 16 (5): 853–55.

Tameris, M. D., M. Hatherill, B. S. Landry, T. J. Scriba, M. A. Snowden, and others. 2013. "Safety and Efficacy of MVA85A, A New Tuberculosis Vaccine, in Infants Previously Vaccinated with BCG: A Randomised, Placebo-Controlled Phase 2b Trial." *The Lancet* 381 (9871): 1021–28.

Temprano ARNS Study Group. 2015. "A Trial of Early Antiretrovirals and Isoniazid Preventative Therapy in Africa." *New England Journal of Medicine* 373 (9): 808–22.

Theron, G., H. E. Jenkins, F. Cobelens, I. Abubakar, A. J. Khan, and others. 2015. "Data for Action: Collection and Use of Local Data to End Tuberculosis." *The Lancet* 386 (10010): 2324–33.

Theron, G., L. Zijenah, D. Chanda, P. Clowes, A. Rachow, and others. 2014. "Feasibility, Accuracy, and Clinical Effect of Point-of-Care Xpert MTB/RIF Testing for Tuberculosis in Primary-Care Settings in Africa: A Multicentre, Randomised, Controlled Trial." *The Lancet* 383 (9915): 424–35.

Thye, T., E. Owusu-Dabo, F. O. Vannberg, R. van Crevel, J. Curtis, and others. 2012. "Common Variants at 11p13 Are Associated with Susceptibility to Tuberculosis." *Nature Genetetics* 44 (3): 257–59.

Toczek, A., H. Cox, P. du Cros, G. Cooke, and N. Ford. 2013. "Strategies for Reducing Treatment Default in Drug-Resistant Tuberculosis: Systematic Review and Meta-Analysis [Review Article]." *International Journal of Tuberculosis and Lung Disease* 17 (3): 299–307.

Tornee, S., J. Kaewkungwal, W. Fungladda, U. Silachamroon, P. Akarasewi, and others. 2005. "The Association between Environmental Factors and Tuberculosis Infection among Household Contacts." *Southeast Asian Journal of Tropical Medicine and Public Health* 36 (Suppl 4): 221–24.

Toungoussova, O. S., G. Bjune, and D. A. Caugant. 2006. "Epidemic of Tuberculosis in the Former Soviet Union: Social and Biological Reasons." *Tuberculosis* 86 (1): 1–10.

Trajman, A., M. L. Bastos, M. Belo, J. Calaça, J. Gaspar, and others. 2016. "Shortened First-Line TB Treatment in Brazil: Potential Cost Savings for Patients and Health Services." *BMC Health Services Research* 16: 27.

Travis, P., S. Bennett, A. Haines, T. Pang, Z. Bhutta, and others. 2004. "Overcoming Health-Systems Constraints to Achieve the Millennium Development Goals." *The Lancet* 364 (9437): 900–906.

Trébucq, A., D. Enarson, C. Y. Chiang, A. Van Deun, A. D. Harries, and others. 2011. "Xpert® MTB/RIF for National Tuberculosis Programmes in Low-Income Countries: When, Where and How?" *International Journal of Tuberculosis and Lung Disease* 15 (12): 1567–72.

Trunz, B. B., P. Fine, and C. Dye. 2006. "Effect of BCG Vaccination on Childhood Tuberculous Meningitis and Miliary Tuberculosis Worldwide: A Meta-Analysis and Assessment of Cost-Effectiveness." *The Lancet* 367 (9517): 1173–80.

Tseng, C.-L., O. Oxlade, D. Menzies, A. Aspler, and K. Schwartzman. 2011. "Cost-Effectiveness of Novel Vaccines for Tuberculosis Control: A Decision Analysis Study." *BMC Public Health* 11 (1): 55.

Tuberculosis Prevention Trial. 1979. "Trial of BCG Vaccines in South India for Tuberculosis Prevention: First Report." 1979. *Bulletin of the World Health Organization* 57 (5): 819–27.

Tupasi, T. E., R. Gupta, M. I. Quelapio, R. B. Orillaza, N. R. Mira, and others. 2006. "Feasibility and Cost-Effectiveness of Treating Multidrug-Resistant Tuberculosis: A Cohort Study in the Philippines." *PLoS Medicine* 3 (September 12): e352.

Udwadia, Z. F., R. A. Amale, K. K. Ajbani, and C. Rodrigues. 2012. "Totally Drug-Resistant Tuberculosis in India." *Clinical Infectious Diseases* 54 (4): 579–81.

Udwadia, Z. F., L. M. Pinto, and M. W. Uplekar. 2010. "Tuberculosis Management by Private Practitioners in Mumbai, India: Has Anything Changed in Two Decades?" *PLoS One* 5 (8): e12023.

Ukwaja, K. N., O. Modebe, C. Igwenyi, and I. Alobu. 2012. "The Economic Burden of Tuberculosis Care for Patients and Households in Africa: A Systematic Review." *International Journal of Tuberculosis and Lung Disease* 16 (6): 733–39.

UN (United Nations) General Assembly. 2000. "United Nations Millennium Declaration." United Nations General Assembly Resolution A/RES/55/2, UN, New York.

Uplekar, M. W., S. Juvekar, S. Morankar, S. Rangan, and P. Nunn. 1998. "Tuberculosis Patients and Practitioners in Private Clinics in India." *International Journal of Tuberculosis and Lung Disease* 2 (4): 324–29.

Uplekar, M. W., V. Pathania, and M. Raviglione. 2001. "Private Practitioners and Public Health: Weak Links in Tuberculosis Control." *The Lancet* 358 (9285): 912–16.

Uplekar, M. W., and D. S. Shepard. 1991. "Treatment of Tuberculosis by Private General Pracitioners in India." *Tubercle* 72 (4): 284–90. http://www.sciencedirect.com/science/article/pii/004138799190055W.

Uplekar, M. W., D. Weil, K. Lonnroth, E. Jaramillo, C. Lienhardt, and others. 2015. "WHO's New End Tuberculosis Strategy." *The Lancet* 385 (9979): 1799–801.

Uwimana, J., and D. Jackson. 2013. "Integration of Tuberculosis and Prevention of Mother-to-Child Transmission of HIV Programmes in South Africa." *International Journal of Tuberculosis and Lung Disease* 17 (10): 1285–90.

Uwimana, J., D. Jackson, H. Hausler, and C. Zarowsky. 2012. "Health System Barriers to Implementation of Collaborative TB and HIV Activities Including Prevention of Mother to Child Transmission in South Africa." *Tropical Medicine and International Health* 17 (5): 658–65.

Uwinkindi, F., S. Nsanzimana, D. J. Riedel, R. Muhayimpundu, E. Remera, and others. 2014. "Scaling Up Intensified Tuberculosis Case Finding in HIV Clinics in Rwanda." *Journal of Acquired Immune Deficiency Syndromes* 66 (2): e45–49.

Uyei, J., D. Coetzee, J. Macinko, and S. Guttmacher. 2011. "Integrated Delivery of HIV and Tuberculosis Services in Sub-Saharan Africa: A Systematic Review." *The Lancet Infectious Diseases* 11 (11): 855–67.

Uys, P. W., R. Warren, P. D. van Helden, M. Murray, and T. C. Victor. 2009. "Potential of Rapid Diagnosis for Controlling Drug-Susceptible and Drug-Resistant Tuberculosis in Communities Where *Mycobacterium tuberculosis* Infections Are Highly Prevalent." *Journal of Clinical Microbiology* 47 (5): 1484–90.

van der Werf, M. J., M. W. Langendam, E. Huitric, and D. Manissero. 2012. "Multidrug Resistance after Inappropriate Tuberculosis Treatment: A Meta-Analysis." *European Respiratory Journal* 39 (6): 1511–19.

van Rie, A., K. McCarthy, L. Scott, A. Dow, W. D. Venter, and others. 2013. "Prevalence, Risk Factors and Risk Perception of Tuberculosis Infection among Medical Students and Healthcare Workers in Johannesburg, South Africa." *South African Medical Journal* 103 (11): 853–57.

van't Hoog, A. H., K. F. Laserson, W. A. Githui, H. K. Meme, J. A. Agaya, and others. 2011. "High Prevalence of Pulmonary Tuberculosis and Inadequate Case Finding in Rural Western Kenya." *American Journal of Respiratory and Critical Care Medicine* 183 (9): 1245–53.

van't Hoog, A. H., H. K. Meme, K. F. Laserson, J. A. Agaya, B. G. Muchiri, and others. 2012. "Screening Strategies for Tuberculosis Prevalence Surveys: The Value of Chest Radiography and Symptoms." *PLoS One* 7 (7): e38691.

Vassall, A. 2013. "Cost-Effectiveness of Introducing Bedaquiline in MDR-TB Regimens: An Exploratory Analysis." WHO, Geneva.

Vassall, A., S. Bagdadi, H. Bashour, H. Zaher, and P. V. Maaren. 2002. "Cost-Effectiveness of Different Treatment Strategies for Tuberculosis in Egypt and Syria." *International Journal of Tuberculosis and Lung Disease* 6 (12): 1083–90.

Vassall, A., Y. Chechulin, I. Raykhert, N. Osalenko, S. Svetlichnaya, and others. 2009. "Reforming Tuberculosis Control in Ukraine: Results of Pilot Projects and Implications for the National Scale-Up of DOTS." *Health Policy and Planning* 24 (1): 55–62.

Vassall, A., S. van Kampen, H. Sohn, J. S. Michael, K. R. John, and others. 2011. "Rapid Diagnosis of Tuberculosis with the Xpert MTB/RIF Assay in High Burden Countries: A Cost-Effectiveness Analysis." *PLoS Medicine* 8 (11): e1001120.

Verguet, S., R. Laxminarayan, and D. T. Jamison. 2015. "Universal Public Finance of Tuberculosis Treatment in India: An Extended Cost-Effectiveness Analysis." *Health Economics* 24 (3): 318–32.

Verma, G., R. E. Upshur, E. Rea, and S. R. Benatar. 2004. "Critical Reflections on Evidence, Ethics and Effectiveness in the Management of Tuberculosis: Public Health and Global Perspectives." *BMC Medical Ethics* 5 (1): 2.

Verver, S., R. M. Warren, N. Beyers, M. Richardson, G. D. van der Spuy, and others. 2005. "Rate of Reinfection Tuberculosis after Successful Treatment Is Higher than Rate of New Tuberculosis." *American Journal of Respiratory and Critical Care Medicine* 171 (12): 1430–35.

Victor, T., E. Streicher, C. Kewley, A. M. Jordaan, G. D. van der Spuy, and others. 2007. "Spread of an Emerging *Mycobacterium tuberculosis* Drug-Resistant Strain in the Western Cape of South Africa." *International Journal of Tuberculosis and Lung Disease* 11 (2): 195–201.

Villemagne, B., C. Crauste, M. Flipo, A. R. Baulard, B. Déprez, and others. 2012. "Tuberculosis: the Drug Development Pipeline at a Glance." *European Journal of Medicinal Chemistry* 51 (May): 1–16.

Vledder, M., P. Yadav, J. Friedman, M. Sjoblom, amd T. Brown. 2015. "Optimal Supply Chain Structure for Distributing Essential Drugs in Low-Income Countries: Results from a Randomized Experiment." Ross School of Business Paper 1269, University of Michigan, Ann Arbor.

von Mutius, E., N. Pearce, R. Beasley, S. Cheng, O. von Ehrenstein, and others. 2000. "International Patterns of Tuberculosis and the Prevalence of Symptoms of Asthma, Rhinitis, and Eczema." *Thorax* 55 (6): 449–53.

Vynnycky, E., M. Borgdorff, C. C. Leung, C. M. Tam, and P. E. M. Fine. 2008. "Limited Impact of Tuberculosis Control in Hong Kong: Attributable to High Risks of Reactivation Disease." *Epidemiology and Infection* 136 (7): 943–52.

Wallis, R. S., and C. Nacy. 2013. "Early Bactericidal Activity of New Drug Regimens for Tuberculosis." *The Lancet* 381 (9861): 111–12.

Walton, D. A., P. E. Farmer, W. Lambert, F. Léandre, S. P. Koenig, and others. 2004. "Integrated HIV Prevention and Care Strengthens Primary Health Care: Lessons from Rural Haiti." *Journal of Public Health Policy* 25 (2): 137–58.

Walzl, G., K. Ronacher, J. F. D. Siawaya, and H. M. Dockrell. 2008. "Biomarkers for TB Treatment Response: Challenges and Future Strategies." *Journal of Infection* 57 (2): 103–09.

Wandwalo, E., N. Kapalata, S. Egwaga, and S. Morkve. 2004. "Effectiveness of Community-Based Directly Observed Treatment for Tuberculosis in an Urban Setting in Tanzania: A Randomised Controlled Trial." *International Journal of Tuberculosis and Lung Disease* 8 (10): 1248–54.

Wandwalo, E., B. Robberstad, and O. Morkve. 2005. "Cost and Cost-Effectiveness of Community Based and Health Facility Based Directly Observed Treatment of Tuberculosis in Dar es Salaam, Tanzania." *Cost Effectiveness and Resource Allocation* 3 (1): 6.

Weir, R., G. Black, B. Nazareth, S. Floyd, S. Stenson, and others. 2006. "The Influence of Previous Exposure to Environmental Mycobacteria on the Interferon—Gamma Response to Bacille Calmette–Guérin Vaccination in Southern England and Northern Malawi." *Clinical and Experimental Immunology* 146 (3): 390–99.

Weiss, P., W. Chen, V. J. Cook, and J. C. Johnston. 2014. "Treatment Outcomes from Community-Based Drug Resistant Tuberculosis Treatment Programs: A Systematic Review and Meta-Analysis." *BMC Infectious Diseases* 14 (June 17): 333.

Wells, W. A., M. W. Uplekar, and M. Pai. 2015. "Achieving Systemic and Scalable Private Sector Engagement in Tuberculosis Care and Prevention in Asia." *PLoS Medicine* 12 (6): e1001842.

Were, M. C., J. Kariuki, V. Chepng'eno, M. Wandabwa, S. Ndege, and others. 2009. "Leapfrogging Paper-Based Records Using Handheld Technology: Experience from Western Kenya." *Studies in Health Technology and Informatics* 160 (1): 525–29.

WHO (World Health Organization). 1994. "WHO Tuberculosis Programme: Framework for Effective Tuberculosis Control." WHO, Geneva.

———. 1999. *The World Health Report 1999: Making a Difference.* Geneva: WHO.

———. 2000. *The World Health Report 2000: Health Systems, Improving Performance.* Geneva: WHO.

———. 2003. *The World Health Report 2003: Shaping The Future.* Geneva: WHO.

———. 2004. "Interim Policy on Collaborative TB/HIV Activities." WHO, Geneva.

———. 2006. "Improving the Diagnosis and Treatment of Smear-Negative Pulmonary and Extrapulmonary Tuberculosis among Adults and Adolescents." WHO, Stop TB Department, Geneva.

———. 2007. *Global Tuberculosis Control: Surveillance, Planning, Financing.* Geneva: WHO.

———. 2009a. "Global Tuberculosis Control: A Short Update to the 2009 Report." WHO, Geneva.

———. 2009b. "WHO Policy on TB Infection Control in Health-Care Facilities, Congregate Settings, and Households." WHO, Geneva.

———. 2010. "Multidrug and Extensively Drug-Resistant TB: 2010 Global Report on Surveillance and Response." WHO, Geneva.

———. 2011a. "Guidelines for the Programmatic Management of Multidrug Resistant Tuberculosis." WHO, Geneva.

———. 2011b. "Towards Universal Access to Diagnosis and Treatment of Multidrug-Resistant and Extensively Drug-Resistant Tuberculosis by 2015." WHO Progress Report 2011, WHO, Geneva.

———. 2011c. "Tuberculosis Country Profiles: South Africa." WHO, Geneva. http://www.who.int/tb/country/data/profiles/en/index.html.

———. 2012a. *Global Tuberculosis Report*. Geneva: WHO.

———. 2012b. "WHO Policy on Collaborative TB/HIV Activities: Guidelines for National Programmes and Other Stakeholders." WHO, Geneva.

———. 2013a. "Consolidated Guidelines on the Use of Antiretroviral Drugs for Treating and Preventing HIV Infection." WHO, Geneva.

———. 2013b. *Global Tuberculosis Report 2013*. Geneva: WHO.

———. 2013c. *Roadmap for Childhood Tuberculosis*. Geneva: WHO. http://apps.who.int/iris/bitstream/10665/89506/1/9789241506137_eng.pdf.

———. 2013d. "Systematic Screening for Active Tuberculosis: Principles and Recommendations." WHO, Geneva. http://www.who.int/tb/tbscreening.

———. 2013e. "The Use of Bedaquiline in the Treatment of Multidrug-Resistant Tuberculosis: Interim Policy Guidance." WHO, Geneva.

———. 2014a. *Global Status Report on Alcohol and Health 2014*. Geneva: WHO.

———. 2014b. *Global Tuberculosis Report 2014*. Geneva: WHO.

———. 2014c. "Tuberculosis." Fact Sheet 104, WHO, Geneva. http://www.who.int/mediacentre/factsheets/fs104/en/.

———. 2015a. "The End TB Strategy." WHO, Geneva. http://www.who.int/tb/End_TB_brochure.pdf.

———. 2015b. *Global Tuberculosis Report*. Geneva: WHO.

———. 2015c. "The End TB Strategy." Fact Sheet, WHO, Geneva. http://www.who.int/tb/post2015_TBstrategy.pdf?ua=1.

———. 2016a. *Global Tuberculosis Report 2016*. Geneva: WHO.

———. 2016b. *WHO Treatment Guidelines for Drug-Resistant Tuberculosis. 2016 Update*. Geneva: WHO. http://www.who.int/tb/MDRTBguidelines2016.pdf.

———. n.d. "The Five Elements of DOTS." WHO, Geneva. http://www.who.int/tb/dots/whatisdots/en/.

Wilkinson, R. J., M. Llewelyn, Z. Toossi, P. Patel, and G. Pasvol. 2000. "Influence of Vitamin D Deficiency and Vitamin D Receptor Polymorphisms on Tuberculosis among Gujarati Asians in West London: A Case-Control Study." *The Lancet* 355 (9204): 618–21.

Willingham, F. F., T. L. Schmitz, M. Contreras, S. E. Kalangi, A. M. Vivar, and others. 2001. "Hospital Control and Multidrug-Resistant Pulmonary Tuberculosis in Female Patients, Lima, Peru." *Emerging Infectious Diseases* 7 (1): 123.

Wolfe, F., K. Michaud, J. Anderson, and K. Urbansky. 2004. "Tuberculosis Infection in Patients with Rheumatoid Arthritis and the Effect of Infliximab Therapy." *Arthritis and Rheumatism* 50 (2): 372–79.

Wood, R., S. D. Lawn, J. Caldwell, R. Kaplan, K. Middelkoop, and others. 2011. "Burden of New and Recurrent Tuberculosis in a Major South African City Stratified by Age and HIV-Status." *PLoS One* 6 (10): e25098.

Wood, R., S. D. Lawn, S. Johnstone-Robertson, and L.-G. Bekker. 2011. "Tuberculosis Control Has Failed in South Africa: Time to Reappraise Strategy." *South African Medical Journal* 101 (2): 111–14.

Wood, R., S. Johnstone-Robertson, P. Uys, J. Hargrove, K. Middelkeep, and others. 2010. "Tuberculosis Transmission to Young Children in a South African Community: Modeling Household and Community Infection Risks." *Clincal Infectious Diseases* 51 (4): 401–8.

Wood, R., K. Middelkoop, L. Myer, A. D. Grant, A. Whitelaw, and others. 2007. "Undiagnosed Tuberculosis in a Community with High HIV Prevalence: Implications for Tuberculosis Control." *American Journal of Respiratory and Critical Care Medicine* 175 (1): 87–93.

Woolhouse, M. E., C. Dye, J.-F. Etard, T. Smith, J. D. Charlwood, and others. 1997. "Heterogeneities in the Transmission of Infectious Agents: Implications for the Design of Control Programs." *Proceedings of the National Academy of Sciences* 94 (1): 338–42.

World Bank. 1993. *World Development Report 1993: Investing in Health*. Washington, DC: World Bank.

Wu, P., E. H. Y. Lau, B. J. Cowling, C.-C. Leung, C.-M. Tam, and others. 2010. "The Transmission Dynamics of Tuberculosis in a Recently Developed Chinese City." *PLoS One* 5 (May 3): e10468.

Yadav, P. 2010. "In-Country Supply Chains: The Weakest Link in the Health System." *Global Health Magazine* 5 (Winter): 18–20.

———. 2015. "Health Product Supply Chains in Developing Countries: Diagnosis of the Root Causes of Underperformance and an Agenda for Reform." *Health Systems and Reform* 1 (2): 142–54.

Yadav, P., O. Stapleton, and L. Van Wassenhove. 2013. "Learning from Coca-Cola." *Stanford Social Innovation Review* (Winter): n.p.

Yadav, P., H. L. Tata, and M. Babaley. 2011. *The World Medicines Situation 2011: Storage and Supply Chain Management*. Geneva: WHO.

Yin, X., X. Tu, Y. Tong, R. Yang, Y. Wang, and others. 2012. "Development and Validation of a Tuberculosis Medication Adherence Scale." *PLoS One* 7 (12): e50328.

Yokoyama, T., R. Sato, T. Rikimaru, R. Hirai, and H. Aizawa. 2004. "Tuberculosis Associated with Gastrectomy." *Journal of Infection and Chemotherapy* 10 (5): 299–302.

Yuen, C. M., F. Amanullah, A. Dharmadhikari, E. A. Nardell, J. A. Seddon, and others. 2015. "Turning Off the Tap: Stopping Tuberculosis Transmission through Active Case-Finding and Prompt Effective Treatment." *The Lancet* 386 (10010): 2334–43.

Zachariah, R., M.-P. L. Spielmann, C. Chinji, P. Gomani, V. Arendt, and others. 2003. "Voluntary Counselling, HIV Testing, and Adjunctive Cotrimoxazole Reduces Mortality in Tuberculosis Patients in Thyolo, Malawi." *AIDS* 17 (7): 1053–61.

Zak, D., A. Penn-Nicholson, T. Scriba, E. Thompson, S. Suliman, and others. 2016. "A Blood RNA Signature for Tuberculosis Disease Risk: A Prospective Cohort Study." *The Lancet* 387 (10035): 2312–22.

Zar, H. J., M. F. Cotton, S. Strauss, J. Karpakis, G. Hussey, and others. 2007. "Effect of Isoniazid Prophylaxis on Mortality and Incidence of Tuberculosis in Children with HIV: Randomised Controlled Trial." *BMJ* 334 (7585): 136.

Zelner, J., M. B. Murray, M. C. Becerra, J. Galea, L. Lecca, and others. 2016. "Identifying Hotspots of Multidrug Resistant Tuberculosis Transmission Using Spatial and Molecular Genetic Data." *Journal of Infectious Diseases* 213 (2): 287–94.

Zhao, Y., S. Xu, L. Wang, D. P. Chin, S. Wang, and others. 2012. "National Survey of Drug-Resistant Tuberculosis in China." *New England Journal of Medicine* 366 (23): 2161–70.

Zumla, A., P. Nahid, and S. T. Cole. 2013. "Advances in the Development of New Tuberculosis Drugs and Treatment Regimens." *Nature Reviews Drug Discovery* 12 (5): 388–404.

Zwarenstein, M., L. R. Fairall, C. Lombard, P. Mayers, A. Bheekie, and others. 2011. "Outreach Education for Integration of HIV/AIDS Care, Antiretroviral Treatment, and Tuberculosis Care in Primary Care Clinics in South Africa: PALSA PLUS Pragmatic Cluster Randomised Trial." *BMJ* 342 (April 21): d2022.

Zwerling, A., G. B. Gomez, J. Pennington, F. Cobelens, A. Vassall, and D. W. Dowdy. 2016. "A Simplified Cost-Effectiveness Model to Guide Decision-Making for Shortened Anti-Tuberculosis Treatment Regimens." *International Journal of Tuberculosis and Lung Disease* 20 (2): 257–60.

Chapter 12

Malaria Elimination and Eradication

Rima Shretta, Jenny Liu, Chris Cotter, Justin Cohen,
Charlotte Dolenz, Kudzai Makomva, Gretchen Newby,
Didier Ménard, Allison Phillips, Allison Tatarsky,
Roly Gosling, and Richard Feachem

INTRODUCTION

The world has made tremendous progress in the fight against malaria in the past 15 years. According to the *World Malaria Report*, malaria case incidence was reduced by 41 percent and malaria mortality rates were reduced by 62 percent between 2000 and 2015 (WHO 2016c). At the beginning of 2016, malaria was considered to be endemic in 91 countries and territories, down from 108 in 2000.

Despite this progress, malaria continues to place a heavy toll on the world. In 2015, 212 million cases occurred globally, leading to 429,000 deaths, most of which occurred in children under age five years in Africa. These estimates are likely to be conservative, as adult deaths from malaria might well be underestimated in Africa and India (Adjuik and others 2006; Bawah and Binka 2007; Dhingra and others 2010; Gupta and Chowdhury 2014).

More than 100 countries have eliminated malaria in the past century. Of the 106 countries with ongoing transmission in 2000, 57 reduced malaria incidence more than 75 percent by 2015, in line with the World Health Assembly target for 2015 of reducing the malaria burden by 75 percent. An additional 18 countries reduced incidence by more than 50 percent (WHO 2015e), also achieving target 6C of the Millennium Development Goals, which called for halting and beginning to reverse the global incidence of malaria by 2015.

An increasing number of countries are moving toward the elimination of malaria. Since 2000, 12 countries have eliminated malaria; 4 were certified as malaria free by the World Health Organization (WHO) between 2007 and 2013 (Armenia, Morocco, Turkmenistan, and the United Arab Emirates); an additional 8 moved into the WHO's prevention-of-reintroduction phase after sustaining at least three years of zero local malaria transmission (Argentina, the Arab Republic of Egypt, Iraq, Georgia, the Kyrgyz Republic, Oman, the Syrian Arab Republic, and Uzbekistan); and 5 interrupted local transmission (Azerbaijan, Costa Rica, Paraguay, Sri Lanka,[1] and Turkey). The WHO European Region reported zero indigenous cases for the first time in 2015, in line with the goal of the Tashkent Declaration to eliminate malaria from the region by 2015.

According to the WHO (2016a), an additional 21 countries are in a position to achieve at least one year of zero indigenous cases of malaria by 2020.[2] These dramatic declines can be attributed to the scale-up of effective malaria control tools and technologies coupled with renewed political leadership and financial commitment.

Bolstered by these successes, most national malaria programs now consider elimination to be an

Corresponding author: Rima Shretta, University of California, San Francisco, Global Health Sciences, San Francisco, California, United States; Rima.Shretta@ucsf.edu.

Table 12.1 Global Milestones and Targets for Elimination

Goal	Milestones		Target
	2020	2025	2030
Reduce malaria mortality rates globally compared with 2015.	At least 40%	At least 75%	At least 90%
Reduce malaria case incidence globally compared with 2015.	At least 40%	At least 75%	At least 90%
Eliminate malaria from countries in which malaria was transmitted in 2015.	At least 10 countries	At least 20 countries	At least 35 countries
Prevent reestablishment of malaria in all countries that are malaria free.	Reestablishment prevented	Reestablishment prevented	Reestablishment prevented

Sources: RBM Partnership 2015; WHO 2015a.

attainable goal, and the idea of eradication is once again on the global health agenda. Many countries have developed national elimination goals, and regional networks have been formed to facilitate collaboration (Newby and others 2016). Leaders from the Asia Pacific Leaders Malaria Alliance and the African Leaders Malaria Alliance endorsed regional goals for malaria elimination by 2030 in November 2014 and January 2015, respectively, galvanizing support for elimination and eradication (APLMA 2015; United Nations 2015).

In this context, two new global malaria policy and advocacy documents supporting elimination and eradication were released in 2015: the Roll Back Malaria (RBM) Partnership's *Action and Investment to Defeat Malaria 2016–2030* and the WHO's *Global Technical Strategy for Malaria 2016–2030*. The *Global Technical Strategy* (GTS), which the WHO ratified in May 2015, calls for at least another 40 percent reduction in malaria-related mortality and morbidity between 2015 and 2020. Other goals and targets are illustrated in table 12.1. A third document, launched in September 2015, *From Aspiration to Action: What Will It Take to End Malaria?*, outlines the resources and strategies needed for global eradication by 2040, calling by 2020 commit to eradication in the next five years (Gates and Chambers 2015).

Despite these advances, malaria elimination and eradication face significant technical, operational, and financial challenges. About 3.2 billion people remain at risk of malaria; in 2015 alone, there were an estimated 214 million new cases of malaria and more than 400,000 malaria-related deaths. Global progress in malaria control and elimination is marked by vast disparities between and within countries, with vulnerable groups that have poor access to health services continuing to be marginalized. The Sub-Saharan Africa region shoulders the heaviest burden, with two countries—the

Democratic Republic of Congo and Nigeria—accounting for more than 35 percent of global malaria deaths. In these areas, malaria control programs aim to maximize the reduction of malaria cases and deaths; elimination will likely require more potent tools and stronger health systems.

A few countries that have successfully reduced malaria transmission are struggling to maintain their gains. An increased number of cases has recently been reported from a number of countries, including Cambodia, Djibouti, Madagascar, Uganda, and República Bolivariana de Venezuela (WHO 2015e). Furthermore, as the global malaria burden declines, emerging biological threats have the potential to critically weaken malaria responses in several parts of the world. In 2014, 60 countries reported resistance of mosquitoes to at least one insecticide used in vector control strategies; resistance of parasites to artemisinin, the cornerstone of malaria chemotherapy, has been detected in five countries in the Greater Mekong subregion, posing a serious threat to global health security.

This chapter summarizes the literature on malaria elimination; describes the progress made; and discusses malaria epidemiology, interventions, and challenges. In addition, it presents empirical information on financing and economics, including cost information from various settings. It concludes with a discussion of the economic basis for eradication and recommendations for research.

WHAT ARE ELIMINATION AND ERADICATION?

In areas of moderate to high transmission that are implementing malaria control, interventions are deployed on a large scale to reduce the public health burden of the disease. In elimination settings, targeted interventions aim to interrupt local transmission in the specific places where it becomes increasingly concentrated, that is, small geographic areas or special subpopulations that may be harder and costlier to reach. The key decisions facing policy makers in low- and moderate-transmission settings are when to embark on malaria elimination (Sabot and others 2010); which interventions to implement and where and when; and at what levels of intensity and reach. Critical to this debate are the political and financial commitments that are needed long after the disease stops being a public health burden.

Malaria elimination involves stopping indigenous transmission through active control measures (Cohen and others 2010; Smith and others 2009). The complete absence of local incidence is very unlikely to be achieved in places with high intrinsic potential for transmission and elevated importation of cases (Cohen and others 2010). For example, even the United States, a relatively low transmission risk area, identified 156 locally acquired cases between 1957 and 2003 (Filler and others 2006). Even countries that do not contiguously border endemic neighbors experience considerable importation annually: Sri Lanka reported 49 confirmed imported malaria cases in 2014, and in Tanzania, Zanzibar's estimated importation of 1.6 cases per 1,000 residents could potentially produce 1,300 incident cases (Le Menach and others 2011). Transmission from imported cases may lead to first degree *introduced* cases; a second degree of transmission from an introduced case produces an *indigenous* case: both are products of *local* transmission. Elimination accordingly requires preventing all indigenous cases, but introduced cases may continue to occur sporadically.

As more countries and regions eliminate malaria and implement measures to prevent reintroduction, fewer imported infections will occur, and eradication will become increasingly feasible. See box 12.1 for the WHO definitions of control, elimination, and eradication.

Box 12.1

Definitions of Control, Elimination, and Eradication

The path to malaria-free status is characterized by four distinct programmatic phases: control, pre-elimination, elimination, and prevention of reintroduction. The terms *elimination* and *eradication* are often used interchangeably. For example, *eradication* was previously used to describe what is now defined as elimination (Feachem and others 2010). To compare programs across these phases, it is important to adhere to agreed-upon terms and definitions.

Malaria control is the reduction of disease incidence, prevalence, morbidity, or mortality to a locally acceptable level as a result of deliberate efforts. Continued intervention is required to sustain control.

Malaria elimination is the interruption of local transmission (that is, reducing the rate of malaria cases to zero) of a specified parasite in a defined geographic area. Continued measures are required to prevent the reestablishment of transmission.

WHO certification of elimination[a] is the WHO certification of a country's malaria-free status. It confirms to the international community that the country, at that time, has halted local transmission of malaria by *Anopheles* mosquitoes and has created an adequate system for preventing reestablishment

of the disease. The WHO grants this certification when a country has proved, beyond reasonable doubt, that the chain of local malaria transmission by *Anopheles* mosquitoes has been interrupted nationwide for at least three consecutive years. Certification of malaria elimination is managed by the WHO Global Malaria Programme. The process is voluntary and can be initiated only after a country has submitted an official request to the WHO. The burden of proof falls on the country requesting certification. The final decision on granting a certification of malaria elimination rests with the WHO director-general.

Malaria eradication is a permanent reduction to zero of the worldwide incidence of infection caused by human malaria parasites as a result of deliberate efforts. Once eradication has been achieved, intervention measures would no longer be needed.

Source: WHO 2016a.
a. Since the early 1960s, the WHO has maintained an official register of areas where malaria elimination has been achieved. The WHO also maintains a supplementary list to the official register, listing countries where malaria never existed or disappeared years or decades ago and where full WHO certification of malaria elimination is not needed. The first supplementary list was published in 1963 and included 23 countries. The most recent list was published in 2012 and included 62 countries (WHO 2012d).

PROGRESS TOWARD MALARIA ELIMINATION

Elimination in the Twentieth Century

Until the mid-nineteenth century, malaria was endemic in most countries across the globe. Countries that did not have malaria included the Pacific islands east of the longitude of Vanuatu (the Buxton line) (Mendis and others 2009), which have no *Anopheles* mosquitoes; or countries that were too high in elevation or too cold in temperature (map 12.1).

Between 1900 and 1945, only nine countries in Europe eliminated malaria (Feachem, Phillips, and Targett 2009). Sparked by the availability of chloroquine for treatment and dichloro-diphenyl-trichloroethane (DDT) for vector control, the WHO launched the Global Malaria Eradication Program (GMEP) in 1955 to interrupt transmission in all endemic areas outside of Africa (Najera 1999). The program relied on vector control—mainly indoor residual spraying—and systematic detection and treatment of cases. The campaign succeeded in eliminating malaria in 37 of the 143 countries or economies where it was endemic in 1950 (Wernsdorfer and Kouznetzov 1980), including some lower-income areas with tropical climates such as Maldives; Mauritius; Réunion; Taiwan, China; much of the Caribbean; Brunei Darussalam; most of China; Hong Kong SAR, China; Singapore (Feachem and others 2010).[3] In many other countries, the burden of disease and deaths from malaria was greatly reduced. For example, in India, the number of malaria cases declined from an estimated 110 million in 1955 to fewer than 1 million in 1968, and in Sri Lanka, the incidence of malaria declined from an estimated 2.8 million cases in 1946 to just 18 cases in 1966 (Mendis and others 2009).

However, failure to sustain strong funding for the program, particularly in the face of increasing costs due to mounting drug and insecticide resistance, led to the effective end of the GMEP in 1969 (WHO 1969) when the World Health Assembly recommended that countries not yet ready for "eradication" focus on controlling malaria as a first step toward the ultimate goal of getting rid of malaria altogether. Multilateral agencies withdrew their support for malaria programs in favor of general health programs. In the ensuing years, although most countries that had eliminated malaria continued to remain malaria free, the scaling back of control efforts in malarious countries led to a global resurgence of the disease during the 1970s and 1980s and a complete reversal of progress in some countries, such as Sri Lanka and Pakistan (Abeyasinghe and others 2012; Cohen and others 2012).

The experience of the GMEP provides critical lessons for contemporary elimination programs about the need to maintain vigilance and sustain investments during the latter stages of elimination efforts.

Elimination in the Twenty-First Century

The adoption of the Global Malaria Control Strategy in 1992 (WHO 1993) and the launch of the Roll Back Malaria initiative in 1998 (Nabarro and Taylor 1998) stimulated increased interest and financial investment in malaria control. Increased investment in research and development resulted in highly effective malaria control tools—notably, long-lasting insecticide-treated nets (LLINs), rapid diagnostic tests, and artemisinin-based combination therapies (ACTs). The creation of the Global Fund to Fight AIDS, Tuberculosis, and Malaria; the President's Malaria Initiative; and other financing mechanisms allowed for the wide-scale deployment of these new tools. The first Global Malaria Action Plan for a malaria-free world 2008–2015 served as a valuable guide for countries and partners to mobilize resources. Between 2005 and 2014, global investment for malaria control increased from US$960 million to US$2.5 billion annually, leading to dramatic declines in the global malaria burden and rapid shrinking of the malaria map. With the end of the Millennium Development Goals in 2015 and the transition to the era of the Sustainable Development Goals, the malaria community has once again committed to the vision of a malaria-free world.

Table 12.2 summarizes the countries and territories that eliminated malaria between 1900 and 2015.

Currently 35 countries are moving from low-endemic malaria to elimination (Newby and others 2016). These countries fit into one of two categories: (1) countries that have assessed the feasibility of elimination, declared a national evidence-based goal, and launched a malaria elimination strategy; or (2) those that are strongly considering an evidence-based national elimination goal as determined by expert opinion, have made substantial progress in spatially progressive elimination (by eliminating malaria from specific islands or geographic areas), and are greatly reducing malaria nationwide. These 35 countries have elimination goals ranging from 2013 to 2035, with the majority aiming for, and likely to achieve, elimination by 2020 (annex 12A).

Five countries—Argentina, the Kyrgyz Republic, Paraguay, Sri Lanka, and Uzbekistan—recently achieved three consecutive years of zero local transmission. All but Uzbekistan have initiated the WHO process for malaria-free certification. Three other countries have achieved zero local transmission but have not yet sustained it for three consecutive years: Azerbaijan, Costa Rica, and Turkey.

Lessons Learned and Planning for Success

Lessons learned from the GMEP highlight the fact that a single strategy is unlikely to be successful everywhere

Map 12.1 Malaria Transmission Worldwide, 1900, 1990, and 2015

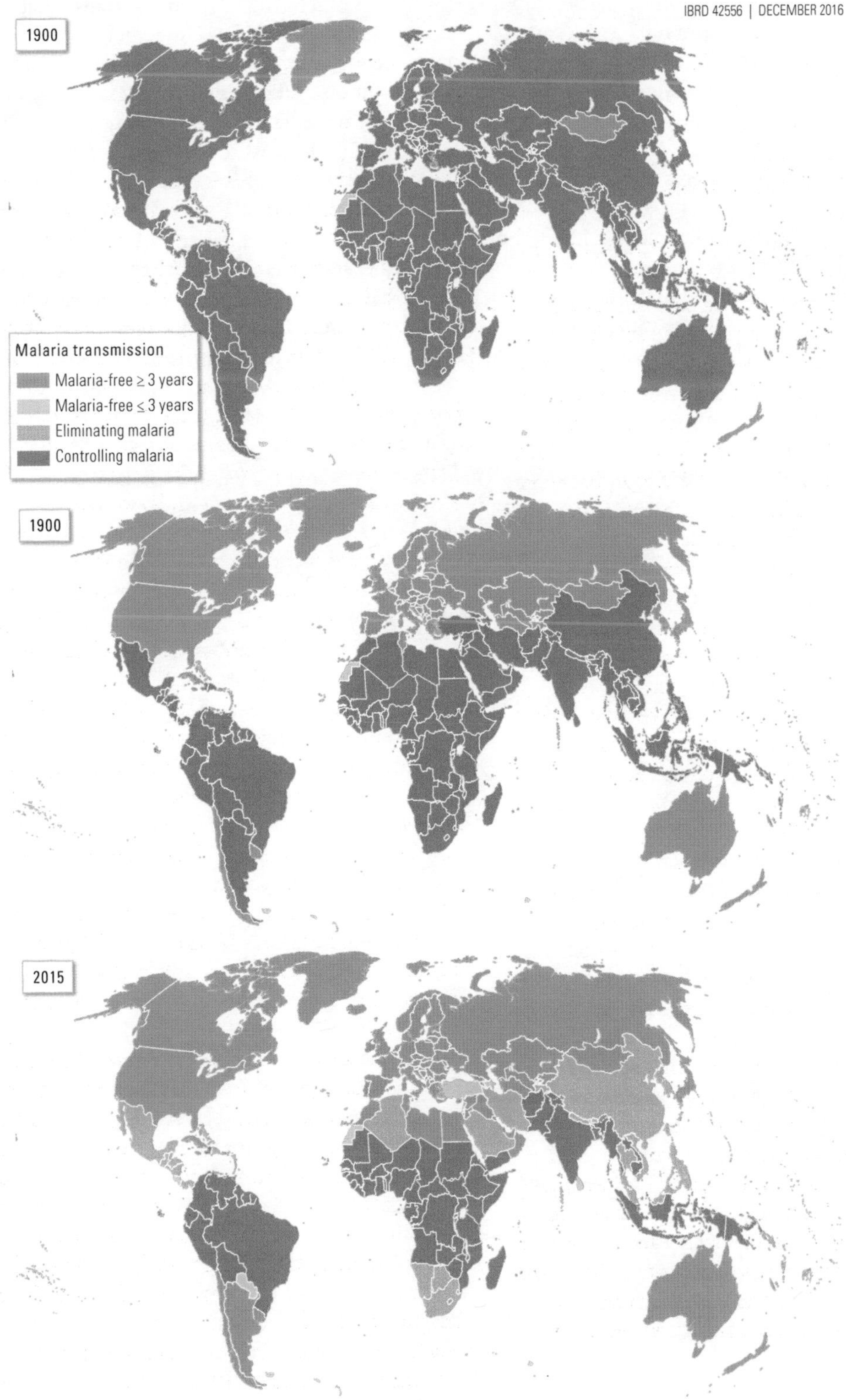

IBRD 42556 | DECEMBER 2016

1900

Malaria transmission
- Malaria-free ≥ 3 years
- Malaria-free ≤ 3 years
- Eliminating malaria
- Controlling malaria

1900

2015

Source: Global Health Group 2016, unpublished data.

given the complexities of malaria transmission systems, and given that a long-term commitment with a flexible strategy that includes community involvement, integration with health systems, and the development of agile surveillance systems with supporting infrastructure is needed (Najera, Gonzalez-Silva, and Alonso 2011). A review conducted at the GMEP's conclusion cited the lack of robust assessments to determine the feasibility of malaria eradication programs (WHO 1968; see box 12.2), including an assessment of the technical and operational evidence and government commitment to sustain funding. Attempting to eliminate malaria before it is feasible to do so can raise expectations, damage the credibility of the public health sector (Moonen and

others 2009), and require prolonged expenditure (Sabot and others 2010). Reducing transmission without sufficiently sustainable interventions to maintain those reductions may also lead to epidemics and resurgence. Out of 49 discontinued programs during GMEP, resurgence was reported in 36 programs following cessation, usually because of an inability to maintain sufficient financial resources (Cohen and others 2012). Countries should assess the technical, operational, and financial feasibility of achieving their goals (discussed further in the section titled Prospects for Malaria Eradication) before embarking on a costly restructuring of their programs (Moonen, Cohen, Tatem, and others 2010; WHO 2014a).

Table 12.2 Number of Countries and Territories That Eliminated Malaria, by Region, 1900–2015

Indicator	Americas and Caribbean	South Asia and East Asia and Pacific	Europe and Central Asia	Middle East and North Africa	Sub-Saharan Africa	Total
Total number of countries	46	39	58	23	45	211
Malaria free						
1900	2	13	3	1	1	20
1900–49	0	0	9	0	0	9
1950–78	23	5	35	4	1	68
1979–90	0	1	2	2	1	6
1991–2015	2	1	9	6	0	18
Total number of malaria-free countries	27	20	58	13	3	121

Box 12.2

Challenges to Elimination: Select Examples

Despite the recent successes in eliminating malaria, challenges remain. The following discussion highlights these challenges and provides examples of some actions taken to overcome them:

• *Lack of sustained funding.* India implemented a widely successful program through DDT spraying that reduced the malaria burden from an estimated 100 million annual cases in the early 1900s to about 100,000 cases in 1965. However,

when U.S. assistance ended, India was unable to maintain its vector control activities. Resurgence over the next decade led to nearly 6 million cases. A key priority identified in India's current *National Framework for Malaria Elimination 2016–2030* is funding its elimination plan with sustained domestic resources and innovative financing models, including cost-sharing partnerships and integration with other government departments (Government of India 2016).[a]

box continues next page

Box 12.2 (continued)

- *Political instability and conflict.* By 1975, malaria was eliminated throughout the former Soviet Union. However, after its collapse in the early 1990s, efforts were disrupted by a lack of funding. Civil wars broke out in several of the former territories, such as Azerbaijan and Tajikistan, contributing to resurgence and reintroduction. Overall strengthening of national health systems and creation of national malaria control programs in 1998 and 1997, respectively, after gaining independence and achieving political stability allowed the malaria situation to be brought under control rapidly in both countries.

- *Weak program vigilance.* Mauritius achieved malaria-free certification in 1973. However, when the program was integrated into preventive health services, the malaria surveillance system was weakened. Vector control activities and screening were reduced, contributing to resurgence associated with an influx of migrant workers. Through the combination of an active surveillance program that screened visitors from malarious areas, an integrated vector management strategy, and a strong health system for detecting and responding to missed cases of imported or introduced malaria, Mauritius has remained malaria free since 1998.

- *Drug and insecticide resistance.* With few replacement options, drug and insecticide resistance is a major threat to elimination. Multidrug resistance emerged and spread rapidly within and outside the Greater Mekong subregion (Cambodia, the Lao People's Democratic Republic, Myanmar, Thailand, Vietnam, and China's Yunnan Province), threatening effective treatment everywhere. In the Greater Mekong subregion, the WHO is leading an urgent, multipartner effort to eliminate *P. falciparum* transmission by 2025.

    At the same time, resistance to pyrethroids, the active ingredients used in insecticide-treated nets, is expanding rapidly in Sub-Saharan Africa. In 2014, 27 countries had reported insecticide resistance (Strode and others 2014). To combat insecticide resistance, the Innovative Vector Control Consortium and UNITAID have recently partnered to improve access to new insecticides for indoor residual spraying in 16 countries across Africa. Their US$65 million Next Generation Indoor Residual Spray Project will work with multiple partners to make alternative insecticides more affordable.

- *Importation.* Four countries in southern Africa— Botswana, Namibia, South Africa, and Swaziland— are seeking to eliminate indigenous transmission within the next five years, but many of their neighbors have much higher malaria burdens. Mobile (moving within a country or coming back from abroad) and migrant (coming from elsewhere into the area) populations are primary sources of imported cases, driving secondary transmission. As a result, the number of cases and deaths between 2012 and 2013 rose in all four countries. Cross-border initiatives are essential to addressing these challenges.

    In September 2015, the Global Fund approved US$17.8 million for the eight countries in southern Africa (Angola, Botswana, Mozambique, Namibia, South Africa, Swaziland, Zambia, and Zimbabwe) termed the "Elimination 8" or "E8," designed to serve as a platform for joint planning, negotiation, and accountability toward a regionally synchronized malaria elimination effort. The main thrust of the E8 regional program is to expand access to early diagnosis and treatment for mobile and underserved populations and to enhance surveillance in the border areas.

- *Weak health systems and program capacity.* The Solomon Islands and Vanuatu have had difficulty maintaining robust malaria elimination programs as a result of weak health systems and limited program capacity to deliver effective diagnosis and treatment to populations in remote areas. Both have experienced periodic spikes in cases that have proved challenging to bring under control.

Sources: Cohen and others 2012; Manguin, Carnevale, and Mouchet 2008; Tatarsky and others 2011.

a. Sustaining domestic and international funding as the malaria burden declines is a serious concern for most malaria-eliminating countries, 15 of which are now upper-middle income and thus no longer eligible for donor funding.

CHALLENGES AND THREATS TO SUCCESS

In contrast to previous attempts at eradication, current efforts explicitly acknowledge that malaria eradication requires a long-term effort incorporating multiple activities and embracing multiple interventions, disciplines, approaches, and organizations. Success will be built largely on a series of effective national and subregional elimination programs, driving global eradication from the bottom up, with countries integrating malaria surveillance, transmission interruption, and treatment programs into their national health systems. Nevertheless, challenges exist.

Eliminating *P. vivax*

In countries where both *P. falciparum* and *P. vivax* are transmitted (mainly outside of Sub-Saharan Africa), as *P. falciparum* malaria declines, the proportion of infections due to *P. vivax* often rises.

P. vivax accounts for more than 70 percent of malaria cases in low-transmission countries (those with fewer than 5,000 cases). Elimination is more difficult for *P. vivax* than for *P. falciparum* because of the presence of persistent liver-stage infections (hypnozoites), the dormant form of the parasite responsible for relapses after months or even years. In addition, gametocytes appear earlier in *P. vivax* than in *P. falciparum*, making onward transmission more likely and more challenging to contain, because eliminating *P. vivax* requires repeated blood-stage treatment or reliable approaches for dealing with the hypnozoite. *P. vivax* therefore persists as the main challenge to malaria elimination, particularly in the late stages.

Despite these difficulties, *P. vivax* has been eliminated in many countries, including China, Mexico, Morocco, Turkey, Turkmenistan, and most recently Sri Lanka, through well-organized deployment of vector control and effective treatment (El Khyari 2001; Shamuradova and others 2012). In 2015, the WHO published a technical brief on the control and elimination of *P. vivax* highlighting the need for international donors and governments to invest in additional measures to control, eliminate, and prevent its reestablishment (WHO 2015c).

Reaching High-Risk Populations

In malaria-eliminating settings, parasite reservoirs are increasingly clustered in high-risk populations or in geographically restricted foci of transmission (Sturrock and others 2013). As transmission decreases, incidence shifts from young children and pregnant women to all age groups, including older children and men. In Asia, this shift is exacerbated by occupational and behavioral risk factors—such as collecting firewood, farming, hunting, or fighting in armed conflict—that put these groups in contact with infective vectors (Bhumiratana and others 2013; Chuquiyauri and others 2012; Hiwat and others 2012; Ngomane and de Jager 2012; Tobgay, Torres, and Na-Bangchang 2011). Adult men often act as parasite reservoirs, with many low-density asymptomatic infections that, if left untreated and carried for long periods, contribute to seasonal transmission outbreaks and epidemics (Harris and others 2010). High-risk populations, such as ethnic or political minorities or mobile tribes, are also often hard to reach. These groups rarely seek treatment and face substantial barriers to accessing health care, including service delivery, and may be missed by disease surveillance systems (Hiwat and others 2012).

As local transmission declines, the threat of secondary transmission from importation becomes increasingly important. The greatest risk for importation is from travel to and from neighboring or well-connected high-endemic areas (Cohen and others 2012; Tao and others 2011; Tatarsky and others 2011). Knowledge of the dynamics of population migration, both domestic and international, and cross-border transmission is crucial for developing appropriate surveillance and response mechanisms. Researchers have used mobile phone data to infer patterns of human movement (Tatem and others 2014; Wesolowski and others 2012) and identify sources and sinks of transmission; some programs are implementing spatial decision support systems (Le Menach and others 2011; Marston and others 2014; Tatem and others 2014).

In some elimination settings, at a given time many malaria infections either are asymptomatic or cause only minor symptoms (Lindblade and others 2013). Passive surveillance misses those individuals who act as parasite reservoirs that are infectious to mosquitoes, causing onward transmission (Sturrock and others 2013). A substantial proportion of infections may also be subpatent or submicroscopic, that is, the density of parasites is lower than the threshold for detection by microscopy or rapid diagnostic tests. These infections account for 20 percent to 50 percent of all transmission occurrences in low-endemic settings (Mosha and others 2013; Okell and others 2012). Draining this asymptomatic reservoir is thus important for elimination. There is, however, growing certitude that curing all symptomatic infections will automatically shrink this asymptomatic reservoir.

Addressing Artemisinin Resistance

Resistance of parasites to artemisinin derivatives, the mainstay of malaria treatment, is a mounting problem. Delayed parasite clearance times following artemisinin monotherapy or ACT were first detected in Western Cambodia in 2007 and soon after along the Thai-Burmese, the Thai-Cambodian, and the Cambodian-Vietnamese borders (Carrara and others 2013; Dondorp and others 2009; Hien and others 2012; Phyo and others 2012). *Plasmodium falciparum* artemisinin resistance is evident in five countries in the Greater Mekong subregion (WHO 2015b), most recently in Myanmar, just 25 kilometers from the Indian border (map 12.2). Delayed parasite clearance times are correlated with some specific mutations (580C→Y, 539R→T, 543I→T, 493Y→H, and 446F→I) in the propeller domain of a Kelch protein gene located on chromosome 13 (PF3D7_1343700) (Ariey and others 2014; Straimer and others 2015). K13 mutant parasites associated with artemisinin resistance are currently prevalent throughout mainland South-East Asia from southern Vietnam to central Myanmar (Ashley and others 2014; Ménard and others 2016; Takala-Harrison and others 2015).

This development has major implications for malaria elimination: First, parasites susceptible to artemisinin will be eliminated earliest, and the remaining parasites in low-transmission areas will be resistant and the hardest to kill (Maude and others 2009). Second, artemisinin-resistant parasites are selected for concomitant resistance to ACT partner drugs, resulting in high late-treatment failure rates, as observed in Cambodia with dihydroartemisinin-piperaquine (Amaratunga and others 2016; Duru and others 2015; Leang and others 2013; Leang and others 2015; Lon and others 2014; Saunders and Lon 2016; Spring and others 2015) and along the Thai-Myanmar border with artesunate-mefloquine (Carrara and others 2013). Although innovative compounds with different modes of action are in development, they will not be ready for deployment before 2020 (Wells and Hooft van Huijsduijnen 2015; Wells, Hooft van Huijsduijnen, and Van Voorhis 2015). Therefore, novel strategies and regimens using available antimalarial drugs need to be further evaluated. These strategies may include drug rotation between different ACTs, extension of the three-day ACT course to five or seven days, and the triple combination of artemisinin derivatives with two partner drugs in a three-day therapy.

Map 12.2 Frequency Distribution of the Wild-Type K13 Allele in Asia and Worldwide

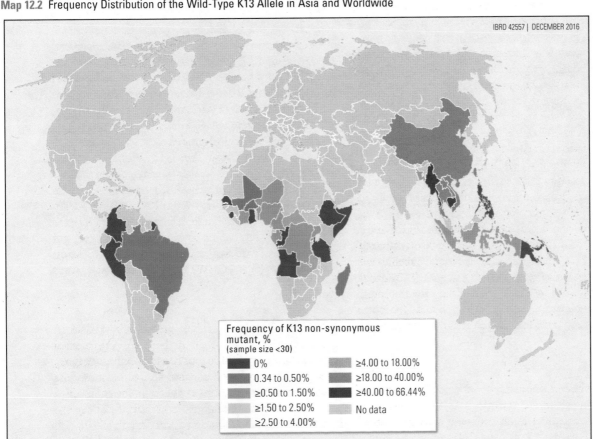

Source: Ménard and others 2016.

The WHO (2012a, 2015d) has labeled multidrug-resistant malaria in the Greater Mekong subregion as a regional public health disaster with the potential for severe global consequences. In March 2015, the WHO concluded that eliminating malaria in this subregion is the only way to extend the lifespan of artemisinin derivatives as an effective treatment and outlined a strategy for elimination by 2030 (WHO 2015d).

The potential spread of artemisinin resistance poses a substantial risk to global health security and economic development. Widespread resistance could increase global malaria mortality by an estimated 25 percent, with an annual economic impact of more than US$0.5 billion (Lubell and others 2014). These increases in mortality and in costs could undermine years of investments, making the case for preventing the spread of resistance even more compelling. Geospatial and temporal mapping of the emergence and spread of parasite resistance allows policy makers to mobilize resources efficiently and to adopt more

efficacious treatment regimens (Ashley and others 2014; Ménard and others 2016; Takala-Harrison and others 2015).

MALARIA ELIMINATION INTERVENTIONS AND STRATEGIES

Elimination and control rely on similar interventions: high-quality case management, vector control, and surveillance. However, while high coverage rates are desirable in control programs, interventions in elimination programs must be highly targeted and tailored, and the right tool needs to be selected according to vector and human behavior (table 12.3). Redistributing resources toward elimination-specific interventions, such as strengthening surveillance systems to identify and investigate transmission foci, may produce economic efficiencies. However, continued investments in enhanced program and managerial capacity are needed.

Table 12.3 Key Differences between Interventions for Malaria Control and Elimination

Indicator	Malaria control	Malaria elimination
Epidemiological setting	High and medium transmission	Low transmission, localized, and seasonal
Population at risk	Entire population(s) considered to be at risk	Populations living in transmission foci, high-risk groups, migrants, and mobile populations
Vector control		
Long-lasting insecticide-treated nets	Widespread coverage	At-risk areas and populations; travelers to endemic areas
Indoor residual spraying	Widespread coverage	At-risk areas and populations
Larval control		
Larviciding	Appropriate in specific circumstances where breeding sites can be identified and regularly targeted; supplement to insecticide-treated nets and indoor residual spraying; may be better suited to urban areas	Appropriate in specific circumstances where breeding sites can be identified and regularly targeted
Environmental management	Not feasible in most high-transmission settings where the specific cases cannot be targeted	Feasible in targeted areas
Case management		
Diagnosis	All suspected cases should undergo diagnostic testing with rapid diagnostic tests or microscopy; goal is to have a confirmed diagnosis; clinical diagnosis not recommended; diagnosis should distinguish between parasite species; quality assurance protocols should be implemented	Rapid diagnostic tests, microscopy, or both with confirmatory diagnostics; quality assurance protocols implemented; highly sensitive molecular diagnostic (polymerase chain reaction, loop-attenuated isothermal amplification) may be considered for quality assurance; diagnostic should distinguish between parasite species
Treatment	*P. falciparum:* ACT	*P. falciparum:* ACT plus single low dose primaquine (0.25mg/kg)

table continues next page

Table 12.3 Key Differences between Interventions for Malaria Control and Elimination (continued)

Indicator	Malaria control	Malaria elimination
	P. vivax:	*P. vivax:*
	Blood-stage infections, chloroquine-sensitive areas: Chloroquine or ACT	Chloroquine-sensitive areas: Chloroquine or ACT for blood-stage infections plus primaquine (0.25–0.5 mg/kg) for 14 days to ensure clearance of liver-stage infection (gametocytes)
	Blood-stage infections, chloroquine-resistant areas: ACT or quinine during pregnancy	
	To prevent relapse: primaquine (0.25–0.5 mg/kg) for 14 days	Prophylaxis for travelers
	G6PD deficiency: primaquine 0.75 mg/kg once a week for 8 weeks	
	Prophylaxis for travelers	
	Intermittent preventive treatment for pregnant women and infants	n.a.
Mass drug administration	Seasonal malaria chemoprevention	High-risk groups in geographic or demographic clusters Trials have used DHA/PIP and artemether lumefantrine accompanied by single low dose of primaquine.
Surveillance		
Passive	Monthly reporting of aggregate, confirmed cases to a central level	Rapid or weekly reporting, ideally electronically, of individual cases classified by origin to a central level
Active	Not feasible because of high number of cases	Includes case investigation, reactive case detection, proactive case detection (which may include mass screening), and foci investigation
Program management		
Program structure	Increased investment in integrated programming in the general health system	Vertical programming investment needed; flexibility needed between vertical and integrated systems
Human resources	Large teams of dedicated staff for specific interventions; specialized skills training	Dedicated managers; basic skills maintained among cadre of integrated staff
High-level commitment	National reduction of disease burden (morbidity, mortality)	National or subnational goals of elimination; may feed into regional elimination goal; regional collaboration encouraged for controlling imported cases

Source: Gosling and others 2014; RBM Partnership 2008; WHO 2012c.
Note: ACT = artemisinin-based combination therapy; DHA/PIP = dihydroartemisinin-piperaquine; mg/kg = milligrams per kilogram; n.a. = not applicable.

Vector Control

Vector control, a key intervention for preventing malaria transmission by *Anopheles* mosquitoes, includes indoor residual spraying with insecticide, use of LLINs, larviciding, and environmental management to remove breeding sites (WHO 2006). The massive gains in malaria control in the past 15 years are attributed largely to the scale-up of these interventions, notably LLINs (Bhatt and others 2015). LLINs have been most widely deployed in Africa, which has the highest proportion of the population at risk of malaria and has malaria vectors most amenable to control with LLINs. The proportion of the population sleeping under LLINs in Sub-Saharan Africa increased from 2 percent in 2000 to an estimated 55 percent in 2015 (WHO 2015e).

However, there are threats to the sustainability of these interventions. First, LLINs must be replaced at least every three years, and maintaining consistent use is difficult, especially when the perceived risks of malaria decline (Hsiang and others 2012). The WHO estimates that as many as 300 million new nets may be required each year to ensure that all populations at risk have access to LLINs in countries where LLINs are the primary vector control strategy (WHO 2015e). Second, mosquitoes are becoming resistant to insecticides: most countries in Sub-Saharan Africa have detected resistance to pyrethroids, the main class of insecticides for indoor residual spraying and LLINs (Ranson and others 2011). While researchers and product development partners are developing and deploying new insecticides, country malaria programs must implement strategies to mitigate resistance by rotating insecticides and using alternative vector control tools (Hemingway and others 2016).

Residual Transmission and New Tools for Control

Despite high coverage of LLINs and indoor residual spraying, transmission persists in many areas because of *residual transmission,* defined as transmission sustained by vectors that evade contact with these two indoor interventions and that rest outdoors and bite humans or animals (Killeen 2014). Residual transmission poses a particular challenge to elimination and eradication and requires efficient tools to target malaria vectors.

Measures such as topical and spatial insect repellants (Ogoma, Moore, and Maia 2012; Wilson and others 2014), insecticide-treated hammocks (Magris and others 2007), and insecticide-treated textile products (Kimani and others 2006; Rowland and others 1999; Thang and others 2009) may be more effective for protecting individuals outdoors (Katz, Miller, and Hebert 2008). Innovative indoor methods such as durable wall liners and insecticidal paint could replace indoor residual spraying, and mosquito-proofed housing (using window screens) and housing modifications (closing eaves and using insecticide-treated eave tubes) may be effective supplemental interventions (Ngufor and others 2014; Oxborough and others 2015; Tusting and others 2015). Space spray and attract-and-kill mechanisms could target adult vectors outdoors, and topical and systemic insecticide treatments for livestock can be effective for vectors that also feed on animals (Matowo and others 2013; Poché and others 2015; Pooda and others 2015; Rowland and others 2001; Shono and others 1991). Researchers are also examining new approaches such as attractive toxic sugar baits and swarm spraying to exploit intrinsic mosquito sugar feeding and mating behaviors, respectively (Müller and others 2010; Qualls and others 2015).

More aggressive approaches to targeting immature stages of vectors, including aerial and ground larviciding and breeding source reduction through environmental management, are the mainstays of mosquito control programs in high-resource settings such as Australia and the United States and can be considered for malaria control and elimination in lower-resource settings (Floore 2006). Research to develop genetic and biological control of adult malaria vectors is ongoing and may be one of the long-term solutions for malaria eradication (Blanford

2012; Helinski and others 2008; Howard and others 2011). As an example, work to develop gene drive systems that either suppress or replace vector populations is proceeding (Hammond and others 2016).

Ultimately, the use of an integrated approach to vector control based on entomological surveillance to understand and target unique vector behaviors and the development of new tools to target different mosquito life stages, habitats, and behaviors are essential for the effective control of malaria vectors (Durnez and Coosemans 2013).

Entomological Surveillance and Integrated Vector Management

Robust entomological surveillance and monitoring is critical to guiding vector control interventions. Information on local vector species, their behaviors, and their susceptibility to insecticides as well as on coverage, usage, quality, and durability of vector control tools is needed to inform decision making and shape local vector control strategies. Entomological expertise was the backbone of successful elimination programs in the past (Mauritius, Sri Lanka, and the United States) and should inform and direct future vector control strategies (Tanner and others 2015).

Evidence-based programming and decision making and entomological intelligence are key components and the foundation of integrated vector management (IVM). IVM is an approach to integrated vector control that optimizes available resources and encourages ecological soundness and sustainability. Other features of the IVM approach include multisectoral collaboration, community and stakeholder engagement, and integrated tools and structures to control disease vectors more effectively and efficiently (WHO 2012b).

Maintenance of Low Transmission

The rate of progress toward elimination and the level of interventions required to interrupt transmission depend on the strength of the health system to detect and respond to cases; the level of investment in malaria programs; and various other factors, including biological determinants, the environment, and the social, demographic, political, and economic realities in the particular country. Two important factors determine the risk of reestablishment of malaria: vulnerability and receptivity. Vulnerability is determined by the importation rate of malaria into malaria-free areas; receptivity is the probabilistic risk of local mosquitos and strategies needed for global becoming infected with malaria parasites and subsequently transmitting the infection to humans. In Canada, Europe, and the United States, vulnerability is high, but receptivity is low. Thousands of imported malaria cases arrive each year, but local mosquitoes rarely become infected and transmit the infection onward. In contrast, the risk of reestablishment is high in countries where both vulnerability and receptivity are high, such as Oman and Sri Lanka, which have previously had high rates of transmission and also receive visitors infected with malaria. In these settings, imported cases must be detected rapidly to prevent onward transmission to the local community.

The success of achieving and sustaining elimination is largely dependent on the receptivity of an area to malaria or "the abundant presence of anopheline vectors and the existence of other ecological and climatic factors favouring malaria transmission" (WHO 2007, 84). Vector control is a key strategy for reducing vectorial capacity—the efficiency of the vector in transmitting malaria based on mosquito density, survival, human biting rates, and parasite incubation period (Brady 2016). In addition, understanding the ecological and climatic factors that cause an increase in receptivity and responding with tailored, effective vector control will be critical to elimination and eradication.

Diagnosis and Treatment

At present, the WHO considers quality-assured microscopy the gold standard for diagnosing clinical malaria. However, microscopy and RDTs are less sensitive at detecting low-density and subpatent infections, which can contribute a sizable proportion of secondary cases and onward transmission. Nucleic acid amplification techniques such as polymerase chain reaction are more sensitive than microscopy and RDTs and are increasingly being used in epidemiological studies; however, they are not yet field friendly and require considerable start-up costs and staff training. Lab-based polymerase chain reaction assays through pooling techniques can provide a high-throughput approach for detecting low parasitemias (Hsiang and others 2012; Imwong and others 2014). However, they do not provide immediate results, and conducting them is capital intensive. Similarly, loop-attenuated isothermal amplification can detect all species of infection at low density and high throughput, is available at a relatively low marginal cost, and involves less lab equipment, but it still requires staff capacity (Surabattula and others 2013). The WHO recommends that the use of highly sensitive diagnostic tools should be considered only in low-transmission settings where malaria diagnostic testing and treatment are already widely used (WHO 2014b).

ACT is the frontline therapy for uncomplicated *P. falciparum* and has been widely deployed globally. The WHO currently recommends five ACT combinations,

and a few others are in the pipeline, although they are not expected to be available in the near future.

Eliminating countries also face significant threat from *P. vivax*. Despite long being regarded as benign, acute cases can have severe consequences. *P. vivax* infections are treated with chloroquine in areas where it remains effective (treatment failure with chloroquine for *P. vivax* malaria has been observed in 24 countries and confirmed in 10 countries) or with ACT where it is not. Primaquine, the only medicine currently available to treat hypnozoites, requires a long course of treatment (7–14 days or even 8 weeks), and poor adherence can lower its efficacy (John and others 2012). Furthermore, the risk of life-threatening hemolysis in patients with glucose-6-phosphate dehydrogenase (G6PD) deficiency, a common blood disorder present in about 8 percent of the population in malaria-endemic areas (Howes and others 2012), limits its use. A reliable point-of-care test to detect G6PD deficiency is not yet widely available (Baird 2015). Tafenoquine, a promising single-dose medicine against hypnozoites and relapses, is likely to be available in 2018 (Eziefula and others 2012; Llanos-Cuentas and others 2014), but it has severe side effects in G6PD-deficient patients. Therefore, solving the problem of G6PD diagnosis and making more sensitive, field-deployable diagnostics more widely available have great potential for eliminating *P. vivax*.

Mass Drug Administration

Interest in the empiric administration of a therapeutic antimalarial regimen to an entire population at the same time, otherwise known as mass drug administration (MDA), has recently been renewed. Proactive MDA has been successfully deployed against several infectious diseases, including lymphatic filariasis, onchocerciasis, schistosomiasis (Hotez 2009), and malaria (Bruce-Chwatt 1959; Newby and others 2015; Poirot and others 2013). The goal is to interrupt transmission by treating all parasitemia in the population. MDA can potentially reduce malaria mortality and morbidity through its direct therapeutic effect on individuals who receive a treatment dose of antimalarials. It also can reduce transmission rates by reducing parasitemia prevalence and interrupting various stages of the parasite lifecycle, and it can inhibit the sporogonic cycle in the mosquito, reducing its vectorial capacity. If every member of a given population were treated by antimalarial MDA, the prevalence of asexual parasites in the population would immediately decline.

However, knowledge gaps remain, especially regarding optimal size of the target population, methods to improve coverage, selection of drug-resistant parasites, and primaquine safety. Malaria elimination programs will likely use MDA in targeted ways to accelerate the impact of vector control and ongoing diagnosis and treatment. Current trials use a full course of dihydroartemisinin-piperaquine or artemether-lumefantrine and a single low dose of primaquine (Eckhoff, Gerardin, and Wenger 2015; White 2013). A key issue is that medicines such as ACTs and primaquine have been registered by drug regulatory authorities based on a clinical indication and a demonstrated risk-benefit ratio in symptomatic patients. The evidence base for its use in asymptomatic or noninfected subjects will need renewed attention. In addition, many medicines considered for MDA are not known to be safe in the first trimester of pregnancy, which presents additional problems if the medicines are deployed in Africa, where pregnancies are rarely reported in the first trimester.

The long-term use of MDA in low-transmission settings faces several challenges. The optimum combination of products and the timing, frequency, and duration of use will depend on the endemicity, seasonality, and rate of importation (Newby and others 2015). For example, MDA, preferably using treatments with a long half-life, is sensible where populations are static and the risk of importation is low (Cohen and others 2013; Gosling and others 2011). To minimize drug pressure on ACTs, a complete course of treatment is needed, and the regimen used for MDA should differ from frontline treatment. At least three "rounds" of administration are needed to affect transmission (Maude and others 2012), requiring adequate resources and political commitment.

The WHO has issued guidelines for implementation of MDA in different epidemiological settings (WHO 2016a). The WHO recommends the use of MDA for the elimination of *P. falciparum* malaria in areas approaching interruption of transmission where there is good access to treatment, effective implementation of vector control and surveillance, and minimal risk of reintroduction of infection, as well as for epidemic control and in exceptional circumstances such as complex emergencies. Like most interventions, MDA is designed to accompany other interventions, including active surveillance and vector control.

Epidemiological Surveillance

Robust and responsive surveillance systems that identify and eliminate transmission foci are critical for the success of malaria control and elimination. (Ohrt and others 2015). An ideal malaria elimination surveillance system swiftly collects and transmits data about individual cases, classified by the origin of infection; integrates it with information on program activities; and analyzes

the information on an ongoing basis to guide rapid response strategies.

In elimination settings, the WHO recommends investigation of all malaria cases to determine if they are imported or the first- (introduced) or second- (indigenous) degree results of local transmission. Passive detection of cases must be complemented with some form of active case detection. Active case detection might take the form of mass screening of high-risk individuals (GHG 2013; Smith Gueye and others 2013; WHO 2013), targeted testing of specific high-risk groups, or household visits seeking febrile or infected individuals. Active case detection typically costs more than passive surveillance; however, the relative cost-effectiveness has not been assessed (Sturrock and others 2013). Less-demanding approaches are being explored, such as surveying children in vaccination clinics, women in antenatal clinics, or children attending school.

Some programs proactively screen at-risk populations on a periodic basis or screen the contacts of index cases for related infections (Moonen, Cohen, Snow, and others 2010; Wickremasinghe and others 2014). For example, migrant laborers and returning military may be screened when entering a malaria-eliminating country, or a village may be screened before and during the malaria season to detect cases before transmission begins. Focal screening and treatment of high-risk communities and mass screening and treatment of whole populations may be used, but these approaches miss infected subjects who are not screened (Hoyer and others 2012) or persons with subpatent infections. In islands or in countries with few entry points, visitors from endemic areas can be screened to prevent reintroduction; however, such screening is difficult to sustain. For any of these methods to be effective, diagnostic tests have to be reliable and able to detect low levels of infection, or presumptive treatment (treatment without a diagnostic test) can be used (WHO 2014b).

Use of serology to measure past exposure could help identify at-risk populations, especially in low-transmission settings where infections are relatively rare (Hsiang and others 2012). Combining serology with conventional diagnostic testing in geospatial models to produce accurate risk maps at finer scales can improve the targeting of interventions (Corran and others 2007; Hsiang, Greenhouse, and Rosenthal 2014; Kelly and others 2012; Lindblade and others 2013; Sissoko and others 2015; Sturrock and others 2014).

Malaria should be made a notifiable disease (required by law to be reported to government authorities) once incidence is low enough that malaria surveillance teams can investigate and report every individual case (Moonen, Cohen, Snow, and others 2010). China and Swaziland have made malaria a notifiable disease to try to increase reporting and encourage more sectors to use the surveillance system (Cohen and others 2013; Hemingway and others 2016). Other approaches to capturing cases that present outside the public sector include restricting access to antimalarials and incorporating private health facilities into the surveillance system (Moonen, Cohen, Tatem, and others 2010).

After elimination has been achieved, passive surveillance at health facilities, including in the informal private sector, is needed to detect and treat introduced infections.

Vaccines

Malaria vaccines include pre-erythrocytic vaccines that aim to prevent blood-stage infection, blood-stage vaccines that clear parasitemia and prevent clinical disease, and transmission-blocking vaccines that prevent infection of mosquitoes and interrupt transmission (Horton 2015). RTS,S, a pre-erythrocytic vaccine to prevent clinical *P. falciparum* in children, is the first malaria vaccine to have completed a Phase 3 clinical trial and was approved by the European Medicines Agency in June 2015. Clinical trials demonstrated a vaccine efficacy for clinical malaria of 28 percent in children ages 5–17 months, but only 18 percent in infants, the target population (RTSS Clinical Trials Partnership 2015) and

36 percent and 26 percent, respectively, after a booster dose administered 18 months after the primary series. In January 2016, the WHO released a position paper recommending further evaluation of the malaria vaccine in a series of pilot implementations before considering wider country-level introduction (WHO 2016b).

An ideal vaccine would be more effective than RTS,S at protecting individuals against infection and at stopping transmission of both *P. falciparum* and *P. vivax* (Nikolaeva, Draper, and Biswas 2015; Tran and others 2015). Such combinations will likely not be commercially available for at least another decade.

Program Management

Reorienting a program from control toward elimination involves retraining staff, developing strong surveillance capacity, building a data architecture that can monitor and direct activities, instituting managerial practices that ensure a capable and ready workforce, and changing program tasks from curative services to preventive community action. These activities involve securing political and financial commitment for at least 6–10 years after elimination has been achieved, as demonstrated by the experiences of Turkmenistan and Sri Lanka, described in boxes 12.3 and 12.4 (Feachem and others 2010).

Box 12.3

Eliminating Malaria in Turkmenistan: Going the Last Mile

Key lessons learned:

- Use regional goals to drive country progress.
- Build and sustain human resource capacity.
- Maintain a dedicated budget even as priorities shift.

Turkmenistan eliminated malaria in the 1950s during the Global Malaria Eradication Program. Over the next four decades, imported cases were detected rapidly through a robust surveillance system. However, population movement after the dissolution of the former Soviet Union in the 1990s led to increases in local vulnerability and imported cases that escaped detection. Two *P. vivax* outbreaks (1998–99 and 2002–03) spurred the Turkmenistan Ministry of Health and Medical Industry to reorient

its program toward eliminating transmission. The goal was reinforced by the 2005 Tashkent Declaration, a commitment to achieving regional elimination by 2015 (WHO 2005). The last local malaria case in Turkmenistan was documented in 2004.

After securing high-level political and financial commitment, a revised elimination strategy was launched in 2007, and malaria-free status was achieved in 2010 (WHO 2010). The prevention-of-reintroduction strategy emphasized intensified surveillance at the Afghanistan border, rapid case investigation, and standardized reporting. Even as health priorities shifted away from malaria, Turkmenistan maintained dedicated funding for human resources, surveillance, monitoring and evaluation, and advocacy.

Sources: Turkmenistan Ministry of Health and Medical Industry, WHO, and University of California, San Francisco, Global Health Group 2012; WHO 2005, 2010.

Eliminating Malaria in Sri Lanka: Flexibility under Fire

Key lessons learned:

- Creativity and flexibility in implementation enabled practical problem solving
- Collaboration and coordination with a range of stakeholders improved program access and efficiency even during conflict.

Malaria has declined substantially in Sri Lanka in the past 15 years, from 264,549 cases in 1999 to no cases in 2012. This success is particularly remarkable given the 1983–2009 civil war, which displaced large populations and disrupted local health services in eight malaria-endemic districts. Malaria cases peaked in 1999, with nearly 60 percent occurring in conflict districts.

The Anti-Malaria Campaign, working with the Ministry of Defense, sent essential supplies by land and sea. Local staff conducted mobile clinics when conditions were safe and, in some areas, enlisted the cooperation of resistance fighters whose troops were affected by malaria. A local nongovernmental organization with extensive presence in the conflict areas was enlisted to distribute long-lasting insecticide-treated nets and provide prevention education through volunteers.

Parasitological and entomological surveillance began in 2008. By the end of the conflict in 2009, the number of cases had dropped to 558 and continued to decline until 2012, when the last indigenous case was recorded. Sri Lanka applied for WHO certification after having achieved three years without autochthonous transmission as of October 2015.

Sources: Sri Lanka Ministry of Health 2014; WHO and GHG 2012.

Despite the need for intensified surveillance and response capabilities during the elimination phase, governments and external donors typically reduce funding as incidence declines (Cohen and others 2012). Program activities are often integrated into the local health system to increase efficiency (Liu and others 2013; Tatarsky and others 2011). A review of managerial experiences with disease elimination suggests that dedicated staff should run and oversee some tasks (vector control and rapid case investigation), while local health teams could oversee others (case management, surveillance, and reporting) (Gosling and others 2014).

Regional collaboration can further reinforce collective goals and foster positive cross-border externalities and financing (Barclay, Smith, and Findeis 2012; Gosling and others 2015; Moonen, Cohen, Snow, and others 2010). For a description of regional initiatives, see annex 12B.

ECONOMICS AND FINANCING OF MALARIA ELIMINATION

One of the strongest arguments against eliminating or eradicating any disease involves the costs associated with finding and treating a decreasing number of cases (Lines, Whitty, and Hanson 2007). These final few cases will likely require an outlay of resources that appear to be disproportional to the marginal return. Maintaining a high level of financial support when transmission has been reduced to low levels remains a challenge. Policy makers have to decide whether to maintain control activities indefinitely or whether to actively pursue elimination.

Articulating the costs of elimination and the relative benefits of investment in elimination versus control will help inform these decisions. Three methods can be used to assess the incremental costs and associated benefits of malaria elimination:

- Analyzing the costs and benefits of an elimination program, summarized using a benefit-cost ratio
- Determining the financial cost savings of an elimination campaign relative to alternative scenarios (for example, control or resurgence costs)
- Evaluating the macroeconomic impact of malaria control and elimination against the economic burden that malaria places on society

Costs and Benefits

Since the conclusion of the GMEP in the 1960s, several studies have reported the costs and consequences of malaria elimination and control, but few benefit-cost

Table 12.4 Benefit-Cost Ratios Associated with Malaria Elimination Programs

Country or setting	Study period	Focus (control or elimination)	Benefit-cost ratio	Source
Global	2010–30	Elimination	6.11	Purdy and others 2013
Greece	1946–49	Elimination	17.09[a]	Livadas and Athanassatos 1963
Iraq	1958–67	Elimination	6.3[a]	Niazi 1969
Paraguay	1965	Elimination	2.6–3.3	Ortiz 1968
India	1953–54,	Control[b]	9.22	Ramaiah 1980
	1976–77	Control	4.14	
Philippines	Unspecified	Control[b]	2.4	Barlow and Grobar 1986
Sri Lanka	1947–55	Control[b]	146.3	Barlow and Grobar 1986
	2014	Prevention of reintroduction	14.3	Shretta and others 2016
West Pakistan	1960	Control[b]	4.9	Barlow and Grobar 1986

a. Calculated based on reported benefits and costs.
b. Although the assessments considered these to be control interventions, they were conducted during the Global Malaria Eradication Program era.

analyses have been conducted (table 12.4). Beyond the direct benefits on health, the main economic benefit considered in the studies is increased labor productivity resulting from reductions in absenteeism. Other benefits include gains from the migration of labor into previously malarial areas and lower treatment costs. Most studies assume a 10-year elimination campaign, and only two (Ortiz 1968; Ramaiah 1980) used empirical data.

All studies showed positive benefit-cost ratios, indicating sizable benefits relative to costs. Benefit-cost ratios ranged from 2.4 in the Philippines (Mills, Lubell, and Hanson 2008), 4.14 and 9.22 for control in India (Prakash and others 2003; Ramaiah 1980), 17.09 for elimination in Greece (Livadas and Athanassatos 1963), to 146.3 and 14.3 for control and prevention of reintroduction, respectively, in Sri Lanka (Barlow and Grobar 1986). Of these countries, Greece continues to report outbreaks as a result of imported cases, despite having eliminated malaria, and Sri Lanka is in the process of seeking WHO malaria-free certification (Samaraweera 2015).

Benefits

Many of the economic benefits associated with malaria interventions extend beyond health to include larger macroeconomic and demographic effects. Investments reduce private out-of-pocket expenditures on prevention and treatment (Chuma, Thiede, and Molyneux 2006; Guiguemdé and Guy 2012), increase productivity, and increase agricultural output via reclaimed land (Gallup and Sachs 2001; Mills, Lubell, and Hanson 2008; Utzinger and others 2002). Lower child mortality may reduce fertility (Aksan and Chakraborty 2013), increase literacy and human capital (Lucas 2010), and eventually increase labor productivity. Domestic and foreign investment may be channeled to formerly malarious areas, contributing to fiscal growth.

Comparing the marginal benefits of control to those of elimination is difficult. Elimination can improve health equity because the last remaining foci of infection are often concentrated within poor or marginalized populations (Feachem, Phillips, and Targett 2009). Prevention of reintroduction also protects against resurgences. Furthermore, eliminating malaria within a single country may confer substantial regional externalities and global public good, fostering collaboration. Elimination may also confer threshold benefits by permanently reducing the receptivity of an area to the reestablishment of local transmission (Chiyaka and others 2013; Sabot and others 2010; Smith Gueye and others 2013), but methods to measure the value of the diminished resurgence risk have yet to be established. Some studies have examined the relationship between elimination and tourism demand in the Dominican Republic, Mauritius, and South Africa, but with little success because of confounding factors such as the overall increase in global travel (Maartens and others 2007; Modrek and others 2012). As benefits become less tangible, they are more difficult to measure. Gaining an understanding of the larger set of economic benefits will require better macroeconomic models that quantify the links between elimination and other outcomes (Mills, Lubell, and Hanson 2008).

Costs and Cost Comparisons

Much of the debate regarding elimination concerns the government's costs of delivering services. However, programmatic costs are only part of the picture—individuals, households, and employers also incur costs for treatment and prevention. From a programmatic perspective, costs increase as control interventions are scaled up, because interventions are often provided for free to increase coverage and to shift costs from individuals to programs.

Analyses of program expenditures are limited to a few studies primarily in Africa and Asia. A systematic literature review identified 21 studies on the costs of malaria elimination with known data sources (Shretta and others 2016). Program expenditures were divided by the cost per capita to account for differences in intended coverage and benchmarked to the first year of data for each country. The reported costs ranged from US$0.18 in Mexico in 1971 (Suarez Torres 1970a) to US$27 in Vanuatu (Kahn and others 2009) (all in 2013 U.S. dollars). Barring a few exceptions, reported costs per capita were generally lowest in East Asia and Pacific and Mexico (Suarez Torres 1970b) and highest in African countries, such as Mauritius (Tatarsky and others 2011), São Tomé and Príncipe (Kahn and others 2009), Swaziland (Kahn and others 2009; Sabot and others 2010), and Zanzibar (Sabot and others 2010). Only Mauritius seeks to prevent reintroduction by screening passengers at ports of entry and using targeted vector control, which may account for the high costs.

Costs for elimination have varied but have generally been low. In the 1960s they were less than US$1 per person-year. Estimates from Nepal and Thailand ranged from US$0.64 to US$1.33 per person-year in the 1980s (in 2006 U.S. dollars) (Mills, Lubell, and Hanson 2008). A retrospective study reports elimination expenditures (including from nongovernmental funders) in Jordan, Lebanon, and Syria of US$0.96, US$0.73, and US$1.69 per person-year, respectively (de Zulueta and Muir 1972). These estimates are lower than those from more recent studies, and it is unclear how directly comparable they are because of variable inputs and the availability of new and more costly tools as well as the rise of new challenges, such as insecticide and artemisinin resistance and human migration (figure 12.1).

Financial Cost Savings of Elimination Relative to Alternative Scenarios

To generate results most relevant to policy, malaria elimination requires a comparison of cost with a counterfactual scenario of malaria control, the costs of which vary substantially with the level of control. Scenarios may encompass a range of alternatives, from a null state of disease without intervention to a state of controlled low-endemic malaria (Sabot and others 2010), to scenarios illustrating the costs of doing "business as usual" with a relatively stable control state punctuated by spikes of epidemics or resurgence when efforts are slowed.

In practice, while an abundance of literature examines the costs of comprehensive control, studies comparing the costs of elimination to the costs of control to determine the financial cost savings of an elimination program relative to control or resurgence are scarce. Nevertheless, once malaria is reduced to a level at which it is no longer a public health threat, reorienting the program from control to elimination is likely to require a significant one-time investment (Sabot and others 2010). One study that projected costs to a 20- to 50-year timeline for Hainan and Jiangsu provinces in China and in Mauritius, Swaziland, and Zanzibar found that elimination is likely to be more costly than control in the short term and is likely to remain more expensive than control at substantially longer timeframes (depending on the inputs of the post-elimination program).

Programs can also be integrated, making disease programs more efficient as well as creating a platform for mobilizing resources, even if malaria is no longer considered a priority. For example, in Singapore, integrating dengue and malaria surveillance facilitated interagency collaboration and reduced transmission of both diseases (Luckhart and others 2010). When transmission decreases and eventually ceases, costs are likely to decline and eventually stabilize as efforts turn to preventing reintroduction primarily through surveillance, vector control, and emergency response. Private out-of-pocket expenditures are also likely to become negligible as the number of cases declines. Two studies (figure 12.2) with empirical data on expenditures over multiple programmatic phases found that expenditures declined when moving from elimination to prevention-of-reintroduction (Abeyasinghe and others 2012; Smith Gueye and others 2014). A study in Sri Lanka estimated the financial cost of prevention of reintroduction activities to cost US$0.37 in 2014 (Shretta and others 2016), less than a quarter of the expenditures in previous years (Abeyasinghe and others 2012).

Elimination should therefore not be justified on the basis of short-term cost savings alone. A focus only on relative cost savings ignores many other factors (for example, population growth, economic development, reductions in malaria in neighboring countries) that could permanently alter the epidemiology of the area, reduce transmission, accelerate the elimination timeline, and decrease costs (Smith and others 2013).

Macroeconomic Gains from Malaria Elimination

Several studies have explored the association between malaria and economic productivity (Audibert, Mathonnat, and Henry 2003; Badiane and Ulimwengu

Figure 12.1 Costs of Malaria Elimination, by Country, Various Years

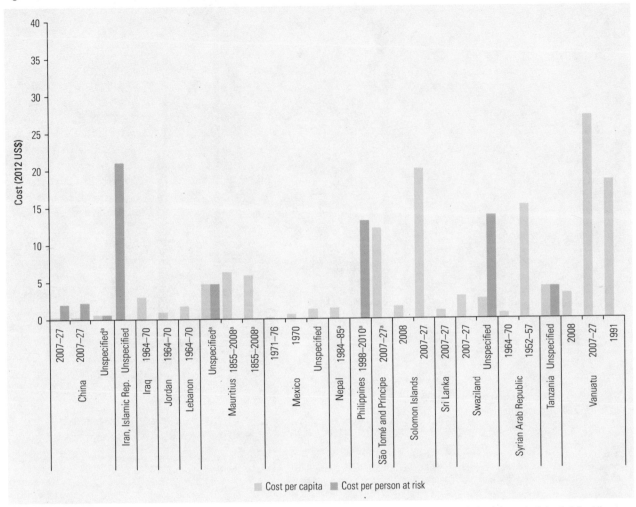

Sources: China: Jackson, Sleigh, and Liu 2002; Sabot and others 2010; the Islamic Republic of Iran: Rezaei-Hemami and others 2013; Iraq, Jordan, Lebanon, the Syrian Arab Republic: de Zulueta and Muir 1972; Mauritius: Tatarsky and others 2011; Mexico: Suarez Torres 1970a, 1970b; Nepal: Kondrashin 1992; the Philippines: Liu and others 2013; São Tomé and Príncipe: Kahn and others 2009; the Solomon Islands: Beaver 2011; Sri Lanka: Abeyasinghe and others 2012; Swaziland and Tanzania (Zanzibar): Sabot and others 2010; Vanuatu (Aneityum Island): Kaneko and others 2000.
a. Multiple costs per capita were reported in the original article; only the highest cost is presented in the figure.

2013; Girardin and others 2004) and can be used to build the investment case. Khan (1966) estimated the cost of decreased efficiency attributable to malaria for Pakistan at more than US$53 million in 1960, while Dua and others (1997) estimated more than US$347,000 in production losses in one Indian industrial complex in 1985. In the United States in 1914, one day lost to malaria was equal to US$119 in production losses (in 2013 U.S. dollars). Many costs of malaria, such as the long-term effects of chronic malaria infection on lowering educational attainment, have yet to be estimated (Chen and others 2016).

Economic modeling using data from Ghana (Asante and Asenso-Okyere 2003), Uganda (Orem and others 2012), and across several countries (Gallup and Sachs 2001; McCarthy, Wolf, and Wu 2000; Okorosobo and others 2011) found that malaria is associated with losses in gross domestic product (GDP) growth. Using cross-country regressions, Gallup and Sachs (2001) demonstrated that countries with intensive malaria lost 1.3 percent of GDP growth per person per year between 1965 and 1990. Similarly, McCarthy, Wolf, and Wu (2000), using WHO morbidity data, estimated that many high-burden countries lost at least 0.25 percent of GDP growth per year from malaria. GDP losses of between 0.41 percent and 8.9 percent or US$4.2 million have been reported in Africa (Okorosobo and others 2011). The annual monetary cost of these losses was as

Figure 12.2 Malaria Program Expenditures in Select Countries, by Phase

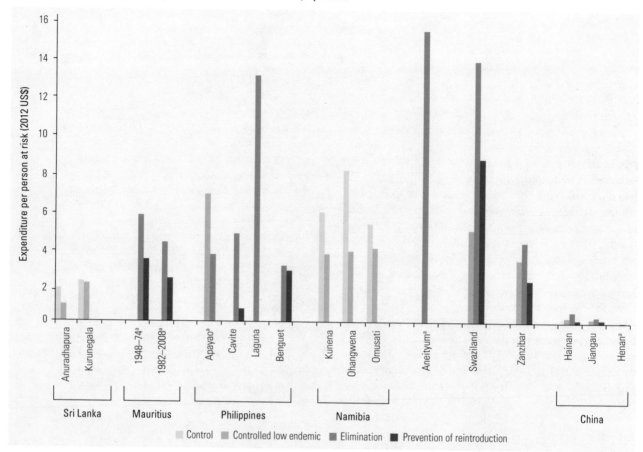

Sources: Sri Lanka: Abeyasinghe and others 2012; Mauritius: Tatarsky and others 2011; the Philippines: Liu and others 2013; Namibia: Smith Gueye and others 2014; Vanuatu (Aneityum Island): Kaneko and others 2000; Swaziland, Zanzibar, and Hainan and Jiangsu, China: Sabot and others 2010; Henan, China: Jackson, Sleigh, and Liu 2002.
a. Multiple costs per capita were reported in the original article; only the highest cost is presented in the figure.

high as US$13.1 million in Mali (Okorosobo and others 2011) to US$10 billion in Nigeria (Okorosobo and others 2011). In Thailand, the economic cost of malaria was valued at US$280 million over five years (Kühner 1971).

Several studies estimated a country's total economic loss by examining expenditures for malaria prevention, control, and treatment, as well as the opportunity cost of caregiving, debility, and premature death. For example, the loss for India was estimated to be between US$856 million and US$1.6 billion a year (Sharma 1996). Losses were estimated to be US$415 million for the Philippines (Barlow and Grobar 1986) and US$133.9 for Pakistan (Khan 1966). However, many of these historical studies are not population based and use secondary sources or expert opinion to calculate the burden of malaria, limiting their contemporary use.

Exposure to malaria in childhood has been associated with lower incomes and a greater likelihood of poverty in adulthood in South America (Barreca 2010;

Bleakley 2003, 2010; Hong 2011). It has also been associated with chronic diseases in later years and an inability to work (Hong 2013), decreased property accumulation in Côte d'Ivoire (Audibert, Mathonnat, and Henry 2003), and decreased spending overall (Somi and others 2009).

The *GTS for Malaria* (WHO 2015a) and Action and Investment to Defeat Malaria (RBM Partnership 2015) use transmission modeling and cost projections to estimate the total cost of reducing the global burden of malaria to 90 percent of its current level by 2030. The estimated cost would be about US$100 billion, resulting in a US$208.6 billion increase in economic output. This figure is in line with a global analysis reporting that malaria reduction and elimination between 2013 and 2035 would produce a benefit whose net present value is US$208.6 billion and a benefit-cost ratio of 6.11 (Purdy and others 2013). Gates and Chambers (2015) estimate that eradication could unlock US$2 trillion in economic benefits at a cost of about US$90 billion to US$120 billion between 2015 and 2040, yielding a return on investment of about 17:1.

Financing and Efficiency

Development assistance for malaria quadrupled between 2007 and 2013. However, the proportion of development assistance directed toward malaria-eliminating countries declined more than 80 percent and continues to decline (figure 12.3). Securing funding for a disease that occurs infrequently is challenging. Malaria-eliminating countries typically have lower disease burdens and are often middle-income countries; therefore, they are a lower priority for donors. The Global Fund to Fight AIDS, Tuberculosis, and Malaria has historically allocated about 7 percent of its portfolio to malaria-eliminating countries but, under its new funding model, now allocates about 5 percent, representing a projected decrease of 31 percent in national funding allocation—a serious shortfall at a time when maintaining national gains and advancing the elimination agenda are essential (GHG 2014; Zelman and others 2016).

Eliminating countries finance about 80 percent of their malaria programs (CEPA 2013), and this spending has been increasing steadily since 2000. However, spending still falls short of the US$8 billion per year needed to reach the 2030 targets (WHO 2015a).

Greater emphasis is being placed on building the capacity of countries to fund their own programs through increased government spending as well as innovative financing mechanisms. Box 12.5 and annex 12C describe some mechanisms that are being implemented or considered and their applicability to malaria programs.

Figure 12.3 Overseas Development Assistance Commitments for Malaria, 2007–13

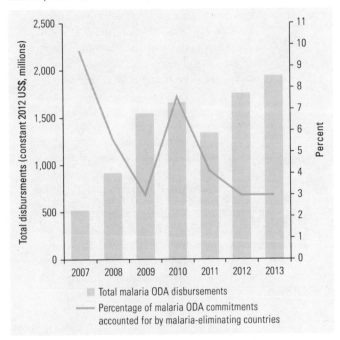

Source: Unpublished data from Global Health Group.
Note: ODA = Overseas Development Assistance.

Box 12.5

New Financing Mechanisms to Support Malaria Elimination

Earmarked travel and airline taxes. Given the direct link between travel and the risk of malaria transmission and resurgence in Zanzibar (Le Menach and others 2011), the local government is considering implementing a tax on airplane tickets. A survey finds that visitors are willing to pay a tourist airline tax (Zanzibar Ministry of Health 2012).

Endowment funds. Endowments are created as a permanent financial asset that generates interest into perpetuity or for as long as the funds are invested. Endowments are ideal for financing long-term activities, such as elimination and prevention of reintroduction, but they require a sizable initial investment (Adams and Victurine 2011). Few endowment funds exist in the health sector, and ministries of health would benefit from further guidance on the investment, finance, and legal aspects of this mechanism.

Cash on delivery. Cash on delivery, wherein countries receive funding once they have achieved a predetermined target (Pertakis and Savedoff 2014), has been included in two regional Global Fund grants to provide incentives to some Sub-Saharan African countries to reduce malaria cases to zero or maintain incidence cases below a certain threshold (CEPA 2013). This model could also be used to encourage countries to achieve elimination or maintain malaria-free status.

Tools for Identifying Efficiency Gains

Receptivity risk maps. Maps of the transmission intensity that would likely occur in the absence of interventions can be generated based on predictions from statistical relationships between disease occurrence and environmental or ecological risk factors, and they can help direct interventions to the places where they will have the greatest impact—and can help withdraw interventions in places where they are not needed.

Elimination scenario planning tool. To guide policy and planning, elimination scenario planning applies a comprehensive framework to assessing the technical, operational, and financial feasibility of moving toward elimination (WHO 2014a).

Self-assessment tool. "Malaria Program Efficiency Analysis Tool" (MPEAT) can help identify programmatic inefficiencies in malaria elimination programs and can help guide policy responses and strategies to achieve better value for money (GHG 2017).

Efficiency in the portfolio and delivery of interventions will ultimately increase cost-effectiveness. More efficient deployment of resources, however, requires a robust surveillance platform in which high-quality data can be collected and analyzed so that measures of response can be adjusted in a timely manner (box 12.6).

PROSPECTS FOR MALARIA ERADICATION

The benefits of achieving and maintaining elimination include a strong public good component—an incremental contribution to global malaria eradication. While many argue that eradication is unlikely given existing tools (Greenwood 2008; Tanner and de Savigny 2008), particularly for high-burden countries in Africa, the global pipeline for new products has never been stronger, supporting the mounting optimism that global eradication is plausible. The technical and operational feasibility of eradication, the operational complexity, and the political appetite need to be considered when assessing the prospects for eradication.

Technical and Operational Feasibility

Determining feasibility involves assessing both the technical challenge—the transmission intensity and the effectiveness of the tools available to reduce it—and the operational capacity to complete the task. Other disease eradication campaigns suggest that eradication has only been considered after many countries have eliminated the disease. For example, when the goal of smallpox eradication was announced, the disease had been eliminated in all high-income countries and was endemic in only 59 low-income countries (Barrett 2007; Henderson 1987). Similarly, the poliomyelitis eradication initiative was launched in 1998 only after polio had been eliminated in the Americas and all high-income countries, with indigenous transmission remaining in 125 countries (Aylward and others 2003; Bart, Foulds, and Patriarca 1996; Khan and Ehreth 2003). Malaria has been eliminated within many local borders, but the overall burden remains high and widespread. As burdens of *P. falciparum* and *P. vivax* decrease, new strategies to diagnose, treat, and interrupt transmission of lesser-studied malaria species, including *P. malariae, ovale,* and *knowlesi,* will be needed. The true burdens of these species are largely unknown because identification by microscopy or rapid diagnostic tests is not reliable (Baltzell and others 2013; Oguike and others 2011; Steenkeste and others 2010).[4]

Eradication of any species only succeeds if the last carrier of disease is isolated, treated, and prevented from causing further transmission. Understanding of transmission between animal and human hosts relevant for zoonotic reservoirs has only recently gained attention. For example, *P. knowlesi,* carried by the macaque monkey, is increasingly being reported in South-East Asia (Baird 2009; Rajahram and others 2012).

Lessons from other campaigns suggest that for eradication to be feasible, a vaccine or an equivalent means is needed to convey long-term protection, as in the case of smallpox (Barrett 2007, 2013).[5] However, no such measure exists for malaria. Even if other measures could be implemented to confer protection similar to a vaccine, many challenges remain. Drug resistance is on the rise, and pyrethroid resistance has emerged after large-scale distribution of LLINs (John, Ephraim, and Andrew 2008; Trape and others 2011; Tulloch and others 2013).

Operational Complexity

The smallpox and polio eradication campaigns implemented eradication-specific management systems that could be integrated into existing health systems (Aylward and others 2003), used performance indicators to measure management processes, trained adequate numbers of staff and gave them incentives to execute eradication-specific tasks, developed a robust surveillance system, and expanded financing to support a stronger health care system (Henderson 1987). Through implementation of the smallpox, polio, and guinea-worm programs, innovative breakthroughs were made in organizing large-scale nationwide campaigns; in devising new methods for approaching and mobilizing communities; in developing effective national surveillance networks and using the data to support better strategies; in fostering effective and relevant research programs to facilitate disease control; and in mobilizing support at international, national, and local levels. Lessons learned from these efforts are critical for malaria eradication. Building programs capable of proactively mitigating the risk of transmission requires careful planning rather than reactive emergency response measures.

Political and Financial Commitment

In 1939, Boyd summarized the prevailing public health point of view and emphasized that "malaria control should not be a campaign—it should be a policy, a long-term program. It cannot be accomplished or maintained by spasmodic effort. It requires the adoption of a practicable program, the reasonable continuity of which will be sustained for a long term of years" (Boyd 1939, 5).

The success of malaria eradication will depend on the ability to mobilize collective action. At a minimum, universal political commitment to achieving an agreed-on target is required, as are financial resources to sustain that commitment. Although countries may be willing to eliminate the disease within their borders, the last country to eliminate it has little incentive to do so on its own, given the larger interests of all other countries (Barrett 2004). The smallpox eradication program nearly failed because of lack of political commitment (Barrett 2007), and the GMEP was cut short for the same reason. Although global attitudes have shifted toward malaria elimination and eradication, political and financial support is needed to bolster the goal of global eradication, should that goal be adopted for malaria.

There are concerns that concentrating resources in areas with lower burdens of disease may divert resources from lower-income countries with higher burdens of disease (Shah 2010); however, progress in low-burden countries is likely to drive global progress toward eradication (Newby and others 2016). In addition, because malaria-free countries stand to benefit from eradication, they have an incentive to offer financial assistance if they are assured that the last countries will work toward elimination (Barrett 2007; Taylor, Cutts, and Taylor 1997).

See box 12.7 for future research priorities.

Box 12.7

Priorities for Research

While achievements made in the past 15 years give reason for optimism, some gaps and priorities for research remain (Tanner and others 2015):

- Detection of emergence and spread of drug-resistant parasites using geospatial and temporal mapping of drug resistance
- Epidemiologically and economically effective and efficient mixes of interventions in different contexts
- Serological tests to detect individual-level recent infections
- Sensitive clinical field diagnostic tests
- New tools for eliminating *P. vivax*, including the identification of asymptomatic hypnozoite carriers
- Effective approaches for mass drug administration in different contexts

- Improved vector control strategies that target residual transmission
- Continued research and development for a combination vaccine
- Appropriate models for private sector and community-based surveillance and response
- Capacity building in program and health system management
- Estimates of costs to identify and secure laboratory specimens of malaria parasites and to stockpile diagnostic, treatment, and vaccine production capabilities in the future
- Advocacy for engagement in the eradication agenda
- Sustained investments in malaria elimination and eradication, including innovative financing mechanisms.

CONCLUSIONS

Despite the absence of a highly efficacious vaccine, many countries around the globe have successfully eliminated malaria and prevented its reintroduction. As malaria elimination progresses in more areas, the case for global eradication is likely to become more compelling. Promising new tools are already in the product development pipeline, including radical treatments, sensitive rapid diagnostic tests, and next-generation vector control methods. Piloting the effective use of these innovations will ensure that they can be scaled up safely and effectively. The introduction of game-changing innovations—including anti-infection or transmission-blocking vaccines and novel mosquito control strategies—could substantially accelerate this next phase. As new technologies and advances occur, the cost of elimination may decline as efficiencies are realized and targeting becomes increasingly focused. Elimination may become progressively easier with new drug therapies, simplified treatment regimens, and more effective vaccines. With smallpox, the targeted nature of surveillance and containment and improved needle technology for vaccinations contributed significantly to the success of the eradicaton campaign.

Malaria eradication calls for a long-term investment that will yield dividends over time. If successful, countries would no longer need to implement prevention measures, thereby reaping an "eradication dividend" and accruing substantial economic benefits for all countries. However, eliminating malaria transmission worldwide will require renewed focus in several areas. Strengthening the human resource capacity of programs is essential. Combating the threat of importation will require collaborative regional surveillance efforts that reach communities and the private sector. In addition, as new tools become available, support will be required for their adoption and rapid uptake to combat the effects of drug and insecticide resistance. These actions all require sustained political and financial commitment to ensure success. While increasing numbers of countries are moving toward financing their own programs, external assistance to the last affected countries will be essential—possibly through a dedicated "last-mile fund"—to ensure that the resources required to complete eradication are available in the final phase.

ANNEXES

The following annexes to this chapter are as follows. They are available at http://www.dcp-3.org/infectiousdiseases.

- Annex 12A. Status and Goals of Elimination Countries, by Region
- Annex 12B. Regional Initiatives to Eliminate Malaria
- Annex 12C. Potential Financing Mechanisms for Malaria Elimination

NOTES

World Bank Income Classifications as of July 2014 are as follows, based on estimates of gross national income (GNI) per capita for 2013:

- Low-income countries (LICs) = US$1,045 or less
- Middle-income countries (MICs) are subdivided:
  (a) lower-middle-income = US$1,046 to US$4,125
  (b) upper-middle-income (UMICs) = US$4,126 to US$12,745
- High-income countries (HICs) = US$12,746 or more.

1. Sri Lanka obtained WHO certification as a malaria-free country in September 2016.
2. Algeria, Belize, Bhutan, Botswana, Cabo Verde, China, Comoros, Costa Rica, Ecuador, El Salvador, the Islamic Republic of Iran, Republic of Korea, Malaysia, Mexico, Nepal, Paraguay, Saudi Arabia, South Africa, Suriname, Swaziland, Timor-Leste.
3. Despite a highly receptive environment in Taiwan, China, intensive spraying combined with improved housing and socioeconomic conditions, better environmental management, and strong case management reduced morbidity to very low levels, and the WHO certified Taiwan, China, as being malaria free in 1965 (Yip 2000).
4. Polymerase chain reaction testing in African and Asian settings shows a higher proportion of both *P. malariae* and *P. ovale* infections than was previously thought (Baltzell and others 2013; Barrett 2007; Oguike and others 2011).
5. In the case of smallpox, there were no long-term carriers, survivors gained lifetime immunity, infections were easily detected, only symptomatic persons could transmit the disease, and vaccination of only 80 percent of the population was necessary to eliminate transmission (Barrett 2007).

REFERENCES

Abeyasinghe, R. R., G. N. Galappaththy, C. Smith Gueye, J. G. Kahn, and R. G. Feachem. 2012. "Malaria Control and Elimination in Sri Lanka: Documenting Progress and Success Factors in a Conflict Setting." *PLoS One* 7 (8): e43162.

Adams, J. S., and R. Victurine. 2011. "Permanent Conservation Trusts: A Study of the Long-Term Benefits of Conservation Endowments." Wildlife Conservation Society, Bronx, NY. http://www.dcnanature.org/wp-content/uploads /fundraising/Permanent-Conservation-Endowments.pdf.

Adjuik, M., T. Smith, S. Clark, J. Todd, A. Garrib, and others. 2006. "Cause-Specific Mortality Rates in Sub-Saharan Africa and Bangladesh." *Bulletin of the World Health Organization* 84 (3): 181–88.

Aksan, A.-M., and S. Chakraborty. 2013. "Childhood Disease and the Precautionary Demand for Children." *Journal of Population Economics* 26 (3): 855–85.

Amaratunga, C., P. Lim, S. Suon, S. Sreng, S. Mao, and others. 2016. "Dihydroartemisinin-Piperaquine Resistance in *Plasmodium falciparum* Malaria in Cambodia: A Multisite Prospective Cohort Study." *The Lancet Infectious Diseases* 16 (3): 357–65.

APLMA (Asia Pacific Leaders Malaria Alliance). 2015. "Asia-Pacific at the Forefront of a Global Movement to Eliminate Malaria." *APLMA Blog*, October 7. http://aplma .org/blog/22/asia-pacific-at-the-forefront-of-a-global -movement-to-eliminate-malaria/.

Ariey, F., B. Witkowski, C. Amaratunga, J. Beghain, A.-C. Langlois, and others. 2014. "A Molecular Marker of Artemisinin-Resistant *Plasmodium falciparum* Malaria." *Nature* 505 (7481): 50–55.

Asante, F. A., and K. Asenso-Okyere. 2003. *Economic Burden of Malaria in Ghana*. Geneva: WHO, African Regional Office.

Ashley, E. A., M. Dhorda, R. M. Fairhurst, C. Amaratunga, P. Lim, and others. 2014. "Spread of Artemisinin Resistance in *Plasmodium falciparum* Malaria." *New England Journal of Medicine* 371: 411–23.

Audibert, M., J. Mathonnat, and M. C. Henry. 2003. "Malaria and Property Accumulation in Rice Production Systems in the Savannah Zone of Côte d'Ivoire." *Tropical Medicine and International Health* 8 (5): 471–83.

Aylward, R. B., A. Acharya, S. England, M. Agocs, and J. Linkins. 2003. "Global Health Goals: Lessons from the Worldwide Effort to Eradicate Poliomyelitis." *The Lancet* 362 (9387): 909–14.

Badiane, O., and J. Ulimwengu. 2013. "Malaria Incidence and Agricultural Efficiency in Uganda." *Agricultural Economics* 44 (1): 15–23.

Baird, J. K. 2009. "Malaria Zoonoses." *Travel Medicine and Infectious Disease* 7 (5): 269–77.

———. 2015. "Point-of-Care G6PD Diagnostics for *Plasmodium vivax* Malaria Is a Clinical and Public Health Urgency." *BMC Medicine* 13 (December): 296.

Baltzell, K. A., D. Shakely, M. Hsiang, J. Kemere, A. S. Ali, and others. 2013. "Short Report: Prevalence of PCR Detectable Malaria Infection among Febrile Patients with a Negative *Plasmodium falciparum* Specific Rapid Diagnostic Test in Zanzibar." *American Journal of Tropical Medicine and Hygiene* 88 (2): 289–91.

Barclay, V., R. Smith, and J. Findeis. 2012. "Surveillance Considerations for Malaria Elimination." *Malaria Journal* 11: 304.

Barlow, R., and L. M. Grobar. 1986. "Costs and Benefits of Controlling Parasitic Diseases." Technical Note PHN 8517, Population, Health, and Nutrition Department, World Bank, Washington, DC.

Barreca, A. I. 2010. "The Long-Term Economic Impact of In Utero and Postnatal Exposure to Malaria." *Journal of Human Resources* 45 (4): 865–92.

Barrett, S. 2004. *Eradication versus Control: The Economics of Global Infectious Disease Policies*. Geneva: WHO.

———. 2007. "The Smallpox Eradication Game." *Public Choice* 130 (1): 179–207.

———. 2013. "Economic Considerations for the Eradication Endgame." *Philosophical Transactions of the Royal Society B: Biological Sciences* 368 (1623): 20120149.

Bart, K. J., J. Foulds, and P. Patriarca. 1996. "Global Eradication of Poliomyelitis: Benefit-Cost Analysis." *Bulletin of the World Health Organization* 74 (1): 35–45.

Bawah, A. A., and F. N. Binka. 2007. "How Many Years of Life Could Be Saved if Malaria Were Eliminated from a Hyperendemic Area of Northern Ghana?" *American Journal of Tropical Medicine & Hygiene* 77 (Suppl 6): 145–52.

Beaver, C. 2011. "Application of a Remoteness Index: Funding Malaria Programs." *International Journal of Geoinformatics* 7 (1).

Bhatt, S., D. J. Weiss, E. Cameron, D. Bisanzio, B. Mappin, and others. 2015. "The Effect of Malaria Control on *Plasmodium falciparum* in Africa between 2000 and 2015." *Nature* 526 (7572): 207–11.

Bhumiratana, A., P. Sorosjinda-Nunthawarasilp, W. Kaewwaen, P. Maneekan, and S. Pimnon. 2013. "Malaria-Associated Rubber Plantations in Thailand." *Travel Medicine and Infectious Disease* 11 (1): 37–50.

Blanford, S., N. E. Jenkins, A. F. Read, and M. B. Thomas. 2012. "Evaluating the Lethal and Pre-Lethal Effects of a Range of Fungi against Adult *Anopheles stephensi* Mosquitoes." *Malaria Journal* 11: 365.

Bleakley, H. 2003. "Disease and Development: Evidence from the American South." *Journal of the European Economic Association* 1 (2–3): 376–86.

———. 2010. "Malaria Eradication in the Americas: A Retrospective Analysis of Childhood Exposure." *American Economic Journal: Applied Economics* 2 (2): 1–45.

Boyd, M. F. 1939. "Malaria: Retrospect and Prospect." *American Journal of Tropical Medicine and Hygiene* 19: 1–6.

Brady, O. 2016. "Vectorial Capacity and Vector Control: Reconsidering Sensitivity to Parameters for Malaria Elimination." *Transactions of the Royal Society of Tropical Medicine and Hygiene* 110 (2): 107–17.

Bruce-Chwatt, L. J. 1959. "Malaria Research and Eradication in the USSR: A Review of Soviet Achievements in the Field of Malariology." *Bulletin of the World Health Organization* 21: 737–72.

Carrara, V., K. Lwin, A. Phyo, E. Ashley, J. Wiladphaingern, and others. 2013. "Malaria Burden and Artemisinin Resistance in the Mobile and Migrant Population on the Thai-Myanmar Border, 1999–2011: An Observational Study." *PLoS One* 10 (3): e1001398.

CEPA (Cambridge Economic and Policy Associates). 2013. "Financing for Malaria Elimination." CEPA and Global Health Group, University of California, San Francisco, CA.

Chen, I., S. E. Clarke, R. Gosling, B. Hamainza, G. Killeen, and others. 2016. "'Asymptomatic' Malaria: A Chronic and Debilitating Infection That Should Be Treated." *PLoS Medicine* 13 (1): e1001942.

Chiyaka, C., A. J. Tatem, J. M. Cohen, P. W. Gething, G. Johnston, and others. 2013. "The Stability of Malaria Elimination." *Science* 339 (6122): 909–10.

Chuma, J. M., M. Thiede, and C. S. Molyneux. 2006. "Rethinking the Economic Costs of Malaria at the Household Level: Evidence from Applying a New Analytical Framework in Rural Kenya." *Malaria Journal* 5: 76.

Chuquiyauri, R., M. Paredes, P. Penataro, S. Torres, S. Marin, and others. 2012. "Socio-Demographics and the Development of Malaria Elimination Strategies in the Low-Transmission Setting." *Acta Tropica* 121 (3): 292–302.

Cohen, J. M., S. Dlamini, J. M. Novotny, D. Kandula, S. Kunene, and others. 2013. "Rapid Case-Based Mapping of Seasonal Malaria Transmission Risk for Strategic Elimination Planning in Swaziland." *Malaria Journal* 12: 61.

Cohen, J. M., B. Moonen, R. W. Snow, and D. L. Smith. 2010. "How Absolute Is Zero? An Evaluation of Historical and Current Definitions of Malaria Elimination." *Malaria Journal* 9: 213.

Cohen, J. M., D. L. Smith, C. Cotter, A. Ward, G. Yamey, and others. 2012. "Malaria Resurgence: A Systematic Review. and Assessment of Its Causes." *Malaria Journal* 11: 122.

Corran, P., P. Coleman, E. Riley, and C. Drakeley. 2007. "Serology: A Robust Indicator of Malaria Transmission Intensity?" *Trends in Parasitology* 23 (12): 575–82.

de Zulueta, J., and D. A. Muir. 1972. "Malaria Eradication in the Near East." *Transactions of the Royal Society of Tropical Medicine and Hygiene* 66 (5): 679–96.

Dhingra, N., P. Jha, V. P. Sharma, A. A. Cohen, R. M. Jotkar, and others. 2010. "Adult and Child Malaria Mortality in India: A Nationally Representative Mortality Survey." *The Lancet* 376 (9754): 1768–74.

Dondorp, A. M., F. Nosten, P. Yi, D. Das, A. P. Phyo, and others. 2009. "Artemisinin Resistance in *Plasmodium falciparum* Malaria." *New England Journal of Medicine* 361: 455–67.

Dua, V., S. Sharma, A. Srivastava, and V. Sharma. 1997. "Bioenvironmental Control of Industrial Malaria at Bharat Heavy Electricals Ltd., Hardwar, India: Results of a Nine-Year Study (1987–95)." *Journal of the American Mosquito Control Association* 13 (3): 278–85.

Durnez, L., and M. Coosemans. 2013. "Residual Transmission of Malaria: An Old Issue for New Approaches." In Anopheles *Mosquitoes: New Insights into Malaria Vectors,* edited by S. Manguin, 671–704. Rijeka: InTech.

Duru, V., N. Khim, R. Leang, S. Kim, A. Domergue, and others. 2015. "*Plasmodium falciparum* Dihydroartemisinin-Piperaquine Failures in Cambodia Are Associated with Mutant K13 Parasites Presenting High Survival Rates in Novel Piperaquine In Vitro Assays: Retrospective and Prospective Investigations." *BMC Medicine* 13: 305.

Eckhoff, P., J. Gerardin, and E. Wenger. 2015. "Mass Campaigns with Antimalarial Drugs: A Modelling Comparison of Artemether-Lumefantrine and DHA-Piperaquine with and without Primaquine as Tools for Malaria Control and Elimination." *BMC Infectious Diseases* 15: 144.

El Khyari, T. 2001. *Malaria Elimination Strategy in Morocco: Plan and Elements of Evaluation.* Unpublished report, Morocco Ministry of Health.

Eziefula, A. C., R. Gosling, J. Hwang, M. S. Hsiang, T. Bousema, and others. 2012. "Rationale for Short Course Primaquine in Africa to Interrupt Malaria Transmission." *Malaria Journal* 11 (1): 360.

Feachem, R. G., A. A. Phillips, J. Hwang, C. Cotter, B. Wielgosz, and others. 2010. "Shrinking the Malaria Map: Progress and Prospects." *The Lancet* 376 (9752): 1566–78.

Feachem, R. G., A. A. Phillips, and G. A. T. Targett, eds. 2009. *Shrinking the Malaria Map: A Prospectus on Malaria Elimination.* San Francisco, CA: Global Health Group, University of California San Francisco.

Filler, S. J., J. R. MacArthur, M. Parise, R. Wirtz, M. J. Eliades, and others. 2006. *Locally Acquired Mosquito-Transmitted Malaria: A Guide for Investigations in the United States.* Atlanta, GA: Centers for Disease Control and Prevention.

Floore, T. G. 2006. "Larval Control Practices: Past and Present." *Journal of the American Mosquito Control Association* 22 (3): 527–33.

Gallup, J. L., and J. D. Sachs. 2001. "The Economic Burden of Malaria." *American Journal of Tropical Medicine and Hygiene* 64 (Suppl 1–2): 85–96.

Gates, B., and R. Chambers. 2015. *From Aspiration to Action: What Will It Take to End Malaria?* Seattle, WA: Bill and Melinda Gates Foundation.

GHG (Global Health Group). 2013. "Malaria-Eliminating Country Briefings." GHG, University of California, San Francisco, CA.

———. 2014. "The Impact of the Global Fund's New Funding Model on the 34 Malaria-Eliminating Countries." GHG, University of California, San Francisco, CA.

———. 2016. "Analysing Technical Efficiency in Malaria Elimination Programs: A Self-Help Toolkit." Unpublished.

Girardin, O., D. Dao, B. G. Koudou, C. Esse, G. Cisse, and others. 2004. "Opportunities and Limiting Factors of Intensive Vegetable Farming in Malaria Endemic Côte d'Ivoire." *Acta Tropica* 89 (2): 109–23.

Gosling, J., P. Case, J. Tulloch, D. Chandramohan, C. Smith Gueye, and others. 2014. "Program Management Issues in Implementation of Elimination Strategies." GHG, University of California, San Francisco, CA.

Gosling, J., P. Case, J. Tulloch, D. Chandramohan, J. Wegbreit, and others. 2015. "Effective Program Management: A Cornerstone of Malaria Elimination." *American Journal of Tropical Medicine and Hygiene* 93 (1): 135–38.

Gosling, R. D., L. Okell, J. Mosha, and D. Chandramohan. 2011. "The Role of Antimalarial Treatment in the Elimination of Malaria." *Clinical Microbiology and Infection* 17 (11): 1617–23.

Government of India, Ministry of Health and Family Welfare. 2016. *National Framework for Malaria Elimination in India (2016–2030).* New Delhi: Directorate of National Vector Borne Disease Control Programme. http://www.searo.who .int/india/publications/national.

Greenwood, B. M. 2008. "Control to Elimination: Implications for Malaria Research." *Trends in Parasitology* 24 (10): 449–54.

Guiguemdé, W. A., and R. K. Guy. 2012. "An All-Purpose Antimalarial Drug Target." *Cell Host and Microbe* 11 (6): 555–57.

Gupta, I., and S. Chowdhury. 2014. "Economic Burden of Malaria in India: The Need for Effective Spending." *South-East Asia Journal of Public Health* 3 (1): 95–102.

Hammond, A., R. Galizi, K. Kyrou, A. Simoni, C. Siniscalchi, and others. 2016. "A CRISPR-Cas9 Gene Drive System

Targeting Female Reproduction in the Malaria Mosquito Vector *Anopheles gambiae*." *Nature Biotechnology* 34 (4): 78–85.

Harris, I., W. W. Sharrock, L. M. Bain, K. A. Gray, A. Bobogare, and others. 2010. "A Large Proportion of Asymptomatic Plasmodium Infections with Low and Sub-Microscopic Parasite Densities in the Low-Transmission Setting of Temotu Province, Solomon Islands: Challenges for Malaria Diagnostics in an Elimination Setting." *Malaria Journal* 9: 254.

Helinski, M., M. Hassan, W. El-Motasim, C. A. Malcolm, B. G. Knols, and B. El-Sayed. 2008. "Towards a Sterile Insect Technique Field Release of *Anopheles arabiensis* Mosquitoes in Sudan: Irradiation, Transportation, and Field Case Experimentation." *Malaria Journal* 7: 65.

Hemingway, J., R. Shretta, T. N. C. Wells, D. Bell, A. A. Djimdé, and others. 2016. "Tools and Strategies for Malaria Control and Elimination: What Do We Need to Achieve a Grand Convergence in Malaria?" *PLoS Biology* 12 (3): e1002380.

Henderson, D. A. 1987. "Principles and Lessons from the Smallpox Eradication Programme." *Bulletin of the World Health Organization* 65 (4): 535–46.

Hien, T. T., N. T. Thuy-Nhien, N. H. Phu, M. F. Boni, N. V. Thanh, and others. 2012. "In Vivo Susceptibility of *Plasmodium falciparum* to Artesunate in Binh Phuoc Province, Vietnam." *Malaria Journal* 11: 355.

Hiwat, H., L. S. Hardjopawiro, W. Takken, and L. Villegas. 2012. "Novel Strategies Lead to Pre-Elimination of Malaria in Previously High-Risk Areas in Suriname, South America." *Malaria Journal* 11: 10.

Hong, S. C. 2011. "Malaria and Economic Productivity: A Longitudinal Analysis of the American Case." *Journal of Economic History* 71 (3): 654–71.

———. 2013. "Malaria: An Early Indicator of Later Disease and Work Level." *Journal of Health Economics* 32 (3): 612–32.

Horton, R. 2015. "Vaccines: A Step Change in Malaria Prevention?" *The Lancet* 385 (9978): 1591.

Hotez, P. J. 2009. "Mass Drug Administration and Integrated Control for the World's High-Prevalence Neglected Tropical Diseases." *Clinical Pharmacology and Therapeutics* 85 (6): 659–64.

Howard, A. F., R. N'Guessan, C. J. Koenraadt, A. Asidi, M. Farenhorst, and others. 2011. "First Report of the Infection of Insecticide-Resistant Malaria Vector Mosquitoes with an Entomopathogenic Fungus under Field Conditions." *Malaria Journal* 10: 24.

Howes, R. E., F. B. Piel, A. P. Patil, O. A. Nyangiri, P. W. Gething, and others. 2012. "G6PD Deficiency Prevalence and Estimates of Affected Populations in Malaria Endemic Countries: A Geostatistical Model-Based Map." *PLoS Medicine* 9 (11): e1001339.

Hoyer, S., S. Nguon, S. Kim, N. Habib, N. Khim, and others. 2012. "Focused Screening and Treatment (FSAT): A PCR-Based Strategy to Detect Malaria Parasite Carriers and Contain Drug-Resistant *P. Falciparum*, Pailin, Cambodia." *PLoS One* 7 (1): e45797.

Hsiang, M. S., B. Greenhouse, and P. J. Rosenthal. 2014. "Point of Care Testing for Malaria Using LAMP, Loop Mediated Isothermal Amplification." *Journal of Infectious Diseases* 210 (8): 1167–69.

Hsiang, M. S., J. Hwang, S. Kunene, C. Drakeley, D. Kandula, and others. 2012. "Surveillance for Malaria Elimination in Swaziland: A National Cross-Sectional Study Using Pooled PCR and Serology." *PLoS One* 7 (1): 329550.

Imwong, M., S. Hanchana, B. Malleret, L. Renia, N. P. Day, and others. 2014. "High-Throughput Ultrasensitive Molecular Techniques for Quantifying Low-Density Malaria Parasitemias." *Journal of Clinical Microbiology* 52 (9): 3303–9.

Jackson, S., A. C. Sleigh, and X. L. Liu. 2002. "Cost of Malaria Control in China: Henan's Consolidation Programme from Community and Government Perspectives." *Bulletin of the World Health Organization* 80 (8): 653–59.

John, G. K., N. M. Douglas, L. von Seidlein, F. Nosten, J. K. Baird, and others. 2012. "Primaquine Radical Cure of *Plasmodium vivax*: A Critical Review of the Literature." *Malaria Journal* 11: 280.

John, R., T. Ephraim, and A. Andrew. 2008. "Reduced Susceptibility to Pyrethroid Insecticide Treated Nets by the Malaria Vector *Anopheles gambiae s. l.* in Western Uganda." *Malaria Journal* 7: 92.

Kahn, J. G., S. Basu, C. Boyle, M. S. Hsiang, D. T. Jamison, and others. 2009. "Financing Elimination." In *Shrinking the Malaria Map: A Prospectus on Malaria Elimination*, edited by R. G. Feachem, A. A. Phillips, and G. A. Targett, 61–80. San Francisco, CA: GHG, University of California.

Kaneko, A., G. Taleo, M. Kalkoa, S. Yamar, T. Kobayakawa, and A. Bjorkman. 2000. "Malaria Eradication on Islands." *The Lancet* 356 (9241): 1560–64.

Katz, T. M., J. H. Miller, and A. A. Hebert. 2008. "Insect Repellents: Historical Perspectives and New Developments." *Journal of the American Academy of Dermatology* 58 (5): 865–71.

Kelly, G. C., M. Tanner, A. Vallely, and A. Clements. 2012. "Malaria Elimination: Moving Forward with Spatial Decision Support Systems." *Trends in Parasitology* 28 (7): 297–304.

Khan, M. J. 1966. "Estimate of Economic Loss due to Malaria in West Pakistan." *Pakistan Journal of Health* 16 (3): 187–93.

Khan, M. M., and J. Ehreth. 2003. "Costs and Benefits of Polio Eradication: A Long-Run Global Perspective." *Vaccine* 21 (7–8): 702–5.

Killeen, G. F. 2014. "Characterizing, Controlling and Eliminating Residual Transmission." *Malaria Journal* 13: 330.

Kimani, E. W., J. M. Vulule, I. W. Kuria, and F. Mugisha. 2006. "Use of Insecticide-Treated Clothes for Personal Protection against Malaria: A Community Trial." *Malaria Journal* 5: 63.

Kondrashin, A. V. 1992. "Malaria in the WHO Southeast Asia Region." *Indian Journal of Malariology* 29 (3): 129–60.

Kühner, A. 1971. "The Impact of Public Health Programs on Economic Development: Report of a Study of Malaria in Thailand." *International Journal of Health Services* 1 (3): 285–92.

Leang, R., A. Barrette, D. M. Bouth, D. Ménard, R. Abdur, and others. 2013. "Efficacy of Dihydroartemisinin-Piperaquine for Treatment of Uncomplicated *Plasmodium falciparum* and *Plasmodium vivax* in Cambodia, 2008 to 2010." *Antimicrobial Agents and Chemotherapy* 57 (2): 818–26.

Leang, R., W. R. Taylor, D. M. Bouth, L. Song, J. Tarning, and others. 2015. "Evidence of *Plasmodium falciparum* Malaria Multidrug Resistance to Artemisinin and Piperaquine in Western Cambodia: Dihydroartemisinin-Piperaquine Open-Label Multicenter Clinical Assessment." Antimicrobial Agents and Chemotherapy 59 (8): 4719–26.

Le Menach, A., A. J. Tatem, J. M. Cohen, S. I. Hay, H. Randell, and others. 2011. "Travel Risk, Malaria Importation, and Malaria Transmission in Zanzibar." *Scientific Reports* 1 (93): 1–7.

Lindblade, K. A., L. Steinhardt, A. Samuels, S. P. Kachur, and L. Slutsker. 2013. "The Silent Threat: Asymptomatic Parasitemia and Malaria Transmission." *Expert Review of Anti-Infective Therapy* 11 (6): 623–39.

Lines, J., C. J. M. Whitty, and K. Hanson. 2007. *Prospects for Eradication and Elimination of Malaria*. London: London School of Hygiene and Tropical Medicine.

Liu, J. X., G. Newby, A. Brackery, C. Smith Gueye, C. J. Candari, and others. 2013. "Determinants of Malaria Program Expenditures during Elimination: Case Study Evidence from Select Provinces in the Philippines." *PLoS One* 8 (9): e73352.

Livadas, G., and D. Athanassatos. 1963. "The Economic Benefits of Malaria Eradication in Greece." *Rivista de Malariologia* 42 (December): 177–87.

Llanos-Cuentas, A., M. V. Lacerda, R. Rueangweerayut, S. Krudsood, S. K. Gupta, and others. 2014. "Tafenoquine Plus Chloroquine for the Treatment and Relapse Prevention of *Plasmodium vivax* Malaria (Detective): A Multicentre, Double-Blind, Randomised, Phase 2b Dose-Selection Study." *The Lancet* 383 (9922): 1049–58.

Lon, C., J. E. Manning, P. Vanachayangkul, M. So, D. Sea, and others. 2014. "Efficacy of Two Versus Three-Day Regimens of Dihydroartemisinin-Piperaquine for Uncomplicated Malaria in Military Personnel in Northern Cambodia: An Open-Label Randomized Trial." *PLoS One* 9 (3): e9313

Lubell, Y., A. Dondorp, P. Guerin, T. Drake, S. Meek, and others. 2014. "Artemisinin Resistance: Modelling the Potential Human and Economic Costs." *Malaria Journal* 13: 452.

Lucas, A. M. 2010. "The Impact of Malaria Eradication on Fertility and Education." Department of Economics, Wellesley College, Wellesley, MA.

Luckhart, S., S. W. Lindsay, A. A. James, and T. W. Scott. 2010. "Reframing Critical Needs in Vector Biology and Management of Vector-Borne Disease." *PLoS Neglected Tropical Diseases* 4 (2): e566.

Maartens, F., B. Sharp, B. Curtis, J. Mthembu, and I. Hatting. 2007. "The Impact of Malaria Control on Perceptions of Tourists and Tourism Operators Concerning Malaria Prevalence in Kwazulu-Natal, 1999/2000 versus 2002/2003." *Journal of Travel Medicine* 14 (2): 96–104.

Magris, M., Y. Rubio-Palis, N. Alexander, B. Ruiz, N. Galván, and others. 2007. "Community-Randomized Trial of Lambdacyalothrin-Treated Hammock Nets for Malaria Control in Yanomami Communities in the Amazon Region of Venezuela." *Tropical Medicine and International Health* 13 (3): 392–402.

Manguin, S., P. Carnevale, and J. Mouchet. 2008. *Biodiversity of Malaria in the World.* London: John Libbey Eurotext.

Marston, L., G. C. Kelly, E. Hale, A. C. Clements, A. Hodge, and others. 2014. "Cost Analysis of the Development and Implementation of a Spatial Decision Support System for Malaria Elimination in Solomon Islands." *Malaria Journal* 13: 325.

Matowo, N. S., J. Moore, S. Mapua, E. P. Madumla, I. R. Moshi, and others. 2013. "Using a New Odour-Baited Device to Explore Options for Luring and Killing Outdoor-Biting Malaria Vectors: A Report on Design and Field Evaluation of the Mosquito Landing Box." *Parasites and Vectors* 6 (May): 137.

Maude, R., W. Pontavornpinyo, S. Saralamba, R. Aguas, S. Yeung, and others. 2009. "The Last Man Standing Is the Most Resistant: Eliminating Artemisinin-Resistant Malaria in Cambodia." *Malaria Journal* 8: 31.

Maude, R. J., D. Socheat, C. Nguon, P. Saroth, P. Dara, and others. 2012. "Optimising Strategies for *Plasmodium falciparum* Malaria Elimination in Cambodia: Primaquine, Mass Drug Administration and Artemisinin Resistance." *PLoS One* 7 (5): e37166.

McCarthy, F. D., H. Wolf, and Y. Wu. 2000. "The Growth Costs of Malaria." NBER Working Paper, National Bureau of Economic Research, Cambridge, MA.

Ménard, D., N. Khim, J. Beghain, A. A. Adegnika, M. Shafiul Alam, and others. 2016. "A Worldwide Map of *Plasmodium falciparum* K13-Propeller Polymorphisms." *New England Journal of Medicine* 374: 2453–64.

Mendis, K., A. Rietveld, M. Warsame, A. Bosman, G. Greenwood, and others. 2009. "From Malaria Control to Eradication: The WHO Perspective." *Tropical Medicine and International Health* 14 (7): 802–9.

Mills, A., Y. Lubell, and K. Hanson. 2008. "Malaria Eradication: The Economic, Financial, and Institutional Challenge." *Malaria Journal* 7 (Suppl 1): S11.

Modrek, S., J. Liu, R. Gosling, and R. G. Feachem. 2012. "The Economic Benefits of Malaria Elimination: Do They Include Increases in Tourism?" *Malaria Journal* 11: 244.

Moonen, B., S. Barrett, J. Tullock, and D. T. Jamison. 2009. "Making the Decision." In *Shrinking the Malaria Map: A Prospectus on Malaria Elimination,* edited by R. G. Feachem, A. A. Phillips, and G. Targett. San Francisco, CA: GHG, University of California.

Moonen, B., J. M. Cohen, R. W. Snow, L. Slutsker, C. Drakeley, and others. 2010. "Operational Strategies to Achieve and Maintain Malaria Elimination." *The Lancet* 376 (9752): 1592–603.

Moonen, B., J. M. Cohen, A. J. Tatem, J. Cohen, S. I. Hay, and others. 2010. "A Framework for Assessing the Feasibility of Malaria Elimination." *Malaria Journal* 9: 322.

Mosha, J. F., H. J. Sturrock, B. Greenhouse, B. Greenwood, C. J. Sutherland, and others. 2013. "Epidemiology of Subpatent *Plasmodium falciparum* Infection: Implications for Detection of Hotspots with Imperfect Diagnostics." *Malaria Journal* 12: 2221.

Müller, G. C., J. C. Beier, S. F. Traore, M. B. Toure, M. M. Traore, and others. 2010. "Successful Field Trial of Attractive Toxic Sugar Bait (ATSB) Plant-Spraying Methods against Malaria Vectors in the *Anopheles gambiae* Complex in Mali, West Africa." *Malaria Journal* 9: 210.

Nabarro, D. N., and E. M. Taylor. 1998. "The Roll Back Malaria Campaign." *Science* 280 (5372): 2062–68.

Najera, J. A. 1999. "Malaria Control Achievements, Problems, and Strategies." WHO and Roll Back Malaria Partnership, Geneva.

Najera, J. A., M. Gonzalez-Silva, and P. L. Alonso. 2011. "Some Lessons for the Future from the Global Malaria Eradication Programme (1955–1969)." *PLoS Medicine* 8 (1): e1000412. doi:10.1371/journal.pmed.1000412.

Newby, G., A. Bennett, E. Larson, C. Cotter, R. Shretta, and others. 2016. "The Path to Eradication: A Progress Report on the Malaria-Eliminating Countries." *The Lancet* 387 (10029): 177–84.

Newby, G., J. Hwang, K. Koita, I. Chen, B. Greenwood, and others. 2015. "Review of Mass Drug Administration for Malaria and Its Operational Challenges." *American Journal of Tropical Medicine and Hygiene* 93 (1): 125–34.

Ngomane, L., and C. de Jager. 2012. "Changes in Malaria Morbidity and Mortality in Mpumalanga Province, South Africa (2001–2009): A Retrospective Study." *Malaria Journal* 11: 19.

Ngufor, C., M. Chouaïbou, E. Tchicaya, B. Loukou, N. Kesse, and others. 2014. "Combining Organophosphate-Treated Wall Linings and Long-Lasting Insecticidal Nets Fails to Provide Additional Control over Long-Lasting Insecticidal Nets Alone against Multiple Insecticide-Resistant *Anopheles gambiae* in Côte d'Ivoire: An Experimental Hut Trial." *Malaria Journal* 13: 396.

Niazi, A. D. 1969. "Approximate Estimates of the Economic Loss Caused by Malaria with Some Estimates of the Benefits of M.E.P." *Bulletin of Endemic Diseases* 11 (1): 28–39.

Nikolaeva, D., S. J. Draper, and S. Biswas. 2015. "Toward the Development of Effective Transmission-Blocking Vaccines for Malaria." *Expert Review of Vaccines* 14 (5): 653–80.

Ogoma, S. B., S. H. Moore, and M. Maia. 2012. "A Systematic Review of Mosquito Coils and Passive Emanators: Defining Recommendations for Spatial Repellency Testing Methodologies." *Parasites and Vectors* 5 (1): 287.

Oguike, M. C., M. Betson, M. Burke, D. Nolder, J. R. Stothard, and others. 2011. "*Plasmodium ovale curtisi* and *Plasmodium ovale wallikeri* Circulate Simultaneously in African Communities." *International Journal of Parasitology* 41 (6): 677–83.

Ohrt, C., K. W. Roberts, H. J. Sturrock, J. Wegbreit, B. Y. Lee, and others. 2015. "Surveillance Systems for Malaria Elimination." GHG, University of California, San Francisco, CA.

Okell, L. C., T. Bousema, J. T. Griffin, A. L. Ouedraogo, A. C. Ghani, and others. 2012. "Factors Determining the Occurrence of Submicroscopic Malaria Infections and Their Relevance for Control." *Nature Communications* 3: 1237.

Okorosobo, T., F. Okorosobo, G. Mwabu, J. N. Orem, and J. M. Kirigia. 2011. "Economic Burden of Malaria in Six Countries of Africa." *European Journal of Business and Management* 3 (6): 42–62.

Orem, J. N., J. M. Kirigia, R. Azairwe, I. Kasirye, and O. Walker. 2012. "Impact of Malaria Morbidity on Gross Domestic Product in Uganda." *International Archives of Medicine* 5: 12.

Ortiz, J. R. 1968. "Estimación del costo de un programa de erradicación del paludismo." *Boletín de la Oficina Sanitaria Panamericana* 64 (2): 110–15.

Oxborough, R. M., J. Kitau, F. W. Mosha, and M. W. Rowland. 2015. "Modified Veranda-Trap Hut for Improved Evaluation of Vector Control Interventions." *Medical and Veterinary Entomology* 29 (4): 371–79.

Pertakis, R., and W. D. Savedoff. 2014. *An Introduction to Cash on Delivery: Aid for Funders.* Washington, DC: Center for Global Development.

Phyo, A. P., S. Nkhoma, K. Stepniewska, E. A. Ashley, S. Nair, and others. 2012. "Emergence of Artemisinin-Resistant Malaria on the Western Border of Thailand: A Longitudinal Study." *The Lancet* 379 (9830): 1960–66.

Poché, R. M., D. Burruss, L. Polyakova, D. M. Poché, and R. B. Garlapati. 2015. "Treatment of Livestock with Systemic Insecticides for Control of *Anopheles arabiensis* in Western Kenya." *Malaria Journal* 14: 351. doi:10.1186/s12936-015-0883-0.

Poirot, E., J. Skarbinski, D. Sinclair, S. P. Kachur, L. Slutsker, and others. 2013. "Mass Drug Administration for Malaria." *Cochrane Database of Systematic Reviews* 12: CD008846.

Pooda, H. S., J. B. Rayaisse, D. F. de Sale Hien, T. Lefèvre, S. R. Yerbanga, and others. 2015. "Administration of Ivermectin to Peridomestic Cattle: A Promising Approach to Target the Residual Transmission of Human Malaria." *Malaria Journal* 14: 496.

Prakash, A., D. R. Bhattacharyya, P. K. Mohapatra, U. Barua, A. Phukan, and others. 2003. "Malaria Control in a Forest Camp in an Oil Exploration Area of Upper Assam." *National Medical Journal of India* 16 (3): 135–38.

Purdy, M., M. Robinson, K. Wei, and D. Rublin. 2013. "The Economic Case for Combating Malaria." *American Journal of Tropical Medicine and Hygiene* 89 (5): 819–23.

Qualls, W., G. Müller, S. Traore, M. M. Traore, K. L. Arheart, and others. 2015. "Indoor Use of Attractive Toxic Sugar Bait (ATSB) to Effectively Control Malaria Vectors in Mali, West Africa." *Malaria Journal* 14: 301.

Rajahram, G. S., B. E. Barber, T. William, J. Menon, N. M. Anstey, and others. 2012. "Deaths Due to *Plasmodium knowlesi* Malaria in Sabah, Malaysia: Association with Reporting as *Plasmodium malariae* and Delayed Parenteral Artesunate." *Malaria Journal* 11: 284.

Ramaiah, T. 1980. *Cost-Benefit Analysis of Malaria Control and Eradication Programme in India.* Ahmedabad: Public Systems Group, Indian Institute of Management.

Ranson, H., R. N'Guessan, J. Lines, N. Moiroux, Z. Nkuni, and others. 2011. "Pyrethroid Resistance in African Anopheline Mosquitoes: What Are the Implications for Malaria Control?" *Trends in Parasitology* 27 (2): 91–98.

Rezaei-Hemami, M., A. Akbari-Sari, A. Raiesi, H. Vatandoost, and R. Majdzadeh. 2013. "Cost Effectiveness of Malaria

Interventions from Preelimination through Elimination: A Study in Iran." *Journal of Arthropod-Borne Diseases* 8 (1): 43.

RBM (Roll Back Malaria) Partnership. 2008. "The Global Malaria Action Plan: For a Malaria-Free World." WHO, Geneva.

———. 2015. *Action and Investment to Defeat Malaria 2016–2030: For a Malaria-Free World*. Geneva: WHO on behalf of the RBM Partnership Secretariat.

Rowland, M., N. Durrani, S. Hewitt, N. Mohammed, M. Bouma, and others. 1999. "Permethrin-Treated Chaddars and Top-Sheets: Appropriate Technology for Protection against Malaria in Afghanistan and Other Complex Emergencies." *Transactions of the Royal Society of Tropical Medicine and Hygiene* 93 (5): 465–72.

Rowland, M., N. Durrani, M. Kenward, N. Mohammed, H. Urahman, and others. 2001. "Control of Malaria in Pakistan by Applying Deltamethrin Insecticide to Cattle: A Community-Randomised Trial." *The Lancet* 357 (9271): 1837–41.

RTSS Clinical Trials Partnership. 2015. "Efficacy and Safety of RTS,S/AS01 Malaria Vaccine with or without a Booster Dose in Infants and Children in Africa: Final Results of a Phase 3, Individually Randomised, Controlled Trial." *The Lancet* 386 (9988): 31–45.

Sabot, O., J. M. Cohen, M. S. Hsiang, J. G. Kahn, S. Basu, and others. 2010. "Costs and Financial Feasibility of Malaria Elimination." *The Lancet* 376 (9752): 1604–15.

Samaraweera, K. 2015. "Sri Lanka Eligible for WHO Malaria-Free Certification." *The Nation*, October 3.

Saunders, D., and C. Lon. 2016. "Combination Therapies for Malaria Are Failing—What Next?" *The Lancet Infectious Diseases* 16 (3): 274–75.

Shah, N. K. 2010. "Assessing Strategy and Equity in the Elimination of Malaria." *PLoS Medicine* 7 (8): e1000312.

Shamuradova, L., S. Alieva, R. Kurdova-Mintcheva, A. Rietveld, R. Cibulskis, and others. 2012. "Achieving Malaria Elimination and Certification in Turkmenistan." *Malaria Journal* 11: O11.

Sharma, V. P. 1996. "Malaria: Cost to India and Future Trends." *Southeast Asian Journal of Tropical Medicine and Public Health* 27 (1): 4–14.

Shono, Y., V. Jean-Francois, Y. Saint Jean, and T. Itoh. 1991. "Field Evaluation of Ultra-Low Volume Applications with a Mixture of D-Allethrin and D-Phenothrin for Control of *Anopheles albimanus* in Haiti." *Journal of the American Mosquito Control Association* 7 (3): 494–95.

Shretta, R., A. L. V. Avancena, and A. Hatefi. 2016. "The Economics of Malaria Control and Elimination: A Systematic Review." *Malaria Journal* 15: 593.

Shretta, R., R. Baral, A. L. Avancena, K. Fox, A. P. Dannoruwa, and others. 2017. "An Investment Case for Preventing the Re-Introduction of Malaria in Sri Lanka." *American Journal of Tropical Medicine & Hygiene* 96 (3): 602–15.

Sissoko, M. S., L. L. Van Den Hoogen, Y. Samake, A. Tapily, A. Z. Diarra, and others. 2015. "Spatial Patterns of *Plasmodium falciparum* Clinical Incidence, Asymptomatic Parasite Carriage and *Anopheles* Density in Two Villages in Mali." *American Journal of Tropical Medicine and Hygiene* 3 (4): 790–97.

Smith, D. L., J. M. Cohen, C. Chiyaka, G. Johnston, P. W. Gething, and others. 2013. "A Sticky Situation: The Unexpected Stability of Malaria Elimination." *Philosophical Transactions of the Royal Society of London, Series B Biological Sciences* 368 (1623): 20120145.

Smith, D. L., S. I. Hay, A. M. Noor, and R. W. Snow. 2009. "Predicting Changing Malaria Risk after Expanded Insecticide-Treated Net Coverage in Africa." *Trends in Parasitology* 25 (11): 511–16.

Smith Gueye, C., M. Gerigk, G. Newby, C. Lourenco, P. Uusiku, and others. 2014. "Namibia's Path toward Malaria Elimination: A Case Study of Malaria Strategies and Costs along the Northern Border." *BMC Public Health* 14: 1190.

Smith Gueye, C., K. C. Sanders, G. N. Galappaththy, C. Rundi, T. Tobgay, and others. 2013. "Active Case Detection for Malaria Elimination: A Survey among Asia Pacific Countries." *Malaria Journal* 12: 358.

Somi, M. F., J. R. Butler, F. Vahid, J. D. Njau, and S. Abdulla. 2009. "Household Responses to Health Risks and Shocks: A Study from Rural Tanzania Raises Some Methodological Issues." *Journal of International Development* 21 (2): 200–11.

Spring, M. D., J. T. Lin, J. E. Manning, J. P. Vanachayangkul, S. Somethy, and others. 2015. "Dihydroartemisinin-Piperaquine Failure Associated with a Triple Mutant Including Kelch13 C580Y in Cambodia: An Observational Cohort Study." *The Lancet Infectious Diseases* 15 (6): 683–91

Sri Lanka Ministry of Health. 2014. "National Malaria Strategic Plan for Elimination and Prevention of Re-Introduction 2014–2018." Anti-Malaria Campaign, Colombo.

Steenkeste, N., W. O. Rogers, L. Okell, I. Jeanne, S. Incardona, and others. 2010. "Sub-Microscopic Malaria Cases and Mixed Malaria Infection in a Remote Area of High Malaria Endemicity in Rattanakiri Province, Cambodia: Implication for Malaria Elimination." *Malaria Journal* 9: 108.

Straimer, J., N. F. Gnadig, B. Witkowski, C. Amaratunga, V. Duru, and others. 2015. "Drug Resistance: K13-Propeller Mutations Confer Artemisinin Resistance in *Plasmodium falciparum* Clinical Isolates." *Science* 347 (6220): 428–31.

Strode, C., S. Donegan, P. Garner, A. A. Enayati, and J. Hemingway. 2014. "The Impact of Pyrethroid Resistance on the Efficacy of Insecticide-Treated Bed Nets against African Anopheline Mosquitoes: Systematic Review and Meta-Analysis." *PLoS Medicine* 11 (3): e1001619. doi:10.1371/journal.pmed.1001619.

Sturrock, H. J., M. S. Hsiang, J. M. Cohen, D. L. Smith, B. Greenhouse, and others. 2013. "Targeting Asymptomatic Malaria Infections: Active Surveillance in Control and Elimination." *PLoS Medicine* 10 (6): e1001467.

Sturrock, H. J., K. Roberts, J. Wegbreit, C. Ohrt, and R. Gosling. 2014. "Effective Responses to Malaria Importation." GHG, University of California, San Francisco, CA.

Suarez Torres, G. 1970a. "El programa de erradicación del paludismo: Plan de seis años." *Salud Pública Mexicana* 12 (6): 751–73.

———. 1970b. "El programa de erradicación del paludismo: Resumen del plan con incremento regional de operaciones en parte de la vertiente del Golfo de México y en la Península de Yucatán." *Salud Pública Mexicana* 12 (6): 745–50.

Surabattula, R., M. P. Vejandla, P. C. Mallepaddi, K. Faulstich, and R. Polavarapu. 2013. "Simple, Rapid, Inexpensive Platform for the Diagnosis of Malaria by Loop Mediated Isothermal Amplification (LAMP)." *Experimental Parasitology* 134 (3): 333–40.

Tanner, M., and D. de Savigny. 2008. "Malaria Eradication Back on the Table." *Bulletin of the World Health Organization* 86 (2): 82.

Tanner, M., B. Greenwood, C. Whitty, E. K. Ansah, R. N. Price, and others. 2015. "Malaria Eradication and Elimination: Views on How to Translate a Vision into Reality." *BMC Medicine* 13: 167.

Takala-Harrison, S., C. G. Jacob, C. Arze, M. P. Cummings, J. C. Silva, and others. 2015. "Independent Emergence of Artemisinin Resistance Mutations among *Plasmodium falciparum* in Southeast Asia." *Journal of Infectious Diseases* 211 (5): 670–79.

Tao, Z. Y., H. Y. Zhou, H. Xia, S. Xu, H. W. Zhu, and others. 2011. "Adaptation of a Visualized Loop-Mediated Isothermal Amplification Technique for Field Detection of *Plasmodium vivax* Infection." *Parasites and Vectors* 4: 115.

Tatarsky, A., S. Aboobakar, J. M. Cohen, N. Gopee, A. Bheecarry, and others. 2011. "Preventing the Reintroduction of Malaria in Mauritius: A Programmatic and Financial Assessment." *PLoS One* 6 (9): e23832.

Tatem, A. J., Z. Huang, C. Narib, U. Kumar, D. Kandula, and others. 2014. "Integrating Rapid Risk Mapping and Mobile Phone Call Record Data for Strategic Malaria Elimination Planning." *Malaria Journal* 13: 52.

Taylor, C. E., F. Cutts, and M. E. Taylor. 1997. "Ethical Dilemmas in Current Planning for Polio Eradication." *American Journal of Public Health* 87 (6): 922–25.

Thang, N. D., A. Erhart, N. Speybroeck, N. X. Xa, N. N. Thanh, and others. 2009. "Long-Lasting Insecticidal Hammocks for Controlling Forest Malaria: A Community-Based Trial in a Rural Area of Central Vietnam." *PLoS One* 4 (10): e7369.

Tobgay, T., C. E. Torres, and K. Na-Bangchang. 2011. "Malaria Prevention and Control in Bhutan: Successes and Challenges." *Acta Tropica* 117 (3): 225–28.

Tran, T. M., S. Portugal, S. J. Draper, and P. D. Crompton. 2015. "Malaria Vaccines: Moving forward after Encouraging First Steps." *Current Tropical Medicine Reports* 2 (1): 1–3.

Trape, J. F., A. Tall, N. Diagne, O. Ndiath, A. B. Ly, and others. 2011. "Malaria Morbidity and Pyrethroid Resistance after the Introduction of Insecticide-Treated Bednets and Artemisinin-Based Combination Therapies: A Longitudinal Study." *The Lancet Infectious Diseases* 11 (12): 925–32.

Tulloch, J., B. David, R. D. Newman, and S. Meek. 2013. "Artemisinin-Resistant Malaria in the Asia-Pacific Region." *The Lancet* 381 (9881): e16–17.

Turkmenistan Ministry of Health and Medical Industry, WHO (World Health Organization), and the University of California, San Francisco, Global Health Group. 2012. "Eliminating Malaria: Case-Study 1: Achieving Elimination in Turkmenistan." Geneva: WHO.

Tusting, L. S., M. M. Ippolito, B. A. Willey, I. Kleinschmidt, G. Dorsey, and others. 2015. "The Evidence for Improving Housing to Reduce Malaria: A Systematic Review and Meta-Analysis." *Malaria Journal* 14 (1): 209.

United Nations. 2015. "African Leaders Call for Elimination of Malaria by 2030." Office of the UN Secretary-General's Special Envoy for Financing the Health Millennium Development Goals and for Malaria. MDG Health Envoy-News, February 3. http://www.mdghealthenvoy.org/african-leaders-call-for-elimination-of-malaria-by-2030/.

Utzinger, J., Y. Tozan, F. Doumani, and B. H. Singer. 2002. "The Economic Payoffs of Integrated Malaria Control in the Zambian Copperbelt between 1930 and 1950." *Tropical Medicine and International Health* 7 (8): 657–77.

Wells, T. N., and R. Hooft van Huijsduijnen. 2015. "Ferroquine: Welcome to the Next Generation of Antimalarials." *The Lancet Infectious Diseases* 15 (12): 1365–66.

Wells, T. N., R. Hooft van Huijsduijnen, and W. C. Van Voorhis. 2015. "Malaria Medicines: A Glass Half Full?" *Nature Reviews Drug Discovery* 14 (6): 424–42.

Wernsdorfer, W. H., and R. L. Kouznetzov. 1980. "Drug Resistant Malaria: Occurrence, Control and Surveillance." *Bulletin of the World Health Organization* 58 (3): 342–352.

Wesolowski, A., N. Eagle, A. J. Tatem, D. L. Smith, A. M. Noor, and others. 2012. "Quantifying the Impact of Human Mobility on Malaria." *Science* 338 (6104): 267–70.

White, N. J. 2013. "Primaquine to Prevent Transmission of *falciparum* Malaria." *The Lancet Infectious Diseases* 13 (2): 175–81.

WHO (World Health Organization). 1968. "WHO Expert Committee on Malaria: Fourteenth Report." WHO Technical Report Series, Geneva: WHO.

———. 1969. "Re-examination of the Global Strategy of Malaria Eradication." Twenty-Second World Health Assembly, Part I. WHO official records number 176, annex 13, 106–26.

———. 1993. "A Global Malaria Control Strategy." WHO, Geneva.

———. 2005. "The Tashkent Declaration: The Move from Malaria Control to Elimination." WHO Regional Office for Europe, Copenhagen.

———. 2006. *Malaria Vector Control and Personal Protection: Report of a WHO Study Group.* WHO Technical Report Series 936. Geneva: WHO.

———. 2007. *Malaria Elimination: A Field Manual for Low and Moderate Endemic Countries.* Geneva: WHO.

———. 2010. "Turkmenistan Certified Malaria-Free." WHO Regional Office for Europe, Copenhagen.

———. 2012a. "Drug Resistance Threatens Malaria Control." WHO, Geneva.

———. 2012b. *Handbook for Integrated Vector Management.* Geneva: WHO.

———. 2012c. "The Role of Larviciding for Malaria Control in Sub-Saharan Africa." WHO, Geneva.

———. 2012d. *World Malaria Report 2012.* Geneva: WHO.

———. 2013. *World Malaria Report 2013.* Geneva: WHO.

———. 2014a. *From Malaria Control to Malaria Elimination: A Manual for Elimination Scenario Planning.* Geneva: WHO.

———. 2014b. "Policy Brief on Malaria Diagnostics in Low-Transmission Settings." WHO, Geneva. http://www.who

.int/malaria/publications/atoz/malaria-diagnosis-low
-transmission-settings-sep2014.pdf.

———. 2015a. *Global Technical Strategy for Malaria 2016–2030.* Geneva: WHO.

———. 2015b. "Q&A on Artemisinin Resistance." WHO, Geneva. http://who.int/malaria/media/artemisinin_resistance_qa/en/.

———. 2015c. "Recommendations on the Role of Mass Drug Administration, Mass Screening and Treatment, and Focal Screening and Treatment for Malaria." WHO, Geneva. http://www.who.int/malaria/publications/atoz/role-of -mda-for-malaria/en/index.html.

———. 2015d. *Strategy for Malaria Elimination in the Greater Mekong Subregion (2015–2030).* Geneva: WHO.

———. 2015e. *World Malaria Report 2015.* Geneva: WHO.

———. 2016a. "Eliminating Malaria." WHO, Geneva. http:// www.who.int/malaria/publications/atoz/eliminating -malaria/en/.

———. 2016b. "Malaria Vaccine." WHO Position Paper, WHO, Geneva.

———. 2016c. *World Malaria Report 2016.* Geneva: WHO.

——— and GHG (Global Health Group). 2012. *Eliminating Malaria: Case-Study 3; Progress towards Elimination in Sri Lanka.* Geneva: WHO.

Wickremasinghe, R., S. D. Fernando, J. Thillekaratne, P. M. Wijeyaratne, and A. R. Wickremasinghe. 2014. "Importance of Active Case Detection in a Malaria Elimination Programme." *Malaria Journal* 13: 186.

Wilson, A. L., V. Chen-Hussey, J. G. Logan, and S. W. Lindsay. 2014. "Are Topical Insect Repellents Effective against Malaria in Endemic Populations? A Systematic Review and Meta-Analysis." *Malaria Journal* 13: 446.

Yip, K. 2000. "Malaria Eradication: The Taiwan Experience." *Parassitologia* 42 (1–2): 117–26.

Zanzibar Ministry of Health. 2012. "Willingness to Pay for a Tourism Levy on International Arrivals." Unpublished.

Zelman, B., M. Melgar, E. Larson, A. Phillips, and R. Shretta. 2016. "Global Fund Financing to the 34 Malaria-Eliminating Countries under the New Funding Model 2014–2017: An Analysis of National Allocations and Regional Grants." *Malaria Journal* 15: 118.

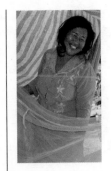

Chapter **13**

Malaria Control

Fabrizio Tediosi, Christian Lengeler, Marcia Castro,
Rima Shretta, Carol Levin, Tim Wells, and Marcel Tanner

INTRODUCTION

This chapter reviews the strategies for malaria control and empirical evidence on the costs and cost-effectiveness of interventions. It then focuses on a systemic approach to malaria control and elimination, describing the relevance of social and environmental determinants, as well as the health system factors that deliver effective coverage of malaria interventions. Finally, it reviews the tools and technologies being developed for malaria control and their potential contribution to integrated strategies. The chapter uses the terminology endorsed by the World Health Organization (WHO) (see WHO 2016a).

Natural History

The ancient Romans knew that draining swamps could prevent disease. Today we know that malaria, a disease that has afflicted humans since the earliest records, is caused by *Plasmodium spp.* parasites, which, following Nobel Prize–winning studies in 1897 by Sir Ronald Ross, are now known to be transmitted by mosquitoes (Smith and others 2012).

Malaria can be transmitted—with varying degrees of efficiency—by more than 100 species of *Anopheles* mosquitoes, a genus that is abundant worldwide. Gametocytes produced in malaria patients represent the *Plasmodium* stage that infects mosquitoes, when female insects (which need the nutrients in vertebrate blood to produce eggs)

take a blood meal. These gametocytes mate and develop in the insect into motile sporozoites. This *Plasmodium* stage enters the host bloodstream during the next blood meal and migrates to the liver, where sporozoites develop into liver schizonts. These rupture and produce merozoites, which invade red blood cells where they reproduce asexually. When large numbers of parasites are produced, patients experience high fever, anemia, and other symptoms. When capillaries in the brain or other vital organs (lungs) are clogged by red blood cells with altered deformabilities, complications may occur (cerebral and complicated or severe malaria), sometimes resulting in death. During the replication phase in red blood cells, gametocytes are produced as well.

There are two main malaria species in humans: *Plasmodium falciparum* and *P. vivax*. *P. falciparum* is restricted to tropical and subtropical (wet season) regions. The disease was called "quotidian fever" because the fever spikes with synchronized release of parasites from infected red blood cells every 24 hours. The parasites' escape to higher latitudes is not prevented by a shortage of mosquitoes but by the fact that their development in the insects is highly dependent on ambient temperatures; in temperate climates, this maturation quickly exceeds the average mosquito life span of two to three weeks. *P. falciparum* is also the deadliest form of malaria, because of its propensity to become severe; 92 percent of all malaria deaths occur in Sub-Saharan Africa. *P. vivax* has found a way to avoid this climate trap

Corresponding author: Fabrizio Tediosi, Department of Epidemiology and Public Health, Swiss Tropical and Public Health Institute, Basel, Switzerland; Fabrizio.tediosi@unibas.ch.

by remaining dormant in the liver, as hypnozoites, for months or even years. This form of malaria, called "tertian fever" for its 48-hour periodicity, was spread globally until the middle of the 20th century and had traveled with Renaissance Europeans to the Americas. In Sub-Saharan Africa, *P. vivax* is not widespread because most of the populations are genetically negative for Duffy, a red blood cell receptor that *P. vivax* requires for infection; these populations are therefore resistant. Other genetic variations, mostly affecting red blood cell function, attest to the enormous effect that malaria has had on human evolution.

Plasmodium parasites are eminently adapted to successfully achieve their host-switching lifecycle. The flip side of this specialization is that the parasite species that infect humans appear unable to choose other mammalian hosts. This lack of a wildlife reservoir is clearly an advantage in malaria eradication campaigns.

Burden of Malaria

P. falciparum and *P. vivax* are by far the most prevalent of the five species of parasites that infect humans; *P. knowlesi*, *P. malariae*, and *P. ovale* are less common. Both *P. falciparum* and *P. vivax* can be found in most regions: *P. falciparum* has the highest rates in Sub-Saharan Africa, where *P. vivax* is almost absent, whereas *P. vivax* is the predominant species in the Asia-Pacific region, accounting for 52 percent of infections (Price and others 2007). *P. falciparum* traditionally accounts for the majority of deaths and cases of severe malaria, but the effect of *P. vivax* on severe morbidity is not to be underestimated.

Despite substantial progress, more than 1 billion people still live in areas where malaria can be transmitted (WHO 2014). In 2015, an estimated 212 million cases of malaria occurred worldwide (uncertainty interval [UI]: 148 million–304 million) (WHO 2016c). Most of the cases in 2015 were in the WHO African Region (90 percent), followed by the WHO South-East Asia Region (7 percent), and the WHO Eastern Mediterranean Region (2 percent). About 4 percent of estimated cases globally are due to *P. vivax*; outside of the African continent, the share of *P. vivax* infections is 41 percent. The incidence rate of malaria is estimated to have decreased globally by 41 percent between 2000 and 2015, and by 21 percent between 2010 and 2015 (WHO 2016c). The massive burden in Sub-Saharan Africa is due mainly to *P. falciparum*. The Democratic Republic of Congo and Nigeria are the most populated states with high levels of transmission. Three Asian countries (India, Indonesia, and Pakistan) account for more than 80 percent of *P. vivax* cases (WHO 2014).

In high-burden countries, the most vulnerable populations at risk for malaria tend to be women and children, marginalized populations, and people living in poverty. Young children are especially at risk, because they have not yet built up the partial immune protection that adults acquire from multiple, sustained infections. Pregnant women are at risk because of placental infection; 30 million women living in Sub-Saharan Africa are at risk, leading to 10,000 maternal deaths (Marchesinig and Crawley 2004) and 200,000 newborn deaths each year (WHO 2016c). Malaria and HIV (human immunodeficiency virus) co-infections occur in more than 3 million cases annually and result in 65,000 additional deaths (Hochman and Kim 2009; WHO 2016c). Economically, countries with a high burden of malaria have growth rates that are 1.3 percent less per person per year than low- and malaria-free countries (Gallup and Sachs 2001; WHO 2016c).

Global Initiatives

Between 1955 and 1970, the WHO led a global initiative to eradicate malaria (Nájera, González-Silva, and Alonso 2011). Control interventions were developed to mitigate the spread of the disease, starting with environmental sanitation measures and the use of dichlorodiphenyl-trichloroethane (DDT) in the 1950s and 1960s. Many countries, particularly in North America and Europe, were successful in substantially reducing malaria transmission and even eliminating it. However, DDT was abandoned because of environmental concerns, and the world's higher-burden countries lacked the necessary tools, approaches, and technical assistance to eliminate the disease without the use of DDT. The goal of worldwide eradication was quietly abandoned around 1970, although many countries continued to drive down the disease rates and some extinguished malaria. The WHO malaria eradication resolution of 1955 was never recalled and formally remains in force.

Decades later, the Millennium Development Goals and Roll Back Malaria (RBM) Partnership's first Global Malaria Action Plan (GMAP) (RBM Partnership 2008) led to a renewed commitment to the fight against malaria and to a substantial increase in resources. In 2007, while considering the then current state of control as well as the potential of new tools and approaches, the global health community at the Malaria Forum of the Bill & Melinda Gates Foundation officially declared that the new goal was elimination (Roberts and Enserink 2007). Consequently, the RBM Partnership (2008) compiled the GMAP, and national control and elimination strategies were established and began being implemented. As a result of this important shift in paradigms and approaches and the insight gained from experiences from 2007 to 2015, the two guiding documents for the control, elimination, and, ultimately, eradication of malaria were developed and approved by the WHO member countries at the World Health Assembly 2015: (1) the WHO's (2015a) *Global Technical Strategy for Malaria 2016–2030 (Global Technical Strategy)* and (2) RBM Partnership's (2015) complementary *Action and Investment to Defeat Malaria 2016–2030 (AIM)*. Both documents were approved by WHO member countries in 2015.

Effective interventions, such as insecticide-treated nets (ITNs) (effective because mosquitoes bite almost exclusively between dusk and dawn) and indoor residual spraying (IRS), have been massively scaled up since 2000, using improved insecticides. The proportion of the population at risk in Sub-Saharan Africa sleeping under an ITN for mosquitoes or being protected by IRS rose from an estimated 37 percent in 2010 (UI: 25–48 percent) to 57 percent in 2015 (UI: 44–70 percent) (WHO 2016c). The proportion of the population at risk protected by IRS declined from a peak of 5.7 percent globally in 2010 to 3.1 percent in 2015 and from 10.5 percent in 2010 to 5.7 percent in 2015 in Sub-Saharan Africa (WHO 2016c).

The recent initiatives were made possible mainly by the massive funding increase that began in 2002, particularly by the Global Fund to Fight AIDS, Tuberculosis and Malaria; the U.S. President's Malaria Initiative; the Bill & Melinda Gates Foundation; and other donors (WHO 2016b). As a direct consequence, global malaria mortality rates were nearly halved between 2000 and 2015 (Bhatt and others 2015). Globally, 95 countries report ongoing transmission, and 6 are working to prevent reintroduction (WHO 2016b).

MALARIA CONTROL INTERVENTIONS: EFFECTIVENESS, COSTS, AND COST-EFFECTIVENESS

Effectiveness and Coverage by Geographical Area

In 2008, the first GMAP helped accelerate progress in malaria control and elimination (RBM Partnership 2008). The strategy included three parts, designed to be executed concurrently (RBM Partnership 2008):

- Aggressive control in the malaria heartland, mainly Sub-Saharan Africa, to lower morbidity and mortality rates
- Progressive elimination from the endemic margins to reduce the number of countries that have to invest in fully developed malaria control programs

- Continued research and development to provide new tools.

Vector Control

The development and validation of ITNs was a major breakthrough for vector control. Further developments led to the long-lasting insecticidal nets (LLINs). Current vector control relies largely on either ITNs, especially LLINs, or IRS. The evidence from randomized controlled trials indicates that ITNs reduce cases by an estimated 50 percent, and they reduce all-cause mortality rates in children under age five years in Sub-Saharan Africa by 18 percent (Lengeler 2004).

The WHO recommends that all persons at risk for malaria be protected by ITNs, using roughly one net per two people. As a result of rapidly increasing coverage, LLINs have been responsible for nearly 70 percent of the gains made against malaria over the past 15 years, in combination with IRS. This progress averted an estimated 663 million malaria cases in Sub-Saharan Africa alone (Bhatt and others 2015), emphasizing the central role of vector control in the control and eradication agenda (malERA Consultative Group on Vector Control 2011).

The use of insecticides—such as DDT, pyrethroids, carbamates, and organophosphates in the form of IRS—has been widely adopted around the world. In Sub-Saharan Africa, only countries in Southern Africa and those supported by the U.S. President's Malaria Initiative are conducting IRS activities on a large scale. Unfortunately, insect resistance to pyrethroids has dramatically increased, including among the three major malaria vectors: *Anopheles gambiae ss, A. arabiensis*, and *A. funestus* (Badolo and others 2012; Mulamba and others 2014). Resistance to the other main classes of insecticides—carbamates, organochlorines, and organophosphates—is on the rise as well (Quinones and others 2015). The rapid spread of resistance of *Anopheles* mosquitoes to pyrethroids is raising the cost of IRS substantially in many endemic areas. Two problems with surveying resistance—beyond weaknesses in the entomological monitoring capabilities in endemic settings—are the great variability in the resistance mechanisms and the lack of suitable markers and related diagnostic tests. All of these factors seriously hamper effective monitoring.

These concerns have been addressed in a five-point Global Plan for Insecticide Resistance Management in malaria vector control proposed by the WHO (Mnzava and others 2015). Anecdotal evidence suggests control failure is occurring in some parts of Sub-Saharan Africa. This was confirmed recently by a five-year study conducted in five countries by the WHO.[1]

Diagnostics

The WHO recommends testing all suspected malaria cases by rapid diagnostic test (RDT) or microscopy. RDTs have substantially changed the individual- and community-based strategies for test-and-treat campaigns, and they form the backbone of the WHO-promoted test-treat-track strategy. The strategy has the following elements:

- Following up and testing every suspected malaria case
- Treating every confirmed case
- Reporting every case in a timely manner through surveillance systems.

The quality of RDTs has continuously improved, mainly because of a quality assurance program developed by the Foundation for Innovative New Diagnostics and the WHO Global Malaria Programme. RDTs for *P. falciparum* are highly sensitive, but their sensitivity for *P. vivax* still needs to be improved. Moreover, health care workers lack the means to diagnose hypnozoite carriers,[2] which prevents the elimination of *P. vivax*. RDT use, primarily to detect *P. falciparum*, has been scaled up substantially in the public sector, especially in Africa; the testing rate in suspected malaria cases increased from 40 percent to 62 percent from 2010 to 2013. However, testing before prescribing or selling treatments remains a challenge in the private sector throughout the world; in Africa, antimalarials are often sold and used without proper diagnosis (WHO 2014).

Treatments

Access to effective treatments—with WHO-recommended artemisinin-based combination therapies (ACTs) for *P. falciparum* and either chloroquine (where still efficacious) or ACTs plus primaquine for *P. vivax*—is crucial to control efforts. Between 2005 and 2013, the number of ACT treatment courses procured by the public and private sectors increased from 11 million to nearly 1 billion (WHO 2016b). During that timeframe, countries in Sub-Saharan Africa reported treating 50–100 percent of malaria patients with an ACT. Using combination treatments in malaria is essential to prevent losing effective medicines to resistance, as happened repeatedly in the 20th century. The Latin American and Eastern Mediterranean regions reported sufficient distribution of medicines to treat all patients in public health facilities.

Surveillance

Finding and detecting cases are important aspects of a national control program aimed at mitigating the spread of malaria. Surveillance becomes critical when a country moves from control to elimination and even more so when it has achieved elimination. Surveillance systems need to be closely interlinked with a public health response, namely, the availability of tailored, integrated response packages that interrupt transmission as soon as the surveillance system identifies existing, new, or reemerging pockets of transmission.

The concept of surveillance and response has evolved. Today, surveillance and response more effectively link the activities to detect, report, analyze, and interpret the public health action through integrated packages tailored to specific settings with the primary goal of stopping transmission and treating all infected people. Surveillance response systems focus on what minimal essential data are required to detect pockets of transmission or reintroduction. This approach differs from the classical monitoring and evaluation based on gathering all possible data, which too often leads to information overflow with no feedback and therefore no rapid effective public health action.

Although surveillance was always a cornerstone of the initial GMAP, the *Global Technical Strategy* (WHO 2015a) now builds on surveillance–response as one of its key determinants for elimination and prevention of reintroduction. Currently, all efforts are made to operationalize surveillance–response approaches fully in national control and elimination programs. In 2015, malaria surveillance systems detected an estimated 19 percent of cases that occur globally (UI: 16–21 percent) (WHO 2016c).

Costs and Cost-Effectiveness of Interventions

The costs and cost-effectiveness of malaria control interventions have been extensively evaluated, and a systematic review found that in most settings, malaria interventions are among the best buys in global health based on relevant indicators (White and others 2011). Nevertheless, the literature varies widely in the range of unit costs and cost-effectiveness ratios; these variations are related to differences in the interventions evaluated, the type of costs included, and, most important, the methodologies adopted.

Annexes 13A and 13B tabulate the costs and cost-effectiveness results of studies published between 2010 and 2015, presented in 2012 US$. The cost of malaria control interventions is relatively low in all countries, but varies widely:

- The financial cost per severe malaria case ranges from US$30 to US$200 in most countries; exceptions were observed in two studies in Myanmar and South Africa, which reported much higher costs.

- Various studies estimated only the costs of medicines for uncomplicated malaria, thereby reporting low estimates. For most of the studies that included outpatient services, the costs varied between US$4.50 and US$30.00; the costs were higher in the few studies that included services in hospital settings. Most of these cost estimates do not include diagnostic tests, which are rather high—on average, around US$10.90 per person—again with wide variations.
- The costs of preventive treatments in infants, children, and pregnant women were low (on average US$2.20, US$2.90, and US$2.60, respectively), except in analyses that estimated the full economic costs, including the noncompliant individuals in all population strata.

Most of the studies available indicate rather low cost-effectiveness ratios. The cost per disability-adjusted life year (DALY) averted for intermittent preventive treatment for children ranged from US$13 to US$35, and that for preventive treatment in pregnant women was estimated to be less than US$2. Slightly higher, but still relatively low costs per DALYs averted were reported for case management (from less than US$2.00 to US$42.00) and for ITNs (US$4.50 to US$128.00). The costs per DALYs averted by IRS were estimated to be higher at US$163 to US$183.

Several studies assessed the costs and potential cost-effectiveness of the RTS,S/AS01 vaccine. This agent, which is well tolerated and partially and temporarily effective, is being considered for implementation in endemic Africa. These studies showed that, conditional on assumptions of price and coverage, adding RTS,S to routine malaria control interventions could be highly cost-effective (Galactionova and others 2017; Penny and others 2016).

The costs of vector control interventions were of the same order of magnitude as treatment costs, with wide variations, depending on the setting and the type of study. The economic costs per person protected with ITNs ranged from US$2.70 to US$9.20 in low-income countries and up to US$19.00 in upper-middle-income countries. These costs approximate those for IRS, whereas the costs for insect larval source management are available only per intervention.

Additionally, recent estimates of the costs and potential returns on investments to achieve the 2030 *Global Technical Strategy* goals indicated a global return of up to 40:1. This return is due to averting 3 billion malaria cases and 10 million malaria deaths and to increasing productivity by US$4 trillion (RBM Partnership 2015; WHO 2015a).

Malaria control and elimination efforts in any setting need to be understood in the context of prevailing ecological and social systems. These highly interconnected systems are the key drivers of control and elimination efforts.

Environmental and Social Determinants of Malaria

Environmental, health, and social system factors affect the transmission intensity, seasonality, and geographical distribution of malaria. Social factors—such as demographics, culture, behavior, migration patterns, socioeconomic characteristics, and politics—affect the uptake and effectiveness of control and elimination interventions. Access to health care and related behavioral factors determine the vulnerability of individuals and communities to infection. These factors have positive and negative effects, which can be modified, depending on how they interact.

In addition, many of these factors adapt to novel local conditions, bringing about additional challenges to control efforts. Relevant examples include the development of drug and insecticide resistance, vector (Awolola and others 2007; Chinery 1984; Sattler and others 2005) and human behavior (Maheu-Giroux and Castro 2013), and environmental changes (Castro and Singer 2011; Gething and others 2010; Hahn and others 2014; Keiser and others 2004; Yamana and Eltahir 2013).

Environmental Determinants
Environmental determinants fall into two broad categories:

- **Natural environment:** temperature, humidity, rainfall, soil quality, elevation and slope, land cover, and hydrography
- **Human environment:** land use, land change, deforestation, housing conditions, infrastructure (water, sanitation, and waste collection), urbanization, development projects (such as roads, railways, dams, irrigation, mining, resettlement projects, and oil pipelines), and disasters abetted by human changes.

Strategies that alter the environmental characteristics associated with malaria transmission were among the earliest interventions tested, validated, and applied at larger scale (Stromquist 1920). Environmental interventions (killing mosquitoes and destroying their habitats) were crucial for the elimination of malaria in European countries and the United States, and they significantly reduced the burden of the disease elsewhere (Boyd 1926; Neiva 1940; Pomeroy 1920). Case studies documenting sustained success include the construction of the Panama Canal (Gorgas 1915), copper mining in Zambia (Utzinger and others 2002; Watson 1953), and rubber production in Malaysia (Watson 1921). A specific, but enlightening, example is the story of malaria-transmitting *Anopheles* mosquitoes breeding in the small water bodies created in *Bromelia* plants. Bromeliads are epiphytes (plants that grow on trees, mainly in tropical South America) that typically provide space for small reservoirs of water in which frogs and insects, including *Anopheles* species, may breed. Malaria was eliminated from southern Brazil by the removal of bromeliads from urban areas and the introduction of eucalyptus trees on which bromeliads do not grow (Deane 1988; Pinotti 1951).

Housing improvements, first introduced by the Italian hygienist Angelo Celli at the end of the 19th century, were a crucial intervention in Europe and the United States; the screening of barracks during recent wars was a successful intervention (Carter and Mendis 2002; Lindsay, Emerson, and Charlwood 2002). The use of intermittent irrigation strategies for control of malaria around rice paddies continues to be an important strategy in China (Baolin 1988; Singer and Castro 2011). The numerous historical examples of the successful use of environmental management show the crucial nature of designing integrated interventions and tailoring them to given socioecological settings (Keiser, Singer, and Utzinger 2005; Konradsen and others 2004).

Environmental management often has a low priority in endemic areas (Lindsay, Emerson, and Charlwood 2002), although the opportunities for its adoption are excellent. Housing improvements—such as screening doors, windows, and eaves; closing eaves; installing ceilings; improving roofs; sealing cracks in walls; using higher-quality building materials; creating new housing designs; and installing eave tubes (Knudsen and von Seidlein 2014; Lindsay, Emerson, and Charlwood 2002; Ogoma and others 2009; Tusting and others 2015)—are applicable in many endemic areas, especially those experiencing rapid economic development. Construction and maintenance of drainage systems in expanding urban areas that often lack proper infrastructure will improve mosquito control effectiveness, as well as the control of other vector-borne diseases, such as dengue and lymphatic filariasis.

Social Determinants

Key social determinants for local populations include age, economic activity, education, cultural beliefs, population density, migratory patterns, personal behavior, and knowledge about malaria. Behavior particularly affects the effectiveness of vector control (for example, ITN and LLIN use). Behavior change communication (BCC) strategies are often used to promote malaria prevention and treatment behaviors (RBM Partnership 2012) and can substantially increase the return on investment in malaria control (Koenker and others 2014). Although many malaria-endemic countries have a BCC strategy, a gap in the literature exists with respect to the effectiveness of BCC in promoting behavior change and ultimately reducing malaria transmission. The design, implementation, and evaluation of locally adapted BCC strategies, founded in solid behavior change theory, are especially important in promoting effective and sustainable changes, but they remain challenging for many national malaria control programs.

Health System Factors for Effective Coverage of Malaria Control Interventions

The scale-up of malaria interventions during the past decade highlights the importance of strong health systems (Stratton and others 2008). Effective treatment provides individual benefits by curing infection and preventing progression to severe disease stages. It also provides community-level benefits by reducing the infectious reservoir and averting the emergence and spread of drug resistance (WHO 2012).

Ensuring effective coverage of malaria treatment is particularly problematic and requires simultaneously addressing both supply-side and demand-side challenges in health systems that are often weak. Efficacious therapy is available, but many patients with malaria do not have access to treatment or delay seeking treatment. Providers do not always comply with treatment guidelines, so patients do not necessarily receive the correct regimen or instructions, which may lead to adherence problems. Even when the correct regimen is communicated and administered, some patients will not adhere to it. Others may be treated with counterfeit or otherwise substandard medication. All of these factors lead to treatment failures and potentially to the development and spread of drug resistance.

Recent analyses of the effectiveness of malaria service delivery have assessed supply-side determinants, including diagnosis, staff training, and availability of antimalarial medicines at the health facility level (Berendes and others 2011; McPake and others 1999; Mikkelsen-Lopez and others 2013; Obrist and others 2007; Rao, Schellenberg, and Ghani 2013a, 2013b; Zurovac and others 2008). Other studies assessed patient awareness and perception of illness, affordability of treatment, and adherence to the treatment regimen (Littrell and others 2013; Mumba and others 2003; Webster and others 2014). These studies estimated the proportion of fever or malaria cases treated in the public sector according to the national guidelines, with estimates generated for the region as a whole (Berendes and others 2011; Zurovac and Rowe 2006) and for given countries (Alonso and others 2011; Khatib and others 2013; Littrell and others 2013; Mikkelsen-Lopez and others 2013; Sumba and others 2008; Webster and others 2014). Consistently, these evaluations revealed substantial inefficiencies in malaria-related service delivery.

A recent comprehensive analysis of available data on effective coverage of malaria case management for 43 countries in Sub-Saharan Africa (Galactionova and others 2015) found considerable international variations. Effective national coverage for malaria case management was found to range from 8 percent to 72 percent in the Sub-Saharan Africa region, for a variety of reasons. Interestingly, the correlation between effective coverage and economic development was weak, indicating that resource constraints play only a limited role. Such patterns of intercountry variation suggest that many system failures are amenable to change. Priority areas for malaria control and eradication policies include identifying the reasons for poor health system performance, intervening to address them, and implementing the respective strategies in program activities.

NEW TOOLS AND TECHNOLOGIES FOR MALARIA CONTROL

Therapies

ACTs have become the mainstay for the case management of uncomplicated malaria over the past decade, and child-friendly versions of most of these agents have become available (Bassat and others 2015). For cases of severe and life-threatening malaria, where oral treatments are not an option, the key data from two pivotal trials in Asia (Dondorp and others 2005) and Africa (Dondorp and others 2013) demonstrated the superiority of injected artesunate over injected quinine. However, the adoption and scale-up of injectable artesunate have been slow. The challenge is to ensure the wide availability of injectable artesunate at affordable prices. The reasons for using parenteral artesunate rather than oral ACTs are, first, that patients are often unconscious and, second, that reduction of the parasitemia quickly and profoundly saves lives in these emergency situations. Where injectable artesunate is not available, particularly where medical facilities are lacking, rectal artesunate suppositories are recommended by the World Health Organization to achieve a similar rapid reduction in parasitemia as occurs with injected artesunate (WHO 2015b). This recommendation is supported, particularly in children, by a large multisite (including Africa and Asia) randomized trial (Gomes and others 2009). Substantial potential exists to improve access to these treatments for the initial treatment of severe malaria.

New agents are needed for the treatment and prevention of all types of malaria, mainly because of the emergence and spread of drug resistance. Numerous new chemical series and compounds have been identified over the past decade (Wells, van Huijsduijnen, and Van Voorhis 2015). Several key characteristics are important for new molecules, described as target candidate profiles (TCPs) (Burrows and others 2017):

- **Molecules that kill the blood-stage parasites (the cause of clinical symptoms):** In practice, most of the new molecules appear to have killing rates as fast as current or recent drugs and deliver an active plasma concentration from a single dose.
- **New medicines that prevent the relapse of hepatic hypnozoites of *P. vivax* and other recurrent malarias:** The current standard is a 14-day course of primaquine, an 8-aminoquinoline (8-AQ). A newer 8-AQ, tafenoquine, was shown to be highly active in preventing relapse after single dosing in phase II studies (Llanos-Cuentas and others 2014). However, all drugs in the class carry a risk of hemolysis in G6PD (glucose-6-phosphate dehydrogenase)–deficient individuals. G6PD deficiency is frequent (around 10 percent) in tropical Africa (Carter and others 2011) because it is thought to afford some resistance against malaria. A roadmap for finding new chemical entities without such a risk factor has recently been published (Campo and others 2015).
- **Agents that block transmission:** The other activity of 8-AQs, including primaquine, is blocking transmission of *P. falciparum* by killing gametocytes (TCP3b). In its most recent treatment guidelines, the WHO recommends a reduced single dose of 0.25 mg/kg (WHO 2015b), which is assumed to be safer than its previous recommendation of a single 0.75 mg/kg dose, following a recommendation of the WHO's Malaria Policy Advisory Committee. New agents without potential risks to G6PD-deficient individuals are needed.
- **Chemoprevention:** As the eradication agenda proceeds, it becomes increasingly important to protect against initial infection with agents active against hepatic schizonts. New agents of this type are needed particularly by people entering areas of high transmission from low-transmission areas.

The drug development pipeline is relatively rich in new molecules and targets for the rapid killing of parasites (Wells, van Huijsduijnen, and Van Voorhis 2015) (figure 13.1). The recent availability of efficient controlled human malaria infection (CHMI) models (McCarthy and others 2011) has allowed the assessment of new molecules at an early stage. In these models, volunteers are infected with low (asymptomatic) densities of parasites, whose proliferation is monitored by PCR (polymerase chain reaction). Following administration of experimental drugs, a minimum inhibitory concentration (in blood) and a rate of parasite reduction can be calculated, both of which are highly predictive of the effects in patients.

New medicines that are fully active against emerging resistant strains and that are administered via three-day

regimens can likely be developed. However, among the eradication goals is the availability of a simplified form of therapy, ideally, a single-exposure radical cure (Burrows and others 2017). This ambitious goal makes development of effective new agents more difficult. A new medicine will be a combination of two or more active ingredients; any new molecule that enters a combination must be powerful enough by itself to kill a reasonable number of parasites in the patient, preferably all of them, so that efficacy is ensured even when some parasites are resistant to one of the partner ingredients.

The *Global Technical Strategy* (WHO 2015a) and the *AIM* (RBM Partnership 2015) foresee a 90 percent reduction in case mortality by 2030, underlining the need for new classes of medicines over the next 20 years

Figure 13.1 Current Portfolio of the Global Malaria Medicines Development Effort

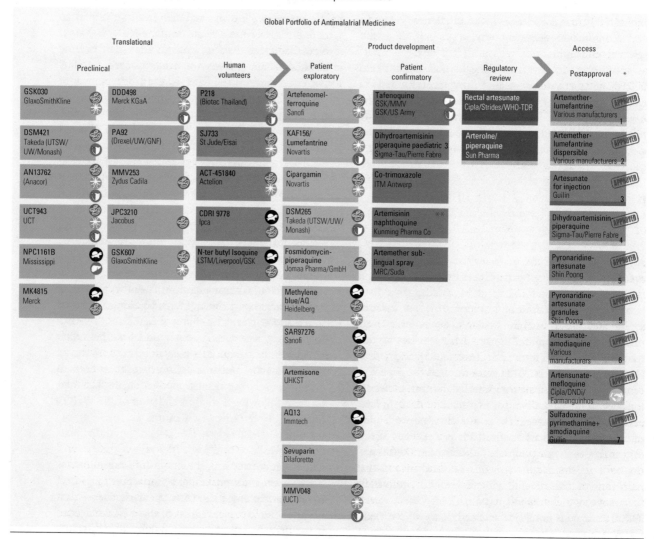

figure continues next page

Figure 13.1 Current Portfolio of the Global Malaria Medicines Development Effort (continued)

Footnotes: Global Portfolio

Target Product Profiles and Target Candidate Profiles
MMV has defined Target Product Profiles and Target Candidate Profiles for medicines to support the eradication campaign.
Burrows, J., R. H. van Huijsduijnen, J. J. Mohrle, C. Oeuvray, and T. N. C. Wells. 2013. "Designing the Next Generation of Medicines for Malaria Control." *Malaria Journal* 12: 187, which is being updated for publication in 2017.

Target Product Profiles
indicated by bars at the bottom of
each compound box

- 3-day cure, artemisinin-based combination therapies
- Combinations aiming at a new single exposure radical cure (TPP–1)
- Severe malaria and prereferral treatment
- Intermittent/seasonal malaria chemoprevention
- Products targeting prevention of relapse for *P. vivax*
- There are currently no products in the development portfolio meeting the single-exposure chemoprotection (SEC) TPP-2

Footnotes for generic names on Global Portfolio
1. First approval: Novartis (Brand name: Coartem®). Generics by Ajanta, Cipla, Ipca, Strides, Macleods, Mylan.
2. First approval: Novartis (Brand name: Coartem® *Dispersible*). Generic by Ajanta.
3. Brand name: Artesun®.
4. Brand name: Eurartesim®.
5. Brand name: Pyramax® tablets and granules.
6. First approval fixed-dose combination: Sanofi/DNDi (brand name: ASAQ Winthrop). Generics by Ajanta, Cipla, Guilin, Ipca, Strides.
7. Brand name: SPAQ-CO™.

Target Candidate Profiles
Activities for each individual molecule, indicated by symbols added to each compound in the translational portfolio

		Burrows and others 2013	Burrows and others 2017
	Asexual blood stages	(TCP-1,2)	TCP-1
	Relapse prevention	(TCP-3a)	TCP-3
	Transmission reduction	(TCP-3b)	TCP-5
	Chemoprevention	(TCP-4)	TCP-4

Additional Symbols on Global Portfolio

- Brought into portfolio after approval; collaborations with DNDi
- No progress report in the past two years
- * Pending review or approval by WHO prequalification or by regulatory bodies that are ICH members or observers
- ** Approved in several countries but not approved by WHO prequalification or regulatory bodies that are ICH members or observers

Note: This figure is constructed from available information using Internet searches, Thomson Reuters Cortellis database (http://lifesciences.thomsonreuters.com/products/cortellis), and searches of the patent and published literature. It represents the portfolio of data as of December 2016. A new version is produced quarterly and is available at Medicines for Malaria Venture, http://www.mmv.org/research-development/rd-portfolio. DNDi = Drugs for Neglected Diseases initiative; ICH = International Council for Harmonisation of Technical Requirements for Pharmaceuticals for Human Use; MMV = Medicines for Malaria Venture; TCP = target candidate profile; TPP = target product profile; WHO = World Health Organization.

if the precious gains against malaria are not to be lost in the future.

Transmission-Blocking Medicines
The primary drug discovery screens have been conducted against blood-stage forms of the parasite. However, many of the compounds show promising activity against the sexual stages (gametocytes) and in membrane-feeding assays (feeding mosquitoes in special devices with blood from patients) (Bolscher and others 2015; Upton and others 2015). The CHMI model has been modified to also allow the production and characterization of gametocytes (Pasay and others 2016) and hence may provide an effective means of testing transmission-blocking treatments.

P. vivax infections are rising: *P. vivax* develops dormant forms or hypnozoites, which result in multiple malaria episodes from a single infection. The ideal medicine for treatment would therefore have activity against the asexual and sexual blood stages of the parasite as well as against the hypnozoites where present (*P. vivax* and *P. ovale*) (Hemingway and others 2016).

Medicines for Long-Term Chemoprotection
The goal of providing chemoprotection has long been one of the mainstays of malaria research and development. Historically, chemoprotection has been targeted at tourists and nonimmune military personnel in times of conflict. More recent developments involve medicines to protect children (Wilson and on behalf of the IPTc Taskforce 2011). Studies of intermittent preventive treatment of children (IPTc) show a remarkable effect when used throughout the rainy malaria season; the medicines

reduced the rate of infection by more than 80 percent and the rate of all-cause mortality by 57 percent. The cost of such medicine is relatively low: sulfadoxine-pyrimethamine in combination with amodiaquine costs less than US$0.70 for one year's treatment. In light of these data, several groups have proposed using ACTs, such as DHA (dihydroartemisinin-piperaquine), for chemoprotection south of the equator, in regions where sulfadoxine-pyrimethamine is ineffective. However, doing so would mean that the same active ingredients would be used for treatment and prevention, which is far from ideal. The WHO recommends against this approach because of the risks of resistance and treatment failure.

Currently available agents are far from idea. Cycloguanil pamoate (Camolar), for example, was developed by Parke Davis in the 1960s as a long-acting form of cycloguanil. This low-solubility salt was developed for intramuscular use in primates, but it required a slow injection through a 20-gauge needle over a 90-second period because the optimal crystal size was large and the vehicle was oleaginous (viscous) (Schmidt and Rossan 1984). These large particle sizes were needed to achieve a drug release over 200 days. Initial trials in humans provided a duration of protection from nonresistant strains of four to six months (Elslager 1969). This formulation is hardly child friendly, requiring four 1 mL intramuscular injections through a 21-gauge needle.

New medicines for chemoprotection are urgently needed because all drugs currently used in treating malaria suffer from resistance. Two compounds in phase II studies, KAF156 (White and others 2016) (acting against the un-annotated CARL locus, a part of the genome with unknown function), and DSM265 (McCarthy and others 2017; Sulyok and others 2017) (an inhibitor of the enzyme dihydroorotate dehydrogenase, which is essential for the DNA synthesis of the parasites), have also shown good activity against the liver schizont stages and could be used in chemoprevention. Studies in CHMI models with insect challenges are needed to validate whether the preclinical activity can be replicated in human subjects. They are also needed to help decide if these medicines would require daily, weekly, or even less frequent administration.

Malaria Vaccine: The Pace Quickens

The agenda for malaria vaccines was originally presented in the 2006 global malaria technology roadmap. By 2015, the landmark roadmap was to have registered a first-generation vaccine with a protective efficacy of more than 50 percent against severe disease and death and with a duration of protection greater than one year. The current frontrunner is the subunit vaccine RTS,S

in combination with a proprietary adjuvant, AS01 (produced by GlaxoSmithKline and the Malaria Vaccine Initiative). The results for the phase III study involving 15,460 children in 11 centers in 7 countries in Sub-Saharan Africa showed a reduction of 18–28 percent against all malaria episodes without a booster, and a reduction of 26–36 percent with a booster at month 20. The protection was slightly less for severe malaria episodes: a 1.1–10.0 percent reduction without booster and 17.0–32.0 percent reduction with a booster at month 20 (RTS,S/AS01 Clinical Trials Partnership 2012). The vaccine received a positive scientific opinion in July 2015 from the Committee for Medicinal Products for Human Use of the European Medicines Agency.

An analysis of the vaccine's protection and its long-term public health effect for 43 African countries reported a rate of initial protection of 80 percent against infection in children ages 5–17 months and a rate of initial protection of 65 percent in infants ages 6–12 weeks (Olotu and others 2013). Despite observed and predicted protection of the RTS,S vaccine being short lived, when used in combination with other malaria control strategies, such as ITNs, the vaccine has the potential to avert up to 700,000 deaths over a 10-year period. After considering all of the safety data from the clinical trials, the WHO issued a positive policy recommendation for starting to plan a series of large-scale implementation programs (Penny and others 2015; WHO Malaria Policy Advisory Committee and Secretariat 2015).

The WHO, working with the Malaria Vaccine Funders Group, updated the *Malaria Vaccine Technology Roadmap* in 2013 to present the organization's goals until 2030 (Malaria Vaccine Funders Group 2013; Tanner and Alonso 2010). Specifically, by 2030, vaccines will be launched that target *P. falciparum* and *P. vivax*, that have a protective efficacy of at least 75 percent against clinical malaria, that are suitable for administration to appropriate at-risk groups in malaria-endemic areas, that reduce transmission of the parasite, and that thereby substantially reduce the incidence of human malaria infection.

These new goals are in line with the Malaria Elimination/Eradication Roadmap (Tanner and Alonso 2010), which introduced the further concept of vaccines that interrupt malaria transmission (VIMT). These VIMT include classical transmission-blocking vaccines that target the sexual and mosquito stages, as well as pre-erythrocytic and asexual stages that have an effect on transmission. More recently, this terminology has been extended to VIMT through the sexual, sporogonic, or mosquito stages of the parasite (Nunes and others 2014). The current malaria vaccine pipeline from the WHO summary is shown in figure 13.2.

The present challenges to vaccine development are as follows:

- A careful selection of antigens to ensure protection against both *P. vivax* and *P. falciparum* is needed.
- A vaccine that costs around US$1 per dose would be most attractive. However, if the ideal vaccine may have multiple antigens to target different parasite stages, its production costs may increase. The cost-benefit tradeoffs must be evaluated early to avoid producing a vaccine that might be very effective but is too expensive for widespread adoption.
- Better and more specific adjuvants (which increase antigenicity) are lacking.
- Improved understanding of why acquired immunity to *Plasmodium* is slow to develop, incomplete, and short-lived is needed; this is essential to improve the likelihood of finding a fully protective vaccine.

The challenge is considerable, because protozoan parasites have evolved multiple strategies to evade attacks from the mammalian immune system, such as encoding and switching between dozens of genes that encode different cell surface proteins. Almost all successful vaccines are directed against viruses, very few act against bacteria, and almost none act against protozoans.

Several vaccines are in human volunteer studies or early field trials. The probability of early success in malaria vaccines as a whole at this stage is quite high (Pronker and others 2013). The combination of a wealth of candidates and a poor success rate highlights the importance of having standardized processes for comparing candidates. The Malaria Vaccine Roadmap underscores this point and recommends standardized CHMI models. These same models are being used to benchmark chemoprotective medicines, giving the additional advantage that chemoprotective medicines and vaccines can be compared side by side.

Most of the current vaccine candidates are blood-stage vaccines and specific for one species. Again, community portfolio management is needed to ensure that vaccines with the potential to fulfill the aspirations of the roadmap receive priority. The development of transmission-blocking vaccines has received much attention, because they would

Figure 13.2 Current Portfolio of the Global Malaria Vaccines Development Effort

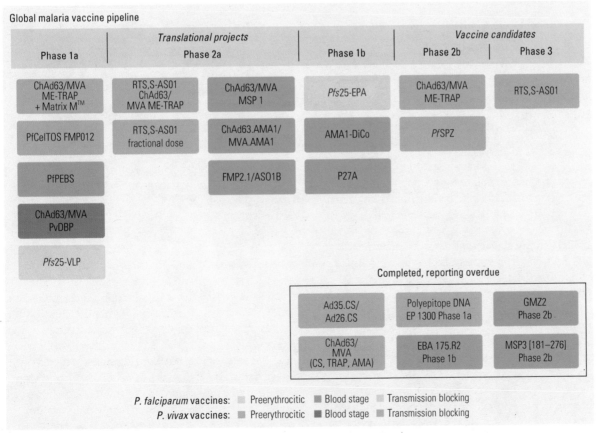

Source: World Health Organization, http://www.who.int/immunization/research/development/Rainbow_tables/en (March 2016).

substantially affect eradication efforts. The regulatory pathway for such vaccines and drugs, which would protect communities rather than individuals, has been complicated; progress is being made in discussions among members of the vaccine community such as developers, clinical epidemiologists involved in trials, and regulatory agencies (Delrieu and others 2015). There is still a paucity of antigens under study. The major exception and very promising approach is the sporozoite vaccine from Sanaria, Inc., which is being tested in early volunteer studies in Africa (Seder and others 2013). Studies using more than 50,000 attenuated, aseptic, purified, cryopreserved *P. falciparum* sporozoites delivered in four intravenous injections are ongoing in endemic areas and for short-term visitors and travelers (Richie and others 2015).

Finally, the timescales are important. RTS,S/AS01 started phase II (field exploratory) studies over a decade ago; the time to complete the confirmatory studies,

ensure two-year follow up, and submit regulatory documentation was approximately six years. A review of the regulatory lessons from this process is critical to future efforts to shorten some of these timelines.

Vector Control

Success of LLINs under Threat from Insecticide Resistance

An essential requirement for effective resistance management is to speed up the development of new active insecticidal ingredients, as well as alternative vector control approaches. The Innovative Vector Control Consortium, a public-private partnership established in 2005, is managing a portfolio of novel insecticide candidates that are expected to deliver new public health insecticides by 2020–22. In addition to new active ingredients, the current development pipeline of vector control products (figure 13.3) contains repurposed and reformulated

Figure 13.3 Current Portfolio of the Global Malaria Vector Control Development Effort

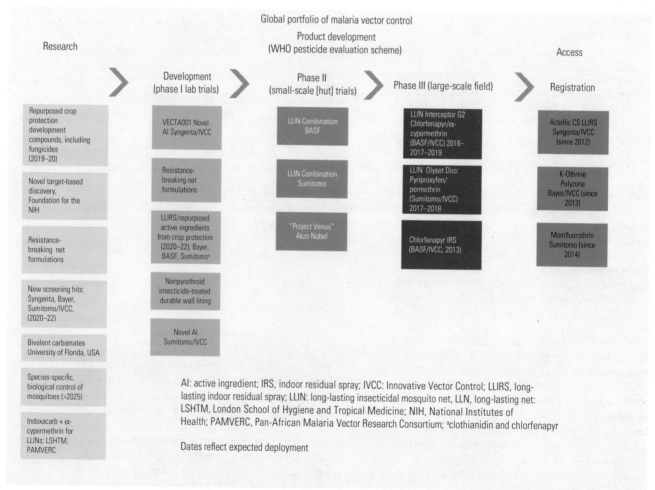

AI: active ingredient; IRS, indoor residual spray; IVCC: Innovative Vector Control; LLIRS, long-lasting indoor residual spray; LLIN: long-lasting insecticidal mosquito net, LLN, long-lasting net; LSHTM, London School of Hygiene and Tropical Medicine; NIH, National Institutes of Health; PAMVERC, Pan-African Malaria Vector Research Consortium; [a]clothianidin and chlorfenapyr

Dates reflect expected deployment

Source: IVCC 2016.

existing insecticides, such as the microencapsulated organophosphate insecticide pirimiphos-methyl.

Finally, the pipeline also includes noninsecticidal new paradigms for vector control. As a stopgap measure to rapidly address the pyrethroid resistance issue, nets have been designed that combine an insecticide (usually a pyrethroid) with a second chemical (usually piperonyl butoxide), which helps reduce enzymatic resistance in *Anopheles* mosquitoes. These combination nets are being field tested and may prove to be effective in areas with high levels of pyrethroid resistance in malaria vectors. As new insecticides with new modes of action become available, nets should regain their effectiveness. Ideally, future nets should be treated with a combination of insecticides representing various modes of action, thereby reducing the risk of resistance. This combination strategy has worked well for antimalarials and should be chosen for vector control strategies as well.

Mosquito Population Modification Strategies

A promising potential intervention is the use of genetically modified mosquitoes. The recent demonstration that CRISPR (clustered regularly interspaced short palindromic repeats)/Cas9 gene-editing technology can be used efficiently to generate genetically modified insects (Gantz and Bier 2015) has raised hopes for future development of malaria-resistant mosquitoes. Another encouraging finding is the recent discovery that genetic modification of certain bacteria (especially *Wolbachia sp.*) from the mosquito microbiota (paratransgenesis) can lead to a dramatic reduction of mosquito vectorial competence (Shaw and others 2016). However, many challenges remain with these approaches, which to date have been largely confined to the laboratory. The issue of driving new genes sustainably into wild mosquito populations remains a major obstacle to widespread implementation, as is testing of the efficacy and the public acceptance of such approaches (WHO/TDR and Foundation for the National Institutes of Health 2014).

Other Noninsecticidal Vector Control Approaches

New vector control tools being developed do not rely on insecticidal action for their effectiveness, thereby providing a welcome alternative at a time of widespread resistance. Spatial repellents have the potential to significantly decrease the entry of malaria vectors into human dwellings (Lambrechts and others 2015; Ogoma and others 2014) and are being tested in large-scale trials around the world. Topical repellents, in contrast, have proven largely disappointing as a malaria control tool, primarily because of compliance problems (Sluydts and others 2016).

Another potential approach is the use of attractive toxic sugar baits, which take advantage of the fact that every female mosquito needs to take one or more sugar meals in addition to blood meals to produce offspring. Such baits attract mosquitoes to artificial sugar sources that are toxic to the mosquito (Qualls and others 2015).

Finally, the careful and evidence-based combination of multiple vector control tools is likely to provide the best avenue to reduce further transmission in currently endemic areas in which either LLINs or IRS is already implemented at high coverage (Okumu and Moore 2011). One such combination, a spatial repellent that protects houses, is associated with attractive traps located at the periphery of villages, using the "push-pull strategy" (Wagman and others 2015).

CONCLUSIONS

Malaria control is one of the great success stories of global public health. Unprecedented success has been and is being achieved for a disease that, by one estimate, may have killed half of all the people who ever lived (Whitfield 2002). Even a high-transmission setting such as the Democratic Republic of Congo has been able to halve the prevalence and incidence rates in the past 15 years (WHO 2016b). These successes have provided the impetus for the world to move forward to attain the goal of eradication. However, substantial threats to these achievements exist. Drug and insecticide resistance top the list of biological and epidemiological problems, while the lack of political will and sustainable financing top the list of external dangers.

In summary, several conclusions emerge:

- Many new malaria control tools are being developed, thanks to product development partnerships for drugs (Medicines for Malaria Venture), diagnostics (Foundation for Innovative New Diagnostics), and vector control tools (Innovative Vector Control Consortium). New strategies are being devised that use existing tools, with countries attempting to become more specific and evidence driven in their strategic plans (WHO 2015a).
- The regulatory landscape for drugs and vaccines is not equipped to evaluate treatments meant to drive low-to-zero malaria transmission. When placing this outlook into the overall context of *AIM* (RBM Partnership 2015) and the Sustainable Development Goals, one can no longer calculate the payoff of tools introduced to drive elimination from low-to-zero transmission only in terms of present and future

cases averted; a broader economic perspective of productivity gained, as well as the transmission effect, is needed. This enhanced perspective focused on return on investments is essential to evaluate the relative merits of the various tools and to prioritize and select their deployment in multiple settings.

- Consequently, there is a growing need to decide how new control approaches are to be applied in an optimal combination and an integrated way in a world with differing levels of malaria transmission and with contrasting malaria endemicity, even within the same country. Addressing this heterogeneity entails adapting the *Global Technical Strategy* (WHO 2015a) to national and even subnational levels and rigorously implementing surveillance–response strategies and systems.

Given that all activities are based on partnership approaches across the public, private, and charitable sectors, the roles and responsibilities of the partnerships must be well defined at each level. The task of malaria control and elimination calls for more than joint actions. Rather, it requires better, well-defined, and assigned tasks and responsibilities, accompanied by the required power and authority to implement the responsibilities within national strategies and coordinated operational plans.

ANNEXES

The annexes to this chapter are available at http://www .dcp-3.org/infectiousdiseases.

- Annex 13A. Dataset of Costs Studies.
- Annex 13B. Dataset of Cost-Effectiveness Studies.

NOTES

World Bank Income Classifications as of July 2014 are as follows, based on estimates of gross national income (GNI) per capita for 2013:

- Low-income countries (LICs) = US$1,045 or less
- Middle-income countries (MICs) are subdivided:
  (a) lower-middle-income = US$1,046–US$4,125
  (b) upper-middle-income (UMICs) = US$4,126–US$12,745
- High-income countries (HICs) = US$12,746 or more.

1. For more information on the study, visit http://www.who .int/malaria/news/2016/llins-effective-tool-malaria-fight/en/.
2. *P. vivax* and *P. ovale* infections can form hypnozoites that can cause relapses months and even years after the initial infection.

REFERENCES

Alonso, P. L., D. Bell, K. Hanson, K. Mendis, R. D. Newman, and others. 2011. "A Research Agenda for Malaria Eradication: Health Systems and Operational Research." *PLoS Medicine* 8: e1000397.

Awolola, T. S., A. O. Oduola, J. B. Obansa, N. J. Chukwurar, and J. P. Unyimadu. 2007. "*Anopheles gambiae s.s.* Breeding in Polluted Water Bodies in Urban Lagos, Southwestern Nigeria." *Journal of Vector Borne Diseases* 44 (4): 241–44.

Badolo, A., A. Traore, C. M. Jones, A. Sanou, L. Flood, and others. 2012. "Three Years of Insecticide Resistance Monitoring in *Anopheles gambiae* in Burkina Faso: Resistance on the Rise?" *Malaria Journal* 11: 232. http:// dx.doi.org/10.1186/1475-2875-11-232.

Baolin, L. 1988. "Environmental Management for the Control of Ricefield-Breeding Mosquitoes in China." International Rice Research Institute in collaboration with the World Health Organization/Food and Agriculture Organization of the United Nations/United Nations Environment Programme Panel of Experts on Environmental Management for Vector Control, Manila.

Bassat, Q., B. Oqutu, A. Djimde, K. Stricker, and K. Hamed. 2015. "Tailoring a Pediatric Formulation of Artemether-Lumefantrine for Treatment of *Plasmodium falciparum* Malaria." *Antimicrobial Agents and Chemotherapy* 59: 4366–74.

Berendes, S., P. Heywood, S. Oliver, and P. Garner. 2011. "Quality of Private and Public Ambulatory Health Care in Low and Middle Income Countries: Systematic Review of Comparative Studies." *PLoS Medicine* 8 (4): e1000433.

Bhatt, S., D. J. Weiss, E. Cameron, D. Bisanzio, B. Mappin, and others. 2015. "The Effect of Malaria Control on *Plasmodium falciparum* in Africa between 2000 and 2015." *Nature* 526 (7572): 207–11. http://dx.doi.org/10.1038/nature15535.

Bolscher, J. M., K. M. Koolen, G. J. Van Gemert, M. G. van de Vegte-Bolmer, T. Bousema, and others. 2015. "A Combination of New Screening Assays for Prioritization of Transmission-Blocking Antimalarials Reveals Distinct Dynamics of Marketed and Experimental Drugs." *Journal of Antimicrobial Chemotherapy* 70 (50): 1357–66.

Boyd, M. F. 1926. "The Influence of Obstacles Unconsciously Erected against Anophelines (Housing and Screening) upon the Incidence of Malaria." *American Journal of Tropical Medicine and Hygiene* 6 (2): 157–60.

Burrows, J. N., S. Duparc, W. E. Gutteridge, R. H van Huijsduijnen, W. Kaszubska, and others. 2017. "New Developments in Anti-Malarial Target Candidate and Product Profiles." *Malaria Journal* 16: 26. http://www.ncbi .nlm.nih.gov/pmc/articles/PMC5237200/.

Campo, B. F., O. Vandal, D. L. Wesche, and J. N. Burrows. 2015. "Killing the Hypnozoite—Drug Discovery Approaches to Prevent Relapse in *Plasmodium vivax*." *Pathogens and Global Health* 109 (3): 107–22.

Carter, N., A. Pamba, S. Duparc, and J. N. Waitumbi. 2011. "Frequency of Glucose-6-Phosphate Dehydrogenase Deficiency in Malaria Patients from Six African Countries Enrolled in Two Randomized Anti-Malarial Clinical Trials."

Malaria Journal 10: 241. http://www.ncbi.nlm.nih.gov /pmc/articles/PMC3188486/.

Carter, R., and K. N. Mendis. 2002. "Evolutionary and Historical Aspects of the Burden of Malaria." *Clinical Microbiology Reviews* 15 (4): 564–94.

Castro, M. C., and B. H. Singer. 2011. "Malaria in the Brazilian Amazon." In *Water and Sanitation-Related Diseases and the Environment: Challenges, Interventions, and Preventive Measures,* edited by J. M. H. Selendy, 401–20. Hoboken, NJ: Wiley-Blackwell.

Chinery, W. A. 1984. "Effects of Ecological Changes on the Malaria Vectors *Anopheles funestus* and the *Anopheles gambiae* Complex of Mosquitoes in Accra, Ghana." *Journal of Tropical Medicine and Hygiene* 87 (2): 75–81.

Deane, L. M. 1988. "Malaria Studies and Control in Brazil." *American Journal of Tropical Medicine and Hygiene* 38 (2): 223–30.

Delrieu, I., D. Leboulleux, K. Ivinson, and B. D. Gessner. 2015. "Design of a Phase III Cluster Randomized Trial to Assess the Efficacy and Safety of a Malaria Transmission Blocking Vaccine." *Vaccine* 33 (13): 1518–26.

Dondorp, A., C. I. Fanello, I. C. Hendriksen, E. Gomes, A. Seni, and others. 2013. "Artesunate versus Quinine in the Treatment of Severe Falciparum Malaria in African Children (AQUAMAT): An Open-Label, Randomised Trial." *The Lancet* 376 (9753): 1647–57. http://www.science-direct.com/science/article/pii/S0140673610619241.

Dondorp, A., F. F. Nosten, K. F. Stepniewska, N. F. Day, and N. White. 2005. "Artesunate versus Quinine for Treatment of Severe Falciparum Malaria: A Randomised Trial." *The Lancet* 366 (9487): 717–25.

Elslager, E. F. 1969. "Progress in Malaria Chemotherapy. 1. Repository Antimalarial Drugs." *Progress in Drug Research* 13: 170–216.

Galactionova, K., F. Tediosi, F. Camponovo, T. A. Smith, P. W. Gething, and others. 2017. "Country-Specific Predictions of the Cost-Effectiveness of Malaria Vaccine RTS,S/AS01 in Endemic Africa." *Vaccine* 35 (1): 53–60.

Galactionova, K., F. Tediosi, D. de Savigny, T. Smith, and M. Tanner. 2015. "Effective Coverage and Systems Effectiveness for Malaria Case Management in Sub-Saharan African Countries." *PLoS One* 10 (5): e0127818. http:// dx.doi.org/10.1371/journal.pone.0127818.

Gallup, J. L., and J. D. Sachs. 2001. "The Economic Burden of Malaria." *American Journal of Tropical Medicine and Hygiene* 64 (Suppl 1–2): 85–96.

Gantz, V. M., and E. Bier. 2015. "The Mutagenic Chain Reaction: A Method for Converting Heterozygous to Homozygous Mutations." *Science* 348 (6233): 442–44. http://science .sciencemag.org/content/348/6233/442.abstract.

Gething, P. W., D. L. Smith, A. P. Patil, A. J. Tatem, R. W. Snow, and others. 2010. "Climate Change and the Global Malaria Recession." *Nature* 465: (7296): 342–45.

Gomes, M. F., M. A Faiz, J. O. Gyapong, M. Warsame, T. Agbenyega, and others. 2009. "Pre-Referral Rectal Artesunate to Prevent Death and Disability in Severe Malaria: a Placebo-Controlled Trial." *The Lancet* 373 (9663): 14–20.

Gorgas, G. W. C. 1915. *Sanitation in Panama.* New York: D. Appleton and Co.

Hahn, M. B., R. E. Gangnon, C. Barcellos, G. P. Asner, and J. A. Patz. 2014. "Influence of Deforestation, Logging, and Fire on Malaria in the Brazilian Amazon." *PLoS One* 9 (1).

Hemingway, J., H. Ranson, A. Magill, J. Kolaczinski, C. Fornadel, and others. 2016. "Averting a Malaria Disaster: Will Insecticide Resistance Derail Malaria Control?" *The Lancet* 387 (10029): 1785–88. http://dx.doi.org/10.1016 /S0140-6736(15)00417-1.

Hochman, S., and K. Kim. 2009. "The Impact of HIV and Malaria Coinfection: What Is Known and Suggested Venues for Further Study." *Interdisciplinary Perspectives on Infectious Diseases* 2009: 617954.

IVCC. 2016. "Annual Report 2015/2016." http://www.ivcc .com/download/file/fid/826.

Keiser, J., B. H. Singer, and J. Utzinger. 2005. "Reducing the Burden of Malaria in Different Eco-Epidemiological Settings with Environmental Management: A Systematic Review." *The Lancet Infectious Diseases* 5 (11): 695–708.

Keiser, J., J. Utzinger, M. C. Castro, T. Smith, M. Tanner, and others. 2004. "Urbanization in Sub-Saharan Africa and Implications for Malaria Control." *American Journal of Tropical Medicine and Hygiene* 71 (Suppl 2): 118–27.

Khatib, R. A., M. Selemani, G. A. Mrisho, I. M. Masanja, M. Amuri, and others. 2013. "Access to Artemisinin-Based Anti-Malarial Treatment and Its Related Factors in Rural Tanzania." *Malaria Journal* 12 (1): 155.

Knudsen, J., and L. von Seidlein. 2014. *Healthy Homes in Tropical Zones: Improving Rural Housing in Asia and Africa.* Felbach, Germany: Edition Axel Menges GmbH.

Koenker, H., J. Keating, M. Alilio, A. Acosta, M. Lynch, and F. Nafo-Traore. 2014. "Strategic Roles for Behaviour Change Communication in a Changing Malaria Landscape." *Malaria Journal* 13 (1). http://dx.doi.org/10.1186/1475-2875-13-1.

Konradsen, F., W. van der Hoek, F. P. Amerasinghe, C. Mutero, and E. Boelee. 2004. "Engineering and Malaria Control: Learning from the Past 100 Years." *Acta Tropica* 89 (2): 99–108.

Lambrechts, L., N. M. Ferguson, E. Harris, E. C. Holmes, E. A. McGraw, and others. 2015. "Assessing the Epidemiological Effect of *Wolbachia* for Dengue Control." *The Lancet Infectious Diseases* 15 (7): 862–66. http://dx.doi .org/10.1016/S1473-3099(15)00091-2.

Lengeler, C. 2004. "Insecticide-Treated Bed Nets and Curtains for Preventing Malaria." *Cochrane Database of Systematic Reviews* 2000 (2): CD000363.

Lindsay, S. W., P. M. Emerson, and J. D. Charlwood. 2002. "Reducing Malaria by Mosquito-Proofing Houses." *Trends in Parasitology* 18 (11): 510–14.

Littrell, M., J. Miller, M. Ndhlovu, B. Hamainza, M. Hawela, and others. 2013. "Documenting Malaria Case Management Coverage in Zambia: A Systems Effectiveness Approach." *Malaria Journal* 12 (1): 371. http://www.malariajournal .com/content/12/1/371.

Llanos-Cuentas, A., M. V. Lacerda, R. Rueangweerayut, S. Krudsood, S. K. Gupta, and others. 2014. "Tafenoquine plus Chloroquine for the Treatment and Relapse Prevention of *Plasmodium vivax* Malaria (DETECTIVE): A Multicentre, Double-Blind, Randomised, Phase 2b Dose-Selection Study." *The Lancet* 383 (9922): 1049–58.

Maheu-Giroux, M., and M. C. Castro. 2013. "Do Malaria Vector Control Measures Impact Disease-Related Behaviour and Knowledge? Evidence from a Large-Scale Larviciding Intervention in Tanzania." *Malaria Journal* 12: 422. http://dx.doi.org/10.1186/1475-2875-12-422.

Malaria Vaccine Funders Group. 2013. *Malaria Vaccine Technology Roadmap.* http://www.who.int/immunization/topics/malaria/vaccine_roadmap/TRM_update_nov13.pdf?ua=1.

malERA Consultative Group on Vector Control. 2011. "A Research Agenda for Malaria Eradication: Vector Control." *PLoS Medicine* 8 (1): e1000401. http://www.ncbi.nlm.nih.gov/pmc/articles/PMC3026704/.

Marchesinig, P., and J. Crawley. 2004. "Reducing the Burden of Anemia in Infants and Young Children in Malaria-Endemic Countries of Africa: From Evidence to Action." *American Journal of Tropical Medicine and Hygiene* 71 (Suppl 2): 25–34.

McCarthy, J. S., J. Lotharius, T. Rickle, S. Chalon, J. Phillips, and others. 2017. "Safety, Tolerability, Pharmacokinetics, and Activity of the Novel Long-Acting Antimalarial DSM265: A Two-Part First-in-Human Phase 1a/1b Randomised Study." *The Lancet Infectious Diseases.* 17 (6): 626–35. http://dx.doi.org/10.1016/S1473-3099(17)30171-8.

McCarthy, J. S., S. Sekuloski, P. M. Griffin, S. Elliott, N. Douglas, and others. 2011. "A Pilot Randomised Trial of Induced Blood-Stage *Plasmodium falciparum* Infections in Healthy Volunteers for Testing Efficacy of New Antimalarial Drugs." *PLOS One* 6 (8): e21914. http://dx.doi.org/10.1371/journal.pone.0021914.

McPake, B., D. Asiimwe, F. Mwesigye, M. Ofumbi, L. Ortenblad, and others. 1999. "Informal Economic Activities of Public Health Workers in Uganda: Implications for Quality and Accessibility of Care." *Social Science and Medicine* 49 (7): 849–65.

Mikkelsen-Lopez, I., F. Tediosi, G. Abdallah, M. Njozi, B. Amuri, and others. 2013. "Beyond Antimalarial Stock-Outs: Implications of Health Provider Compliance on Out-of-Pocket Expenditure during Care-Seeking for Fever in South East Tanzania." *BMC Health Services Research* 13: 444. http://dx.doi.org/10.1186/1472-6963-13-444.

Mnzava, A. P., T. B. Knox, E. A. Temu, A. Trett, C. Fornadel, and others. 2015. "Implementation of the Global Plan for Insecticide Resistance Management in Malaria Vectors: Progress, Challenges and the Way Forward." *Malaria Journal* 14: 173. http://www.ncbi.nlm.nih.gov/pmc/articles/PMC4423491/.

Mulamba, C., J. M. Riveron, S. S. Ibrahim, H. Irving, K. G. Barnes, and others. 2014. "Widespread Pyrethroid and DDT Resistance in the Major Malaria Vector *Anopheles funestus* in East Africa Is Driven by Metabolic Resistance Mechanisms." *PLoS One* 9 (10): e110058. http://dx.doi.org/10.1371/journal.pone.0110058.

Mumba, M., J. Visschedijk, M. van Cleef, and B. Hausman. 2003. "A Piot Model to Analyse Case Management in Malaria Control Programs." *Tropical Medicine and International Health* 8 (6): 544–51.

Nájera, J. A., M. González-Silva, and P. L. Alonso. 2011. "Some Lessons for the Future from the Global Malaria Eradication Programme (1955–1969)." *PLoS Med* 8 (1): e1000412. http://www.ncbi.nlm.nih.gov/pmc/articles/PMC3026700.

Neiva, A. 1940. "Profilaxia da malária e trabalhos de engenharia: Notas, comentários, recordações." *Revista do Clube de Engenharia* 6 (70): 60–75.

Nunes, J. K., C. Woods, T. Carter, T. Raphael, M. J. Morin, and others. 2014. "Development of a Transmission-Blocking Malaria Vaccine: Progress, Challenges, and the Path Forward." *Vaccine* 32 (343): 5531–39.

Obrist, B., N. Iteba, C. Lengeler, A. Makemba, C. Mshana, and others. 2007. "Access to Health Care in Contexts of Livelihood Insecurity: A Framework for Analysis and Action." *PLoS Medicine* 4 (10): e308. http://dx.doi.org/10.1371%2Fjournal.pmed.0040308.

Ogoma, S. B., K. Kannady, M. Sikulu, P. Chaki, N. Govella, and others. 2009. "Window Screening, Ceilings and Closed Eaves as Sustainable Ways to Control Malaria in Dar es Salaam, Tanzania." *Malaria Journal* 8: 221.

Ogoma, S. B., H. Ngonyani, E. T. Simfukwe, A. Mseka, J. Moore, and others. 2014. "The Mode of Action of Spatial Repellents and Their Impact on Vectorial Capacity of *Anopheles gambiae* sensu stricto." *PLoS One* 9 (12): e110433. http://dx.doi.org/10.1371%2Fjournal.pone.0110433.

Okumu, F. O., and S. J. Moore. 2011. "Combining Indoor Residual Spraying and Insecticide-Treated Nets for Malaria Control in Africa: A Review of Possible Outcomes and an Outline of Suggestions for the Future." *Malaria Journal* 10 (1): 208–22. http://dx.doi.org/10.1186/1475-2875-10-208.

Olotu, A., G. Fegan, J. Wambua, G. Nyangweso, K. O. Awuondo, and others. 2013. "Four-Year Efficacy of RTS,S/AS01E and Its Interaction with Malaria Exposure." *New England Journal of Medicine* 368 (12): 1111–20. http://dx.doi.org/10.1056/NEJMoa1207564.

Pasay, C. J., R. Rockett, S. Sekuloski, P. Griffin, L. Marquart, and others. 2016. "Piperaquine Monotherapy of Drug-Susceptible *Plasmodium falciparum* Infection Results in Rapid Clearance of Parasitemia but Is Followed by the Appearance of Gametocytemia." *Journal of Infectious Diseases* 214 (1): 105–13. http://dx.doi.org/10.1093/infdis/jiw128.

Penny, M. A., K. Galactionova, M. Tarantino, M. Tanner, and T. A. Smith. 2015. "The Public Health Impact of Malaria Vaccine RTS,S in Malaria Endemic Africa: Country-Specific Predictions Using 18 Month Follow-Up Phase III Data and Simulation Models." *BMC Medicine* 13 (1): 170–90. http://dx.doi.org/10.1186/s12916-015-0408-2.

Penny, M. A., R. Verity, C. A. Bever, C. Sauboin, K. Galactionova, and others. 2016. "Public Health Impact and Cost-Effectiveness of the RTS, S/AS01 Malaria Vaccine: A Systematic Comparison of Predictions from Four Mathematical Models." *The Lancet* 387: 367–75.

Pinotti, M. 1951. "The Biological Basis for the Campaign against the Malaria Vectors in Brazil." *Transactions of the Royal Society of Tropical Medicine and Hygiene* 44 (6): 663–82.

Pomeroy, A. W. J. 1920. "The Prophylaxis of Malaria in Dar es Salaam, East Africa." *Journal of the Royal Army Medical Corps* 35 (1): 44–68.

Price, R. N., E. Tjitra, C. A. Guerra, S. Yeung, N. J. White, and others. 2007. "Vivax Malaria: Neglected and Not Benign." *American Journal of Tropical Medicine and Hygiene* 77 (Suppl 6): 79–87.

Pronker, E. S., T. C. Weenen, H. Commandeur, E. H. Claassen, and A. D. Osterhaus. 2013. "Risk in Vaccine Research and Development Quantified." *PLoS One* 8 (3): e57755. http://dx.doi.org/10.1371%2Fjournal.pone.0057755.

Qualls, W. A., G. C. Müller, S. F. Traore, M. M. Traore, K. L. Arheart, and others. 2015. "Indoor Use of Attractive Toxic Sugar Bait (ATSB) to Effectively Control Malaria Vectors in Mali, West Africa." *Malaria Journal* 14 (1): 301–8. http://dx.doi.org/10.1186/s12936-015-0819-8.

Quinones, M. L., D. E. Norris, J. E. Conn, M. Moreno, T. R. Burkot, and others. 2015. "Insecticide Resistance in Areas under Investigation by the International Centers of Excellence for Malaria Research: A Challenge for Malaria Control and Elimination." *Amerian Journal of Tropical Medicine and Hygiene* 93 (3): 68–78.

Rao, B. V., D. Schellenberg, and A. Ghani. 2013a. "Overcoming Health Systems Barriers to Successful Malaria Treatment." *Trends in Parasitology* 29 (4): 164–80.

———. 2013b. "The Potential Impact of Improving Appropriate Treatment for Fever on Malaria and Non-Malaria Febrile Illness Management in Under-5s: A Decision-Tree Modeling Approach." *PLoS One* 8 (7): e69654.

RBM (Roll Back Malaria) Partnership. 2008. *Global Malaria Action Plan for a Malaria-Free World.* Geneva: World Health Organization.

———. 2012. *The Strategic Framework for Malaria Communication at the Country Level, 2012–2017.* Geneva: RBM Partnership.

———. 2015. *Action and Investment to Defeat Malaria 2016–2030.* Geneva: World Health Organization, http://www.rollbackmalaria.org/about/about-rbm/aim-2016-2030.

Richie, T. L., P. F. Billingsley, B. K. L. Sim, E. R. James, S. Chakravarty, and others. 2015. "Progress with *Plasmodium falciparum* Sporozoite (PfSPZ)–Based Malaria Vaccines." *Vaccine* 33 (52): 7452–61. http://www.sciencedirect.com/science/article/pii/S0264410X15013869.

Roberts, L., and M. Enserink. 2007. "Did They Really Say ... Eradication?" *Science* 318 (5856): 1544–45. http://science.sciencemag.org/content/318/5856/1544.abstract.

RTS,S/AS01 Clinical Trials Partnership. 2012. "A Phase 3 Trial of RTS,S/AS01 Malaria Vaccine in African Infants." *New England Journal of Medicine* 367 (24): 2284–95. http://dx.doi.org/10.1056/NEJMoa1208394.

Sattler, M. A., D. Mtasiwa, M. Kiama, Z. Premji, M. Tanner, and others. 2005. "Habitat Characterization and Spatial Distribution of *Anopheles sp.* Mosquito Larvae in Dar es Salaam (Tanzania) during an Extended Dry Period." *Malaria Journal* 4: 4. http://dx.doi.org/10.1186/1475-2875-4-4.

Schmidt, L. H., and R. N. Rossan. 1984. "Activities of Respository Preparations of Cycloguanil Pamoate and 4,4'-Diacetyldiaminodiphenylsulfone, Alone and in Combination, against Infections with *Plasmodium Cynomolgi* in Rhesus Monkeys." *Antimicrobial Agents and Chemotherapy* 26 (5): 611–42. http://www.ncbi.nlm.nih.gov/pmc/articles/PMC179984/.

Seder, R. A., L. J. Chang. M. E. Enama, K. L. Zephir, U. N. Sarwar, and others. 2013. "Protection against Malaria by Intravenous Immunization with a Nonreplicating Sporozoite Vaccine." *Science* 341 (6152): 1359–65.

Shaw, W. R., P. Marcenac, L. M. Childs, C. O. Buckee, F. Baldini, and others. 2016. "*Wolbachia* Infections in Natural *Anopheles* Populations Affect Egg Laying and Negatively Correlate with *Plasmodium* Development." *Nature Communications* 7: 11772. http://dx.doi.org/10.1038/ncomms11772.

Singer, B. H., and M. C. Castro. 2011. "Reassessing Multiple-Intervention Malaria Control Programs of the Past: Lessons for the Design of Contemporary Interventions." In *Water and Sanitation-Related Diseases and the Environment: Challenges, Interventions, and Preventive Measures*, edited by J. M. H. Selendy, 151–66. Hoboken, NJ: Wiley-Blackwell.

Sluydts, V., L. Durnez, S. Heng, C. Gryseels, L. Canier, and others. 2016. "Efficacy of Topical Mosquito Repellent (Picaridin) plus Long-Lasting Insecticidal Nets Versus Long-Lasting Insecticidal Nets Alone for Control of Malaria: A Cluster Randomised Controlled Trial." *The Lancet Infectious Disease* 16 (10): 1169–77. http://dx.doi.org/10.1016/S1473-3099(16)30148-7.

Smith, D. L., K. E. Battle, S. I. Hay, C. M. Barker, T. W. Scott, and F. E. McKenzie. 2012. "Ross, Macdonald, and a Theory for the Dynamics and Control of Mosquito-Transmitted Pathogens." *PLoS Pathogens* 8 (4): e1002588. http://dx.doi.org/10.1371%2Fjournal.ppat.1002588.

Stratton, L., M. S. O'Neill, M. E. Kruk, and M. L. Bell. 2008. "The Persistent Problem of Malaria: Addressing the Fundamental Causes of a Global Killer." *Social Science and Medicine* 67 (5): 854–62. http://www.sciencedirect.com/science/article/pii/S0277953608002347.

Stromquist, W. G. 1920. "Malaria Control from the Engineering Point of View." *American Journal of Public Health* 10 (6): 497–501.

Sulyok, M., T. Rückle, A. Roth, R. E. Mürbeth, S. Chalon, and others. 2017. "DSM265 for *Plasmodium falciparum* Chemoprophylaxis: A Randomised, Double Blinded, Phase 1 Trial with Controlled Human Malaria Infection." *The Lancet Infectious Diseases* 17 (6): 636–44. http://dx.doi.org/10.1016/S1473-3099(17)30139-1.

Sumba, P. O., L. S. Wong, H. K. Kanzaria, K. A. Johnson, and C. C. John. 2008. "Malaria Treatment-Seeking Behavior and Recovery from Malaria in Highland Area of Kenya." *Malaria Journal* 7: 245.

Tanner, M. and P. L. Alonso. 2010. "Research and Development for the Malaria Elimination/Eradication Roadmap." *Malaria Journal* 9 (Suppl 2): 11.

Tusting, L., M. Ippolito, B. Willey, I. Kleinschmidt, G. Dorsey, and others. 2015. "The Evidence for Improving Housing to Reduce Malaria: A Systematic Review and Meta-Analysis." *Malaria Journal* 14: 209.

Upton, L. M., P. M. Brock, T. S. Churcher, A. C. Ghani, P. W. Gething, and others. 2015. "Lead Clinical and Preclinical Antimalarial Drugs Can Significantly Reduce Sporozoite Transmission to Vertebrate Populations." *Antimicrobial Agents and Chemotherapy* 59 (1): 490–97.

Utzinger, J., Y. Tozan, F. Doumani, and B. H. Singer. 2002. "The Economic Payoffs of Integrated Malaria Control in the Zambian Copperbelt between 1930 and 1950." *Tropical Medicine and International Health* 7 (8): 657–77.

Wagman, J. M., J. P. Grieco, K. Bautista, J. Polanco, I. Brice, and others. 2015. "The Field Evaluation of a Push-Pull System to Control Malaria Vectors in Northern Belize, Central America." *Malaria Journal* 14: 184. http://dx.doi.org/10.1186/s12936-015-0692-5.

Watson, M. 1921. *The Prevention of Malaria in the Federated Malay States: A Record of Twenty Years' Progress.* London: J. Murray.

———. 1953. *African Highway: The Battle for Health in Central Africa.* London: J. Murray.

Webster, J., F. Baiden, J. Bawah, J. Bruce, M. Tivura, and others. 2014. "Management of Febrile Children under Five Years in Hospitals and Health Centers of Rural Ghana." *Malaria Journal* 13: 261.

Wells, T. N. C., R. H. van Huijsduijnen, and W. C. Van Voorhis. 2015. "Malaria Medicines: A Glass Half Full?" *Nature Reviews Drug Discovery* 14 (6): 424–42. http://dx.doi.org/10.1038/nrd4573.

White, M. T., L. Conteh, R. Cibulskis, and A. C. Ghani. 2011. "Costs and Cost-Effectiveness of Malaria Control Interventions: A Systematic Review." *Malaria Journal* 10 (1): 337.

White, N. J., T. T. Duong, C. Uthaisin, F. Nosten, A. P. Phyo, and others. 2016. "Antimalarial Activity of KAF156 in *Falciparum* and *Vivax* Malaria." *New England Journal of Medicine* 375 (12): 1152–60. http://dx.doi.org/10.1056/NEJMoa1602250.

Whitfield, J. 2002. "Portrait of a Serial Killer: A Roundup of the History and Biology of the Malaria Parasite." *Nature.* http://dx.doi.org/10.1038/news021001-6.

WHO (World Health Organization). 2012. *World Malaria Report 2012.* Geneva: WHO.

———. 2014. *World Malaria Report 2014.* Geneva: WHO.

———. 2015a. *Global Technical Strategy for Malaria 2016–2030.* Geneva: WHO. http://apps.who.int/iris/bitstream/10665/176712/1/9789241564991_eng.pdf?ua=1.

———. 2015b. *WHO Malaria Treatment Guidelines.* 3rd ed. Geneva: WHO.

———. 2016a. *WHO Malaria Terminology.* Geneva: WHO. http://apps.who.int/iris/bitstream/10665/208815/1/WHO_HTM_GMP_2016.6_eng.pdf.

———. 2016b. *World Malaria Report 2015.* Geneva: WHO.

———. 2016c. *World Malaria Report 2016.* Geneva: WHO.

WHO Malaria Policy Advisory Committee and Secretariat. 2015. "Malaria Policy Advisory Committee to the WHO: Conclusions and Recommendations of Seventh Biannual Meeting (March 2015)." *Malaria Journal* 14: 295. http://www.ncbi.nlm.nih.gov/pmc/articles/PMC4524000/.

WHO/TDR (Special Programme for Research and Training in Tropical Diseases) and Foundation for the National Institutes of Health. 2014. *Guidance Framework for Testing of Genetically Modified Mosquitoes.* Geneva: WHO.

Wilson, A. L., and on behalf of the IPTc Taskforce. 2011. "A Systematic Review and Meta-Analysis of the Efficacy and Safety of Intermittent Preventive Treatment of Malaria in Children (IPTc)." *PLoS ONE* 6 (2): e16976. http://www.ncbi.nlm.nih.gov/pmc/articles/PMC3038871/.

Yamana, T. K., and E. A. Eltahir. 2013. "Projected Impacts of Climate Change on Environmental Suitability for Malaria Transmission in West Africa." *Environmental Health Perspectives* 121 (10): 1179–86.

Zurovac, D., and A. K. Rowe. 2006. "Quality of Treatment for Febrile Illness among Children at Outpatient Facilities in Sub-Saharan Africa." *Annals of Tropical Medicine and Parasitology* 100 (4): 283–96.

Zurovac, D., J. K. Tibenderana, J. Nankabirwa, J. Ssekitooleko, J. N. Njogu, and others. 2008. "Malaria Case-Management under Artemether-Lumefantrine Treatment Policy in Uganda." *Malaria Journal* 7: 181. http://dx.doi.org/10.1186/1475-2875-7-181.

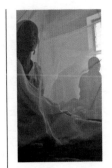

Febrile Illness in Adolescents and Adults

John A. Crump, Paul N. Newton,
Sarah J. Baird, and Yoel Lubell

INTRODUCTION

Fever is one of the most common symptoms reported by patients seeking health care in low-resource areas in the tropics, where it may occur either in isolation or in association with other common symptoms such as cough or diarrhea (Feikin and others 2011; Prasad, Sharples, and others 2015). Fever without localizing features presents a particular challenge to health care workers and health systems because it may be caused by a wide range of bacterial, fungal, parasitic, and viral infections (Crump and others 2013; Mayxay and others 2013), as well as by noninfectious conditions. Clinical assessment has limited accuracy both for identifying the likely cause and for the early recognition of patients who will progress to serious or fatal disease. Compounding the limitations of clinical assessment is the dearth of available epidemiologic data on common causes of fever (Crump 2014) and absence of clinical laboratory services in many areas (Archibald and Reller 2001; Petti and others 2006).

Given its prevalence and severity, malaria has been the common default diagnosis for fever without localizing features in the tropics for decades (WHO 2006). In countries historically highly endemic for malaria, fever is controlled and managed with vertical programs. However, a growing number of fever etiology studies (Prasad, Murdoch, and others 2015; Reyburn and others 2004) and more widespread use of malaria diagnostic tests (WHO 2010b) have served to unmask the problem of malaria

overdiagnosis among febrile patients in many areas. Documented declines in malaria since 2004 (Murray and others 2014; WHO 2013) and expansion of nonmalarial infections such as dengue (Stanaway and others 2016), combined with widespread use of malaria diagnostic tests (WHO 2010b), mean that health care workers face a growing proportion of patients with fever and a negative malaria diagnostic test. This increase is troubling because patients presenting to hospitals with fever not due to malaria are as likely to die as those who have malaria (Reyburn and others 2004). Furthermore, vertical programs exist rarely for febrile illnesses other than malaria.

This chapter identifies key challenges, issues for diagnosis and treatment of relevant infections, and data gaps for health care workers and policy makers regarding nonmalarial fever management and its cost-effectiveness. We highlight the needs for increasing etiologic research, restructuring of burden-of-disease estimates to recognize nonmalarial fever, and development of approaches to evaluating clinical interventions to improve patient outcomes.

BURDEN OF DISEASE FROM NONMALARIAL FEBRILE ILLNESS

No estimate has been made of the global burden of disability and death due to febrile illnesses without localizing features. Consequently, this group of infections has lacked collective prominence. By extension, estimating

Corresponding author: John A. Crump, Centre for International Health, University of Otago, Dunedin, New Zealand; john.crump@otago.ac.nz.

the effect size of interventions for fevers is challenging. Disability-adjusted life years (DALYs), including deaths, from diarrhea and pneumonia are estimated at the syndrome level before being assigned to individual causes by the World Health Organization (WHO) and the Institute for Health Metrics and Evaluation (IHME).[1] However, these sources estimate the individual disease burdens of some causes of fever, such as malaria, dengue, and enteric fever, but not for others, including, for example, chikungunya, leptospirosis, and Q fever.

Thus, the organizational structures of global, national, and academic public health institutions rarely include cross-cutting expertise addressing fever across the range of responsible pathogens. Similarly, fever etiology research has tended to focus on one or a small number of pathogens rather than on a broad range of causes (Prasad, Murdoch, and others 2015).

Also contributing to the difficulty in estimating the global burden of death from febrile illnesses is the inadequacy of autopsy procedures. Verbal autopsy has limited ability to distinguish deaths caused by malaria from other conditions with fever. Verbal autopsy may classify febrile deaths as due to malaria in malaria-endemic areas. Many causes of febrile illness are not available for assignment by verbal autopsy. Even with a positive malaria diagnostic test, deaths assigned to cerebral malaria may be found to be due to other causes on autopsy (Mallewa and others 2007). Complete diagnostic autopsy is not widely available in low-resource areas, but minimally invasive autopsy approaches are being studied as a means to reduce uncertainty regarding causes of death in developing countries (Bassat and others 2013).

NONMALARIAL FEVER IN ADOLESCENTS AND ADULTS

Since 2010, WHO guidelines have recommended that malaria treatment decisions be based on the result of malaria diagnostic tests (WHO 2010b). For patients with positive malaria diagnostic tests, health care workers would prescribe antimalarial treatment and consider co-infections as described in detail in chapter 12 of this volume (Shretta and others 2017). However, for those patients with negative malaria diagnostic tests, health care workers often lack the epidemiological information or laboratory services necessary to support rational diagnostic and management decisions (Crump, Gove, and Parry 2011).

Etiology of Nonmalarial Fever

Annex 14A lists studies conducted from 1980 through 2013 of the etiology of severe febrile illness among, predominantly, adolescents and adults. Key features of studies

undertaken in Africa (N = 16) and South and South-East Asia (N = 11) are described below (Prasad, Murdoch, and others 2015). These studies illustrate both many data gaps and sufficient geographic and seasonal heterogeneity in the etiology of fevers to require subnational empiric treatment guidelines (White and others 2012). The studies also confirm the need for guidelines to respond to changes over time in the etiology of febrile illness and in antimicrobial resistance of relevant pathogens.

Geography

Africa

Considerable data gaps exist in our understanding of the etiology of severe febrile illness in Africa. Few studies investigate more than one or a small group of pathogens, and many countries and some regions lack contemporary studies. Furthermore, standard laboratory-based case definitions are not widely used, and study designs rarely include control groups or other approaches to estimating pathogen-specific attributable fractions.

Reddy, Shaw, and Crump (2010) conducted a systematic review of prospective studies of the etiology of community-acquired bloodstream infection in Africa. Their findings are as follows:

- Of 58,296 patients enrolled in 22 eligible studies in 34 locations from 1984 through 2006, 2,051 (13.5 percent) of 15,166 adolescents and adults had nonmalarial bloodstream infections, yielding 2,078 bloodstream isolates.
- Of these isolates, 1,019 (49.0 percent) were Enterobacteriaceae, including 878 (42.3 percent) *Salmonella enterica*, of which 553 (63.0 percent) were *Salmonella* serovar Typhi, 5 (less than 1.0 percent) *Salmonella* serovar Paratyphi A, and 291 (33.1 percent) nontyphoidal *Salmonella*.
- Among the Enterobacteriaceae, *Salmonella* Typhi predominated in North Africa, whereas nontyphoidal *Salmonella* predominated in East Africa, West and Central Africa, and Southern Africa.
- Among the 141 (6.8 percent) non–*Salmonella* Enterobacteriaceae, *Escherichia coli* accounted for 77 (54.6 percent), *Klebsiella* species (spp.) for 24 (17.0 percent), *Proteus mirabilis* for 17 (12.1 percent), and *Shigella* spp. for 10 (7.1 percent).
- Other Gram-negative organisms caused 341 bloodstream infections (16.4 percent), of which *Brucella* spp. accounted for 275 (80.6 percent), occurring predominantly in North Africa; *Neisseria* spp. for 22 (6.5 percent); *Acinetobacter* spp. for 16 (4.7 percent); and *Pseudomonas* spp. for 15 (4.3 percent).

- Of the 336 (16.2 percent) Gram-positive isolates, *Streptococcus pneumoniae* accounted for 198 (58.9 percent), *Staphylococcus aureus* for 111 (33.0 percent), and other streptococci for 21 (6.3 percent).
- Yeasts caused 39 bloodstream infections (1.9 percent of the total), of which *Cryptococcus* spp. accounted for 31 (79.5 percent) and *Candida* spp. for 5 (12.8 percent). *Histoplasma capsulatum* is sometimes isolated from blood culture (Archibald and others 1998), but urine-antigen testing detects more cases (Lofgren and others 2012).
- Mycobacterial bloodstream infections were found in 173 of the patients tested, of which 166 (96.0 percent) were due to *Mycobacterium tuberculosis* complex, and 2 (1.2 percent) to *M. avium* complex.

The bacterial zoonoses brucellosis, leptospirosis, Q fever, and rickettsial infections are also important causes of febrile illness in Africa. Brucellosis appears to be particularly common in North Africa (Afifi and others 2005; Jennings and others 2007; Reddy, Shaw, and Crump 2010), but it also occurs in Sub-Saharan Africa (Dean and others 2012). Although not often sought, leptospirosis is a common cause of febrile illness in Africa, identified as the cause of fever in up to 20 percent of inpatients in some studies (Parker and others 2007). Q fever was responsible for 2 percent to 9 percent of febrile hospitalizations according to a systematic review of African inpatient studies (Vanderburg and others 2014). Spotted fever group rickettsioses and, in some locations, typhus group rickettsioses are also common among febrile inpatients (Prabhu and others 2011). Viral infections including influenza (Yazdanbakhsh and Kremsner 2009) and arbovirus infections such as chikungunya, dengue, Rift Valley fever, and others also may occur.

South and South-East Asia

Although a relatively large number of studies have examined the epidemiology of single diseases in Asia—for example, typhoid, scrub typhus, and melioidosis—they cover relatively few sites that are concentrated in South-East Asia (Acestor and others 2012). Vast knowledge gaps persist for China and India, with no studies examining the diversity of pathogens stratified by patient age, outpatient or inpatient status, and disease severity.

Deen and others (2012) identified 17 studies of the etiology of community-acquired bloodstream infection in South and South-East Asia. Among those, pathogenic organisms were isolated from 12 percent of adults. Of adults with bloodstream infections, *Salmonella enterica* serotype Typhi was the most common bacterial pathogen (30 percent). Other commonly isolated organisms in adults were *Staphylococcus aureus*, *Escherichia coli*, and

other Gram-negative organisms. China was excluded from the review, and no reports were found from peninsular India, representing an enormous gap in knowledge.

In the Kathmandu Valley of Nepal, Blacksell, Sharma, and others (2007) and Murdoch and others (2004) identified the importance of typhoid, dengue, leptospirosis, scrub typhus, and murine typhus. In Papua, Indonesia, Punjabi and others (2012) found among 227 predominantly adult patients hospitalized with negative malaria diagnostic tests that the most common etiological diagnoses were typhoid, leptospirosis, rickettsioses, and dengue.

In a large study of patients ages 7–49 years at three health centers in rural Cambodia, Mueller and others (2014) identified at least one pathogen in 73.3 percent of febrile patients. The most frequent pathogens were the malaria parasites *Plasmodium vivax* (33.4 percent) and *P. falciparum* (26.5 percent). Others included pathogenic *Leptospira* spp. (9.4 percent), influenza viruses (8.9 percent), dengue viruses (6.3 percent), and *Orientia tsutsugamushi* (3.9 percent). However, in the control group, consisting of nonfebrile persons accompanying febrile patients to health centers, a potential pathogen was identified in 40.4 percent of participants, most commonly malaria parasites and *Leptospira* spp.

In a similar study, but without a control group, Mayxay and others (2013) investigated the etiology of fever in patients ages 5–49 years presenting at two provincial hospitals in rural northern and southern areas of the Lao People's Democratic Republic. They identified at least one pathogen in 41 percent of patients at diagnosis, most commonly dengue (8 percent), scrub typhus (7 percent), Japanese encephalitis virus (JEV) (6 percent), leptospirosis (6 percent), and bacteremia (2 percent). Influenza diagnostics were available for one site, where influenza B was the most frequently detected type (87 percent). However, as described in Cambodia (Kasper and others 2010), 50 percent of cases of influenza B would not have been identified by surveillance for influenza-like illness. In rural Lao PDR, the contribution of bacteremia diagnosed by conventional blood cultures was relatively low (2 percent). The etiologies in children and adults were similar, but the data were not stratified by outpatients and inpatients.

With regard to patient management, Mayxay and others (2013) estimated that azithromycin, doxycycline, ceftriaxone, and ofloxacin would have had substantial efficacy for 13 percent, 12 percent, 8 percent, and 2 percent of patients, respectively. They suggested that empiric treatment with doxycycline for patients with undifferentiated fever and negative rapid diagnostic tests (RDTs) for malaria and dengue could be an appropriate strategy for rural health workers in Lao PDR. Because JEV, usually without encephalitis, was an important cause of fever, JEV vaccination is likely to have a substantial effect on reducing the frequency of patients presenting with fever as well as those developing encephalitis (Mayxay and others 2013).

Despite many data gaps and uncertainties, the evidence highlights the importance of typhoid, dengue, scrub typhus, leptospirosis, and influenza viruses in South and South-East Asia. Relative to Africa, brucellosis and Q fever appear to be less important. Consensus is greatly needed on designing fever studies that emphasize, for example, the inclusion of control groups, especially when sampling sites that are not normally sterile, and standardized reporting. The studies' variation in inclusion criteria and age stratification make summarizing and comparing data between sites difficult. The lack of reports from China and India is especially troubling because, presumably, most persons in Asia developing fevers live in these two countries.

The lack of an evidence base for development and testing of diagnostic accuracy and cost-effectiveness of algorithms of empirical treatment creates much uncertainty for policy makers. A major impediment to better understanding the epidemiology of diverse infections across the continent has been the dearth of quality-assured diagnostic facilities in rural Asia—including the substantial expense and human and technical capacity they would require. The situation suggests that a new model is needed for infectious disease diagnostic facilities in the rural tropics—not one copied from high-income countries (HICs) but a model designed for the local pathogens and environment.

Special Groups

Specific issues arise when considering certain subgroups of patients with fever—particularly pregnant women, individuals infected with the human immunodeficiency virus (HIV), people with diabetes, malaria patients, and people at increased risk for occupational or other types of exposure to certain nonmalarial pathogens. Infections and considerations affecting these special groups are described in table 14.1.

Table 14.1 Febrile Illness Considerations for Special Groups

Group	Disease	Comments	References
Pregnant women	*Plasmodium falciparum* and *Listeria monocytogenes* are more common.	Few data are available on etiology and impact of nonmalarial fevers on mother, fetus, and infant.	Gravett and others 2012; Kourtis, Read, and Jamieson 2014; Louie and others 2010; Machado and others 2013; McGready and others 2010; Say and others 2014
	Hepatitis E and herpes simplex virus disease, malaria, and influenza are more severe.	Some antimicrobials that are important for treatment of bacterial pathogens are contraindicated in pregnancy.	
	Dengue, scrub typhus, and typhoid fever may be more severe.		
	Obstetric sepsis.		
HIV infection	Invasive bacterial and fungal infections, including *Cryptococcus neoformans*, *C. grubii*, nontyphoidal *Salmonella enterica*, and *Mycobacterium tuberculosis* are more common.	Knowledge of patient's HIV infection status assists in differential diagnosis of febrile illness; provider-initiated HIV testing is recommended.	Huson and others 2014; Reddy, Shaw, and Crump 2010; Sanders and others 2014; WHO and UNAIDS 2007
	Acute HIV infection may be common among persons seeking care for fever in areas with concentrated or generalized epidemics.	Few data are available on interaction between HIV and several febrile illnesses.	
Diabetes	Tuberculosis, infections with Enterobacteriaceae, lower respiratory tract infection, urinary tract infection, skin and mucous membrane infection, and melioidosis are more common.	Hyperglycemia impairs antibacterial function of neutrophils and T cell–mediated immune response.	Esper, Moss, and Martin 2009; Faurholt-Jepsen and others 2013; Figueiredo and others 2010; Kapur and Harries 2013; Knapp 2013; Muller and others 2005; Park and others 2011; Suputtamongkol and others 1999; Thomsen and others 2005; Van den Berghe and others 2006
	Poorer outcomes occur with tuberculosis and infections with Enterobacteriaceae.	Few data are available from low-resource settings.	
		Few data are available on interaction between diabetes and several febrile illnesses such as leptospirosis and rickettsial infections.	

table continues next page

Table 14.1 Febrile Illness Considerations for Special Groups (continued)

Group	Disease	Comments	References
Malaria	Nontyphoidal *S. enterica* bloodstream infection and other bacteremias are more common.	Positive malaria film may mean malaria is the cause of current illness, a cofactor in a concurrent infection, or an incidental finding. *P. falciparum* malaria rapid diagnostic tests may remain positive for a month or more after clearance of parasites.	Abba and others 2011; Feasey and others 2012; Kyabayinze and others 2008; Nadjm and others 2010
Occupational and other exposures	Rural residence increases risk for leptospirosis, melioidosis, scrub typhus, and spotted fever group rickettsioses. Pastoralist animal husbandry practices increase risk for brucellosis. Q fever is more common among livestock keepers and abattoir workers. Urban residence is associated with enteric fever and murine typhus.	Knowledge of patient's occupational and exposure history assists in differential diagnosis of febrile illness.	Breiman and others 2012; Cheng and Currie 2005; Shirima and others 2007; Vallée and others 2010; Wardrop and others 2013

Note: HIV = human immunodeficiency virus.

Diagnosis and Treatment of Specific Infections

The initial challenge for managing the febrile patient is deciding whether an antimicrobial agent is indicated and, if so, selecting the most appropriate empiric treatment. Making an etiologic diagnosis allows rationalization and correction of initial treatment. Considerations for diagnosis and treatment of specific infections are summarized in table 14.2.

Other challenges concerning diagnosis and treatment of febrile patients involve the quality of diagnostics and medicines for many of the pathogens considered in this chapter. These issues can be divided into two groups: inadequate diagnostic capacity and poor quality of diagnostics and therapeutic products.

Inadequate Diagnostic Capacity

Because of the relative paucity of investment in and understanding of febrile illnesses, accurate, accessible point-of-care tests (POCTs) are currently inadequate, and evaluations of their diagnostic accuracy and cost-effectiveness are insufficient. Although whole-genome sequencing of pathogens is now commonly performed in research settings in both HICs and low- and middle-income countries (LMICs), no accurate, simple, and affordable diagnostic tests are available for key infections such as typhoid, scrub typhus, and leptospirosis in peripheral health care facilities (Peacock and Newton 2008). This deficiency is in part due to intrinsic difficulties such as low bacterial blood load (Dittrich and others 2014) but also due to a lack of investment in targeted diagnostic research and development. We will not be able to understand and provide evidence to guide health policy without a surge in investment in accurate, simple, and affordable diagnostic tests for these neglected diseases. The success of nonstructural protein 1 (NS1)-based dengue POCTs in assisting with dengue diagnosis in rural facilities suggests that such tests can be developed.

Poor Quality of Diagnostics and Therapeutic Products

The diagnostic tests, vaccines, and medicines necessary to reduce the burden of fevers are often of poor quality, especially in countries with insufficient regulation (Caudron and others 2008; Mori, Ravinetto, and Jacobs 2011; Newton and others 2009). The evidence regarding antimalarials suggests severe quality issues (Tabernero and others 2014), but data regarding diagnostic tests, vaccines, and other classes of medicines are limited.

The only long-term sustainable solution to the poor quality of diagnostics and therapeutic products would be the dramatic strengthening of the authorities that regulate medicines in the 30 percent or so of countries without functional capacity (Newton and others 2009). Health care providers should exercise caution in using diagnostic tests, in case the instructions either inflate the products' claims for diagnostic accuracy or are of poor quality. Furthermore, they should be aware that poor patient outcomes may reflect poor-quality medicines, both substandard and falsified, rather than the disease process itself.

Table 14.2 Nonmalarial Febrile Diseases: Exposure, Diagnosis, Prevention, and Treatment

Disease type	Subgroup	Exposure	Diagnosis	Prevention	Treatment
Arbovirus infections	Dengue	Arthropod vectors	• Detection of antibody and NS1 antigen • Fourfold rise in antibody titer • Demonstration of virus in blood by nucleic acid amplification test	– Mosquito avoidance – Vector control – Vaccine	Supportive
	Japanese encephalitis virus	Arthropod vectors	• Culture or nucleic acid amplification test from serum, cerebrospinal fluid (CSF), or tissue • Detection of virus-specific IgM in CSF confirmed by plaque reduction assay • Demonstration of virus in body fluid by nucleic acid amplification test	– Mosquito avoidance – Vector control – Vaccine	Supportive
	Other (for example, chikungunya)	Arthropod vectors	• Culture or nucleic acid amplification test from serum or tissue • Fourfold rise in antibody titer • Demonstration of virus in tissue by immunohistochemistry or nucleic acid amplification test	– Mosquito avoidance – Vector control	Supportive
Bloodstream infection	Enteric fever	Fecally contaminated water or food	• Blood culture	– Improved water, sanitation, and food safety – Detection and treatment of infected persons – Vaccines	Fluoroquinolones, extended-spectrum cephalosporins, or azithromycin, according to local patterns of susceptibility
	Melioidosis	Exposure to contaminated soil and water	• Blood culture • Culture of throat swab, pus, and other bodily fluids	– Management of exposure to environmental sources – Management of predisposing conditions	• Ceftazidime • Carbapenems (for example, meropenem) usually reserved for severe infections or treatment failures • Amoxicillin-clavulanic acid as second-line therapy; trimethoprim-sulfamethoxazole alone for eradication phase
	Other	Miscellaneous	• Blood culture	– Varies by pathogen	Antimicrobials according to local patterns of susceptibility

table continues next page

Disease type	Subgroup	Exposure	Diagnosis	Prevention	Treatment
Brucellosis	n.a.	Exposure to infected animals and their products	• Fourfold rise in antibody titer by microagglutination test • Nucleic acid amplification test • Blood culture	– Control in animal husbandry – Management of exposure among occupational groups at high risk – Food safety, including pasteurization of dairy products	Doxycycline plus gentamicin or streptomycin, or doxycycline plus rifampin, for six weeks
Leptospirosis	n.a.	Exposure to urine or environments contaminated by the urine of infected animals	• Fourfold rise in antibody titer by microagglutination test • Nucleic acid amplification test • Culture of blood or urine using special media	– Control in animal husbandry and rodent control – Management of exposure among occupational groups at high risk – Management of exposure to environmental sources	Doxycycline, penicillin, cephalosporins
Q fever	n.a.	Exposure to infected animals, their products, and environments	• Fourfold rise in antibody titer by immunofluorescence assay • Nucleic acid amplification test • Culture	– Control in animal husbandry – Management of exposure among occupational groups at high risk – Food safety	Tetracyclines
Rickettsioses	n.a.	Arthropod vectors, vary by pathogen species	• Fourfold rise in antibody titer by immunofluorescence assay • Nucleic acid amplification test • Culture	– Prevention of exposure to vectors – Use of prophylactic tetracyclines in very high risk groups	Tetracyclines

Note: n.a. = not applicable; NS1 = nonstructural protein 1; IgM = immunoglobulin M. "Supportive" treatment refers to measures to prevent, control, or relieve complications.

Integrated Management of Adolescent and Adult Febrile Illness

Management at First-Level Health Facilities

The WHO Integrated Management of Adolescent and Adult Illness (IMAI) guidelines for health workers at first-level facilities, specifically health centers and first-level outpatient clinics, provide guidance on the management of febrile patients (WHO 2009). Management of febrile adolescents and adults at first-level facilities is based on current WHO guidelines for the treatment of malaria (WHO 2010b) and described in detail in chapter 12 of this volume (Shretta and others 2017).

Management at the District Hospital

The WHO IMAI district clinician manual provides guidelines for the hospital care of adolescents and adults in low-resource areas (WHO 2011a). The manual has been subjected to few evaluations to date (Rubach and others 2015). The district clinician manual assumes availability of a minimum level of human resources (medical officer, clinical officer, or senior nurse) and a limited range of essential drugs, equipment, and laboratory and other investigations at the hospital level. Emergency management includes the use of antibacterials (ceftriaxone) and antimalarials (parenteral artesunate) if sepsis or severe malaria is suspected.

Adherence to Guidelines

Considerable evidence indicates that the WHO practice recommendations and diagnostic technologies are often not adopted and used in low-resource areas (English and others 2014). The reasons include poor dissemination, limited training and monitoring, and limited capacity of human and other resources.

Diagnostic Approaches

Laboratory services have been a neglected component of health services in low-resource areas (Archibald and Reller 2001; Petti and others 2006), and patient management has been based predominantly on syndromic approaches (WHO 2009, 2011a). Notable exceptions have been assays in support of programs for the diagnosis and management of HIV, malaria, and tuberculosis (WHO 2010a, 2010b, 2010c). Experts have recommended clinical laboratory services that should be available at various tiers of the health service in low-resource areas (WHO 2008). However, these services remain widely unavailable.

Knowledge of the HIV serostatus of a febrile patient is useful. Many rapid HIV antibody tests have high sensitivity and specificity in established HIV infection (WHO 1997). Further risk stratification for specific HIV co-infections may be based on the results of a CD4-positive T-lymphocyte count when available.[2]

Culture of a sufficient volume of blood is useful for the diagnosis of bloodstream infections (Lee and others 2007). Once available, the results of blood cultures may be used to refine initial antimicrobial management. In addition, aggregate data provide useful information about the local prevalence of pathogens causing bloodstream infection as well as patterns of antimicrobial resistance. Continuously monitored blood culture systems may shorten the time to detection and improve sensitivity compared with manual blood culture methods, but they are more expensive than manual methods. Special blood culture bottles optimize the recovery of organisms with particular growth requirements, including some yeasts, mycobacteria, anaerobes, and leptospires.

Diagnostic tests for many febrile illnesses other than malaria and dengue remain complex, expensive, and limited to a few supranational reference laboratories mostly in HICs. In LMICs, their use has been restricted to a few studies done predominantly in large cities, where conditions differ from those in the vast rural areas (Acestor and others 2012). Newer diagnostics often lack standardization of both operation and interpretation and have not been sufficiently validated in the range of settings in which they will be used.

Independent evaluations of diagnostic tests are vital because key information is often missing from the details provided by the manufacturers, which may claim high sensitivity and specificity without appropriate justification (Blacksell, Bell, and others 2007). For example, high sensitivity and specificity of a dengue POCT has minimal clinical utility for a sample taken seven days after fever onset.

A consensus statement—perhaps linked to the Standards for Reporting of Diagnostic Accuracy (Bossuyt and others 2003) but dedicated to evaluation of infectious disease diagnostic tests, especially POCTs—could help improve the current situation. Because estimates of the sensitivity and specificity of diagnostic tests based on evaluation against a known but imperfect gold standard may be imprecise, Bayesian latent class models may be helpful in their evaluation (Lim and others 2013). Use of filter paper and POCTs as storage matrices for both serological and molecular diagnosis may be a practical way forward in LMICs (Fhogartaigh and others 2015; Smit and others 2014).

Despite these limitations, we would expect that common pathogens, especially if sharing routes of transmission and risk factors, would result in common occurrence of mixed or concurrent infections (Phommasone and others 2013). However, the laboratory diagnosis and management of mixed infections is challenging. Reports of mixed infections often use only serological criteria. However, the problems of antibody persistence and interspecies cross-reaction raise uncertainty about whether these results represent true mixed infections, sequential infections, or cross-reactions. Hence, reports of mixed infections should include explicit discussions of the likely specificity and sensitivity of the diagnostic assays used and the likelihood that the observations represent true concurrent mixed infections (Phommasone and others 2013).

The incidence of mixed infections, including pathogens such as *Salmonella* Typhi and *Streptococcus pneumoniae*, will also be highly influenced by vaccination coverage. The management of mixed infections has received little attention. With regard to bacterial mixed infections, a key consideration is that although doxycycline is likely to be efficacious for pathogens such as scrub typhus and leptospirosis, it would not be for other common pathogens such as *Salmonella* Typhi and *Burkholderia pseudomallei*. Combination therapy may be problematic because of antagonism, such as if bacteriostatic and bactericidal antimicrobials are given in parallel, or adverse reactions.

COSTS OF FEBRILE ILLNESS AND COST-EFFECTIVENESS OF DIAGNOSTICS AND TREATMENTS

This section briefly reviews the evidence on the costs of febrile illness in adolescents and adults and the cost-effectiveness of interventions to improve its management. It then summarizes three new cost-effectiveness evaluations of interventions for the management of fever in hospitals, first-level health facilities, and the community. It concludes with a discussion of how future economic evaluations could improve on common limitations in the existing literature.

Costs to Households and Health Care Providers

As a dominant reason for seeking medical care, febrile illnesses are key drivers of health expenditures and productivity losses. However, no data are available on the economic impact of common diseases such as brucellosis and scrub typhus on either households or health care systems. For other diseases such as melioidosis, limited data are available from hospital settings, where the visible burden of confirmed cases is likely to be a small fraction of the full burden, because pathogens such as *B. pseudomallei* and *Orientia tsutsugamushi* are unlikely to be detected outside well-equipped hospitals.

Although methodological differences among cost-of-illness studies impede comparison of the relative cost burden of different diseases, some general trends can be detected (figure 14.1 and annex 14B). The largest impact is often associated with household productivity losses rather than direct medical costs, a particular concern for adult patients. For melioidosis, the known burden is concentrated among adult agricultural workers; therefore, the economic impact on rural households can be particularly hard. Among hospitalized patients with typhoid fever in India and Indonesia, productivity losses have been as high as 15 percent to 20 percent of annual income (Bahl and others 2004; Poulos and others 2004).

Tellingly, household and provider costs are lower for malaria than for other febrile illnesses among both ambulatory and admitted patients. This finding is evident from both indirect cost-of-illness comparisons and from studies comparing the costs of malaria and nonmalarial cases in the same setting (Ansah and others 2013; Batwala and others 2011; Deressa, Hailemariam, and Ali 2007; Kyaw and others 2014; Morel and others 2008; Mustafa and Babiker 2007; Rammaert and others 2011; Yukich and others 2010). One such study compared household costs for patients diagnosed clinically as having malaria, with and without subsequent confirmation of parasitemia, finding that patients incorrectly diagnosed with malaria were more likely to remain symptomatic at three weeks' follow-up and had a higher risk of reattendance at a health facility (Hume and others 2008). Severe malaria admissions have also been found to be less costly than nonmalarial diseases with similar presentations on the same wards because of lower medication costs and shorter durations of admission (Ayieko and English 2007; Lubell and others 2010).

These differences in cost between malaria and nonmalaria illness could be explained by the concentration of malaria-related studies in low-income Sub-Saharan African countries. However, the differences could also indicate a genuine trend for two reasons. First, with extensive donor support, malaria diagnostics and treatments have become increasingly available across the malaria-endemic world at low cost. Second, the strengthening of distribution mechanisms in the public and private sectors has helped ensure access to rapid diagnosis and effective treatment. Thus, patients suffering from malaria may fare better than those with fever from other causes that often go undiagnosed, or for which effective treatment is unavailable, resulting in a longer duration of illness and higher expenses for repeated seeking of medical care (Reyburn and others 2004).

The high costs of nonmalarial febrile illnesses to households and health care systems suggest considerable scope for cost-effective investment to reduce the impact of these illnesses through prevention, diagnosis, and treatment. Households might also be willing to pay for such interventions should they become available, as has been found regarding a typhoid vaccine in Bangladesh and leptospirosis prevention in the Philippines (Arbiol and others 2013; Cook and others 2009). However, there is virtually no guidance as to the cost-effectiveness of diagnostics and treatments for febrile illnesses other than malaria.

Figure 14.1 Direct and Indirect Costs of Febrile Illnesses in Adolescents and Adults, by Illness, 2012

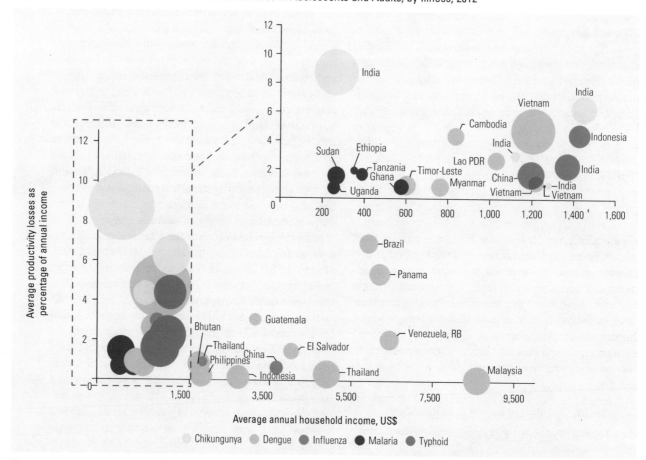

Note: Average household income as reported in the original studies; where not reported, 2012 GDP per capita are used (http://data.worldbank.org/indicator/NY.GDP.PCAP.CD?). Circle size indicates the direct cost of illness, which includes both household and provider direct medical and nonmedical costs per febrile episode relative to household income. The largest circle on the top left, for instance, represents the direct cost of an episode of chikungunya, which in this rural Indian setting is equivalent to 18 percent of annual household income. Most malaria episodes on the bottom left consumed an equivalent of 1 percent to 3 percent of household income, as indicated by the smaller circles. These episodes also resulted in relatively fewer productivity losses, as indicated by their lower vertical positioning. As would be expected, direct costs of illness are regressive, consuming a larger proportion of household income in lower-income settings. However, as indicated by the inverse relationship between household income and productivity losses, these indirect costs also appear to be regressive, with households in lower-income settings losing higher proportions of their income per episode of febrile illness.

Cost-Effectiveness Analyses of Diagnostics and Treatments of Undifferentiated Febrile Illness

Major policy changes by the WHO (WHO 2010b) in the diagnosis and treatment of malaria were well supported by evidence of their cost-effectiveness. For example, the paradigm shift from empiric treatment of fever with anti-malarials toward parasitological confirmation was accompanied by numerous economic evaluations (Ansah and others 2013; Batwala and others 2011; de Oliveira, Castro, and Toscano 2010; Lubell, Hopkins, and others 2008; Shillcutt and others 2008; White and others 2011; Zurovac and others 2006). Several economic evaluations have also compared treatments for uncomplicated malaria, demonstrating the superiority of artemisinin-based combination therapies over preexisting monotherapies (Chanda and others 2007; Wiseman and others 2006) and of

artesunate over quinine for severe malaria (Lubell and others 2009; Lubell and others 2011). Reviews of the cost-effectiveness of preventive interventions for malaria such as insecticide-treated bednets, indoor residual spraying, and intermittent preventive treatment can be found elsewhere (White and others 2011).

Only a few economic evaluations have been carried out on diagnoses and treatments of nonmalarial fevers in the context of LMICs (detailed in annex 14C). This scarcity stems from the dearth of relevant POCTs and treatments that warrant evaluation. Other than dengue and influenza POCTs, no tests have been deemed sufficiently accurate and appropriate for use in routine care. Few advances have been made in recent years for the treatment of nonmalarial fevers, with the exception of new combination therapies for visceral leishmaniasis.

The few available evaluations include cost-effectiveness analyses of the following:

- Leptospirosis tests compared with empiric treatment with doxycycline (Suputtamongkol and others 2010)
- Influenza POCTs for the detection of influenza A (H1N1) in Mexico City (González-Canudas and others 2011)
- Eflornithine compared with melarsoprol for the treatment of human African trypanosomiasis (Robays and others 2008)
- Combination treatments over monotherapy for leishmaniasis (Meheus and others 2010; Olliaro and others 2009)
- Yet-undeveloped prereferral rectal antimicrobial suppositories for severe febrile illness, both alone and in combination with an antimalarial suppository (Buchanan and others 2010).

These studies represent the scant evidence on the cost-effectiveness of diagnostics and treatments for nonmalarial causes of fever. We next extend this limited body of evidence, summarizing three evaluations of diagnostic tools for the management of febrile episodes and sepsis in the hospital, first-level, and community settings.

Surveillance of Bloodstream Infections for Sepsis Management in Low-Resource Settings

A leading cause of mortality among febrile patients in LMICs is bacterial sepsis, but blood culture services are not widely available. Consequently, empiric antimicrobial management of suspected bloodstream infection is based on generic guidelines that are rarely informed by local data on etiology and antimicrobial resistance patterns.

To evaluate the cost-effectiveness of surveillance of bloodstream infections to inform empiric management of suspected sepsis in low-resource areas, Penno, Baird, and Crump (2015) compared costs and outcomes of generic antimicrobial management with management informed by local data on etiology and patterns of antimicrobial resistance across all of Africa. Applying a decision-tree model to a hypothetical population of febrile patients presenting at first-level hospitals in Africa, the authors found that the evidence-based regimen saved an additional 534 lives per 100,000 patients with fever at an increase in cost of US$25.35 per life saved, which corresponded to an incremental cost-effectiveness ratio of US$4,749.[3] Although this number compares favorably to standard cost-effectiveness thresholds, it should ultimately be compared with other relevant policy alternatives to confirm whether routine surveillance for bloodstream infections is a cost-effective strategy in the African context.

POCTs for Sepsis among Patients with Febrile Illnesses in Low-Resource Settings

Similarly, distinguishing patients with sepsis from those with other illnesses remains a challenge. Management decisions are based on clinical assessment using algorithms such as the WHO's IMAI guidelines (WHO 2009, 2011a).

Efforts to develop and evaluate POCTs for sepsis to guide decisions on the use of antimicrobials are under way. To establish the minimum performance characteristics of such a test, Penno, Crump, and Baird (2015) varied the characteristics required for cost-effectiveness of a hypothetical POCT for sepsis and applied similar methods to the bloodstream infection surveillance analysis of Penno, Baird, and Crump (2015). The existing clinical assessment algorithms were compared with POCT-driven management.

Based on a clinical assessment for sepsis with the established sensitivity of 83 percent and specificity of 62 percent, the authors found that a POCT for sepsis with a specificity of 94 percent and a sensitivity of 83 percent was cost-effective, resulting in equivalence with clinical assessment with regard to survival but costing US$1.14 less per life saved. A POCT with sensitivity and specificity of 100 percent, slightly superior to those of the best malaria RDTs, was both cheaper and more effective than clinical assessment. Overall, this work helps establish performance targets for POCTs for sepsis in low-resource areas.

Diagnosis and Treatment Strategies for the Management of Febrile Patients in the Community

Lubell and others (2016) considered the implications of using pathogen-specific tests for dengue and scrub typhus, as compared with testing for a biomarker of host inflammation—C-reactive protein (CRP)—to inform management of fever in the community. Using data on causes of fever in outpatients in rural Lao PDR (Mayxay and others 2013), the proportion of patients that would be correctly treated with an antimicrobial under each of the approaches was estimated as was the cost-effectiveness of the tests.

After accounting for the accuracy of the tests, the following assumptions were made regarding how their results would be used to inform treatment practices:

- Patients with positive dengue test results are not prescribed an antimicrobial.
- Patients with positive scrub typhus test results are prescribed an effective antimicrobial, for example, tetracycline or macrolide.
- Where a pathogen-specific test is negative, antimicrobials are prescribed at random to 38 percent of patients, resembling current practice, with the choice of antibiotic resembling current practice as observed in Mayxay and others (2013).

- Patients with CRP levels below the threshold of 20 milligrams per liter do not receive an antimicrobial; those above the threshold do, with the choice of antibiotic resembling current practice.

The approaches were first evaluated for their ability to classify patients as requiring treatment. Then their ability to guide the choice of antimicrobials, with regard to pathogen susceptibility to the different drugs, was incorporated. Patients with positive scrub typhus tests are therefore assumed to receive doxycycline; for other treated patients, the choice of antimicrobial is made at random based on the frequency of their (often inappropriate) use in current practice.

The analysis suggests that use of either pathogen-specific test offered modest improvements over current practice in the ability to classify patients as requiring an antimicrobial (figure 14.2). The dengue RDT implied a reduction in antimicrobials prescribed for viral infections but a larger proportion of bacterial infections going untreated, while the reverse was true for the scrub typhus test. Use of the CRP test implied both reductions in the use of antimicrobials in viral infections and fewer bacterial infections going untreated. These advantages were consistent despite variation of all model parameters, including the incidence of infections and baseline antimicrobial prescription practices, and when accounting for the

uncertainty surrounding the accuracy of the tests (figure 14.2, panel a).

The incremental costs and DALYs averted from the output of 500 simulations and the corresponding cost-effectiveness acceptability curves are shown in figure 14.3, illustrating that both the scrub typhus and the CRP tests are likely to be cost-effective, despite the considerable uncertainty surrounding many model parameters.

The analysis suggests that pathogen-specific tests can improve the management of nonmalarial fevers, but their utility and cost-effectiveness are highly sensitive to contextual factors such as heterogeneity of fever etiologies and preexisting prescription patterns. Testing for pathogens for which there are no immediate treatment implications, such as dengue, might not offer a direct health benefit over current practice. However, this approach does not account for factors such as patient reassurance in having a confirmed diagnosis, raising of awareness of possible danger signs, outbreak detection, or initiation of measures for vector control. Testing for bacterial pathogens can guide the use of appropriate antimicrobials; therefore, testing could be a cost-effective approach, but cost-effectiveness varies widely depending on local etiology. Testing for biomarkers of inflammation could offer an approach to targeting antimicrobials in rural settings that is cost-effective and robust to heterogeneity in causes of fevers

Figure 14.2 Antimicrobial Targeting Using Lao PDR Data across a Range of Simulated Incidences and Test Accuracies

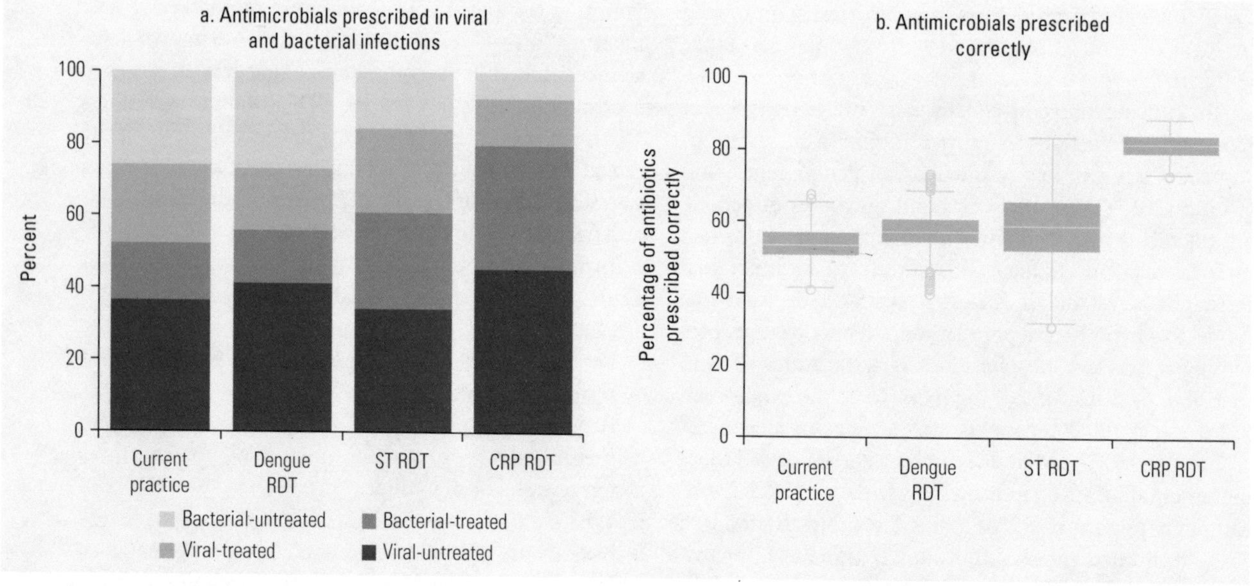

Source: Lubell and others 2016; Mayxay and others 2013.
Note: CRP = C-reactive protein; RDT = rapid diagnostic test; ST = scrub typhus. In panel b, the shaded boxes represent the interquartile ranges of simulated outputs, with the median marked by the mid-way horizontal line. The whiskers represent the simulation outputs closest to 1.5 times the interquartile range, with the remaining outliers shown as independent circles.

Figure 14.3 Cost-Effectiveness Plane and Cost-Effectiveness Probability Curves for the Three Strategies When Compared with a Baseline of Current Practice

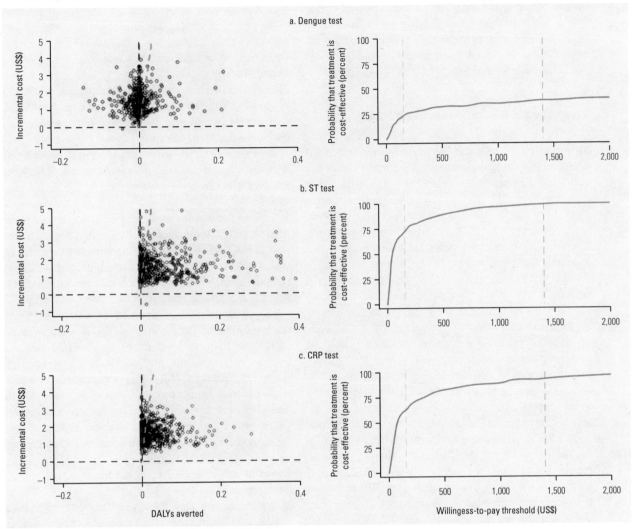

Note: CRP = C-reactive protein; DALY = disability-adjusted life year; ST = scrub typhus. The blue solid lines indicate a willingness-to-pay threshold of US$1,400, approximating Lao PDR's 2012 GDP per capita; the green dashed line is a much more conservative willingness-to-pay threshold of US$150. The dengue test in most instances was associated with worse health outcomes and higher costs. The scrub typhus test averted on average 0.07 DALYs as compared with current practice, and the CRP test averted on average 0.05 DALYs as compared with current practice, with median incremental cost-effectiveness ratios of US$59 and US$110, respectively. When accounting for parameter uncertainty, the scrub typhus and CRP tests are approximately 90 percent and 80 percent likely, respectively, to be cost-effective at a willingness-to-pay threshold of US$1,400.

and host factors typical of the rural tropics, but realizing the full potential gains of this approach requires locally appropriate empirical treatment guidelines.

FUTURE RESEARCH NEEDS

Fever Etiology Research

To provide a clearer picture of the relative importance of relevant causes of nonmalarial febrile illness, fever etiology research is needed that takes into account geographic, seasonal, and ethnic diversity; includes a broad range of treatable or preventable pathogens and their antimicrobial susceptibility patterns; uses standardized case definitions and diagnostic assays; and uses a control group to estimate attributable fractions. The findings of such research would better apprise health care workers about the prior probability of specific infections in their area and would contribute data relevant to burden-of-disease assessments for infections that currently lack robust estimates of illness and death.

Researchers should also consider structuring burden-of-disease estimates for febrile illness without localizing features similarly to estimates for diarrhea and pneumonia. Data from fever etiology research could be applied to the syndrome-wide envelope of DALYs and deaths for febrile illness to develop pathogen-specific estimates. Such an approach would provide the basis for estimating the effects of interventions, including robust cost-effectiveness analyses.

Diagnostic and Clinical Management Studies

POCTs for febrile illnesses can be classified into pathogen-specific tests and biomarker assays that might detect states such as the systemic inflammatory response associated with sepsis. Malaria RDTs demonstrate that a pathogen-specific diagnostic can find an important place in management algorithms for fever in low-resource areas (WHO 2010b). However, current pathogen-specific POCTs for most other causes of fever do not approach the performance of the best malaria RDTs (WHO 2011b). Research priorities for pathogen-specific POCTs should be based on burden-of-disease data and should focus on infections for which potentially lifesaving treatments are available. Biomarker assays that identify a group of patients with severe disease or those likely to develop severe disease could have a role in triage and in the targeting of antimicrobial agents. However, such tests must be at least as sensitive as clinical evaluation to avoid excess deaths and at least as specific as clinical evaluation to avoid antimicrobial overuse and excessive costs.

In addition, clinical management studies are urgently needed to provide a foundation for the best empiric treatment strategies for patients with severe nonmalarial febrile illness (Crump, Gove, and Parry 2011). Studies that support decisions at first-level health care facilities about when to use and when to withhold antimicrobial therapy are essential to optimizing patient outcomes while preserving scarce health care resources and containing antimicrobial resistance.

Necessary Elements for Cost-Effectiveness Analyses

Five elements need to be strengthened for the design of economic evaluations of diagnostics and treatments for febrile illnesses:

- Inclusion of the intervention's implications for all febrile patients rather than for a subset with specific pathogens of interest
- Inclusion of factors affecting the intervention's performance in real-life settings
- Framing of the evaluations within specified etiological contexts and exploration of the implications of heterogeneity

- Extension of the analyses, where appropriate, to include the implications for ongoing pathogen transmission
- Accounting for the intervention's impact on development of antimicrobial resistance.

Inclusion of the Intervention's Implications for All Febrile Patients

An important limitation in many evaluations of malaria diagnostics was the use of malaria-centered outcomes, such as cost per malaria case diagnosed or treated. Such outcomes failed to account for the impact on other nonmalarial diseases—often affecting the majority of patients. What is needed is a clear indication of how the intervention affects the management of febrile patients as a whole.

One of the reasons malaria POCTs were found to be cost-effective was this methodological shift toward inclusion of their potential benefit for other causes of illness, such as the provision of antimicrobials to treatable bacterial infections. In contrast, there was some apprehension that the benefits of malaria POCTs were overestimated in cost-effectiveness analyses, particularly in high-transmission areas, where malaria POCTs could be detrimental to the management of nonmalarial diseases because older children and adults could be carrying malaria parasites to which they are clinically immune while suffering from a potentially severe nonmalarial illness (Bisoffi and others 2011). These considerations will be important in other pathogen-specific tests already on the market for diseases such as dengue and scrub typhus.

Inclusion of Factors Affecting the Intervention's Performance

The performance and impact of the tests in routine settings can be affected by intermediate factors such as interpretation of and adherence to test results, diagnostic test stockouts, and compromised quality due to inadequate storage and handling. For malaria POCTs, the prescribing of antimalarials to patients who had tested negative for malaria was of particular concern, raising the question of whether POCTs were in fact cost-effective in routine care as opposed to in trial settings and model-based evaluations.

An economic evaluation that accounted for compromised adherence demonstrated that although the cost-effectiveness of POCTs was diminished, a substantial degree of nonadherence could be absorbed while use of the tests remained cost-effective (Lubell, Reyburn, and others 2008). Models that incorporate such factors can not only provide a more realistic assessment of the intervention's cost-effectiveness in routine care, but also assist in guiding resources for training and other supportive interventions.

Framing of Evaluations within Specific Etiological Contexts

The diagnostic value of a test is not an inherent characteristic, but one that is strongly influenced by the prior probability of the condition it is designed to detect. This point implies that the suitability of many pathogen-specific tests will vary by etiological setting, both seasonally and spatially. This circumstance is a challenge to effective policy making but also an opportunity to vastly improve the efficient allocation of scarce resources.

Extension of Analyses to Include Implications for Pathogen Transmission

One important concern is the degree to which the analysis should account for the impact of interventions on disease transmission, as opposed to a limited focus on direct costs and benefits to the patient. Although the latter focus can avoid many of the uncertainties that often pervade dynamic transmission models, the more-conservative results of such analyses could unduly penalize an intervention that would be an efficient use of resources if the indirect health benefits associated with reduced transmission were to be considered.

Inclusion of Intervention's Impact on Antimicrobial Resistance

Perhaps most challenging, the evaluations of diagnostics and treatments for fevers could be improved by including the societal costs and consequences associated with antimicrobial resistance (Loubiere and Moatti 2010). The methodological challenges to this approach are considerable and likely explain this glaring omission (Coast, Smith, and Millar 1996). In the absence of such measurements, presumptive treatment will almost always dominate as long as the purchase cost of the drugs is less than that of the diagnostics employed to determine their use, even if this analysis fails to reflect the broader societal costs and consequences of such a strategy (Girosi and others 2006).

Few attempts have been made to define the societal cost per antimicrobial consumed. One such study, in a high-income hospital setting, estimated that each defined daily dose of antimicrobial was associated with a cost of US$7–17 because of its contribution to antimicrobial resistance in that hospital (Kaier and Frank 2010). Despite the difficulties in deriving these values, the inclusion of even highly conservative estimates for these costs in the evaluation of malaria POCTs has been shown to dramatically affect their conclusions (Lubell, Reyburn, and others 2008). If not formally incorporated in the analysis, the implications of their exclusion should at the very least be addressed.

CONCLUSIONS

Declines in malaria in many areas and growing recognition of the problem of malaria overdiagnosis have focused new attention on the problem of management of fevers in low-resource areas. We recommend the following in descending order of priority:

1. Develop accurate pathogen-specific and bacterial disease biomarker POCTs for causes of fever other than malaria.
2. Improve the identification and management of patients with bacterial and fungal sepsis and those with tetracycline-responsive infections to avert morbidity and mortality from febrile illness.
3. Undertake comprehensive, standardized, and coordinated fever etiology research in low-resource areas to identify priorities for improvements in management, such as selection of empiric antimicrobials, and for control of causes of fever other than malaria.
4. Gather more cost and outcome data and improve approaches to cost-effectiveness analyses related to fever to strengthen resource-stratified approaches to adoption and integration of interventions in the emerging field of nonmalarial febrile illness.
5. Support surveillance for bloodstream infections and antimicrobial resistance in low-resource areas.
6. Explore burden-of-disease structures that capture febrile illnesses as a group to estimate the effect size of interventions for fevers.

ANNEXES

The annexes to this chapter are as follows. They are available at http://www.dcp-3.org/infectiousdiseases.

- Annex 14A. Etiology of Severe Febrile Illness: Studies of Adolescents and Adults, by Region, 1980–2013
- Annex 14B. Studies of Febrile Illness Costs to Households and Health Care Providers
- Annex 14C. Studies Reporting the Cost-Effectiveness of Diagnostics and Treatments for Nonmalarial Fevers

NOTES

World Bank Income Classifications as of July 2014 are as follows, based on estimates of gross national income (GNI) per capita for 2013:

- Low-income countries (LICs) = US$1,045 or less
- Middle-income countries (MICs) are subdivided:
  (a) lower-middle-income = US$1,046 to US$4,125
  (b) upper-middle-income (UMICs) = US$4,126 to US$12,745
- High-income countries (HICs) = US$12,746 or more.

1. The WHO estimates the global burden of disease through its Global Health Estimates database, available at http://www.who.int/healthinfo/global_burden_disease/en/. The Institute for Health Metrics and Evaluation (IHME) produces the Global Burden of Diseases, Injuries, and Risk Factors Study. However, some of the IHME's findings have been controversial; for example, it estimated in 2012 that 1.24 million people had died from malaria worldwide in 2010, double the WHO estimate (*The Lancet* 2012).
2. CD4 (cluster of differentiation 4) refers to a T-lymphocyte surface antigen; CD4-positive T-lymphocyte depletion in HIV infection is associated with HIV comorbidities.
3. All costs are in 2012 U.S. dollars.

REFERENCES

Abba, K., J. J. Deeks, P. Olliaro, C. M. Naing, S. M. Jackson, and others. 2011. "Rapid Diagnostic Tests for Diagnosing Uncomplicated *P. falciparum* Malaria in Endemic Countries." *Cochrane Database of Systematic Reviews* 7 (7): CD008122. doi:10.1002/14651858.CD008122.pub2.

Acestor, N., R. Cooksey, P. N. Newton, D. Ménard, P. J. Guerin, and others. 2012. "Mapping the Aetiology of Non-Malarial Febrile Illness in Southeast Asia through a Systematic Review—Terra Incognita Impairing Treatment Policies." *PLoS One* 7 (9): e44269.

Afifi, S., K. Earhart, M. A. Azab, F. G. Youssef, H. El Sakka, and others. 2005. "Hospital-Based Surveillance for Acute Febrile Illness in Egypt: A Focus on Community-Acquired Bloodstream Infections." *American Journal of Tropical Medicine and Hygiene* 73 (2): 392–99.

Ansah, E. K., M. Epokor, C. J. Whitty, S. Yeung, and K. S. Hansen. 2013. "Cost-Effectiveness Analysis of Introducing RDTs for Malaria Diagnosis as Compared to Microscopy and Presumptive Diagnosis in Central and Peripheral Public Health Facilities in Ghana." *American Journal of Tropical Medicine and Hygiene* 89 (4): 724–36.

Arbiol, J., M. Borja, M. Yabe, H. Nomura, N. Gloriani, and others. 2013. "Valuing Human Leptospirosis Prevention Using the Opportunity Cost of Labor." *International Journal of Environmental Research and Public Health* 10 (5): 1845–60.

Archibald, L. K., M. O. den Dulk, K. J. Pallangyo, and L. B. Reller. 1998. "Fatal *Mycobacterium tuberculosis* Bloodstream Infections in Febrile Hospitalized Adults in Dar es Salaam, Tanzania." *Clinical Infectious Diseases* 26 (2): 290–96.

Archibald, L. K., and L. B. Reller. 2001. "Clinical Microbiology in Developing Countries." *Emerging Infectious Diseases* 7 (2): 302–5.

Ayieko, P., and M. English. 2007. "Case Management of Childhood Pneumonia in Developing Countries." *Pediatric Infectious Disease Journal* 26 (5): 432–40.

Bahl, R., A. Sinha, C. Poulos, D. Whittington, S. Sazawal, and others. 2004. "Costs of Illness due to Typhoid Fever in an Indian Urban Slum Community: Implications for Vaccination Policy." *Journal of Health, Population and Nutrition* 22 (3): 304–10.

Bassat, Q., J. Ordi, J. Vila, M. R. Ismail, C. Carrilho, and others. 2013. "Development of a Post-Mortem Procedure to Reduce the Uncertainty Regarding Causes of Death in Developing Countries." *The Lancet Global Health* 1 (3): e125–26.

Batwala, V., P. Magnussen, K. S. Hansen, and F. Nuwaha. 2011. "Cost-Effectiveness of Malaria Microscopy and Rapid Diagnostic Tests versus Presumptive Diagnosis: Implications for Malaria Control in Uganda." *Malaria Journal* 10 (1): 372.

Bisoffi, Z., S. B. Sirima, F. Meheus, C. Lodesani, F. Gobbi, and others. 2011. "Strict Adherence to Malaria Rapid Test Results Might Lead to a Neglect of Other Dangerous Diseases: A Cost Benefit Analysis from Burkina Faso." *Malaria Journal* 10 (1): 226.

Blacksell, S. D., D. Bell, J. Kelley, M. P. Mammen, R. V. Gibbons, and others. 2007. "Prospective Study to Determine Accuracy of Rapid Serological Assays for Diagnosis of Acute Dengue Virus Infection in Laos." *Clinical and Vaccine Immunology* 14 (11): 1458–64.

Blacksell, S. D., N. P. Sharma, W. Phumratanaprapin, K. Jenjaroen, S. J. Peacock, and others. 2007. "Serological and Blood Culture Investigations of Nepalese Fever Patients." *Transactions of the Royal Society of Tropical Medicine and Hygiene* 101 (7): 686–90.

Bossuyt, P. M., J. B. Reitsma, D. E. Bruns, C. A. Gatsonis, P. P. Glasziou, and others. 2003. "Towards Complete and Accurate Reporting of Studies of Diagnostic Accuracy: The STARD Initiative." *BMJ* 326 (7379): 41–44.

Breiman, R. F., L. Cosmas, H. Njuguna, A. Audi, B. Olack, and others. 2012. "Population-Based Incidence of Typhoid Fever in an Urban Informal Settlement and a Rural Area in Kenya: Implications for Typhoid Vaccine Use in Africa." *PLoS One* 7: e29119.

Buchanan, J., B. Mihaylova, A. Gray, and N. White. 2010. "Cost-Effectiveness of Pre-Referral Antimalarial, Antibacterial, and Combined Rectal Formulations for Severe Febrile Illness." *PLoS One* 5 (12): e14446.

Butler, D. 2010. "Verbal Autopsy Methods Questioned." *Nature* 467 (7319): 1015.

Caudron, J. M., N. Ford, M. Henkens, C. Macé, R. Kiddle-Monroe, and others. 2008. "Substandard Medicines in Resource-Poor Settings: A Problem That Can No Longer Be Ignored." *Tropical Medicine and International Health* 13 (8): 1062–72.

Chanda, P., F. Masiye, B. M. Chitah, N. Sipilanyambe, M. Hawela, and others. 2007. "A Cost-Effectiveness Analysis of Artemether Lumefantrine for Treatment of Uncomplicated Malaria in Zambia." *Malaria Journal* 6: 21.

Cheng, A. C., and B. J. Currie. 2005. "Melioidosis: Epidemiology, Pathophysiology, and Management." *Journal of Clinical Microbiology* 18 (2): 383–416.

Coast, J., R. D. Smith, and M. R. Millar. 1996. "Superbugs: Should Antimicrobial Resistance Be Included as a Cost in Economic Evaluation?" *Health Economics* 5 (3): 217–26.

Cook, J., D. Sur, J. Clemens, and D. Whittington. 2009. "Evaluating Investments in Typhoid Vaccines in Two Slums in Kolkata, India." *Journal of Health, Population and Nutrition* 27 (6): 711–24.

Crump, J. A. 2014. "Time for a Comprehensive Approach to the Syndrome of Fever in the Tropics." *Transactions of the Royal Society of Tropical Medicine and Hygiene* 108 (2): 61–62.

Crump, J. A., S. Gove, and C. M. Parry. 2011. "Management of Adolescents and Adults with Febrile Illness in Resource Limited Areas." *BMJ* 343: d4847.

Crump, J. A., A. B. Morrissey, W. L. Nicholson, R. F. Massung, R. A. Stoddard, and others. 2013. "Etiology of Severe Non-Malaria Febrile Illness in Northern Tanzania: A Prospective Cohort Study." *PLoS Neglected Tropical Diseases* 7 (7): e2324.

Dean, A. S., L. Crump, H. Greter, E. Schelling, and J. Zinsstag. 2012. "Global Burden of Human Brucellosis: A Systematic Review of Disease Frequency." *PLoS Neglected Tropical Diseases* 6 (10): e1865.

Deen, J., L. von Seidlein, F. Andersen, N. Elle, N. J. White, and others. 2012. "Community-Acquired Bacterial Bloodstream Infections in Developing Countries in South and Southeast Asia: A Systematic Review." *The Lancet Infectious Diseases* 12 (6): 480–87.

de Oliveira, M. R., G. A. de Castro, and C. M. Toscano. 2010. "Cost Effectiveness of OptiMal® Rapid Diagnostic Test for Malaria in Remote Areas of the Amazon Region, Brazil." *Malaria Journal* 9 (1): 277.

Deressa, W., D. Hailemariam, and A. Ali. 2007. "Economic Costs of Epidemic Malaria to Households in Rural Ethiopia." *Tropical Medicine and International Health* 12 (10): 1148–56.

Dittrich, S., J. Castonguay-Vanier, C. E. Moore, N. Thongyoo, P. N. Newton, and others. 2014. "Loop-Mediated Isothermal Amplification for *Rickettsia typhi* (the Causal Agent of Murine Typhus): Problems with Diagnosis at the Limit of Detection." *Journal of Clinical Microbiology* 52 (3): 832–28.

English, M., D. Gathara, S. Mwinga, P. Ayieko, C. Opondo, and others. 2014. "Adoption of Recommended Practices and Basic Technologies in a Low-Income Setting." *Archives of Disease in Childhood* 99 (5): 452–56.

Esper, A. M., M. Moss, and G. S. Martin. 2009. "The Effect of Diabetes Mellitus on Organ Dysfunction with Sepsis: An Epidemiological Study." *Critical Care* 13 (1): R18.

Faurholt-Jepsen, D., N. Range, G. PrayGod, K. Jeremiah, M. Faurholt-Jepsen, and others. 2013. "Diabetes Is a Strong Predictor of Mortality during Tuberculosis Treatment: A Prospective Cohort Study among Tuberculosis Patients from Mwanza, Tanzania." *Tropical Medicine and International Health* 18 (7): 822–29.

Feasey, N. A., G. Dougan, R. A. Kingsley, R. S. Heyderman, and M. A. Gordon. 2012. "Invasive Non-Typhoidal *Salmonella* Disease: An Emerging and Neglected Tropical Disease in Africa." *The Lancet* 379 (9835): 2489–99.

Feikin, D. R., B. Olack, G. M. Bigogo, A. Audi, L. Cosmas, and others. 2011. "The Burden of Common Infectious Syndromes at the Clinic and Household Level from Population-Based Surveillance in Rural and Urban Kenya." *PLoS One* 6 (1): e16085.

Fhogartaigh, C. N., D. A. Dance, V. Davonga, P. Tannd, R. Phetsouvanha, and others. 2015. "A Novel Technique for Detecting Antibiotic-Resistant Typhoid from Rapid Diagnostic Tests." *Journal of Clinical Microbiology* 53 (5): 1758–60.

Figueiredo, M. A., L. C. Rodrigues, M. L. Barreto, J. W. Lima, M. C. Costa, and others. 2010. "Allergies and Diabetes as Risk Factors for Dengue Hemorrhagic Fever: Results of a Case Control Study." *PLoS Neglected Tropical Diseases* 4 (6): e699.

Girosi, F., S. S. Olmsted, E. Keeler, D. C. Burgess, Y. W. Lim, and others. 2006. "Developing and Interpreting Models to Improve Diagnostics in Developing Countries." *Nature* 444 (Suppl 1): 3–8.

González-Canudas, J., J. M. Iglesias-Chiesa, Y. Romero-Antonio, C. Chávez-Cortes, J. G. Gay-Molina, and others. 2011. "Cost-Effectiveness in the Detection of Influenza H1N1: Clinical Data versus Rapid Tests." *Revista Panamericana de Salud Pública* 29 (1): 1–8.

Gravett, C. A., M. G. Gravett, E. T. Martin, J. D. Bernson, S. Khan, and others. 2012. "Serious and Life-Threatening Pregnancy-Related Infections: Opportunities to Reduce the Global Burden." *PLoS Medicine* 9 (10): e1001324.

Hume, J. C., G. Barnish, T. Mangal, L. Armázio, E. Streat, and others. 2008. "Household Cost of Malaria Overdiagnosis in Rural Mozambique." *Malaria Journal* 7: 33.

Huson, M. A., S. M. Stolp, T. van der Poll, and M. P. Grobusch. 2014. "Community-Acquired Bacterial Bloodstream Infections in HIV-Infected Patients: A Systematic Review." *Clinical Infectious Diseases* 58 (1): 79–92.

Jennings, G. J., R. A. Hajjeh, F. Y. Girgis, M. A. Fadeel, M. A. Maksoud, and others. 2007. "Brucellosis as a Cause of Acute Febrile Illness in Egypt." *Transactions of the Royal Society of Tropical Medicine and Hygiene* 101 (7): 707–13.

Kaier, K., and U. Frank. 2010. "Measuring the Externality of Antibacterial Use from Promoting Antimicrobial Resistance." *Pharmacoeconomics* 28 (12): 1123–28.

Kapur, A., and A. D. Harries. 2013. "The Double Burden of Diabetes and Tuberculosis: Public Health Implications." *Diabetes Research and Clinical Practice* 101 (1): 10–19.

Kasper, M. R., T. F. Wierzba, L. Sovann, P. J. Blair, and S. D. Putnam. 2010. "Evaluation of an Influenza-Like Illness Case Definition in the Diagnosis of Influenza among Patients with Acute Febrile Illness in Cambodia." *BMC Infectious Diseases* 10 (1): 320.

Knapp, S. 2013. "Diabetes and Infection: Is There a Link? A Mini-Review." *Gerontology* 59: 99–104.

Kourtis, A. P., J. S. Read, and D. J. Jamieson. 2014. "Pregnancy and Infection." *New England Journal of Medicine* 370 (23): 2211–18.

Kyabayinze, D. J., J. K. Tibenderana, G. W. Odong, J. B. Rwakimari, and H. Counihan. 2008. "Operational Accuracy and Comparative Persistent Antigenicity of HRP2 Rapid Diagnostic Tests for *Plasmodium falciparum* Malaria in a Hyperendemic Region of Uganda." *Malaria Journal* 7: 221.

Kyaw, S. S., T. Drake, R. Ruangveerayuth, W. Chierakul, N. J. White, and others. 2014. "Cost of Treating Inpatient *falciparum* Malaria on the Thai-Myanmar Border." *Malaria Journal* 13: 416.

Lancet. 2012. "New Estimates of Malaria Deaths: Concern and Opportunity." *The Lancet* 379 (9814): 385.

Lee, A., S. Mirrett, L. B. Reller, and M. C. Weinstein. 2007. "Detection of Bloodstream Infections in Adults: How Many Blood Cultures Are Needed?" *Journal of Clinical Microbiology* 45 (11): 3546–48.

Lim, C., P. Wannapinij, L. White, N. P. Day, B. S. Cooper, and others. 2013. "Using a Web-Based Application to Define the Accuracy of Diagnostic Tests when the Gold Standard Is Imperfect." *PLoS One* 8 (11): e79489.

Lofgren, S. M., E. J. Kirsch, V. P. Maro, A. B. Morrissey, L. J. Msuya, and others. 2012. "Histoplasmosis among Hospitalized Febrile Patients in Northern Tanzania." *Transactions of the Royal Society of Tropical Medicine and Hygiene* 106 (8): 504–7.

Loubiere, S., and J. P. Moatti. 2010. "Economic Evaluation of Point-of-Care Diagnostic Technologies for Infectious Diseases." *Clinical Microbiology and Infection* 16 (8): 1070–76.

Louie, J. K., M. Acosta, D. J. Jamieson, M. A. Honein, and California Pandemic (H1N1) Working Group. 2010. "Severe 2009 H1N1 Influenza in Pregnant and Postpartum Women in California." *New England Journal of Medicine* 362 (1): 27–35.

Lubell, Y., T. Althaus, S. D. Blacksell, D. H. Paris, M. Mayxay, and others. 2016. "Modelling the Impact and Cost-Effectiveness of Biomarker Tests as Compared with Pathogen-Specific Diagnostics in the Management of Undifferentiated Fever in Remote Tropical Settings." *PLoS One* 11 (3): e0152420.

Lubell, Y., H. Hopkins, C. J. Whitty, S. G. Staedke, and A. Mills. 2008. "An Interactive Model for the Assessment of the Economic Costs and Benefits of Different Rapid Diagnostic Tests for Malaria." *Malaria Journal* 7: 21.

Lubell, Y., A. J. Mills, C. J. Whitty, and S. G. Staedke. 2010. "An Economic Evaluation of Home Management of Malaria in Uganda: An Interactive Markov Model." *PLoS One* 5 (8): e12439.

Lubell, Y., H. Reyburn, H. Mbakilwa, R. Mwangi, S. Chonya, and others. 2008. "The Impact of Response to the Results of Diagnostic Tests for Malaria: Cost-Benefit Analysis." *BMJ* 336 (7637): 202–25.

Lubell, Y., A. Riewpaiboon, A. M. Dondorp, L. von Seidlein, O. A. Mokuolu, and others. 2011. "Cost-Effectiveness of Parenteral Artesunate for Treating Children with Severe Malaria in Sub-Saharan Africa." *Bulletin of the World Health Organization* 89 (7): 504–12.

Lubell, Y., S. Yeung, A. M. Dondorp, N. P. Day, F. Nosten, and others. 2009. "Cost-Effectiveness of Artesunate for the Treatment of Severe Malaria." *Tropical Medicine and International Health* 14 (3): 332–27.

Machado, C. R., E. S. Machado, R. D. Rohloff, M. Azevedo, D. P. Campos, and others. 2013. "Is Pregnancy Associated with Severe Dengue? A Review of Data from the Rio de Janeiro Surveillance Information System." *PLoS Neglected Tropical Diseases* 7 (5): e2217.

Mallewa, M., A. R. Fooks, D. Banda, P. Chikungwa, L. Mankhambo, and others. 2007. "Rabies Encephalitis in Malaria-Endemic Area, Malawi, Africa." *Emerging Infectious Diseases* 13(1): 136–39.

Mayxay, M., J. Castonguay-Vanier, V. Chansamouth, A. Dubot-Pérès, D. H. Paris, and others. 2013. "Causes of Non-Malarial Fever in Laos: A Prospective Study." *The Lancet Global Health* 1 (1): e46–54.

McGready, R., E. A. Ashley, V. Wuthiekanun, S. O. Tan, M. Pimanpanarak, and others. 2010. "Arthropod Borne Disease: The Leading Cause of Fever in Pregnancy on the Thai-Burmese Border." *PLoS Neglected Tropical Diseases* 4 (11): e888.

Meheus, F., M. Balasegaram, P. Olliaro, S. Sundar, S. Rijal, and others. 2010. "Cost-Effectiveness Analysis of Combination Therapies for Visceral Leishmaniasis in the Indian Subcontinent." *PLoS Neglected Tropical Diseases* 4 (9): e818.

Morel, C. M., N. D. Thang, N. X. Xa, L. X. Hung, L. K. Thuan, and others. 2008. "The Economic Burden of Malaria on the Household in South-Central Vietnam." *Malaria Journal* 7: 166.

Mori, M., R. Ravinetto, and J. Jacobs. 2011. "Quality of Medical Devices and In Vitro Diagnostics in Resource-Limited Settings." *Tropical Medicine and International Health* 16 (11): 1439–49.

Mueller, T. C., S. Siv, N. Khim, S. Kim, E. Fleischmann, and others. 2014. "Acute Undifferentiated Febrile Illness in Rural Cambodia: A 3-Year Prospective Observational Study." *PLoS One* 9 (4): e95868.

Muller, L. M., K. J. Gorter, E. Hak, W. L. Goudzwaard, F. G. Schellevis, and others. 2005. "Increased Risk of Common Infections in Patients with Type 1 and Type 2 Diabetes Mellitus." *Clinical Infectious Diseases* 41 (3): 281–88.

Murdoch, D. R., C. W. Woods, M. D. Zimmerman, P. M. Dull, R. H. Belbase, and others. 2004. "The Etiology of Febrile Illness in Adults Presenting to Patan Hospital in Kathmandu, Nepal." *American Journal of Tropical Medicine and Hygiene* 70 (6): 670–75.

Murray, C. J., K. F. Ortblad, C. Guinovart, S. S. Lim, T. M. Wolock, and others. 2014. "Global, Regional, and National Incidence and Mortality for HIV, Tuberculosis, and Malaria during 1990–2013: A Systematic Analysis for the Global Burden of Disease Study 2013." *The Lancet* 384 (9947): 1005–70.

Mustafa, M. H., and M. A. Babiker. 2007. "Economic Cost of Malaria on Households during a Transmission Season in Khartoum State, Sudan." *Eastern Mediterranean Health Journal* 13 (6): 1298–307.

Nadjm, B., B. Amos, G. Mtove, J. Ostermann, S. Chonya, and others. 2010. "WHO Guidelines for Antimicrobial Treatment in Children Admitted to Hospital in an Area of Intense *Plasmodium falciparum* Transmission: Prospective Study." *BMJ* 340: c1350. doi:10.1136/bmj.c1350.

Newton, P. N., F. M. Fernandez, M. D. Green, J. Primo-Carpenter, and N. J. White. 2009. "Counterfeit and Substandard Anti-Infectives in Developing Countries." In *Antimicrobial Resistance in Developing Countries*, edited by A. de J. Sosa, D. K. Byarugaba, C. F. Amábile-Cuevas, P.-R. Hsueh, S. Kariuki, and I. N. Okeke, 413–46. New York: Springer.

Olliaro, P., S. Darley, R. Laxminarayan, and S. Sundar. 2009. "Cost-Effectiveness Projections of Single and Combination Therapies for Visceral Leishmaniasis in Bihar, India." *Tropical Medicine and International Health* 14 (8): 918–25.

Park, S.-W., C. S. Lee, C. K. Lee, Y. G. Kwak, C. Moon, and others. 2011. "Severity Predictors in Eschar-Positive Scrub

Typhus and Role of Serum Osteopontin." *American Journal of Tropical Medicine and Hygiene* 85 (5): 924–30.

Parker, T. M., C. K. Murray, A. L. Richards, A. Samir, T. Ismail, and others. 2007. "Concurrent Infections in Acute Febrile Illness Patients in Egypt." *American Journal of Tropical Medicine and Hygiene* 77 (2): 390–92.

Peacock, S. J., and P. N. Newton. 2008. "Public Health Impact of Establishing the Cause of Bacterial Infections in Rural Asia." *Transactions of the Royal Society of Tropical Medicine and Hygiene* 102 (1): 5–6.

Penno, E. C., S. J. Baird, and J. A. Crump. 2015. "Cost-Effectiveness of Surveillance for Bloodstream Infections for Sepsis Management in Low-Resource Settings." *American Journal of Tropical Medicine and Hygiene* 93 (4): 850–60.

Penno, E. C., J. A. Crump, and S. J. Baird. 2015. "Performance Requirements to Achieve Cost-Effectiveness of Point-of-Care Tests for Sepsis among Patients with Febrile Illness in Low-Resource Settings." *American Journal of Tropical Medicine and Hygiene* 93 (4): 841–49.

Petti, C. A., C. R. Polage, T. C. Quinn, A. R. Ronald, and M. A. Sande. 2006. "Laboratory Medicine in Africa: A Barrier to Effective Health Care." *Clinical Infectious Diseases* 42 (3): 377–82.

Phommasone, K., D. H. Paris, T. Anantatat, J. Castonguay-Vanier, S. Keomany, and others. 2013. "Concurrent Infection with Murine Typhus and Scrub Typhus in Southern Laos: The Mixed and the Unmixed." *PLoS Neglected Tropical Diseases* 7 (8): e2163.

Poulos, C., R. Bahl, D. Whittington, M. K. Bhan, J. D. Clemens, and others. 2004. "A Cost-Benefit Analysis of Typhoid Fever Immunization Programmes in an Indian Urban Slum Community." *Journal of Health, Population and Nutrition* 22 (3): 311–21.

Prabhu, M., W. L. Nicholson, A. J. Roche, G. J. Kersh, K. A. Fitzpatrick, and others. 2011. "Q Fever, Spotted Fever Group, and Typhus Group Rickettsioses among Hospitalized Febrile Patients in Northern Tanzania." *Clinical Infectious Diseases* 53 (4): e8–e15.

Prasad, N., D. R. Murdoch, H. Reyburn, and J. A. Crump. 2015. "Etiology of Severe Febrile Illness in Low- and Middle-Income Countries: A Systematic Review." *PLoS One* 10 (6): e0127962.

Prasad, N., K. J. Sharples, D. R. Murdoch, and J. A. Crump. 2015. "Community Prevalence of Fever and Relationship with Malaria among Infants and Children in Low-Resource Areas." *American Journal of Tropical Medicine and Hygiene* 93 (1): 178–80.

Punjabi, N. H., W. R. Taylor, G. S. Murphy, S. Purwaningsih, H. Picarima, and others. 2012. "Etiology of Acute, Non-Malaria, Febrile Illnesses in Jayapura, Northeastern Papua, Indonesia." *American Journal of Tropical Medicine and Hygiene* 86 (1): 46–51.

Rammaert, B., J. Beauté, L. Borand, S. Hem, P. Buchy, and others. 2011. "Pulmonary Melioidosis in Cambodia: A Prospective Study." *BMC Infectious Diseases* 11: 126.

Reddy, E. A., A. V. Shaw, and J. A. Crump. 2010. "Community-Acquired Bloodstream Infections in Africa: A Systematic Review and Meta-Analysis." *The Lancet Infectious Diseases* 10 (6): 417–32.

Reyburn, H., R. Mbatia, C. Drakeley, I. Carneiro, E. Mwakasungula, and others. 2004. "Overdiagnosis of Malaria in Patients with Severe Febrile Illness in Tanzania: A Prospective Study." *BMJ* 329 (7476): 1212–15.

Robays, J., M. E. Raguenaud, T. Josenando, and M. Boelaert. 2008. "Eflornithine Is a Cost-Effective Alternative to Melarsoprol for the Treatment of Second-Stage Human West African Trypanosomiasis in Caxito, Angola." *Tropical Medicine and International Health* 13 (2): 265–71.

Rubach, M. P., V. P. Maro, J. A. Bartlett, and J. A. Crump. 2015. "Etiologies of Illness among Patients Meeting Integrated Management of Adolescent and Adult Illness District Clinician Manual Criteria for Severe Infections in Northern Tanzania: Implications for Empiric Antimicrobial Therapy." *American Journal of Tropical Medicine and Hygiene* 92 (2): 454–62.

Sanders, E. J., P. Mugo, H. A. Prins, E. Wahome, A. N. Thiong'o, and others. 2014. "Acute HIV-1 Infection Is as Common as Malaria in Young Febrile Adults Seeking Care in Coastal Kenya." *AIDS* 28 (9): 1357–63.

Say, L., D. Chou, A. Gemmill, O. Tunçalp, A. B. Moller, and others. 2014. "Global Causes of Maternal Death: A WHO Systematic Analysis." *The Lancet Global Health* 2 (6): e323–33.

Shillcutt, S., C. Morel, C. Goodman, P. Coleman, D. Bell, and others. 2008. "Cost-Effectiveness of Malaria Diagnostic Methods in Sub-Saharan Africa in an Era of Combination Therapy." *Bulletin of the World Health Organization* 86 (2): 101–10.

Shirima, G. M., S. Cleveland, R. R. Kazwala, D. M. Kambarage, N. French, and others. 2007. "Seroprevalence of Brucellosis in Smallholder Dairy, Agropastoral, Pastoral, Beef Ranch and Wildlife Animals in Tanzania." *Bulletin of Animal Health and Production in Africa* 55: 13–21.

Shretta, R., J. Liu, C. Cotter, J. Cohen, C. Dolenz, and others. 2017. "Malaria Elimination and Eradication." In *Disease Control Priorities* (third edition): Volume 6, *Major Infectious Diseases*, edited by K. Holmes, S. Bertozzi, B. Bloom, and P. Jha. Washington, DC: World Bank.

Smit, P. W., I. Elliott, R. W. Peeling, D. Mabey, and P. N. Newton. 2014. "An Overview of the Clinical Use of Filter Paper in the Diagnosis of Tropical Diseases." *American Journal of Tropical Medicine and Hygiene* 90 (2): 195–210.

Stanaway, J. D., D. S. Shepard, E. A. Undurraga, Y. A. Halasa, L. E. Coffeng, and others. 2016. "The Global Burden of Dengue: An Analysis from the Global Burden of Disease Study 2013." *The Lancet Infectious Diseases*. doi:10.1016/S1473-3099(16)00026-8.

Suputtamongkol, Y., W. Chaowagul, P. Chetchotisakd, N. Lertpatanasuwun, S. Intaranongpai, and others. 1999. "Risk Factors for Melioidosis and Bacteremic Melioidosis." *Clinical Infectious Diseases* 29 (2): 408–13.

Suputtamongkol, Y., W. Pongtavornpinyo, Y. Lubell, C. Suttinont, S. Hoontrakul, and others. 2010. "Strategies for Diagnosis and Treatment of Suspected Leptospirosis: A Cost-Benefit Analysis." *PLoS Neglected Tropical Diseases* 4 (2): e610.

Tabernero, P., F. M. Fernández, M. Green, P. J. Guerin, and P. N. Newton. 2014. "Mind the Gaps: The Epidemiology of Poor-Quality Anti-Malarials in the Malarious World: Analysis of the WorldWide Antimalarial Resistance Network Database." *Malaria Journal* 13: 139.

Thomsen, R. W., H. H. Hundborg, H. H. Lervang, S. P. Johnsen, H. C. Schønheyder, and others. 2005. "Diabetes Mellitus as a Risk and Prognostic Factor for Community-Acquired Bacteremia due to Enterobacteria: A 10-Year, Population-Based Study among Adults." *Clinical Infectious Diseases* 40 (4): 628–31.

Vallée, J., T. Thaojaikong, C. E. Moore, R. Phetsouvanh, A. L. Richards, and others. 2010. "Contrasting Spatial Distribution and Risk Factors for Past Infection with Scrub Typhus and Murine Typhus in Vientiane City, Lao PDR." *PLoS Neglected Tropical Diseases* 12: e909.

Van den Berghe, G., A. Wilmer, G. Hermans, W. Meersseman, P. J. Wouters, and others. 2006. "Intensive Insulin Therapy in the Medical ICU." *New England Journal of Medicine* 354 (5): 449–61.

Vanderburg, S., M. P. Rubach, J. E. Halliday, S. Cleaveland, E. A. Reddy, and others. 2014. "Epidemiology of *Coxiella burnetii* Infection in Africa: A OneHealth Systematic Review." *PLoS Neglected Tropical Diseases* 8 (4): e2787.

Wardrop, N. A., C. C. Kuo, H. C. Wang, A. C. Clements, F. F. Lee, and others. 2013. "Bayesian Spatial Modelling and the Significance of Agricultural Land Use to Scrub Typhus Infection in Taiwan." *Geospatial Health* 8 (1): 229–39.

White, L. J., P. N. Newton, R. J. Maude, W. Pan-ngum, J. R. Fried, and others. 2012. "Defining Disease Heterogeneity to Guide the Empirical Treatment of Febrile Illness in Resource Poor Settings." *PLoS One* 7 (9): e44545.

White, M. T., L. Conteh, R. Cibulskis, and A. C. Ghani. 2011. "Costs and Cost-Effectiveness of Malaria Control Interventions: A Systematic Review." *Malaria Journal* 10: 337.

WHO (World Health Organization). 1997. "Joint United Nations Programme on HIV/AIDS (UNAIDS)–WHO Revised Recommendations for the Selection and Use of HIV Antibody Tests." *Weekly Epidemiological Record* 72 (12): 81–88.

———. 2006. *Guidelines for the Treatment of Malaria.* Geneva: WHO.

———. 2008. *Consultation on Technical and Operational Recommendations for Clinical Laboratory Testing Harmonization and Standardization.* Report of consensus meeting of major stakeholders, Maputo, Mozambique, January 22–24.

———. 2009. *Integrated Management of Adolescent and Adult Illness (IMAI) Acute Care: Guidelines for First-Level Facility Health Workers at Health Centre and District Outpatient Clinic.* WHO/CDS/IMAI/2004.1, Rev. 3. Geneva: WHO. http://www.who.int/hiv/pub/imai/acute_care.pdf?ua=1.

———. 2010a. *Antiretroviral Therapy for HIV Infection in Adults and Adolescents. Recommendations for a Public Health Approach: 2010 Revision.* Geneva: WHO.

———. 2010b. *Guidelines for the Treatment of Malaria.* 2nd ed. Geneva: WHO.

———. 2010c. *Guidelines for the Treatment of Tuberculosis.* 4th ed. Geneva: WHO.

———. 2011a. *IMAI District Clinician Manual. Hospital Care for Adolescents and Adults: Guidelines for the Management of Illnesses with Limited Resources.* Geneva: WHO.

———. 2011b. *Malaria Rapid Diagnostic Test Performance. Results of WHO Product Testing of Malaria RDTs: Round 3 (2010–2011).* Geneva: WHO.

———. 2013. *World Malaria Report 2013.* Geneva: WHO.

WHO, and UNAIDS (Joint United Nations Programme on HIV/AIDS). 2007. *Guidance on Provider-Initiated HIV Testing and Counselling in Health Facilities.* Geneva: WHO.

Wiseman, V., M. Kim, T. K. Mutabingwa, and C. J. Whitty. 2006. "Cost-Effectiveness Study of Three Antimalarial Drug Combinations in Tanzania." *PLoS Medicine* 3 (10): e373.

Yazdanbakhsh, M., and P. G. Kremsner. 2009. "Influenza in Africa." *PLoS Medicine* 6 (12): e1000182.

Yukich, J., V. D'Acremont, J. Kahama, N. Swai, and C. Lengeler. 2010. "Cost Savings with Rapid Diagnostic Tests for Malaria in Low-Transmission Areas: Evidence from Dar es Salaam, Tanzania." *American Journal of Tropical Medicine and Hygiene* 83 (1): 61–68.

Zurovac, D., B. A. Larson, W. Akhwale, and R. W. Snow. 2006. "The Financial and Clinical Implications of Adult Malaria Diagnosis Using Microscopy in Kenya." *Tropical Medicine and International Health* 11 (8): 1185–94.

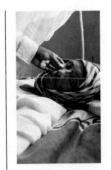

15

Cost-Effectiveness of Strategies for the Diagnosis and Treatment of Febrile Illness in Children

Joseph B. Babigumira, Hellen Gelband, and Louis P. Garrison Jr.

INTRODUCTION

Fever is a common presenting complaint of ill children all over the world. Until recently in Sub-Saharan Africa, fever was synonymous with a presumed diagnosis of malaria. However, malaria is not the only common cause of fever or serious febrile illness (FI) in Sub-Saharan Africa, and the widespread success of malaria control has reduced the region's share of the FI burden. In 2008, 16 percent of the 4.2 million deaths of children in this region were attributed to malaria, 18 percent to pneumonia, and 19 percent to diarrhea (Black and others 2010).

Historically, the response to fever in children in Sub-Saharan Africa was presumptive antimalarial treatment. Cheap, safe, and efficacious antimalarial medications were widely available, and the only method of diagnosis—microscopy—was scarce. The historically inexpensive medicines—chloroquine (CQ) and sulfadoxine/pyrimethamine (SP)—succumbed to the development of drug-resistant malaria parasites; since 2000, these drugs have been replaced as first-line treatment by the more expensive but highly efficacious artemisinin-based combination therapies (ACTs). Rapid diagnostic tests (RDTs) that do not require

laboratory facilities or technical training have become available. In light of these two developments, in 2006 the World Health Organization (WHO) recommended that parasitological confirmation precede malaria treatment except in children in high-transmission settings (WHO 2006), and in 2010 the WHO made the recommendation universal, even for highly exposed children (WHO 2010). Most Sub-Saharan African countries have officially adopted this policy, although few have been able to implement it fully.

The major advantages claimed for pretreatment confirmation of malaria are the following:

- Prevention of unnecessary ACT use, which can save money and reduce drug pressure that could lead to resistance
- More appropriate treatment of nonmalaria fevers
- Improved surveillance and better data for planning.

The appropriateness of the WHO test-and-treat policy is clear in low-endemicity settings; it is not so clear in many high-transmission settings, where all of the supposed advantages have been challenged (D'Acremont and others 2009; English and others 2009; Graz and others 2011).

Corresponding author: Joseph B. Babigumira, Global Medicines Program, Department of Global Health, University of Washington, Seattle, Washington, United States; babijo@uw.edu.

Many economic evaluations have compared malaria RDTs to presumptive treatment and microscopy, using cost-effectiveness methods and measuring the following:

- Cost per correctly diagnosed malaria case (Bualombai and others 2003; Chanda, Castillo-Riquelme, and Masiye 2009; de Oliveira, de Castro Gomes, and Toscano 2010; Fernando and others 2004; Rolland and others 2006)
- Cost per correctly diagnosed and treated malaria case (Batwala and others 2011; Chanda and others 2011; Lubell and others 2007; Ly and others 2010; Rosas Aguirre, Llanos Zavalaga, and Trelles de Belaunde 2009; Willcox and others 2009; Zikusooka, McIntyre, and Barnes 2008)
- Cost per disability-adjusted life year (DALY) averted (Shillcutt and others 2008).

Others have used cost-benefit analysis (Bisoffi and others 2011; Lubell, Hopkins, and others 2008; Lubell, Reyburn, and others 2008).

Most evaluations have found that an RDT test-and-treat approach performs better than a microscopy test-and-treat approach or presumptive treatment below a certain level of malaria endemicity (Batwala and others 2011; Bisoffi and others 2011; Bualombai and others 2003; Chanda, Castillo-Riquelme, and Masiye 2009; Hansen and others 2015; Ly and others 2010; Mosha and others 2010; Msellem and others 2009; Rolland and others 2006; Rosas Aguirre, Llanos Zavalaga, and Trelles de Belaunde 2009; Shillcutt and others 2008; Uzochukwu and others 2009; Zikusooka, McIntyre, and Barnes 2008; Zurovac and others 2008). Microscopy performed better than RDT in Brazil (de Oliveira, de Castro Gomes, and Toscano 2010), Sri Lanka for *Plasmodium vivax* (Fernando and others 2004), and one high-transmission setting (Willcox and others 2009) and about equivalent to RDT in Ghana (Ansah and others 2013).

The most influential factors affecting the results are malaria transmission intensity (Lubell, Hopkins, and others 2008; Zurovac and others 2008), cost and accuracy of the RDTs (Lubell, Hopkins, and others 2008), age (Zikusooka, McIntyre, and Barnes 2008), season (Bisoffi and others 2011), and response to negative test results (Bisoffi and others 2011; Lubell, Reyburn, and others 2008).

The analysis in this chapter assesses the potential cost-effectiveness of RDTs and their role in treatment strategies for overall FI management in children under age five years, taking into account transmission intensity, treatment setting, and relative availability of antibiotic treatment (or no drug treatment) for nonmalaria FI.

It also examines the impact of the availability of different levels of diagnosis on optimal FI management strategy.

METHODOLOGY

Analytic Overview

The reference case for this decision-analytic policy model of FI management is a child under age five years presenting at a point of care (including pharmacies and drug sellers) with fever or history of fever. The model covers a one-month time horizon given the short duration of acute febrile illnesses such as malaria and respiratory tract infections. This chapter presents results for a run of the model using parameters specific to Tanzania, which represent the best estimates from publicly available sources, including the published scientific literature and various reports. The model itself can be adapted to different regions, countries, or settings if local data are available. A key characteristic of the analysis is the planned flexibility of the ranges used for sensitivity analyses, which are varied to reflect current and potential future policy goals or field realities.

The analysis assumes that children with fever may have malaria; treatable nonmalaria febrile illness (T-NMFI), which is illness that responds to appropriate antibiotic treatment; or nontreatable nonmalaria febrile illness (NT-NMFI), which is viral illness. It also assumes that severity assessments are possible at all points of care (which is a simplifying assumption that is not uniformly true) and that, although children may have malaria parasites, the index illness may be caused by something else. (Even in cases of nonclinical malaria infection, it is assumed that eliminating malaria parasites with an antimalarial drug is beneficial.)

The model assesses the costs, effectiveness, and cost-effectiveness of using malaria RDTs and treating children with acute FI with antimalarial drugs, antibiotics, both, or neither. Model parameters include the following: rural versus urban location, type of facility, malaria transmission intensity, etiology of FI, access to diagnostic technology (RDTs and microscopy), antimalarial medications and antibiotics, diagnostic test performance in the field, adherence to negative malaria test results by clinicians or other prescribers, adverse drug events, mortality, and costs (in 2013 U.S. dollars). The analytic framework also allows for the assessment of sequential treatment for FI: children who initially present with mild illness may return with severe illness.

In the base case, malaria diagnosis is by RDTs if available, by microscopy if RDTs are not available, and by no testing if both are unavailable. The base case assumes malaria treatment by ACTs if available, by another antimalarial medicine if ACT is not available, and by a broad-spectrum antibiotic for strategies that include an antibiotic. Differential access to diagnostic tests and drugs is explicitly built into the model, and the base case allows some patients to go without diagnosis or treatment. Variations in the impact of universal access to ACTs and antibiotics are examined using scenario and sensitivity analyses. The main sensitivity analyses assume universal access to ACTs to mirror the likely near-future state of affairs, but this access depends critically on price.

Key scenario and sensitivity analyses are used to answer policy questions that include the impact on optimal FI management strategy of increasing access to diagnostic tests, antimalarial medicines, and antibiotics and whether increasing access to these commodities would have the greatest impact in low- or high-transmission settings, public or private settings, and urban or rural areas. The analytic framework also allows an assessment to be made of the impact of prescriber adherence to negative tests on the optimal strategy. The model calculates the expected probability of survival and costs for different FI management strategies and estimates the optimal strategy from the standpoint of survival, cost, and cost-effectiveness.

Included are the costs of diagnostic technology (RDTs and microscopy), antimalarial medicines, and broad-spectrum antibiotics; the added cost of assessing severity and administering RDTs; the cost of treating mild and severe disease; and the cost of managing adverse events. Direct nonmedical costs incurred by patients and indirect costs due to lost productivity of parents are not included. Health system costs, cost of health worker training, cost of creating demand with behavior change communication, cost of future ACT and antibiotic resistance, and cost of potential RDT use in the private and informal sectors (such as sharps disposal) are not included. This approach constitutes a modified societal perspective for the analysis (Garrison and others 2010).

Comparators: Potential Strategies for Febrile Illness Management

Seven strategies are compared (table 15.1): three presumptive strategies (P-1, P-2, and P-3) and four diagnosis-based strategies (RDT-1, RDT-2, RDT-3, and RDT-4). The strategies were constructed to encompass the following:

- Historical policy options
- Possible policy options given actual conditions in the field
- Pragmatic policy options given system capacity and health workforce issues

Table 15.1 Modeled Febrile Illness Management Strategies

Comparator	RDT administered	Antimalarial given	Antibiotic given
P-1	To none	All	None
P-2	To none	All	If severe illness
P-3	To none	All	All
RDT-1	To all	If RDT positive	None
RDT-2	To all	If RDT positive	If severe illness and malaria, no antibiotic; if severe illness and no malaria, treat with antibiotic
RDT-3	To all	If RDT positive	If no malaria, treat with antibiotic
RDT-4	To all	If RDT positive	If severe illness, treat with antibiotic

Note: P = presumptive treatment; RDT = rapid diagnostic test.

- Potential future options, given improving access to malaria diagnostic technology, ACTs, new bacterial illness diagnostics, and antibiotics.

Some of the strategies are unlikely to be implemented in the real world but have value as historical comparisons or for assessment of the potential impact of poor implementation. In all cases, the diagnostic technology is presumed to be RDT if available, and if RDTs are not available, microscopy if available. The antimalarial is presumed to be an ACT if available, and if an ACT is not available, an alternative antimalarial.

The strategies are as follows:

- *P-1, presumptive treatment with antimalarials only for all children.* Presumptive treatment of FI because malaria was the historical management option in the vast majority of low-income, resource-constrained settings with high malaria endemicity in the pre-RDT era. It remains the default where RDTs are not available and malaria is still common. Under P-1, a child presenting with fever or a history of fever is treated with an ACT if available, another antimalarial if an ACT is not available, and no treatment if ACTs or other antimalarials are not available. P-1 is the base comparator.

- *P-2, presumptive treatment with antimalarials for all children and presumptive treatment with broad-spectrum antibiotics for children with severe illness.* P-2 is modeled around the original version of Integrated Management of Childhood Illness (IMCI), introduced by the WHO in 1997 in response to increasing under-five mortality in low-income countries (WHO 1999). The original version recommended that all children with fever or a history of fever receive a first-line antimalarial drug and be evaluated for signs of other potential causes of fever, such as rapid breathing for pneumonia, followed by appropriate treatment. It did not explicitly recommend parasitological confirmation of malaria.

- *P-3, presumptive treatment with both antimalarials and antibiotics for all children.* P-3 is included as a fallback position in recognition of the difficulty of clinically assessing children for pneumonia and other serious causes of fever. Such assessment is usually not carried out by caregivers making treatment decisions, even in primary care facilities that are understaffed or staffed by poorly trained health care workers.

- *RDT-1, treatment with antimalarials for children who test positive for malaria and no treatment for children who test negative.* RDT-1 is included in the model to demonstrate the potential consequences of untreated T-NMFI. Children with fever are tested for malaria using RDT or microscopy, and those testing positive are treated with an available antimalarial. No antibiotics are prescribed regardless of test result or disease severity.

- *RDT-2, treatment with antimalarials for children who test positive for malaria and presumptive treatment with antibiotics for children with severe illness who test negative.* RDT-2 mirrors the second iteration of IMCI, which recommended that the assessment of children with fever include diagnostic testing for malaria. In the modeling framework, children with fever or a history of fever are tested for malaria using RDT or microscopy and those testing positive are treated with an available antimalarial. Children testing negative are assessed for signs of disease severity (such as fast breathing, dehydration), and those showing signs of severe disease are treated with a broad-spectrum antibiotic in addition to the antimalarial medicine.

- *RDT-3, treatment with antimalarials for children who test positive for malaria and presumptive treatment with broad-spectrum antibiotics for all children who test negative.* RDT-3 is included in the model to demonstrate the potential consequences of presumptive treatment of all NMFI with antibiotics. In the model, children with fever are tested for malaria using RDT or microscopy, and those testing positive

are treated with an available antimalarial. All children testing negative for malaria are treated with a broad-spectrum antibiotic.

- *RDT-4, treatment with antimalarials for children who test positive for malaria and presumptive treatment with broad-spectrum antibiotics for all children with severe disease.* Under RDT-4, children with fever are tested for malaria using RDT or microscopy, and those testing positive are treated with an available antimalarial. All children showing signs of severe disease are treated with a broad-spectrum antibiotic in addition to the antimalarial medicine.

Decision-Analytic Model

The model consists of (1) a "front-end" decision tree that classifies presenting children by their setting of treatment, point of care, diagnostic result, and treatment received, and (2) a "back-end" Markov model that estimates the impact of illness severity, progression, and mortality on costs and outcomes.

The front end of the model is divided into four parts, as shown in figure 15.1: panel a shows FI management strategies, treatment setting, and disease etiology; panel b shows malaria diagnostic test availability and test results (true positive, false negative, false positive, true negative); panel c shows availability and prescription of ACT and antibiotics; and panel d shows availability and prescription of antimalarials (CQ and SP) and antibiotics.

In figure 15.1, panel a, children with FI may present and be treated in rural or urban settings and at one of five points of care: at home by a community health worker, at a general retail outlet, at a drug shop such as duka la dawa baridis in Tanzania or a pharmacy, at a private health facility, or at a public health facility (including nongovernmental organization and faith-based facilities). Children may live and present for treatment in high-transmission-intensity areas (1 or more malaria cases per 1,000 population) or low-transmission-intensity areas (0.051 cases per 1,000 population). Depending on the setting, children may or may not have parasites in their blood. Those who are parasitemic may have clinical malaria or asymptomatic parasitemia, in which case their illness is caused by T-NMFI, usually bacterial infection, or NT-NMFI, usually viral infection. Those who are not parasitemic will similarly have T-NMFI or NT-NMFI. In this analysis, the combined diagnosis of malaria and T-NMFI is modeled, but not the other combined diagnoses such as T-NMFI plus NT-NMFI or malaria plus NT-NMFI.

Figure 15.1 Decision-Analytic Model

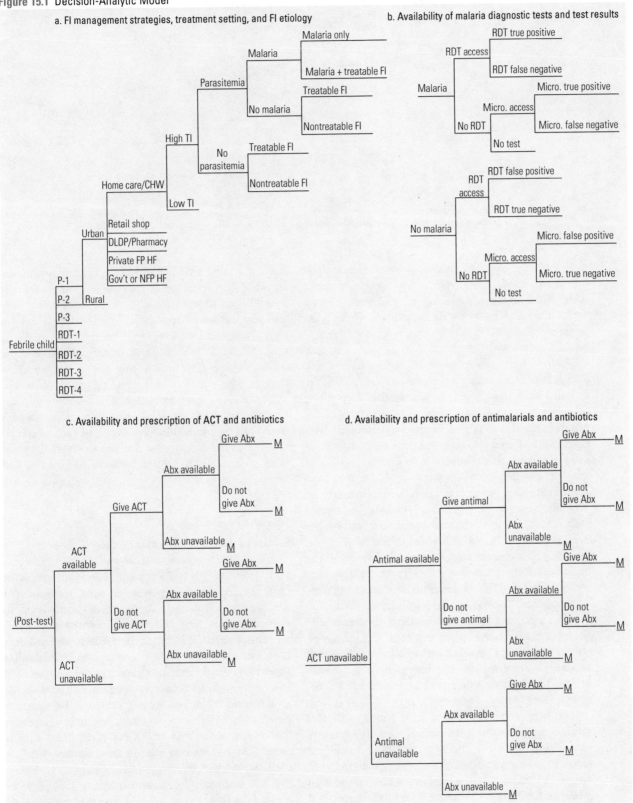

a. FI management strategies, treatment setting, and FI etiology

b. Availability of malaria diagnostic tests and test results

c. Availability and prescription of ACT and antibiotics

d. Availability and prescription of antimalarials and antibiotics

figure continues next page

Figure 15.1 Decision-Analytic Model (continued)

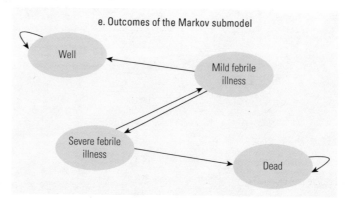

Note: Abx = antibiotics; ACT = artemisinin-based combination therapy; Antimal = antimalarial; CHW = community health worker; DLDB = duka la dawa baridi; FI = febrile illness; FP = for profit; Gov't = government; HF = health facility; M = transition to Markov Model; Micro. = microscopy; NFP = not for profit; RDT = rapid diagnostic test; TI = transmission intensity.

In figure 15.1, panel b, children with malaria (malaria only and malaria plus T-NMFI) as well as children without malaria are subjected to diagnostic testing depending on access to testing technology. At the point of care, malaria RDTs may or may not be available. If available, the model assumes that they are the first choice, but if unavailable, the provider uses microscopy, if available. If microscopy is also unavailable, children are assumed to be treated with an antimalarial. Depending on the performance (sensitivity and specificity) of the malaria test used (RDT or microscopy), patients with malaria are divided into two treatment pools: true positive and false negative. Those without malaria are divided into false positive and true negative pools.

In figure 15.1, panels c and d, following the test and depending on the treatment pool, patients are treated with ACTs, antimalarial medicines, or antibiotics depending on their availability and in line with one of the seven FI management strategies in the model. At the point of care it is assumed that if ACTs are available, they are given, but if ACTS are not available, other antimalarials are given. The model also explicitly considers the provider's decision to give antimalarial medicines and antibiotics in the face of positive or negative malaria test results. In the base case, when no medicines are available, children go untreated. Adverse drug events also occur in the model, depending on the drug given, with consequences for cost but not for mortality.

The Markov model (figure 15.1, panel e) divides acute FI into four health states: well, mild illness, severe illness, and dead. All children start in the mild or severe FI health state. During every cycle, assumed to be one week, children in the mild state may progress to severe and children in the severe state may improve and join the mild state. Children in the mild state may also move to the well state, and children in the severe state

face a mortality risk. The model does not allow mortality other than from the severe state nor complete wellness without moving through the mild state. Both the well and the dead states are absorbing states. The rates of mortality and progression depend on the medicine received and the true diagnosis as defined earlier in the model. Where diagnostic testing results in false negatives or false positives, the model directs patients into incorrect treatment algorithms, which are included in the model. Given that only two transitions are allowed from both the mild and severe states, the rates of transition from mild illness to well and from severe illness to mild are modeled as complements of progression and mortality, respectively.

Tanzania Parameters

Setting of Febrile Illness Management

Tanzania is 26 percent urban and 74 percent rural (Tanzania NBS 2011); 24 percent of children with fever in urban areas and 39 percent in rural areas did not seek fever treatment from health care providers in 2010 (Tanzania NBS and Macro International 2011), an estimate used to represent children under home care, assuming that their point of care is through a pharmacy or drug shop or a community health worker. Information from Kenya is used in the absence of information from Tanzania to estimate the distribution of point of care by different urban facilities (Molyneux and others 1999). For rural areas, a study from Kilosa, Tanzania (Simba and others 2010), is used. An estimated 73 percent of Tanzania's population live in high-transmission-intensity areas, and 27 percent live in low-transmission-intensity areas (WHO 2012b). The model distribution by setting is presented in table 15.2.

Table 15.2 Modeled Distribution of Children with Febrile Illness in Tanzania, by Management Setting, 2013, Based on Best Estimates

Setting	Base case	Reference
Residence		Tanzania NBS 2011
Urban	0.742	
Rural	0.258	
Point of care		
Urban		Molyneaux and others 1999; Tanzania NBS and Macro International 2011
Home care	0.242	
General shop	0.087	
Pharmacy or drug shop	0.270	
Private health facility	0.298	
Government health facility	0.103	
Rural		Simba and others 2010; Tanzania NBS and Macro International 2011
Home care	0.391	
General shop	0.294	
Pharmacy or drug shop	0.092	
Private health facility	0.166	
Government health facility	0.057	
Transmission intensity		WHO 2012b
High	0.730	
Low	0.270	

Table 15.3 Estimated Average Probability of Malaria Parasitemia and Febrile Illness Etiology in Children in Tanzania, 2013

Indicator	Base case	Reference
Parasitemia		
High transmission	0.423	Patrick Kachur and others 2006
Low transmission	0.013	Zanzibar Malaria Control Program and Karolinska Institute 2012
Malaria		
High transmission		Gosoniu and others 2012
Clinical	0.870	
Asymptomatic	0.130	
Low transmission		Assumption
Clinical	0.999	
Asymptomatic	0.001	
NMFI		D'Acremont 2011
Treatable	0.182	
Nontreatable	0.714	
Malaria and treatable NMFI	0.343	D'Acremont 2011

Note: NMFI = nonmalaria febrile illness.

Parasitemia and Etiology of Febrile Illness

In low-transmission areas (Pemba and Zanzibar), the parasite prevalence among children presenting with fever is 0.13 percent (Zanzibar Malaria Control Program and Karolinska Institute 2012), and all patients with parasitemia are expected to have clinical malaria. In high-transmission areas, the parasite prevalence among children with fever is approximately 42 percent (Patrick Kachur and others 2006), and 13 percent of patients with parasitemia are assumed to be asymptomatic (Gosoniu and others 2012).

Table 15.3 presents the parasitemia and etiology of malaria in Tanzania, assuming that 81 percent of acute respiratory infections and 75 percent of other infections of unknown etiology are due to viruses. A treatable co-infection occurs in 34 percent of patients with malaria (D'Acremont 2011).

Availability and Performance of Diagnostic Tests

Table 15.4 differentiates the availability of diagnostic tests between urban and rural settings, assuming at baseline that diagnosis by microscopy is not available in home care, general shops, and duka la dawa baridis. The sensitivity of microscopy in Tanzania is assumed to be 71.4 percent, and specificity is assumed to be 47.3 percent. The sensitivity of RDTs is 97.0 percent, and specificity is 96.8 percent (Kahama-Maro and others 2011).

Availability of Medicines for Febrile Management

In the absence of data from Tanzania, ACT access information from Uganda is used (ACTwatch Group, PACE, and IE Team 2012), combined with published estimates for segments of the population in Tanzania (Simba and others 2010). As an example, in rural areas, access to ACTs is 71 percent in government facilities and 11 percent in private facilities in rural areas (table 15.5).

Prescribing Practices and Prescriber Adherence to Negative Test Results

Based on a randomized trial in Tanzania comparing RDTs with routine microscopy (Reyburn and others 2007), results in table 15.6 assume that all patients who test positive or are not tested receive antimalarials (Lubell, Reyburn, and others 2008).

Table 15.4 Availability and Performance of Rapid Diagnostic Tests and Microscopy in Tanzania, 2013

Indicator	Base case	Reference
RDTs		
Availability		
Urban		
Home care	0.000	Assumption
General shop	0.001	Assumption
Pharmacy or drug shop	0.056	Albertini and others 2012; CPM 2008
Private health facility	0.835	Assumption
Government health facility	0.635	Masanja and others 2012; assumption
Rural		
Home care	0.000	Assumption
General shop	0.000	Assumption
Pharmacy or drug shop	0.000	Assumption
Private health facility	0.635	Assumption
Government health facility	0.435	Masanja and others 2012
Performance		Kahama-Maro and others 2011
Sensitivity	0.970	
Specificity	0.968	
Microscopy		
Availability		
Urban		
Home care	0.000	Assumption
General shop	0.000	Assumption
Pharmacy or drug shop	0.000	Assumption
Private health facility	1.000	Assumption
Government health facility	0.366	Masanja and others 2012; Tanzania NBS and Macro International 2007; assumption
Rural		
Home care	0.000	Assumption
General shop	0.000	Assumption
Pharmacy or drug shop	0.000	Assumption
Private health facility	0.800	Assumption
Government health facility	0.190	Masanja and others 2012
Performance		Kahama-Maro and others 2011; Masanja and others 2012
Sensitivity	0.714	
Specificity	0.473	

Note: RDTs = rapid diagnostic tests.

Table 15.5 Availability of Antimalarial Medicines and Antibiotics in Tanzania, 2013

Indicator	Base case	Reference
ACTs		
Urban		
Home care	0.999	ACTwatch Group, PACE, and IE Team 2012
General shop	0.560	ACTwatch Group, PACE, and IE Team 2012
Pharmacy or drug shop	0.968	ACTwatch Group, PACE, and IE Team 2012
Private health facility	0.791	ACTwatch Group, PACE, and IE Team 2012
Government health facility	0.780	Chimnani and others 2010
Rural		
Home care	0.550	ACTwatch Group, PACE, and IE Team 2012
General shop	0.747	ACTwatch Group, PACE, and IE Team 2012
Pharmacy or drug shop	0.736	Yadav and others 2012
Private health facility	0.110	Simba and others 2010
Government health facility	0.710	Chimnani and others 2010
Other antimalarial drugs		
Urban		
Home care	0.080	ACTwatch Group, PACE, and IE Team 2012
General shop	0.001	ACTwatch Group, PACE, and IE Team 2012
Pharmacy or drug shop	0.995	ACTwatch Group, PACE, and IE Team 2012
Private health facility	0.960	ACTwatch Group, PACE, and IE Team 2012
Government health facility	0.760	Chimnani and others 2010
Rural		
Home care	0.111	ACTwatch Group, PACE, and IE Team 2012
General shop	0.004	ACTwatch Group, PACE, and IE Team 2012
Pharmacy or drug shop	0.999	ACTwatch Group, PACE, and IE Team 2012
Private health facility	0.943	ACTwatch Group, PACE, and IE Team 2012
Government health facility	0.670	Chimnani and others 2010
Antibiotics		
Urban		
Home care	0.000	Assumption
General shop	0.200	Assumption
Pharmacy or drug shop	1.000	Assumption
Private health facility	1.000	Assumption
Government health facility	0.770	Chimnani and others 2010
Rural		
Home care	0.000	Assumption
General shop	0.500	Assumption
Pharmacy or drug shop	1.000	Assumption
Private health facility	1.000	Assumption
Government health facility	0.790	Chimnani and others 2010

Note: ACTs = artemisinin-based combination therapies.

Table 15.6 Average Probability of Prescription of Different Medicines in Tanzania, by Malaria Diagnostic Test Result, 2013

Indicator	Base case	Reference
Antimalarial prescribed		
RDT positive	1.000	Assumption
RDT negative		Reyburn and others 2007
Low transmission	0.697	
High transmission	0.410	
Microscopy positive	1.000	Assumption
Microscopy negative		Reyburn and others 2007
Low transmission	0.626	
High transmission	0.230	
No test	1.000	Assumption
Antibiotic prescribed		
Malaria test positive	0.140	Reyburn and others 2007
Malaria test negative	0.740	Reyburn and others 2007
No test	0.740	Assumption

Note: RDT = rapid diagnostic test.

Table 15.7 Starting Distributions among Markov States in Tanzania, by Diagnosis, 2013

Indicator	Base case	Reference
Well	0.00	
Mild febrile illness		
Malaria		Lubell, Staedke, and others 2011
Low transmission intensity	0.70	
High transmission intensity	0.87	
Treatable febrile illness	0.70	Lubell, Staedke, and others 2011
Nontreatable febrile illness	0.90	Assumption
Severe febrile illness		
Malaria		Lubell, Staedke, and others 2011
Low transmission intensity	0.30	
High transmission intensity	0.13	
Treatable febrile illness	0.30	Lubell, Staedke, and others 2011
Nontreatable febrile illness	0.10	Assumption
Dead	0.00	

Markov Model Parameters

The starting distributions of patients in Markov states, which depend on etiology and, for malaria, on transmission intensity, are summarized in table 15.7. For malaria and treatable nonmalaria FIs, data from a Delphi survey are used (Lubell, Staedke, and others 2011). For nontreatable nonmalaria FI, a 9:1 ratio of mild to severe disease at baseline is assumed.

Adverse Events

For children receiving ACTs and artesunate-mefloquine, 11.3 percent and 63.0 percent, respectively, experience any adverse event (Mueller and others 2006); these figures are used here as the probability of adverse events for other antimalarials; 16 percent experience any adverse event due to amoxicillin (Garbutt and others 2012).

Costs of Diagnosis and Treatment

The costs of RDTs, microscopy, ACTs, other antimalarial medicines, and antibiotics are from ACTwatch (in the absence of data for Tanzania, data from Uganda are used) and from Health Action's *International Medicines Price Workbook* for Tanzania (WHO 2012a). Personnel costs for performing RDTs and for severity assessment are from Uganda. The personnel cost of treating mild disease is estimated for Tanzania to be US$2.66, based on the cost of a single outpatient visit inflated to 2013 costs

(WHO 2011a), and the cost of treating severe disease is estimated to be US$61.07, based on a cost-effectiveness analysis of intravenous artesunate for severe malaria (Lubell, Riewpaiboon, and others 2011). Treating drug-related adverse events is assumed to be equal to the cost of treating mild illness (table 15.8).

Analyses

The base case and the following scenarios were analyzed: (1) universal access to RDTs; (2) universal access to ACTs; (3) universal access to antibiotics; (4) universal access to RDTs and ACTs; (5) universal access to RDTs and antibiotics; (6) universal access to ACTs and antibiotics; and (7) universal access to RDTs, ACTs, and antibiotics. Probabilities were varied by +/− 20 percent, and costs were halved and doubled for sensitivity analyses. TreeAge Pro 2013 was used for the analyses.

RESULTS

In both low- and high-transmission settings and overall, presumptive treatment with ACTs and antibiotics (P-3) leads to the fewest deaths (393 per 10,000 children), and treating only RDT-positive children with an antimalarial alone (RDT-1) leads to the most deaths (484 per 10,000)

Table 15.8 Costs of Diagnosis and Treatment of Febrile Illness in Tanzania

Indicator	Base case (US$)	Reference
RDTs		
Urban		ACTwatch Group, PACE, and IE Team 2012
CHW and home care	1.96	
Public (including PNFP HF)	1.96	
Private FP HF	1.17	
Drug seller (pharmacy or drug shop)	0.98	
General shop or vendor	0.98	
Rural		ACTwatch Group, PACE, and IE Team 2012
CHW and home care	0.78	
Public (including PNFP HF)	0.78	
Private FP HF	1.17	
Drug seller (pharmacy or drug shop)	0.90	
General shop or vendor	0.90	
Microscopy		
Urban		
CHW and home care	—	
Public (including PNFP HF)	0.78	ACTwatch Group, PACE, and IE Team 2012
Private FP HF	0.78	ACTwatch Group, PACE, and IE Team 2012
Drug seller (pharmacy or drug shop)	0.93	ACTwatch Group, PACE, and IE Team 2012
General shop or vendor	—	
Rural		
CHW and home care	—	
Public (including PNFP HF)	0.39	ACTwatch Group, PACE, and IE Team 2012
Private FP HF	0.78	ACTwatch Group, PACE, and IE Team 2012
Drug seller (pharmacy or drug shop)	0.59	ACTwatch Group, PACE, and IE Team 2012
General shop or vendor	—	
ACTs		
Urban		
CHW and home care	0.20	WHO 2011a
Public (including PNFP HF)	4.01	ACTwatch Group, PACE, and IE Team 2012
Private FP HF	9.70	ACTwatch Group, PACE, and IE Team 2012
Drug seller (pharmacy or drug shop)	9.70	ACTwatch Group, PACE, and IE Team 2012
General shop or vendor	9.70	ACTwatch Group, PACE, and IE Team 2012
Rural		
CHW and home care	0.20	WHO 2011a
Public (including PNFP HF)	4.11	ACTwatch Group, PACE, and IE Team 2012

table continues next page

Table 15.8 Costs of Diagnosis and Treatment of Febrile Illness in Tanzania (continued)

Indicator	Base case (US$)	Reference
Private FP HF	9.76	ACTwatch Group, PACE, and IE Team 2012
Drug seller (pharmacy or drug shop)	9.76	ACTwatch Group, PACE, and IE Team 2012
General shop or vendor	9.76	ACTwatch Group, PACE, and IE Team 2012
Non-ACT antimalarials		
Urban		ACTwatch Group, PACE, and IE Team 2012
CHW and home care	0.35	
Public (including PNFP HF)	4.11	
Private FP HF	4.93	
Drug seller (pharmacy or drug shop)	4.93	
General shop and vendor	4.93	
Rural		ACTwatch Group, PACE, and IE Team 2012
CHW and home care	0.35	
Public (including PNFP HF)	2.46	
Private FP HF	4.93	
Drug seller (pharmacy or drug shop)	4.93	
General shop or vendor	4.93	
Antibiotics		
Urban		WHO 2011a
CHW and home care	0.81	
Public (including PNFP HF)	0.78	
Private FP HF	1.86	
Drug seller (pharmacy or drug shop)	1.86	
General shop or vendor	1.86	
Rural		WHO 2011a
CHW and home care	0.81	
Public (including PNFP HF)	0.78	
Private FP HF	1.86	
Drug seller (pharmacy or drug shop)	1.86	
General shop or vendor	1.86	
RDT personnel	0.20	Babigumira and others 2009
Severity assessment	0.30	Babigumira and others 2009
Treatment		
Mild disease	2.66	WHO 2011a
Severe disease	61.07	Lubell, Riewpaiboon, and others 2011
Adverse event	2.66	WHO 2011a

Note: — = not available; ACT = artemisinin-based combination therapy; CHW = community health worker; FP = for profit; HF = health facility; PNFP = private not for profit; RDT = rapid diagnostic test.

(tables 15.9–15.11). In the base case, P-3 is also the least costly strategy (US$251,000 per 10,000 children), but the costs of the strategies vary by less than US$10,000 per 10,000 children in all cases except one (RDT-4—treating RDT-positive children with an antimalarial and all children with severe disease with an antibiotic).

Presumptive treatment with ACTs and antibiotics is the optimal strategy and is highly cost-effective in Tanzania. The ranking of the strategies varies somewhat with endemicity levels, but the leading strategy does not change.

The results are robust to univariate sensitivity analyses. The cost estimates are most sensitive to the

Table 15.9 Survival, Mortality, Costs, and Cost-Effectiveness per 10,000 Children Presenting with Fever in Tanzania

Policy	Survivors	Deaths	Additional lives saved	Cost in 2013 US$	Incremental cost in 2013 US$	Cost-effectiveness
RDT-1	9,516	484	n.a.	258,100	n.a.	Lower than P-1, P-3, RDT-2, and RDT-3
RDT-4	9,562	438	46	263,400	5,300	Lower than P-1, P-2, P-3, RDT-2, and RDT-3
RDT-3	9,563	437	1	255,400	–8,000	Lower than P-1 and P-3
RDT-2	9,563	437	0	256,000	600	Lower than P-1 and P-3
P-1	9,566	434	3	253,500	–2,500	Lower than P-3
P-2	9,606	394	40	258,400	4,900	Lower than P-3
P-3	9,607	393	1	251,000	–7,400	Dominant

Note: n.a. = not applicable.

Table 15.10 Survival, Mortality, Costs, and Cost-Effectiveness per 10,000 Children Presenting with Fever in High-Transmission Areas of Tanzania

Policy	Survivors	Deaths	Additional lives saved	Cost in 2013 US$	Incremental cost in 2013 US$	Cost-effectiveness
RDT-1	9,534	466	n.a.	260,200	n.a.	Lower than P-1, P-3, RDT-2, and RDT-3
RDT-4	9,572	428	38	265,300	5,100	Lower than P-1, P-2, P-3, RDT-2, and RDT-3
RDT-3	9,573	427	1	257,900	–7,400	Lower than P-1 and P-3
RDT-2	9,573	427	0	258,500	600	Lower than P-1 and P-3
P-1	9,587	413	14	255,100	–3,400	Lower than P-3
P-2	9,621	379	34	259,800	4,700	Lower than P-3
P-3	9,622	378	1	252,800	–7,000	Dominant

Note: n.a. = not applicable.

Table 15.11 Survival, Mortality, Costs, and Cost-Effectiveness per 10,000 Children Presenting with Fever in Low-Transmission Areas in Tanzania

Policy	Survivors	Deaths	Additional lives saved	Cost in 2013 US$	Incremental cost in 2013 US$	Cost-effectiveness
RDT-1	9,469	531	n.a.	252,400	n.a.	Lower than P-1, P-3, and RDT-3
P-1	9,508	492	39	249,300	–3,100	Lower than P-3 and RDT-3
RDT-4	9,536	464	28	258,300	9,000	Lower than P-2, P-3, RDT-2, and RDT-3
RDT-3	9,538	462	2	248,700	–9,600	Lower than P-2 and P-3
RDT-2	9,538	462	0	249,500	800	Lower than P-3
P-2	9,566	434	28	254,700	5,200	Lower than P-3
P-3	9,568	432	2	246,100	–8,600	Dominant

Note: n.a. = not applicable.

starting proportion of patients in the severe Markov health state for children with T-NMFI, and mortality is most sensitive to the probability of progression from mild to severe illness for children with T-NMFI.

CONCLUSIONS

Presumptive treatment of all children under age five years with fever, or only those who are severely ill, with both ACTs and a broad-spectrum antibiotic can minimize mortality and is projected to be highly cost-effective by global standards. This result is based on conditions in Tanzania, but it is generalizable to many Sub-Saharan African countries with similar malaria endemicity and health service delivery.

The WHO recommendation of definitive malaria diagnosis before treatment is the clinical practice ideal; physicians aim to make definitive diagnoses before prescribing treatment of any kind. It is a useful goal and should be adopted in clinical settings where a test—microscopy or an RDT—can be conducted reliably. Unfortunately, the places where malaria transmission is highest also tend to be the places where the capacity for testing and reliability are most limited. Drugs are often purchased directly from pharmacies or drug shops or from poorly staffed and provisioned health facilities, both public and private. In these cases, presumptive treatment with antimalarial medicines and antibiotics for all children is the only strategy that prevents the most deaths; it is also optimal from the standpoint of survival and cost-effectiveness. The same conclusion was reached in an independent analysis using a net health benefit approach for six Sub-Saharan African countries (Basu, Modred, and Bendavid 2014).

Price is a major driver of the results of these analyses. If prevailing ACT subsidies were lost and the prices of ACTs were to rise, presumptive treatment would become less attractive from a cost standpoint, but it would not alter the effectiveness side of the equation. Even at a low cost, some individuals are unable to afford ACTs. RDTs have other costs that might further reduce their cost-effectiveness, including the costs of scaling up their use, distribution and storage, sharps disposal, treatment of potential blood-borne infections from needle stick injuries, and behavior change to encourage adherence to test results.

Cost and cost-effectiveness from a model such as this one are but one input into the development of a global treatment policy. This analysis does not monetize certain important externalities, such as the cost of accelerating the development of antibiotic resistance or antimalarial resistance (although the latter may be small). Also important, but impossible to estimate the cost of, is the need to maintain different policies in different areas, even

within the same country. Defining the criteria for delineating the areas where each policy would be appropriate is a hurdle that would be created by having two policies. Even more difficult may be deciding when and how to move from a presumptive to a test-and-treat policy as malaria control continues to lower endemicity levels.

Until primary health care is more widely available, a large proportion of fevers in high-transmission rural areas will be managed in the informal sector, where the analysis suggests that it is more cost-effective to focus on treatment than on diagnostics. In low-transmission-intensity areas and in clinical settings with well-trained practitioners, diagnostics are valuable for targeting treatment. Until the burden of malaria declines more broadly, countries might consider a mixture of strategies tailored to local conditions.

NOTE

World Bank Income Classifications as of July 2014 are as follows, based on estimates of gross national income (GNI) per capita for 2013:

- Low-income countries (LICs) = US$1,045 or less
- Middle-income countries (MICs) are subdivided:
  (a) lower-middle-income = US$1,046 to US$4,125
  (b) upper-middle-income (UMICs) = US$4,126 to US$12,745
- High-income countries (HICs) = US$12,746 or more.

REFERENCES

ACTwatch Group, PACE (Program for Accessible Health, Communication, and Education), and IE (Independent Evaluation) Team. 2012. *ACTwatch Outlet Survey Report 2011 (Round 4). Endline Outlet Survey Report for the Independent Evaluation of Phase 1 of the Affordable Medicines Facility: Malaria (AMFm), Uganda.* Kampala, Uganda: ACTwatch Group, PACE, and IE Team.

Albertini, A., D. Djalle, B. Faye, D. Gamboa, J. Luchavez, and others. 2012. "Preliminary Enquiry into the Availability, Price, and Quality of Malaria Rapid Diagnostic Tests in the Private Health Sector of Six Malaria-Endemic Countries." *Tropical Medicine and International Health* 17 (2): 147–52.

Ansah, E. K., M. Epokor, C. J. Whitty, S. Yeung, and K. S. Hansen. 2013. "Cost-Effectiveness Analysis of Introducing RDTs for Malaria Diagnosis as Compared to Microscopy and Presumptive Diagnosis in Central and Peripheral Public Health Facilities in Ghana." *American Journal of Tropical Medicine and Hygiene* 89 (4): 724–36.

Babigumira, J. B., B. Castelnuovo, M. Lamorde, A. Kambugu, A. Stergachis, and others. 2009. "Potential Impact of Task-Shifting on Costs of Antiretroviral Therapy and Physician Supply in Uganda." *BMC Health Services Research* 9 (192): 192.

Basu, S., S. Modred, and E. Bendavid. 2014. "Comparing Decisions for Malaria Testing and Presumptive Treatment:

A Net Health Benefit Analysis." *Medical Decision Making* 34 (8): 996–1005.

Batwala, V., P. Magnussen, K. S. Hansen, and F. Nuwaha. 2011. "Cost-Effectiveness of Malaria Microscopy and Rapid Diagnostic Tests versus Presumptive Diagnosis: Implications for Malaria Control in Uganda." *Malaria Journal* 10: 372.

Bisoffi, Z., S. B. Sirima, F. Meheus, C. Lodesani, F. Gobbi, and others. 2011. "Strict Adherence to Malaria Rapid Test Results Might Lead to a Neglect of Other Dangerous Diseases: A Cost Benefit Analysis from Burkina Faso." *Malaria Journal* 10: 226.

Black, R. E., S. Cousens, H. L. Johnson, J. E. Lawn, I. Rudan, and others. 2010. "Global, Regional, and National Causes of Child Mortality in 2008: A Systematic Analysis." *The Lancet* 375 (9730): 1969–87.

Bualombai, P., S. Prajakwong, N. Aussawatheerakul, K. Congpoung, S. Sudathip, and others. 2003. "Determining Cost-Effectiveness and Cost Component of Three Malaria Diagnostic Models Being Used in Remote Non-Microscope Areas." *Southeast Asian Journal of Tropical Medicine and Public Health* 34 (2): 322–33.

Chanda, P., M. Castillo-Riquelme, and F. Masiye. 2009. "Cost-Effectiveness Analysis of the Available Strategies for Diagnosing Malaria in Outpatient Clinics in Zambia." *Cost Effectiveness and Resource Allocation* 7: 5.

Chanda, P., B. Hamainza, H. B. Moonga, V. Chalwe, P. Banda, and others. 2011. "Relative Costs and Effectiveness of Treating Uncomplicated Malaria in Two Rural Districts in Zambia: Implications for Nationwide Scale-up of Home-Based Management." *Malaria Journal* 10: 159.

Chimnani, J., J. Kamunyori, E. Bancroft, N. Nazarewicz, N. Kisoka, and others. 2010. *Tanzania: Review of the Health Facility Report and Request Forms at MSD Zonal Stores.* Arlington, VA: USAID Deliver Project.

CPM (Center for Pharmaceutical Management). 2008. *Accredited Drug Dispensing Outlets in Tanzania: Strategies for Enhancing Access to Medicines Program.* Report prepared for the Strategies for Enhancing Access to Medicines Program. Arlington, VA: Management Sciences for Health.

D'Acremont, V. 2011. "Understanding and Improving Malaria Diagnosis in Health Facilities in Dar es Salaam, Tanzania." PhD dissertation, University of Basel.

D'Acremont, V., C. Lengeler, H. Mshinda, D. Mtasiwa, M. Tanner, and others. 2009. "Time to Move from Presumptive Malaria Treatment to Laboratory-Confirmed Diagnosis and Treatment in African Children with Fever." *PLoS Medicine* 6 (1): e252.

de Oliveira, M. R., A. de Castro Gomes, and C. M. Toscano. 2010. "Cost-Effectiveness of OptiMal® Rapid Diagnostic Test for Malaria in Remote Areas of the Amazon Region, Brazil." *Malaria Journal* 9: 277.

English, M., H. Reyburn, C. Goodman, and R. W. Snow. 2009. "Abandoning Presumptive Antimalarial Treatment for Febrile Children Aged Less than Five Years—A Case of Running before We Can Walk?" *PLoS Medicine* 6 (1): e1000015.

Fernando, S. D., N. D. Karunaweera, W. P. Fernando, N. Attanayake, and A. R. Wickremasinghe. 2004. "A Cost Analysis of the Use of the Rapid, Whole-Blood, Immunochromatographic P.f/P.v Assay for the Diagnosis of *Plasmodium vivax* Malaria in a Rural Area of Sri Lanka." *Annals of Tropical Medicine and Parasitology* 98 (1): 5–13.

Garbutt, J. M., C. Banister, E. Spitznagel, and J. F. Piccirillo. 2012. "Amoxicillin for Acute Rhinosinusitis: A Randomized Controlled Trial." *Journal of the American Medical Association* 307 (7): 685–92.

Garrison, L. P., Jr, E. C. Mansley, T. A. Abbott, B. W. Bresnahan, J. W. Hay, and others. 2010. "Good Research Practices for Measuring Drug Costs in Cost-Effectiveness Analyses: A Societal Perspective: The ISPOR Drug Cost Task Force Report—Part II." *Value in Health* 13 (1): 8–13.

Gosoniu, L., A. Msengwa, C. Lengeler, and P. Vounatsou. 2012. "Spatially Explicit Burden Estimates of Malaria in Tanzania: Bayesian Geostatistical Modeling of the Malaria Indicator Survey Data." *PLoS One* 7 (5): e23966.

Graz, B., M. Willcox, T. Szeless, and A. Rougemont. 2011. "'Test and Treat' or Presumptive Treatment for Malaria in High-Transmission Situations? A Reflection on the Latest WHO Guidelines." *Malaria Journal* 10: 136.

Hansen, K. S., E. Grieve, A. Mikhail, I. Mayan, N. Mohammed, and others. 2015. "Cost-Effectiveness of Malaria Diagnosis Using Rapid Diagnostic Tests Compared to Microscopy or Clinical Symptoms Alone in Afghanistan." *Malaria Journal* 14: 217.

Kahama-Maro, J., V. D'Acremont, D. Mtasiwa, B. Genton, and C. Lengeler. 2011. "Low Quality of Routine Microscopy for Malaria at Different Levels of the Health System in Dar es Salaam." *Malaria Journal* 10: 332.

Lubell, Y., H. Hopkins, C. J. Whitty, S. G. Staedke, and A. Mills. 2008. "An Interactive Model for the Assessment of the Economic Costs and Benefits of Different Rapid Diagnostic Tests for Malaria." *Malaria Journal* 7: 21.

Lubell, Y., H. Reyburn, H. Mbakilwa, R. Mwangi, K. Chonya, and others. 2007. "The Cost-Effectiveness of Parasitologic Diagnosis for Malaria-Suspected Patients in an Era of Combination Therapy." *American Journal of Tropical Medicine and Hygiene* 77 (Suppl 6): 128–32.

———. 2008. "The Impact of Response to the Results of Diagnostic Tests for Malaria: Cost-Benefit Analysis." *British Medical Journal* 336 (7637): 202–5.

Lubell, Y., A. Riewpaiboon, A. M. Dondorp, L. von Seidlein, O. A. Mokuolu, and others. 2011. "Cost-Effectiveness of Parenteral Artesunate for Treating Children with Severe Malaria in Sub-Saharan Africa." *Bulletin of the World Health Organization* 89 (7): 504–12.

Lubell, Y., S. G. Staedke, B. M. Greenwood, M. R. Kamya, M. Molyneux, and others. 2011. "Likely Health Outcomes for Untreated Acute Febrile Illness in the Tropics in Decision and Economic Models; A Delphi Survey." *PLoS One* 6 (2): e17439.

Ly, A. B., A. Tall, R. Perry, L. Baril, A. Badiane, and others. 2010. "Use of HRP-2-Based Rapid Diagnostic Test for *Plasmodium falciparum* Malaria: Assessing Accuracy and Cost-Effectiveness in the Villages of Dielmo and Ndiop, Senegal." *Malaria Journal* 9: 153.

Masanja, I., M. Selemani, B. Amuri, D. Kajungu, R. Khatib, and others. 2012. "Increased Use of Malaria Rapid Diagnostic

Tests Improves Targeting of Anti-Malarial Treatment in Rural Tanzania: Implications for Nationwide Rollout of Malaria Rapid Diagnostic Tests." *Malaria Journal* 11 (1): 221.

Molyneux, C. S., V. Mung'Ala-Odera, T. Harpham, and R. W. Snow. 1999. "Maternal Responses to Childhood Fevers: A Comparison of Rural and Urban Residents in Coastal Kenya." *Tropical Medicine and International Health* 4 (12): 836–45.

Mosha, J. F., L. Conteh, F. Tediosi, S. Gesase, J. Bruce, and others. 2010. "Cost Implications of Improving Malaria Diagnosis: Findings from North-Eastern Tanzania." *PLoS One* 5 (1): e8707.

Msellem, M. I., A. Martensson, G. Rotllant, A. Bhattarai, J. Stromberg, and others. 2009. "Influence of Rapid Malaria Diagnostic Tests on Treatment and Health Outcome in Fever Patients, Zanzibar: A Crossover Validation Study." *PLoS Medicine* 6 (4): e1000070.

Mueller, E. A., M. van Vugt, W. Kirch, K. Andriano, P. Hunt, and others. 2006. "Efficacy and Safety of the Six-Dose Regimen of Artemether-Lumefantrine for Treatment of Uncomplicated *Plasmodium falciparum* Malaria in Adolescents and Adults: A Pooled Analysis of Individual Patient Data from Randomized Clinical Trials." *Acta Tropica* 100 (1–2): 41–53.

Patrick Kachur, S., J. Schulden, C. A. Goodman, H. Kassala, B. F. Elling, and others. 2006. "Prevalence of Malaria Parasitemia among Clients Seeking Treatment for Fever or Malaria at Drug Stores in Rural Tanzania 2004." *Tropical Medicine and International Health* 11 (4): 441–51.

Reyburn, H., H. Mbakilwa, R. Mwangi, O. Mwerinde, R. Olomi, and others. 2007. "Rapid Diagnostic Tests Compared with Malaria Microscopy for Guiding Outpatient Treatment of Febrile Illness in Tanzania: Randomised Trial." *British Medical Journal* 334 (7590): 403.

Rolland, E., F. Checchi, L. Pinoges, S. Balkan, J. P. Guthmann, and others. 2006. "Operational Response to Malaria Epidemics: Are Rapid Diagnostic Tests Cost-Effective?" *Tropical Medicine and International Health* 11 (4): 398–408.

Rosas Aguirre, A. M., L. F. Llanos Zavalaga, and M. Trelles de Belaunde. 2009. "Cost-Effectiveness Ratio of Using Rapid Tests for Malaria Diagnosis in the Peruvian Amazon." *Revista Panamericana de Salud Pública* 25 (5): 377–88.

Shillcutt, S., C. Morel, C. Goodman, P. Coleman, D. Bell, and others. 2008. "Cost-Effectiveness of Malaria Diagnostic Methods in Sub-Saharan Africa in an Era of Combination Therapy." *Bulletin of the World Health Organization* 86 (2): 101–10.

Simba, D. O., M. Warsame, D. Kakoko, Z. Mrango, G. Tomson, and others. 2010. "Who Gets Prompt Access to Artemisinin-Based Combination Therapy? A Prospective Community-Based Study in Children from Rural Kilosa, Tanzania." *PLoS One* 5 (8): e12104.

Tanzania NBS (National Bureau of Statistics). 2011. "Tanzania in Figures 2010." NBS, Ministry of Finance, Dar es Salaam, June.

http://www.nbs.go.tz/nbs/takwimu/references/Tanzania_in _Figures2010.pdf.

Tanzania NBS (National Bureau of Statistics) and Macro International. 2007. *Tanzania Service Provision Assessment Survey 2006*. Dar es Salaam: NBS and Macro International.

———. 2011. *Tanzania Demographic and Health Survey 2010*. Dar es Salaam: NBS and Macro International. http://www.measuredhs.com/pubs/pdf/FR243/FR243 [24June2011].pdf.

Uzochukwu, B. S., E. N. Obikeze, O. E. Onwujekwe, C. A. Onoka, and U. K. Griffiths. 2009. "Cost-Effectiveness Analysis of Rapid Diagnostic Test, Microscopy, and Syndromic Approach in the Diagnosis of Malaria in Nigeria: Implications for Scaling-up Deployment of ACT." *Malaria Journal* 8: 265.

WHO (World Health Organization). 1999. *Improving Child Health: Integrated Management of Childhood Illnesses; The Integrated Approach*. Geneva: WHO. http://www.who.int /child_adolescent_health/documents/chd_97_12_Rev_2 /en/index.html.

———. 2006. *Guidelines for the Treatment of Malaria*. Geneva: WHO.

———. 2010. *Guidelines for the Treatment of Malaria*, second edition. Geneva: WHO.

———. 2011. "Estimates of Unit Costs for Patient Services for United Republic of Tanzania." WHO, Geneva. http://www .who.int/choice/country/tza/cost/en/.

———. 2012a. *International Medicines Price Workbook: Part I*. Geneva: WHO and Health Action International/Tanzania.

———. 2012b. *World Malaria Report 2012*. Geneva: WHO. http://www.who.int/malaria/publications/world_malaria _report_2012/wmr2012_full_report.pdf.

Willcox, M. L., F. Sanogo, B. Graz, M. Forster, F. Dakouo, and others. 2009. "Rapid Diagnostic Tests for the Home-Based Management of Malaria, in a High-Transmission Area." *Annals of Tropical Medicine and Parasitology* 103 (1): 3–16.

Yadav, P., J. L. Cohen, S. Alphs, J. Arkedis, P. S. Larson, and others. 2012. "Trends in Availability and Prices of Subsidized ACT over the First Year of the AMFm: Evidence from Remote Regions of Tanzania." *Malaria Journal* 11: 1–11.

Zanzibar Malaria Control Program and Karolinska Institute. 2012. "Malaria in Zanzibar 1999–2011." Presentation by Anders Björkman, May 22. http://www.infektion.net/sites /default/files/pdf/malaria_zanzibar_anders_bjorkman.pdf.

Zikusooka, C. M., D. McIntyre, and K. I. Barnes. 2008. "Should Countries Implementing an Artemisinin-Based Combination Malaria Treatment Policy also Introduce Rapid Diagnostic Tests?" *Malaria Journal* 7: 176.

Zurovac, D., B. A. Larson, J. Skarbinski, L. Slutsker, R. W. Snow, and M. J. Hamel. 2008. "Modeling the Financial and Clinical Implications of Malaria Rapid Diagnostic Tests in the Case-Management of Older Children and Adults in Kenya." *American Journal of Tropical Medicine and Hygiene* 78 (6): 884–91.

Chapter 16

Viral Hepatitis

Stefan Z. Wiktor

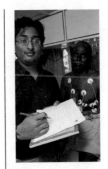

INTRODUCTION

Viral hepatitis is caused by five distinct viruses (hepatitis A, B, C, D, and E), which have different routes of transmission and varying courses of disease (table 16.1). According to the Global Health Estimates, deaths from acute and chronic hepatitis in 2012 were the tenth leading cause of death and the sixteenth leading cause of disability. In 2013, an estimated 1.45 million persons (95 percent uncertainty interval 1.38 million to 1.54 million) died from viral hepatitis; this estimate includes deaths due to acute hepatitis, as well as hepatitis-related liver cancer and cirrhosis (Stanaway and others 2016). Furthermore, while deaths from infectious diseases such as HIV/AIDS, malaria, and tuberculosis are decreasing, deaths from hepatitis increased by 63 percent between 1990 and 2013. Most (96 percent) hepatitis deaths are caused by hepatitis B virus (HBV) and hepatitis C virus (HCV)—these two viruses cause chronic, lifelong infection resulting in progressive liver damage leading to cirrhosis and hepatocellular carcinoma (figure 16.1).

The burden of hepatitis infection is not equally distributed globally. Mortality rates from hepatitis are highest in West Africa and parts of Asia; in absolute numbers, East Asia and South Asia account for the greatest number of people dying from hepatitis—51 percent of the total number of deaths.

Effective interventions exist to prevent transmission of viral hepatitis (table 16.2). Safe and effective vaccines have been developed to prevent hepatitis A, B, and E, and

protection from hepatitis B infection by immunization also prevents hepatitis D.

Hepatitis B and C chronic infections can be treated effectively. The new direct acting antiviral (DAA) medicines for hepatitis C can cure more than 90 percent of those with chronic infection with a two to three month course of treatment. Hepatitis C treatment could also reduce hepatitis C transmission because people who have been cured do not transmit the infection. There is no cure for chronic hepatitis B, but effective antiviral treatments can suppress viral replication and prevent disease progression.

INCIDENCE, PREVALENCE, AND DISTRIBUTION

Because infection with the hepatitis viruses is often asymptomatic, there are no reliable estimates of the incidence of acute and chronic viral hepatitis. An estimated 250 million people live with chronic hepatitis B infection; 80 million have chronic hepatitis C infection (Gower and others 2014; Schweitzer and others 2015).

The prevalence of hepatitis B and C varies considerably in different regions. The areas of highest prevalence for hepatitis B are West Africa, where in some countries more than 8 percent of the population is infected, and East and Central Asia (map 16.1). For hepatitis C infection, the regions with the highest prevalence are West and Central Africa, Eastern Europe, and Central Asia. The prevalence of hepatitis C infection is extremely high in a few countries, most notably,

Corresponding author: Stefan Z. Wiktor, School of Public Health, University of Washington, Seattle, Washington, United States; wiktors@uw.edu.

Table 16.1 Characteristics of Main Types of Viral Hepatitis Infections

	Hepatitis A	Hepatitis B with or without hepatitis D	Hepatitis C	Hepatitis E
Mode of transmission	Contaminated food or water	Blood, sex, mother-to-child		Contaminated food or water
				Undercooked pork and pork liver
Number of chronic infections	0	Approximately 250 million	Approximately 80 million	Very few and mainly in immuno-suppressed persons
Disease outcomes	Fulminant hepatitis	Fulminant hepatitis; cirrhosis and hepatocellular carcinoma		Fulminant hepatitis; maternal mortality

Figure 16.1 Number of Deaths per Year Due to Hepatitis, HIV/AIDS, Tuberculosis, and Malaria, 2000–15

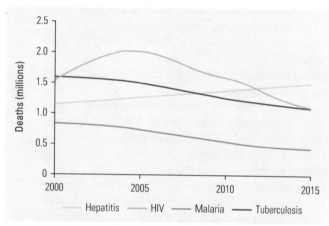

Sources: Hepatitis: GBD 2013 Mortality and Causes of Death Collaborators 2015; HIV: UNAIDS 2015; Malaria: WHO and UNICEF 2015; Tuberculosis: WHO 2015a.
Note: HIV/AIDS = human immunodeficiency virus/acquired immune deficiency syndrome.

Table 16.2 Elements of a Comprehensive Hepatitis Prevention Program

Prevention intervention	Hepatitis virus types
Safe water and food	A, E
Hepatitis A vaccination according to the country's epidemiological situation	A
Hepatitis B vaccination for all children and administration of birth dose; vaccination of health care workers and at-risk adults	B, D
Access to safe blood (universal screening of all blood donations in a quality-assured manner)	B, C, D
Access to sterile injections and other invasive medical equipment in formal and informal health settings	B, C, D
Access to sterile injection equipment and other harm-reduction measures for people who inject drugs	B, C, D
Promotion of safe sex practices	A, B, C

the Arab Republic of Egypt and Pakistan, where high incidence continues, largely the result of weak prevention measures, such as reuse of syringes and needles in health care settings (Ahmed and others 2013; Mostafa and others 2010).

NATURAL HISTORY AND MORTALITY FROM VIRAL HEPATITIS

The natural history of the hepatitis viruses can be categorized based on whether they cause chronic infection. All hepatitis viruses cause acute hepatitis, which can result in fulminant hepatitis in rare cases and may be fatal. Hepatitis B and hepatitis C also can cause chronic infection. Hepatitis D is an incomplete virus that can only replicate and cause infection in the presence of hepatitis B.

The risk of developing chronic hepatitis B infection depends on the age at infection; it declines from more than 90 percent among children infected during the first year to 20 percent to 30 percent for children infected between the ages of 1 and 5 years, and 6 percent for children ages 5 to 15 years (Edmunds and others 1993). For hepatitis C, approximately one-third of individuals will spontaneously clear infection, while the remaining two-thirds will develop chronic infection. For both viruses, chronic infection is marked by continued replication of the virus in the liver, which can lead to cirrhosis, hepatocellular carcinoma, or both (Chen, Iloeje, and Yang 2007; Thein and others 2008). These two conditions account for more than 90 percent of all deaths due to viral hepatitis (figure 16.2) (Stanaway and others 2016). Chronic hepatitis B or hepatitis C infections cause an estimated 78 percent of all liver cancer and 57 percent of all liver cirrhosis (Perz and others 2006). Because of the higher prevalence of hepatitis B and hepatitis C in Asia and Sub-Saharan Africa, countries in these regions, which are least able to deal with these diseases, experience the highest rates of death due to viral hepatitis.

Map 16.1 Hepatitis Mortality Rates and Virus Distribution, by Global Burden of Disease Region, 2013

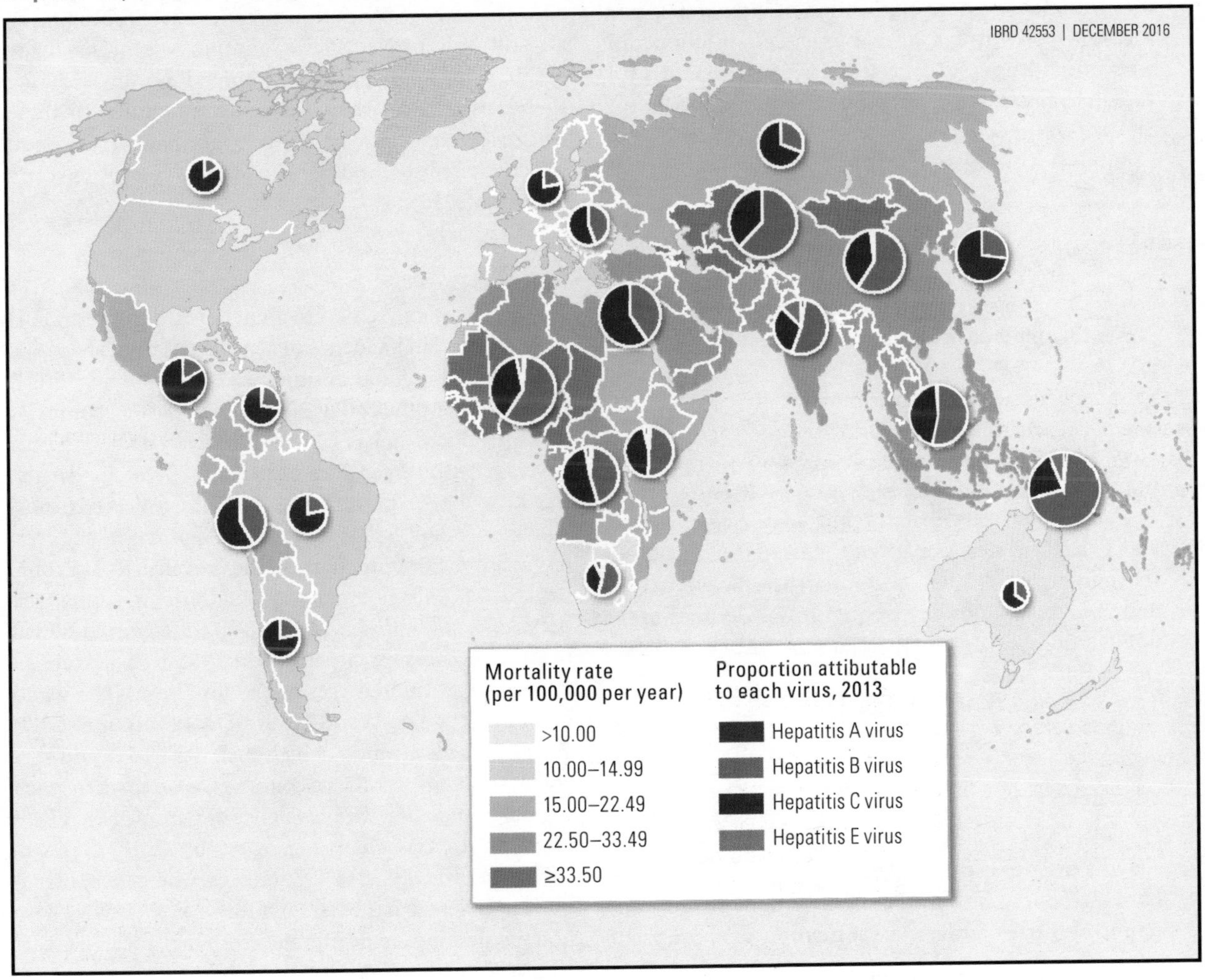

IBRD 42553 | DECEMBER 2016

Mortality rate
(per 100,000 per year)

>10.00

10.00–14.99

15.00–22.49

22.50–33.49

≥33.50

Proportion attibutable
to each virus, 2013

Hepatitis A virus

Hepatitis B virus

Hepatitis C virus

Hepatitis E virus

Source: Stanaway and others 2016.

Figure 16.2 Number of Hepatitis-Related Deaths, by Virus Type, 2013

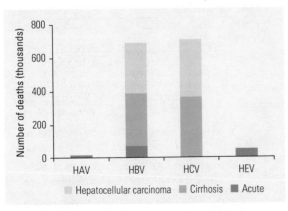

Source: Stanaway and others 2016.

Note: HAV = hepatitis A virus; HBV = hepatitis B virus; HCV = hepatitis C virus; HEV = hepatitis E virus.

TRANSMISSION OF HEPATITIS VIRUSES

Hepatitis A and hepatitis E are transmitted through the fecal-oral route by contact with contaminated food or water. Hepatitis E is also a zoonotic infection that can be spread by eating undercooked or uncooked pork or deer meat (Kamar and others 2012). Sexual transmission of hepatitis A by frequent oral-anal contact is common among men who have sex with men (Jin and others 2007). Hepatitis B, C, and D are transmitted through blood and bodily fluids. Globally, most hepatitis B infections occur through mother-to-child and early-life horizontal transmission between family members. Among adults, transmission occurs through sexual intercourse, as well as through unsafe injection practices and transfusion of unscreened blood and sexual transmission (Goldstein and others 2005). Most infections with HCV occur through unsafe injections, either in medical settings from reuse of medical equipment and substandard application of infection control measures, or through unsafe practices among people who inject drugs. Sexual transmission of hepatitis C is rare in heterosexual couples but more common among HIV/AIDS-infected men who have sex with men (Tohme and Holmberg 2010).

INTERVENTIONS

Table 16.2 summarizes the effective interventions for preventing the transmission of viral hepatitis.

Sanitation

Hepatitis A and E infections can be prevented through improved sanitation. Although no reliable estimates are available, it is likely that the incidence of hepatitis A and E has declined as part of the overall reduction in the number of deaths due to diarrhea. Between 1990 and 2012, all regions experienced major declines in the annual number of diarrheal diseases attributable to inadequate water, sanitation, and hygiene, from 1.8 million to 842,000 (WHO 2014).

Vaccination

Hepatitis A

An effective hepatitis A vaccine exists, and 18 countries have introduced universal childhood hepatitis A vaccination. Whether universal vaccination is appropriate

depends on the socioeconomic status of a country. In countries where sanitation practices are improving as a result of improved socioeconomic conditions, many children escape hepatitis A infection, thus leaving them susceptible when they become adults. In these countries, wide-scale hepatitis A vaccination is likely to be cost-effective and is encouraged (Jacobsen and Wiersma 2010).

Hepatitis B

The most notable achievement in hepatitis prevention is the reduction in incidence of acute and chronic hepatitis B infection as a result of universal childhood hepatitis B vaccination. At the end of 2013, 183 out of 194 countries had introduced universal childhood vaccination; global coverage with three doses of hepatitis B vaccine is estimated to be 81 percent (figure 16.3) (WHO 2015b). Universal infant vaccination with high coverage levels has led to major reductions in the prevalence of chronic hepatitis B infection among children. In China, the prevalence of chronic hepatitis B infection declined from approximately 8 percent in 1992 to 1 percent in 2006 among children ages one to four years (Liang and others 2009). The World Health Organization (WHO) Western Pacific Region, which includes China and several other high-prevalence countries, is on track to reach its goal of reducing the prevalence of chronic hepatitis B infection to less than 1 percent by 2017 (Wiesen, Diorditsa, and Li 2016). Countries where hepatitis B vaccine coverage has been high for several decades have noted reductions in death rates from hepatocellular carcinoma (Hung and others 2015).

Challenges remain to further reductions in incidence. Full protection for children requires that they receive the first vaccine dose within 24 hours of birth; this dose is termed a *birth dose*. Of 194 countries, 94 have introduced the birth dose in the vaccine schedule, and an estimated 38 percent of children globally receive this early dose (WHO 2015c). There are many logistical challenges to the delivery of the birth dose, including that most births occur at home in some countries. Treating pregnant women who have a high viral load of hepatitis B with antiviral medications during pregnancy can prevent mother-to-child transmission of hepatitis B (Pan and others 2016).

Hepatitis E

Outbreaks of hepatitis E occur primarily in Africa and South-East Asia through contaminated drinking water. An effective vaccine has been developed against one of the genotypes of hepatitis E. However, its effectiveness in outbreak settings and among children has not been assessed. For these reasons, the WHO has not made a

Figure 16.3 Global Coverage of Childhood Hepatitis Immunization and Birth Dose, 2000–13

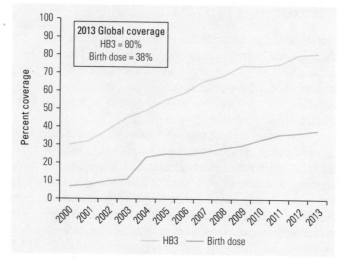

2013 Global coverage
HB3 = 80%
Birth dose = 38%

Source: WHO 2015b.
Note: HB3 = three doses of hepatitis B vaccine.

recommendation for its use in national vaccination programs (WHO 2015c).

Safety of Health Care Injections

In 2000, unsafe health care injections accounted for an estimated 32 percent of hepatitis B infections, 40 percent of hepatitis C infections, and 5 percent of HIV infections acquired in low- and middle-income countries (LMICs) (Hauri, Armstrong, and Hutin 2004). An updated analysis estimated that between 2000 and 2010, the number of infections due to unsafe injections declined by 91 percent for hepatitis B and 83 percent for hepatitis C, primarily attributable to a reduction in the reuse of injection equipment (Pepin and others 2014).

Addressing health care–associated infections, particularly unsafe injections, is difficult because in many countries the health system is fragmented and poorly regulated. In some areas, the health care system overuses injections because of the perception that injected medicines are more effective than oral medicines. The approach to reducing this risk needs to combine raising awareness about the effectiveness of oral medicines with the introduction of needles and syringes with reuse-prevention features (WHO 2015d).

Safety of Blood Supply

The risk of transmission of hepatitis B and C viruses through the transfusion of unsafe blood can be dramatically lowered by appropriate selection of donors and universal, quality-assured testing of blood donations. Many countries, however, still collect a significant proportion of the blood for transfusion from donors who have a high prevalence of hepatitis infection, for example, paid donors, and not all countries screen 100 percent of their blood collections for hepatitis B or C. Accordingly, the risk of transfusion-related transmission of these viruses remains unacceptably high in these settings (WHO 2011).

Harm Reduction Programs

People who inject drugs are the group most highly affected by viral hepatitis. Globally, an estimated 67 percent of people who inject drugs have evidence of hepatitis C infection and 8 percent have hepatitis B (Nelson and others 2011). An effective package of intervention, termed *harm reduction*, has been developed and includes the provision of sterile injecting equipment and opioid substitution therapy (WHO, UNODC, and UNAIDS 2009). Countries that have provided these services as part of a public health response to injecting drug use have been most successful in addressing the epidemics of injecting drug use, hepatitis, and HIV/AIDS (Palmateer and others 2014). Despite solid public health evidence demonstrating the effectiveness of harm reduction interventions, many decision makers remain reluctant to implement or scale up such programs because of their controversial nature. Ongoing dedicated advocacy efforts are still needed to initiate and sustain harm reduction programs across the globe.

Access to Treatment

Even a comprehensive hepatitis prevention program cannot prevent deaths occurring among persons already infected. Fortunately, effective treatment exists to treat persons with chronic hepatitis B and C infections. HBV replication can be suppressed, and therapy is lifelong in most cases (Yapali, Talaat, and Lok 2014). By effectively suppressing the replication of HBV, hepatitis B treatment can result in a reversal of cirrhosis (Marcellin and others 2013). Hepatitis C can be cured in as little as eight weeks by providing treatment with DAA medications. Persons cured of hepatitis C have improved quality of life and lower rates of liver-related and overall mortality (Smith-Palmer, Cerri, and Valentine 2015).

Despite the availability of these medicines, very few people, particularly in LMICs, are treated. The high price of the medicines is an important factor. Prices for DAAs in high-income countries (HICs) generally exceed US$50,000 per person. Through price negotiations, middle-income countries such as Brazil are able to obtain the same medicines for approximately US$7,000 (Andrieux-Meyer and others 2015). In low-income countries, through the introduction of generic medications, the price to treat one person is less than US$500. Hepatitis B medicines are available in generic formulations and prices can be as low as US$4/month. Other important challenges to scaling up are the delay in drug registration of the DAAs and the lack of a workforce trained in hepatitis treatment. An additional important barrier is that most persons with chronic hepatitis infection are still undiagnosed and lack the opportunities to be tested because of the low availability, high complexity, and high cost of diagnostics.

COSTS, COST-EFFECTIVENESS, AND EXTENDED COST-EFFECTIVENESS ANALYSES RESULTS

The quality and availability of data on the cost-effectiveness of the interventions to prevent and treat hepatitis infection vary by intervention and are primarily limited to HICs (table 16.3).

Table 16.3 Cost-Effectiveness of Interventions for Hepatitis

Intervention	Cost-effectiveness and affordability	Sources
Vaccination, hepatitis A	• Universal childhood vaccination is very cost-effective in UMICs and more cost-effective than targeted approaches. • Depending on incidence of hepatitis A infection and vaccination approach, vaccination is sometimes cost-effective or not cost-effective.	Anonychuk and others 2008
Vaccination, hepatitis B	• Universal childhood vaccination is very cost-effective in LMICs and HICs and can be cost saving depending on level of incidence and cost of vaccine administration.	Miller and McCann 2000
Interventions to reduce unnecessary and unsafe injections	• Combination of patient and health care worker education and provision of single-use injection equipment is very cost-effective.	Dziekan and others 2003
Needle- and syringe-exchange programs among people who inject drugs	• Limited data are available and only for HICs, with a range of cost-effectiveness results from not cost-effective to highly cost-effective.	Kwon and others 2012; Pollack 2001
Screening blood transfusion for hepatitis B, C	• No data are available on cost-effectiveness related to hepatitis B or C infection. • Screening is highly cost-effective in preventing HIV/AIDS infections in Sub-Saharan Africa so could be for hepatitis, too.	Creese and others 2002
Hepatitis B treatment	• Treatment is cost-effective in HICs and MICs. • Treatment can be cost saving assuming access to low-cost, generic medicines.	Buti and others 2013; Toy, Hutton, and So 2015
Hepatitis C treatment	• Treatment is cost-effective in HICs, despite very high cost of treatment. • Few studies have been conducted in LMICs. • Treatment is likely to be cost-effective in LICs and some MICs that have negotiated favorable medicine prices or have access to inexpensive generic medicines.	Younossi and Henry 2014

Note: HICs = high-income countries; LICs = low-income countries; LMICs = low- and middle-income countries; MICs = middle-income countries; UMICs = upper-middle-income countries. Definition of very cost-effective and cost-effective follows: If cost per disability-adjusted life year averted is less than the per capita income of the country, the intervention is very cost-effective; if less than three times the per capita income, it is cost-effective.

Immunization

Hepatitis B childhood immunization is the most cost-effective of the interventions to prevent infection, given the high morbidity associated with chronic hepatitis B infection and the low cost of vaccination. The cost-effectiveness of vaccination is directly linked to the population prevalence of infection; according to one analysis, the cost per year of life saved ranged from US$6 to US$51 in LMICs and upper-middle-income countries but was much higher (US$8,712–US$12,197) in HICs because of higher administration costs and lower prevalence of hepatitis B infection. In certain country-specific analyses, for example, in China, universal hepatitis B vaccination is cost saving as is catch-up vaccination of children and adolescents (Hutton, So, and Brandeau 2010; Lu and others 2013). An estimated 5.3 million to 6.0 million future hepatitis B–related deaths could be averted if 90 percent of children in 94 LMICs were vaccinated, compared with no vaccination. The only vaccine with greater estimated impact is that for measles (WHO 2013).

Assessing the cost-effectiveness of hepatitis A vaccination is complicated because the risk of symptomatic disease is linked with increasing age at time of infection. In countries where nearly the entire population is infected in childhood, when most infections are asymptomatic, there is very little morbidity, and thereby cost, associated with hepatitis A infection. In countries where the incidence of infection is lower, analyses show that universal childhood vaccination is more cost-effective than targeted approaches. Hepatitis A vaccination of adults is less cost-effective than for children. In a systematic review, 64 percent of studies assessing universal vaccination in children had cost-effectiveness ratios of less than US$28,606 per year of life saved or quality-adjusted life year (QALY) gained, compared with only 29 percent of studies in adults (Anonychuk and others 2008).

Injection-Associated Infections

Only limited data are available on the economic aspects of the prevention of health care–associated hepatitis infection. An analysis of the cost-effectiveness of measures to reduce unnecessary and unsafe injections resulted in a cost-effectiveness ratio between US$20.02 and US$3,280 per disability-adjusted life year (DALY) averted, depending on the region (Dziekan and others 2003).

Needle- and syringe-exchange programs for people who inject drugs are shown to be effective in preventing HIV/AIDS, but with regard to the effectiveness of these programs in the prevention of hepatitis C infection, the data are more limited and only from HICs. One analysis concluded that the cost to prevent one hepatitis C infection was between US$357,586 and US$1.4 million; a study from Australia assessing the cost-effectiveness of harm reduction to prevent hepatitis C and HIV/AIDS infections found that a needle- and syringe-exchange program resulted in US$801–US$16,840 per QALY gained (Kwon and others 2012; Pollack 2001).

Treatment

The high cost of the new hepatitis C medicines has engendered considerable controversy. Economic analyses concerning treatment have yielded widely varying results, partly because of differences in the assessed treatment regimens; virus genotypes; and types of patient populations, for example, those undergoing treatment for the first time versus those who failed previous treatment. Most of the analyses show that treatment with DAAs for hepatitis C genotype 1 regardless of the stage of liver disease is highly cost-effective in the United States, with an incremental cost-effectiveness ratio of less than US$71,517 (Tice and others 2015). Few studies have assessed the cost-effectiveness of the treatments in LMICs. These analyses are complicated by the varying and rapidly changing prices of DAAs in these countries (Andrieux-Meyer and others 2015).

The economics of treatment for hepatitis B differ from those for hepatitis C. Although the price of medicines is much lower on a per-day basis, treatment is lifelong for most patients with HBV infection; however, analyses show hepatitis B treatment to be cost-effective. In a systematic review, most of the studies conducted in HICs showed that treating compared to not treating resulted in an incremental cost-effectiveness ratio of less than US$70,000 per QALY gained (Buti and others 2013). Several studies have assessed the economics of treatment in China, which has the largest number of persons with chronic hepatitis B infection. In one study, entecavir or tenofovir monotherapy treatment in non-cirrhotic patients would prevent 49 percent to 69 percent of liver-related deaths and 26 percent to 31 percent of hepatocellular carcinoma deaths; treatment would be cost saving at a drug price of less than US$32–US$75 a month (Toy, Hutton, and So 2015).

CONCLUSIONS

The arrival of highly effective treatments for hepatitis B and C and an improved understanding of the attendant burden of disease have resulted in a call for increased action to eliminate hepatitis. In view of the differences in the distribution of hepatitis viruses and the related burden of disease, policy makers will need to develop national plans that are tailored to their epidemiologic patterns and response capacity. The goals of the United Nations 2030 Agenda for Sustainable Development include a goal to combat the epidemic of hepatitis (UN 2015). The WHO has developed a global hepatitis strategy to eliminate hepatitis B and C as major public health threats by 2030 (WHO 2016). The means to achieve these goals exist. What is needed is increased advocacy and country-level investment and action.

NOTE

World Bank Income Classifications as of July 2014 are as follows, based on estimates of gross national income (GNI) per capita for 2013:

- Low-income countries (LICs) = US$1,045 or less
- Middle-income countries (MICs) are subdivided:
  (a) lower-middle-income = US$1,046 to US$4,125
  (b) upper-middle-income (UMICs) = US$4,126 to US$12,745
- High-income countries (HICs) = US$12,746 or more.

REFERENCES

Ahmed, B., T. Ali, H. Qureshi, and S. Hamid. 2013. "Population-Attributable Estimates for Risk Factors Associated with Hepatitis B and C: Policy Implications for Pakistan and Other South Asian Countries." *Hepatology Internatonal* 7 (2): 500–507.

Andrieux-Meyer, I., J. Cohn, E. S. de Araujo, and S. S. Hamid. 2015. "Disparity in Market Prices for Hepatitis C Virus Direct-Acting Drugs." *The Lancet Global Health* 3 (11): e676–77. doi:10.1016/S2214-109X(15)00156-4.

Anonychuk, A. M., A. C. Tricco, C. T. Bauch, B. Pham, V. Gilca, and others. 2008. "Cost-Effectiveness Analyses of Hepatitis A Vaccine: A Systematic Review to Explore the Effect of Methodological Quality on the Economic Attractiveness of Vaccination Strategies." *Pharmacoeconomics* 26 (1): 17–32.

Buti, M., I. Oyaguez, V. Lozano, and M. A. Casado. 2013. "Cost Effectiveness of First-Line Oral Antiviral Therapies for Chronic Hepatitis B: A Systematic Review."

Pharmacoeconomics 31 (1): 63–75. doi:10.1007/s40273-012-0009-2.

Chen, C. J., U. H. Iloeje, and H. I. Yang. 2007. "Long-Term Outcomes in Hepatitis B: The REVEAL-HBV Study." *Clinics in Liver Disease* 11 (4): 797–816, viii.

Creese, A., A. Floyd, A. Alban, and L. Guinness. 2002. "Cost-Effectiveness of HIV/AIDS Interventions in Africa: A Systematic Review of the Evidence." *The Lancet* 359 (9318): 1635–43.

Dziekan, G., D. Chisholm, B. Johns, J. Rovira, and Y. J. Hutin. 2003. "The Cost-Effectiveness of Policies for the Safe and Appropriate Use of Injection in Healthcare Settings." *Bulletin of the World Health Organization* 81 (4): 277–85.

Edmunds, W. J., G. F. Medley, D. J. Nokes, A. J. Hall, and H. C. Whittle. 1993. "The Influence of Age on the Development of the Hepatitis B Carrier State." *Proceedings of the Royal Society: Biological Sciences* 253 (1337): 197–201. doi: 10.1098/rspb.1993.0102.

GBD 2013 Mortality and Causes of Death Collaborators. 2015. "Global, Regional, and National Age-Sex Specific All-Cause and Cause-Specific Mortality for 240 Causes of Death, 1990–2013: A Systematic Analysis for the Global Burden of Disease Study 2013." *The Lancet* 385 (9963): 117–71. doi:10.1016/S0140-6736(14)61682-2.

Goldstein, S. T., F. Zhou, S. C. Hadler, B. P. Bell, E. E. Mast, and others. 2005. "A Mathematical Model to Estimate Global Hepatitis B Disease Burden and Vaccination Impact." *International Journal of Epidemiology* 34 (6): 1329–39. doi:10.1093/ije/dyi206.

Gower, E., C. Estes, S. Blach, K. Razavi-Shearer, and H. Razavi. 2014. "Global Epidemiology and Genotype Distribution of the Hepatitis C Virus Infection." *Journal of Hepatology* 61 (Suppl 1): S45–57. doi:10.1016/j.jhep.2014.07.027.

Hauri, A. M., G. L. Armstrong, and Y. J. Hutin. 2004. "The Global Burden of Disease Attributable to Contaminated Injections Given in Health Care Settings." *International Journal of STD and AIDS* 15 (1): 7–16. doi:10.1258/095646204322637182.

Hung, G. Y., J. L. Horng, H. J. Yen, C. Y. Lee, and L. Y. Lin. 2015. "Changing Incidence Patterns of Hepatocellular Carcinoma among Age Groups in Taiwan." *Journal of Hepatology* 63 (6): 1390–96. doi:10.1016/j.jhep.2015.07.032.

Hutton, D. W., S. K. So, and M. L. Brandeau. 2010. "Cost-Effectiveness of Nationwide Hepatitis B Catch-Up Vaccination among Children and Adolescents in China." *Hepatology* 51 (2): 405–14. doi:10.1002/hep.23310.

Jacobsen, K. H., and S. T. Wiersma. 2010. "Hepatitis A Virus Seroprevalence by Age and World Region, 1990 and 2005." *Vaccine* 28 (41): 6653–57. doi:10.1016/j.vaccine.2010.08.037.

Jin, F., G. P. Prestage, I. Zablotska, R. Rawstone, S. C. Kippax, and others. 2007. "High Rates of Sexually Transmitted Infections in HIV Positive Homosexual Men: Data from Two Community Based Cohorts." *Sexually Transmitted Infections* 83: 397–99.

Kamar, N., R. Bendall, F. Legrand-Abravanel, N. S. Xia, S. Ijaz, and others. 2012. "Hepatitis E." *The Lancet* 379 (9835): 2477–88. doi:10.1016/S0140-6736(11)61849-7.

Kwon, J. A., J. Anderson, C. C. Kerr, H. H. Thein, L. Zhang, and others. 2012. "Estimating the Cost-Effectiveness of Needle-Syringe Programs in Australia." *AIDS* 26 (17): 2201–10. doi:10.1097/QAD.0b013e3283578b5d.

Liang, X., S. Bi, W. Yang, L. Wang, G. Cui, and others. 2009. "Epidemiological Serosurvey of Hepatitis B in China: Declining HBV Prevalence Due to Hepatitis B Vaccination." *Vaccine* 27 (47): 6550–57. doi:10.1016/j.vaccine.2009.08.048.

Lu, S. Q., S. M. McGhee, X. Xie, J. Cheng, and R. Fielding. 2013. "Economic Evaluation of Universal Newborn Hepatitis B Vaccination in China." *Vaccine* 31 (14): 1864–69. doi:10.1016/j.vaccine.2013.01.020.

Marcellin, P., E. Gane, M. Buti, N. Afdhal, W. Sievert, and others. 2013. "Regression of Cirrhosis during Treatment with Tenofovir Disoproxil Fumarate for Chronic Hepatitis B: A 5-Year Open-Label Follow-Up Study." *The Lancet* 381 (9865): 468–75. doi:10.1016/S0140-6736(12)61425-1.

Miller, M. A., and L. McCann. 2000. "Policy Analysis of the Use of Hepatitis B, *Haemophilus influenzae* Type b-, *Streptococcus pneumoniae*-Conjugate and Rotavirus Vaccines in National Immunization Schedules." *Health Economics* 9 (1): 19–35.

Mostafa, A., S. M. Taylor, M. el-Daly, M. el-Hoseiny, I. Bakr, and others. 2010. "Is the Hepatitis C Virus Epidemic Over in Egypt? Incidence and Risk Factors of New Hepatitis C Virus Infections." *Liver International* 30 (4): 560–66. doi:10.1111/j.1478-3231.2009.02204.x.

Nelson, P. K., B. M. Mathers, B. Cowie, H. Hagan, D. Des Jarlais, and others. 2011. "Global Epidemiology of Hepatitis B and Hepatitis C in People Who Inject Drugs: Results of Systematic Reviews." *The Lancet* 378 (9791): 571–83. doi:10.1016/S0140-6736(11)61097-0.

Palmateer, N. E., A. Taylor, D. J. Goldberg, A. Munro, C. Aitken, and others. 2014. "Rapid Decline in HCV Incidence among People Who Inject Drugs Associated with National Scale-Up in Coverage of a Combination of Harm Reduction Interventions." *PLoS One* 9 (8): e104515. doi:10.1371/journal.pone.0104515.

Pan, C. Q., Z. Duan, E. Dai, S. Zhang, G. Han, and others. 2016. "Tenofovir to Prevent Hepatitis B Transmission in Mothers with High Viral Load." *New England Journal of Medicine* 374 (24): 2324–34. doi:10.1056/NEJMoa1508660.

Pepin, J., C. N. Abou Chakra, E. Pepin, V. Nault, and L. Valiquette. 2014. "Evolution of the Global Burden of Viral Infections from Unsafe Medical Injections, 2000–2010." *PLoS One* 9 (6): e99677. doi:10.1371/journal.pone.0099677.

Perz, J. F., G. L. Armstrong, L. A. Farrington, Y. J. Hutin, and B. P. Bell. 2006. "The Contributions of Hepatitis B Virus and Hepatitis C Virus Infections to Cirrhosis and Primary Liver Cancer Worldwide." *Journal of Hepatology* 45 (4): 529–38. doi:10.1016/j.jhep.2006.05.013.

Pollack, H. A. 2001. "Cost-Effectiveness of Harm Reduction in Preventing Hepatitis C among Injection Drug Users." *Medical Decision Making* 21 (5): 357–67.

Schweitzer, A., J. Horn, R. T. Mikolajczyk, G. Krause, and J. J. Ott. 2015. "Estimations of Worldwide Prevalence of Chronic Hepatitis B Virus Infection: A Systematic Review of Data Published between 1965 and 2013." *The Lancet* 386 (10003): 1546–55. doi:10.1016/S0140-6736(15)61412-X.

Smith-Palmer, J., K. Cerri, and W. Valentine. 2015. "Achieving Sustained Virologic Response in Hepatitis C: A Systematic Review of the Clinical, Economic and Quality of Life Benefits." *BMC Infectious Diseases* 15: 19. doi:10.1186/s12879-015-0748-8.

Stanaway, J. D., A. D. Flaxman, M. Naghavi, C. Fitzmaurice, T. Vos, and others. 2016. "The Global Burden of Viral Hepatitis from 1990 to 2013: Findings from the Global Burden of Disease Study 2013." *The Lancet.* doi:10.1016/S0140-6736(16)30579-7.

Thein, H. H., Q. Yi, G. J. Dore, and M. D. Krahn. 2008. "Estimation of Stage-Specific Fibrosis Progression Rates in Chronic Hepatitis C Virus Infection: A Meta-Analysis and Meta-Regression." *Hepatology* 48 (2): 418–31. doi:10.1002/hep.22375.

Tice, J. A., D. A. Ollendorf, H. S. Chahal, J. G. Kahn, E. Marseille, and others. 2015. *The Comparative Clinical Effectiveness and Value of Novel Combination Therapies for the Treatment of Patients with Genotype 1 Chronic Hepatitis C Infection.* A Technology Assessment Final Report. Boston, MA: Institute for Clinical and Economic Review.

Tohme, R. A., and S. D. Holmberg. 2010. "Is Sexual Contact a Major Mode of Hepatitis C Virus Transmission?" *Hepatology* 52 (4): 1497–505. doi:10.1002/hep.23808.

Toy, M., D. W. Hutton, and S. K. So. 2015. "Cost-Effectiveness and Cost Thresholds of Generic and Brand Drugs in a National Chronic Hepatitis B Treatment Program in China." *PLoS One* 10 (11): e0139876. doi:10.1371/journal.pone.0139876.

UN (United Nations). 2015. "United Nations General Assembly Resolution A/RES/70/1 – Transforming Our World: The 2030 Agenda for Sustainable Development." United Nations, New York. http://www.un.org/ga/search/view_doc.asp?symbol=A/RES/70/1&Lang=E.

UNAIDS (Joint United Nations Programme on HIV/AIDS). 2015. *How AIDS Changed Everything. MDG 6: 15 Years, 15 Lessons of Hope from the AIDS Response.* Geneva: UNAIDS. http://www.unaids.org/en/resources/campaigns/HowAIDSchangedeverything.

WHO (World Health Organization). 2011. Global Database on Blood Safety. Blood Transfusion Safety [web page]. WHO, Geneva.

———. 2013. *Global Vaccine Action Plan 2011–2020.* Geneva: WHO.

———. 2014. *Preventing Diarrhoea through Better Water, Sanitation and Hygiene Exposures and Impacts in Low- and Middle-Income Countries.* Geneva: WHO. http://www.who.int/water_sanitation_health/gbd_poor_water/en/.

———. 2015a. *Global Tuberculosis Report 2015.* Geneva: WHO. http://www.who.int/tb/publications/global_report/en/.

———. 2015b. "WHO–UNICEF Estimate of HepB3 Coverage." Web page. http://apps.who.int/immunization_monitoring/globalsummary/timeseries/tswucoveragehepb3.html.

———. 2015c. "Hepatitis E Vaccine: WHO Position Paper. May 2015." *Weekly Epidemiological Record* 90 (18): 185–200.

———. 2015d. "Who Guideline on the Use of Safety-Engineered Syringes for Intramuscular, Intradermal and Subcutaneous Injections in Health-Care Settings." WHO, Geneva. http://www.who.int/injection_safety/global-campaign/injection-safety_guidline.pdf.

———. 2016. *WHO Global Health Sector Strategy on Viral Hepatitis: Towards Ending Viral Hepatitis.* Geneva: WHO. http://apps.who.int/iris/bitstream/10665/246177/1/WHO-HIV-2016.06-eng.pdf?ua=1.

WHO and UNICEF (United Nations Children's Fund). 2015. *Achieving the Malaria MDG Target: Reversing the Incidence of Malaria 2000–2015.* Geneva: WHO and UNICEF.

WHO, UNODC (United Nations Office on Drugs and Crime), and UNAIDS. 2009. *Technical Guide for Countries to Set Targets for Universal Access to HIV Prevention, Treatment and Care for Injecting Drug Users.* Geneva: WHO, Regional Office for Europe, UNAIDS, UNODC.

Wiesen, E., S. Diorditsa, and X. Li. 2016. "Progress towards Hepatitis B Prevention through Vaccination in the Western Pacific, 1990–2014." *Vaccine* 34 (25): 2855–62. doi: 10.1016/j.vaccine.2016.03.060.

Yapali, S., N. Talaat, and A. S. Lok. 2014. "Management of Hepatitis B: Our Practice and How It Relates to the Guidelines." *Clinical Gastroenterology and Hepatology* 12 (1): 16–26.

Younossi, Z., and L. L. Henry. 2014. "The Impact of the New Antiviral Regimens on Patient Reported Outcomes and Health Economics of Patients with Chronic Hepatitis C." *Digestive and Liver Disease* 46 (Suppl 5): S186–96.

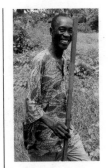

Chapter **17**

An Investment Case for Ending Neglected Tropical Diseases

Christopher Fitzpatrick, Uzoma Nwankwo, Edeltraud Lenk,
Sake J. de Vlas, and Donald A. P. Bundy

Box 17.1

Key Messages

- Neglected tropical diseases (NTDs) together account for a significant and inequitably distributed global disease burden, similar in order of magnitude to those of tuberculosis or malaria at approximately 22 million disability-adjusted life-years (DALYs) in 2012.
- Cost-effective interventions to end NTDs are available for as little as US$3 per DALY averted; these interventions reach the poorest and most marginalized populations and provide an integrated approach to treat multiple diseases.
- Ambitious eradication, elimination, and control targets for individual diseases emerged with the launch of the World Health Organization's NTD roadmap in 2012; the Sustainable Development Goals target "the end of NTDs" by 2030.
- Interventions to end NTDs are affordable globally; estimated treatment costs are US$750 million per year for 2015 to 2020 and US$300 million per year for 2020 to 2030.
- Interventions to end NTDs are affordable for the governments of most endemic countries;

treatment and vector control combined require less than 0.1 percent of domestic health spending. Domestic value for money is enhanced by the unprecedented scale of the London Declaration donation of medicines for nine of the most prevalent NTDs.
- Reaching those targets could avert an estimated 519 million DALYs from 2015 to 2030, compared to 1990 and the beginning of concerted efforts to control NTDs.
- The benefit to affected individuals in terms of averted out-of-pocket health expenditures and lost productivity exceeds US$342 billion over the same period.
- The net benefit to affected individuals is about US$25 for every dollar to be invested by public and philanthropic funders between 1990 and 2030—a 30 percent annualized rate of return.
- The end of NTDs represents a fair and efficient transfer toward universal health coverage and social protection for those who are least well-off.

Corresponding author: Christopher Fitzpatrick, Department of Control of Neglected Tropical Diseases, World Health Organization, Geneva, Switzerland; fitzpatrickc@who.int.

INTRODUCTION

The neglected tropical diseases (NTDs) affect more than 1 billion of the poorest and most marginalized people of the world. These infections are a consequence of the environmental and socioeconomic conditions in which the poor live, and the ill health and disability they cause are a primary factor locking the poor into poverty. They are diseases of the most neglected people who live in countries that lack the basic resources to control them. Yet this chapter demonstrates that the tools to end this neglect already exist, and that there are compelling economic arguments that ending these diseases would be one of the most cost-effective of global public health programs.

The NTD concept was developed to draw attention to this opportunity that was overlooked by the Millennium Development Goals (MDGs). At least 18 diseases are recognized as NTDs by World Health Assembly resolutions; the latest addition is mycetoma (WHO 2013, 2016). The World Health Organization (WHO) has set specific targets for control, elimination, and eradication of a subset of these diseases (table 17.1). These are the NTDs that we focus on in this chapter. The end of NTDs

Table 17.1 Global Targets for Control, Elimination, and Eradication toward "the End of NTDs"

Indicator	Target
Incidence/ prevalence[a]	• Eradication of Guinea worm disease (2015[b]) and yaws (2020)
	• Global elimination of leprosy (2020), lymphatic filariasis (2020), trachoma (2020), onchocerciasis (2025), and human African trypanosomiasis (2020, with zero incidence in 2030)
	• Regional elimination of schistosomiasis (2020), rabies (2020), and visceral leishmaniasis (2020)
	• Regional interruption of intradomiciliary transmission of Chagas disease (2020)
	• 25 percent reduction in the number of cases of dengue (2020, compared with 2010)
Mortality	• 50 percent reduction in number of deaths attributable to dengue (2020, compared with 2010)
Coverage[a]	• 75 percent coverage with preventive chemotherapy for food-borne trematode infections and soil-transmitted helminthiasis (2020)
	• 70 percent of all cases of Buruli ulcer detected and treated (2020)
	• Universal coverage against NTDs[c] (2030)

Source: WHO 2012.

Note: NTDs = neglected tropical diseases.

a. Reaching the incidence and coverage targets should result in at least a 90 percent reduction in the number of people requiring interventions against NTDs between 2015 and 2030; this is the combined NTD indicator that will be monitored under Sustainable Development Goal target 3.3.

b. Target year for Guinea worm eradication has not been updated; only 22 cases were reported in 2015.

c. 80 percent service coverage and 100 percent financial protection of people requiring at least one of five key interventions against NTDs: preventive chemotherapy; innovative and intensified disease management; vector ecology and management; veterinary public health: water, sanitation, and hygiene.

is now firmly embedded within the Sustainable Development Goals (SDGs) for 2030, under target 3.3, reflecting the promise to "leave no one behind."

This chapter reaffirms the case that NTDs account for a significant and unfairly distributed global disease burden, cost-effective interventions exist to reduce that burden, these interventions are affordable, and they are good investments in universal health coverage and social protection. It builds on the second edition of the *Disease Control Priorities (DCP2)* project (Hotez and others 2006) with new data and analysis. It also takes into account new strategies and tools that have been introduced since 2006 and the increasingly ambitious elimination and eradication targets for individual diseases that have emerged since 2012, including the unprecedented donation by the pharmaceutical industry under the London Declaration of more than a billion medicines annually to treat nine of the most important NTDs. Finally, it helps provide a longer-term perspective on SDG target 3.3 and the 2030 goals.

This chapter is structured around three key NTD interventions, rather than individual NTDs, in recognition of the increasingly integrated delivery of interventions to the poorest, most remote, and otherwise most marginalized communities of the world. These interventions are as follows:

- Preventive chemotherapy by mass drug administration
- Innovative and intensified disease management
- Vector ecology and management.

For simplicity of analysis, we focus on a subset of the NTDs recognized by the WHO. We do not provide a full analysis of veterinary public health interventions against zoonotic NTDs or of water, sanitation, and hygiene (WASH). These conditions are beyond the scope of this chapter, but WASH is addressed in chapter 9 in volume 7 of the third edition of *Disease Control Priorities* (Hutton and Chase 2017). Chapter 13 in volume 8 (Bundy and others 2017) discusses mass deworming programs, and chapter 29 (Ahuja and others 2017) in volume 8 analyzes the economics of such programs.

BURDEN OF NTDs

The MDGs evolved around HIV/AIDS malaria, and tuberculosis (TB); other diseases were overlooked and not prioritized for funding. The focus was on mortality. These three diseases accounted for about 3.9 million deaths in 2000, including about 875,000 for malaria; NTDs accounted for about 242,000 deaths (Horton 2012; Hotez and others 2014). Several of the NTDs do not kill; they do, however, disable, disfigure, and even impair the cognitive development of children. Today, the focus of the SDGs has broadened to include healthy lives and well-being for all at all ages.

The disability-adjusted life year (DALY) is meant to account for years of life lost because of premature death, as well as years of life lived with disability. In practice, it tends to underestimate the burden of NTDs in part because of gaps in the data from low- and middle-income countries (LMICs). Even so, in 2012, the NTDs accounted for approximately 22 million DALYs globally, which amounts to about 40 percent of the DALYs for malaria and about 1 percent of the global total. The contribution of individual NTDs to the total is shown in table 17.2.

This burden is heavy, especially for regions and countries where NTDs are most endemic. In several countries in Sub-Saharan Africa, NTDs make up more than 6 percent of the total burden of disease.

However, the NTDs are not only a concern of low-income countries (LICs) in Sub-Saharan Africa. A significant burden is shouldered by the poorest and most marginalized communities of middle-income countries, as evidenced by figure 17.1. Indeed, environmental change and population movement have redefined

tropical diseases. Dengue has reemerged in high-income countries that had not seen cases in decades. Chagas disease now affects migrant populations across North America and Europe. Today, a majority of the poor lives in countries assessed as middle income or above.

With national income and other secular trends being generally upward in the LMICs where NTDs are most prevalent, the overall burden of disease has been coming down since at least 2000. However, the persistence of NTDs in middle- and even high-income countries indicates that some communities have been left behind by the macroeconomic development of the past decades. A review found that more than 60 percent of studies reveal inequalities in the prevalence of NTDs across socioeconomic groups (Houweling and others 2016). For example, in rural Nigeria, the prevalence of ascariasis among children ranges from 10 percent when both parents have at least primary education, to 31 percent when only the mother does, 53 percent when only the father does, and 96 percent when neither parent does (Ugbomoiko and others 2009).

In Ethiopia, trichiasis cases (a consequence of trachoma) are more likely to occur in poorer households, whether measured by asset ownership,

Table 17.2 Disease Burden (Mortality and Morbidity) of Malaria and NTDs, 2012

	DALYs (thousands)	%	YLD (thousands)	%	YLL (thousands)	%
Parasitic and vector diseases	72,006	2.62	11,697	1.58	60,309	3.01
Malaria	55,111	2.01	4,301	0.58	50,810	2.54
Trypanosomiasis	1,264	0.05	9	0.00	1,256	0.06
Chagas disease	528	0.02	326	0.04	202	0.01
Schistosomiasis	4,026	0.15	3,179	0.43	848	0.04
Leishmaniasis	3,374	0.12	128	0.02	3,245	0.16
Lymphatic filariasis	2,839	0.10	2,839	0.38	0	0.00
Onchocerciasis	598	0.02	598	0.08	0	0.00
Leprosy[a]	257	0.01	6	0.00	251	0.01
Dengue	1,445	0.05	12	0.00	1,432	0.07
Trachoma	299	0.01	299	0.04	0	0.00
Rabies	2,265	0.08	0	0.00	2,265	0.11
Intestinal nematode infections	5,266	0.19	5,057	0.68	209	0.01
Ascariasis	1,355	0.05	1,146	0.15	209	0.01
Trichuriasis	666	0.02	666	0.09	0	0.00
Hookworm disease	3,246	0.12	3,246	0.44	0	0.00
Total excluding malaria	22,161	0.81	12,453	1.68	9,708	0.48

Source: World Health Organization, http://www.who.int/healthinfo/global_burden_disease/estimates/en/index2.html.

Note: NTDs = neglected tropical diseases. Cause-specific disability-adjusted life year (DALYs), years of life lost (YLLs), and years lived with disability (YLDs). Percentages are expressed relative to the global total.

a. Leprosy is formally not a parasitic disease, it is caused by a mycobacterium. Furthermore, we suspect that the YLD and YLL numbers for leprosy may have been inverted; we nonetheless report them here as in the original source.

Figure 17.1 Disease Burden of NTDs, by Country Income Group, 2012

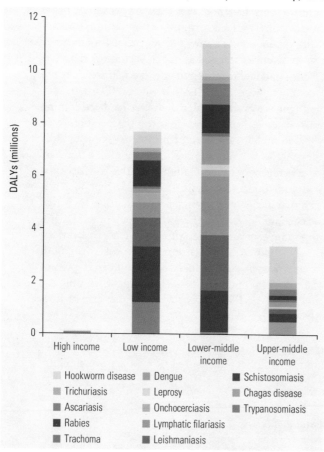

Source: WHO 2014a.
Note: DALYs = disability-adjusted life years; NTDs = neglected tropical diseases.

Table 17.3 Economic Burden (Lost Productivity) of Selected NTDs

NTD	Sequela	Annualized loss in productive input (%)[a]
Chagas disease	General (excluding severe heart failure)	2–5
Leprosy	Disfigurement	28
Lymphatic filariasis	Hydrocele	14–19
	Lymphedema	2–23
Onchocerciasis	Visual impairment	14–38
	Blindness	79–100
Schistosomiasis	General	1–23
Soil-transmitted helminthiasis	Anemia	0.1–6.0
Trachoma	Visual impairment	25
	Blindness	60–100
Visceral leishmaniasis	General (treated)	6–30

Sources: Ibe and others 2015; Lenk and others 2016.
Note: NTD = neglected tropical disease.
a. Minimum and maximum from the available literature.

self-rated wealth, or peer-rated wealth (the odds range from 2.8 to 8.2) (Habtamu and others 2015). Compared with controls, those with trichiasis are also significantly less likely to participate in economically productive activities, more likely to report difficulty in performing activities, and more likely to receive assistance in performing productive activities (Habtamu and others 2015).

In addition to the disease burden is the heavy economic burden that NTDs impose on patients and their families. Most of the economic cost comes in lost productivity, usually working time (and wages), but also agricultural land, lost to morbidity and disability. The extent of loss of productive inputs depends on the type and severity of the NTD as well as where it occurs (table 17.3). The particularly high economic cost of blindness motivated the World Bank's first investments in health, with the creation of the Onchocerciasis Control Programme in West Africa in 1975.

Added to the productivity losses are the direct medical costs of diagnosis and treatment and, even if tests and medicines are offered free of charge, direct nonmedical costs associated with accessing or adhering to treatment. The latter include transportation, accommodation, and food. Altogether, costs can easily exceed 20 percent of annual household income, a threshold for so-called catastrophic cost that can propel a previously stable household into penury and unsupportable debt (Ruan and others 2016). Protection against this risk requires further public sector investment in finding cases early, treating patients free of charge, and, as required, other social protection to cover transport and other nonmedical and indirect costs. These are some well-documented examples:

Buruli ulcer. In Cameroon, the cost of hospitalization attibutable to Buruli ulcer (caused by *Mycobacterium ulcerans*) has been estimated to be 25 percent of household annual earnings, despite treatment being available free of charge. In Ghana, medical costs made up less than 4 percent of total direct costs; the largest cost (81 percent of direct costs) is transportation to treatment (WHO 2015b).

Chagas disease. The cost of Chagas disease (caused by *Trypanosoma cruzi*) was estimated in 2013 to be about US$7 billion per year, including lost productivity (Lee and others 2013). Health care costs accounted for slightly less than 9 percent of this total. The cost of treatment ranges from less than US$200 to more than US$30,000 per person per year in endemic countries, and exceeds US$40,000 in the United States (WHO 2015b).

Dengue. In Cambodia and Vietnam, "between half and two-thirds of affected households have incurred debt as a result of treatment for dengue" (WHO 2015b, 82). The economic burden of the disease is measured in the billions of dollars annually; urbanization and climate change are conspiring to raise the cost even higher (Constenla, Garcia, and Lefcourt 2015; Martelli and others 2015; Shepard, Undurraga, and Halasa 2013; Shepard and others 2011; Shepard and others 2014; Undurraga and others 2015).

Human African trypanosomiasis. In the Democratic Republic of Congo, the cost to affected households in a typical rural community represents more than 40 percent of annual household income. New and more effective melarsoprol-free treatment has increased the average cost to treat one patient with second-stage gambiense sleeping sickness from US$30 in 2001 to US$440 in 2010 (WHO 2015b).

Leprosy. Erythema nodosum leprosum is a common immune-mediated complication of leprosy. In a district of West Bengal, India, the total household cost of erythema nodosum leprosum was about 28 percent of monthly household income (Chandler and others 2015). Direct costs accounted for 35 percent of this total. Total household costs exceeded 40 percent of household income for more than one-third of cases.

Visceral leishmaniasis. In Bihar, India, 83 percent of affected households belong to the two lowest wealth quintiles (the poorest 40 percent) (Boelaert and others 2009). In Bangladesh, India, Nepal, and Sudan, 25 percent to 75 percent of affected households experience some type of financial catastrophe in obtaining a diagnosis and treatment, even when tests and medicines are provided free of charge (Anoopa and others 2006; Meheus and others 2013; Ozaki and others 2011; Sundar and others 2010; Uranw and others 2013).

In addition to the health (death and disability) and economic burden, there is also the social and psychological (mental health) burden of NTDs because of stigma. Reasons given for stigmatization include appearance, fear of contagion, burden on family, hereditary etiology, promiscuity, and performance impediment. This burden is harder to quantify, but there is evidence that no less than 10 NTDs are associated with stigma, with especially strong evidence related to leprosy, lymphatic filariasis, Buruli ulcer, onchocerciasis, and leishmaniasis (Hofstraat and van Brakel 2016). The visible impact of NTDs has been shown to be an important determinant of stigma; disease management should therefore have a positive effect on stigma.

PROOF OF CONCEPT FOR ENDING NTDs

Despite being sidelined in the MDGs, an integrated approach to the prevention and control of NTDs began to take shape during the MDG era, and by the end, NTD interventions had delivered a number of successes. These successes include a reduction of 80 percent in new human African trypanosomiasis (HAT) cases between 2000 and 2014, to an estimated less than 4,000 cases; and a reduction of 75 percent in the number of cases of visceral leishmaniasis (kala-azar) in Bangladesh, India, and Nepal between 2005 (when a regional program was launched) and 2014, to a reported 10,209 cases. In 2000, there were more than 130,000 cases of dracunculiasis (Guinea worm); in 2015, there were only 22 reported cases, reflecting near-eradication (figure 17.2). Map 17.1 shows the reported numbers of cases of these three NTDs targeted for elimination or eradication.

For other NTDs, especially those for which cases are not routinely reported to the WHO, country-level progress has been made toward the interruption of transmission. For example, by 2014, 18 countries reported having been able to stop preventive chemotherapy for lymphatic filariasis, and 8 countries have stopped mass antibiotic treatment for trachoma, because the set targets had been reached.

Other NTDs that have been eliminated in certain countries or that are under surveillance for verification

Figure 17.2 Reported Number of Cases of Three Neglected Tropical Diseases Targeted for Elimination or Eradication, 2000–15

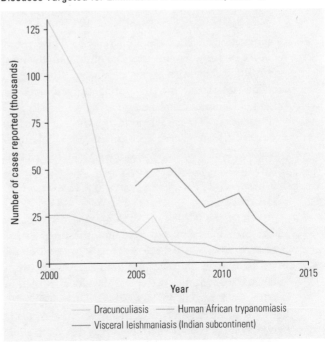

Source: WHO Global Health Observatory, (http://apps.who.int/gho/data/node.main.A1629?lang=en).

IBRD 42555 | OCTOBER 2016

NTDs that have been eliminated since 2000

- Dracunculiasis
- Onchocerciasis
- Trachoma
- Yaws
- Lymphatic filariasis
- Rabies
- Visceral leishmaniasis

Source: WHO Global Health Observatory, (http://apps.who.int/gho/data/node.main.A1629?lang=en).
Note: NTD = neglected tropical disease.

of elimination are illustrated in figure 17.3. Those countries are already reaping the economic and financial rewards that come with having eliminated a disease and stopping treatment, thereby freeing up resources for other public health priorities.

Progress on NTD-related mortality includes a reduction in deaths caused by visceral leishmaniasis, rabies, schistosomiasis, HAT, Chagas disease, and soil-transmitted helminthiases (that is, ascariasis, collectively estimated to be 142,000 deaths in 2012, down from about 220,000 in 2000 (WHO 2014a).

Much of the burden of NTDs occurs in morbidity rather than mortality, and here, too, the progress has been good, albeit somewhat less dramatic, with a decrease of 19 percent in the total number of DALYs between 2000 and 2012, from 1 percent of the global burden of disease to 0.8 percent (WHO 2014a). There have been logistical challenges, of course, that have differed greatly between diseases and between countries. However, elimination of dracunculiasis, for example, has been achieved in some of the most difficult settings in the world.

INTERVENTIONS TO END NTDs

The WHO recommends five interventions for the control, elimination, and eradication of the NTDs: preventive chemotherapy by mass drug administration; innovative and intensified disease management; vector ecology and management; veterinary public health services; and the provision of safe water, sanitation, and hygiene (WHO 2010; see the discussion in volume 7 of this series [Hutton and Chase 2017]). We review the evidence for all but the last two of these interventions.

Delivering Large-Scale Preventive Treatment to Entire Communities

Preventive chemotherapy involves the large-scale delivery of medicines to eligible populations at regular intervals. Medicines donated to and distributed through the WHO are quality assured and safe for administration by non-health workers. Table 17.4 provides the disease-specific details of how preventive chemotherapy is delivered. In many areas, these diseases do not occur exclusive of each other, but are co-endemic. A combination of medicines is recommended in this scenario. Integrated delivery of treatments for more than one disease is now the norm in several countries, with resulting cost savings (WHO 2015b).

Preventive chemotherapy is effective toward elimination only if the threshold coverage is sustained annually for at least three years or longer, depending on the disease. The WHO has set clear thresholds for effective program coverage, by disease (table 17.4), meaning delivery of medicines to a minimum percentage of eligible individuals during approximately the same time period, with 100 percent geographic coverage of endemic areas. If the threshold coverage is not met, the disease burden is reduced but will return when preventive chemotherapy is stopped. If threshold coverage is met, countries can stop mass treatment, or at least reduce its frequency, and shift resources to integrated disease surveillance and other public health priorities.

The global population in need of preventive chemotherapy is reported to be 1.7 billion as of 2014, of which 851 million people actually received treatment, leaving a coverage gap of approximately 50 percent (WHO 2015c).

Figure 17.3 Update on the Global Status of Implementation of Preventive Chemotherapy, 2008–20

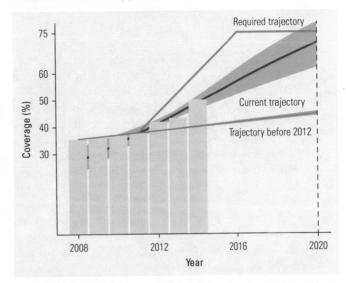

Source: WHO (http://www.who.int/neglected_diseases/preventive_chemotherapy/PC_Update.pdf?ua=1).
Note: Analysis includes current and projected percentage of people receiving preventive chemotherapy for at least one of these diseases (including lymphatic filariasis, onchocerciasis, schistosomiasis, and soil-transmitted helminthiases) out of the estimated number of people requiring preventive chemotherapy. The required trajectory assumes a linear scale-up to 75 percent, the minimum target coverage indicated in table 17.4.

Table 17.4 Selected NTDs Targeted by Preventive Chemotherapy

Disease	Causative organism and transmission	Medicine, single dose	Target population (minimum effective coverage)	Frequency and duration of intervention
Lymphatic filariasis	Parasites (*Wuchereria bancrofti, Brugia malayi, Brugia timori*) transmitted by mosquito	Albendazole 400 mg with ivermectin (150–200 μg/kg) or with diethylcarbamazine 6 mg/kg	Ivermectin: ≥ age 5 years Diethlycarbamazine: ≥ age 2 years (65%)	Annually for at least 5 years
Onchocerciasis	Parasites (*Onchocerca volvulus*) transmitted by blackfly	Ivermectin 150 μg/kg or mcg/kg	> age 5 years (80%)[c]	Annually for at least 10–15 years
Schistosomiasis	People are infected by parasites (*S. haematobium, S. mansoni, S. japonicum*) when exposed to freshwater infested by cercariae released by intermediate host snails.	Praziquantel 40 mg/kg	SAC (ages 5–14 years) and adults at risk (75%)	Once a year, or every two to three years, depending on community prevalence, for variable or unknown duration[a]
Soil-transmitted helminthiases	The main parasites that infect people are the roundworm (*Ascaris lumbricoides*), the whipworm (*Trichuris trichiura*) and the hookworms (*Necator americanus and Ancylostoma duodenale*)	Albendazole 400 mg Mebendazole 500 mg	Pre-SAC (< age 5 years) and SAC (age 5–14 years) (75%)	Once or twice a year depending on community prevalence, for variable or unknown duration[a]
Trachoma	Bacterial infection (*Chlamydia trachomatis*) through contact with infected people or spread by flies	Azithromycin 20 mg/kg to a maximum of 1g (This is given as part of a SAFE[b] strategy)	> age 6 months (80%)	Annually, with the number of rounds given before review dependent on the prevalence of disease at last estimate.

Source: WHO (http://apps.who.int/iris/bitstream/10665/43545/1/9241547103_eng.pdf).
Note: g = gram; kg = kilograms; mg = milligrams; SAC = school-age children; μg or mcg = micrograms.
a. Treatment is geared toward reducing the intensity of infection in individuals. The frequency of treatment may be reduced over time, but ultimately, the duration will depend on improved water, sanitation, and hygiene.
b. SAFE strategy comprises: S-eyelid surgery for trichiasis, A-antibiotics, F- facial cleanliness, and E-environmental improvement.
c. 80% of the eligible population is roughly equivalent to 65% of the total population.

Still, it is important to acknowledge the tremendous progress that has been made in shifting the trajectory in coverage up from the levels of 2000–11 (figure 17.3). In 2012, the WHO NTD Roadmap (WHO 2012) and subsequent London Declaration drove the pivot from the trajectory in 2011 (green line) to the current trajectory (dark blue line). It also remains clear that the current trajectory is not sufficient to meet the required level of coverage of 75 percent (light blue line) early enough (2016) to ensure that treatment can be stopped or its frequency reduced by 2020 (WHO 2012).

Morbidity management and disability prevention is a related intervention for those for whom preventive chemotherapy has arrived too late, particularly for those with a long history of infection with lymphatic filariasis or trachoma, now suffering the chronic consequences. Adult filarial worms lodge in the lymphatic system and disrupt the immune system, resulting in swelling of the scrotum and lower limbs. Repeated reinfection with *Chlamydia trachomatis* gives rise to trichiasis, in which eyelashes rub on the eyeball, leading to corneal opacification and blindness. Hydrocele and trichiasis surgery, as well as lymphedema management, are complementary to measures to reduce infection prevalence—the benefits being more visible than those from the distribution of drugs.

The pharmaceutical industry has expressed its commitment to meet medicine requirements. A full list of medicines donated by the pharmaceutical industry is available in annex 5 of the third global report on NTDs (WHO 2015b). These are highly effective medicines—most of which are on the WHO's list of essential medicines—being provided for free. Logistic constraints have, however, hindered the ability of NTD programs to ensure universal access to these medicines. The delivery network has been heavily subsidized by communities. Members are selected as community drug distributors and paid in kind or with cash incentives by their communities. This approach has worked well in small-scale projects, but many communities are overstretched. Bridging the coverage gap will require investment in delivery chains within endemic countries; how much is needed and what the return will be are described later in the chapter.

Preventing the Transmission of NTDs by Vectors

Vectors are living organisms that can transmit infectious diseases between humans or from animals to humans (and vice versa). Many of these vectors are bloodsucking insects that ingest disease-producing microorganisms during a blood meal from an infected host (human or animal) and later inject it into a new host during their subsequent blood meal. Mosquitoes are the best known vector, transmitting malaria as well as lymphatic filariasis. Others include blackflies (onchocerciasis), sandflies (leishmaniasis), and triatomine bugs (Chagas disease).

Vector ecology and management aims to control the transmission of the causative pathogens of insect-borne NTDs with proven interventions that are applied in an ecologically friendly manner. The WHO's integrated vector management strategy has found use in areas with multiple vector-borne diseases or where preventive chemotherapy is contraindicated because of the risk of severe adverse events (for example, in areas of onchocerciasis and *Loa* co-endemicity) and where there is no other intervention to control infection (for example, dengue, chikungunya). NTDs targeted primarily by vector management are listed in table 17.5.

Table 17.5 Selected NTDs Targeted by Vector Ecology and Management Interventions

Disease (vector)	Description of vector management intervention
Chagas disease (hematophagous triatomine or "kissing bug")	Spray homes and surroundings with residual insecticides
	Improve walls and roofs of dwellings
	Use bednets and other personal control measures
Dengue, chikungunya (female mosquitos *Aedes aegypti* and *Aedes albopictus*)	Individual and household protection
	Vector surveillance
	Biological, chemical, and environmental control (including insecticides)
	Outbreak preparedness and response
Visceral leishmaniasis or kala-azar (female sandflies)	In areas of the Indian subcontinent where vector control is not already being undertaken by malaria programs:
	Vector surveillance
	Indoor residual spraying and use of bednets

Note: NTDs = neglected tropical diseases. Vector control interventions also exist for onchocerciasis, human African trypanosomiasis, and lymphatic filariasis; however, these are not discussed here. There is little recent evidence on their cost-effectiveness or, in the case of lymphatic filariasis, evidence is limited to areas that are co-endemic with malaria.

Coverage with vector management for the prevention of Chagas disease and dengue remains uneven. More than 100 million people still require an attack phase of vector control for the interruption of intradomiciliary transmission of Chagas disease in Latin America. This intensive phase involves residual insecticide spraying by specialized mobile teams two times with a six-month intermediate period (to kill all insects, including the ones coming from eggs) and dwelling or house hygiene and improvement (plastering) to avoid reinfestation.

Although 2 billion to 4 billion people are at risk of dengue or chikungunya, only a handful of counties offer coverage with sustained vector management involving biological, environmental, and chemical measures adapted to the needs of the communities. Most countries only respond to dengue outbreaks when it is too late to make much of a difference (Stahl and others 2013). However, sustained vector control interventions could make a very large difference, not only for dengue and chikungunya, but also for other diseases transmitted by *Aedes aegypti* and *Aedes albopictus*.

Progress toward elimination of visceral leishmaniasis as a public health problem on the Indian subcontinent provides evidence of the impact that vector management can have. In 2005, the governments of Bangladesh, India,

and Nepal launched a comprehensive strategy including integrated vector management. In Nepal elimination has been achieved in 12 districts. In Bangladesh, the number of hyperendemic subdistricts (*upazilas*) decreased from eight in 2012 to two in 2014, with elimination achieved in about 90 percent of endemic upazilas (WHO 2015d).

Providing Treatment and Care to Individuals

Not all NTD cases can be prevented by preventive chemotherapy and vector management, for example, because the drugs are too toxic. A complementary approach focuses on the innovative and intensified clinical management of diseases. Innovation and intensification refer to a shift from passive management to active surveillance, early diagnosis, and treatment, with the aim to eliminate or control, not just to manage. Treatment of Buruli ulcer, for example, has evolved from late-stage surgical removal of infected or dead tissue and correction of deformity to the early-stage use of antibiotics (a combination of rifampicin and streptomycin or amikacin). The gains go beyond health benefits to include reductions in the cost of hospitalization to health systems and to individuals. The NTDs for which the primary intervention is disease management are listed in table 17.6.

Table 17.6 Selected NTDs Targeted by Disease Management Interventions

Disease (agent)	Disease management intervention
Buruli ulcer (*Mycobacterium ulcerans*)	Early case detection and antibiotic treatment, including rifampicin and streptomycin, or rifampicin and clarithromycin
	Surgical removal of dead skin and grafting
	Rehabilitation for deformities
Chagas disease (*Trypanosoma cruzi*)	Early case detection and treatment with nifurtimox and benznidazole
	Adequate screening of blood for transfusion
	Screening (testing) of organ, tissue, or cell donors and receivers
	Screening of newborns and other children of infected mothers to provide early diagnosis and treatment
	Other morbidity-specific treatment
Human African trypanosomiasis (*Trypanosoma*)	Early case detection and treatment with pentamidine or suramin or nifurtimox-eflornithine combination treatment (NECT), depending on the stage of the disease
Leishmaniases (*Leishmania spp*)	Early case detection
	For visceral leishmaniasis, treatment options include: sodium stibogluconate, meglumine antimonite, paromomycin, liposomal amphotericin B or miltefosine, depending on the parasite species and the endemic region
	For cutaneous leishmaniasis, management options include local or systemic treatments with antileishmanial drugs or local procedures with cryotherapy, thermotherapy
Leprosy (*Mycobacterium leprae*)	Early case detection and treatment with multidrug regimen (combination of rifampicin, dapsone, and clofazimine) and management of morbidity and prevention of disability
Yaws (*Treponema pallidum pertenue*)	Formerly, identification of the population at risk of infection by case finding (active and passive) and treatment with injectable penicillin
	Currently, Total Community Treatment followed by Total Targeted Treatment of confirmed cases and their contacts with single dose of azithromycin

Note: NTDs = neglected tropical diseases.

The inclusion here of yaws warrants an explanation, given the recent shift in strategy from individual treatment with injectable penicillin to mass treatment with single-dose azithromycin. While the risk is thought to be low in populations with little previous antibiotic exposure, surveillance is undertaken to guard against antimicrobial resistance. This mass treatment for yaws is similar to preventive chemotherapy but is known as Total Community Treatment. In keeping with the convention within the NTD community, this chapter considers Total Community Treatment as separate from preventive chemotherapy.

COST AND COST-EFFECTIVENESS OF INTERVENTIONS TO END NTDS

This section is a synthesis and update of the review of the cost and cost-effectiveness conducted for the WHO's NTD report (WHO 2015b) and subsequent systematic reviews.

Preventive Chemotherapy

Unit Cost of Delivery

Advocacy around preventive chemotherapy has typically put the cost per person treated at less than US$0.50. While useful for advocacy, the focus on a single number misrepresents the complexity of delivering "free" donated medicines to more than 1 billion people across the world.

There is now a rich literature—34 studies of 23 countries and at least 91 sites over 19 years—documenting the cost per person treated in diverse settings (Fitzpatrick and others, forthcoming). The average unit cost is US$0.40 (in 2015 U.S. dollars) in financial terms, but the average unit cost increases to US$0.70 in studies that also consider the economic cost of ministry of health staff time and assets. About half of the available estimates of the economic unit cost fall between US$0.30 and US$1.00, but they range from a low of US$0.02 in large-scale programs to US$2.9 in smaller projects. Benchmarking tools can help assess the value for money in mass treatment campaigns (WHO 2015b).

Cost-Effectiveness

Hotez and others (2006) described preventive chemotherapy as one of the most cost-effective interventions available in public health. The large and unprecedented donation of NTD medicines in the London Declaration in 2012 strengthens that case from the perspective of national health systems. Indeed, reviews continue to show that preventive chemotherapy remains cost-effective, even with an expansion beyond the traditional zones of focus, or with an increase in treatment frequency to accelerate progress (Keating and others 2014).

Some of the more recent cost-effectiveness analyses are presented in table 17.7, with results standardized for prices in 2012.

Table 17.7 Recent Cost-Effectiveness Analyses of Preventive Chemotherapy

Disease	Study	Intervention	Setting	Target population	2012 US$ per DALY averted, relative to doing nothing
Lymphatic filariasis	Turner and others 2016	Albendazole + ivermectin	Global	All	28[a]
Onchocerciasis	Turner and others 2014	Ivermectin, annual	Africa	Mesoendemic (microfilarial prevalence: 40%)	15
				Hyperendemic (60%)	6
				Highly hyperendemic (80%)	3
Schistosomiasis and STH	Turner and others 2015	Albendazole + praziquantel	Global	School-age children	5-80
	Lo and others 2015		Côte d'Ivoire	School-age children	114
Trachoma	Baltussen and Smith 2012	Mass treatment with azithromycin + trichiasis surgery	Sub-Saharan Africa	95% coverage	22–83[b]

Note: DALY = disability-adjusted life year; STH = soil-transmitted helminthiasis.

a. Stone and others (2016) do not report the number of DALYs averted relative to a null (do nothing) scenario; they report the incremental costs and effects of a hypothetical eradication program over the baseline elimination program.

b. This estimate is based on Baltussen and Smith (2012) using median purchasing-power-parity exchange rates for Sub-Saharan Africa in 2012 to convert from international dollars of 2000. Baltussen and Smith (2012) used 2012 market prices for azithromycin; an assumption of zero cost would be closer to the reality of the current situation. See text for further comment.

Annual mass treatment with ivermectin is estimated to cost 2012 US$3–US$15 per DALY averted, depending on the degree of onchocerciasis endemicity; biannual mass treatment would cost an additional 2012 US$12–US$36 per DALY averted in hyperendemic areas (Turner and others 2014). This does not take into account the substantial collateral reduction in DALYs attributable to the impact of ivermectin on lymphatic filariasis, soil-transmitted helminthiasis (STH), and scabies (Krotneva and others 2015).

With regard to STH, there has been a recent controversy about the extent to which it is possible to detect population-level benefit from mass treatment. However, there is no doubt that infected persons are at risk of disease and require treatment; the WHO recommendation is for mass treatment in communities where prevalence exceeds 20 percent (see Bundy and others 2017 for a discussion of these issues). A recent review finds that most studies present results within the range of being highly cost-effective according to World Bank thresholds (Turner and others 2015). Mass treatment of school-age children in Côte d'Ivoire for STH and schistosomiasis together costs 2014 US$118 (2012 US$114) per DALY averted relative to doing nothing (Lo and others 2015). Mass treatment of the entire community would also be cost-effective, at 2014 US$167 (2012 US$161) per DALY averted relative to school-age children only (Lo and others 2015). Combination with other interventions is also possible. Mass treatment for STH costs 2012 US$13 per DALY averted when added to a vitamin A supplementation campaign for children ages 6 months to 14 years in Uganda (Fiedler and Semakula 2014).

Of the medicines delivered as preventive chemotherapy, azithromycin, a broad-spectrum antibiotic, has the greatest market value. The cost-effectiveness of preventive chemotherapy for trachoma (relative to other interventions for the prevention of blindness) depends crucially on assumptions about the cost of azithromycin. There is no market price for azithromycin for use in global trachoma elimination. Applying the market price of azithromycin for use in smaller-scale programs, mass treatment combined with trichiasis surgery costs about 2012 US$83 per DALY averted in Sub-Saharan Africa, relative to doing nothing (Baltussen and Smith 2012). In practice, azithromycin is available as a free donation to trachoma-elimination programs worldwide, and the cost per DALY averted is lower than the cost using market pricing. An earlier study suggested a 73 percent decrease in the cost per DALY averted with donated azithromycin (Baltussen and others 2005). Therefore, the cost per DALY averted is probably closer to 2012 US$22.

All of the cost-effectiveness ratios described above are well below the threshold of one times gross domestic product (GDP) per capita, implying that they are very cost-effective (WHO-CHOICE 2012). Even so, they may be overstated. Integrated delivery of more than one medicine at a time is safe and there is evidence that it will reduce cost (Evans and others 2011; Leslie and others 2013).

Vector Ecology and Management

Chagas Disease

The cost-effectiveness of vector control for Chagas disease in the Argentinean Chaco region has been estimated to be 2004 US$45–US$132 per human case averted, depending on the strategy chosen (Vazquez-Prokopec and others 2009). A mixed strategy—vertical (centralized) attack phase followed by a horizontal (community-led) surveillance phase—is thought to be the most cost-effective option. A comparison of vector control policies for Chagas disease in Colombia to a do-nothing policy revealed net benefits for all considered villages at a willingness to pay of 2004 US$631 (2012 US$940) per DALY averted (Castillo-Riquelme and others 2008).

Dengue

For dengue, DCP2 put the cost per DALY averted by vector control at US$1,992–US$3,139 (Cattand and others 2006). Since then, the dengue economics literature suggests lower cost-effectiveness ratios that range from 2005 US$227 (2012 US$334) per DALY averted by larval control in Cambodia to 2009 US$615–US$1,267 (2012 US$779–US$1,604) per DALY averted by adult mosquito control in Brazil (Suaya and others 2007; Luz and others 2011). Environmental change, including urbanization and climate change, strengthen the investment case for sustained vector control, which is cost-effective even in the era of a low-cost, medium-efficacy vaccine. If benefits for the control of chikungunya and Zika virus (transmitted by the same vector) were taken into account, the cost per DALY averted would be even lower.

Disease Management

Cutaneous Leishmaniasis

The cost-effectiveness of interventions for cutaneous leishmaniasis was not specifically discussed in DCP2. The difficulty with assessing their cost-effectiveness is that this form of the disease is not fatal and disability weights may not fully reflect the social stigma associated with disfigurement. Nonetheless, recent economic evaluations suggest that interventions for early diagnosis and treatment can be cost-effective, ranging from 2010 US$156 (2012 US$218) per DALY averted in Argentina to 2003 US$1,200 (2012 US$3,000) per DALY averted by treatment in a complex emergency setting in Afghanistan (Orellano, Vazquez, and Salomon 2013; Reithinger and Coleman 2007).

Visceral Leishmaniasis

Liposomal amphotericin B (AmBisome) has been found to be the most effective treatment option available for the Indian subcontinent for visceral leishmaniasis (Meheus and Boelaert 2010). Recent donations of AmBisome have also made it the most cost-effective treatment option from the health system perspective. In Bangladesh, a comprehensive elimination program involved active case detection, single-dose treatment with donated AmBisome, indoor residual spraying, long-lasting insecticide treated nets, and environmental vector management. It was the most cost-effective option available at thresholds above 50 percent of GDP per capita, and cost far less than 50 percent of GDP per capita per DALY averted relative to doing nothing (Federici and others, forthcoming).

Human African Trypanosomiasis

The latest economic evaluations identified in a recent review focused on the Democratic Republic of Congo and Angola, of which the Democratic Republic of Congo makes up most of the remaining burden of HAT in the world (Sutherland and others 2015). Case detection, diagnosis, and treatment were considered cost-effective at 2002 US$17 (2012 US$79) per DALY averted in the Democratic Republic of Congo. However, the current treatment, nifurtimox-eflornithine combination therapy (NECT), has not yet been evaluated for cost-effectiveness. Given that NECT too is donated and has efficacy in excess of 90 percent, we would anticipate at least similar ratios.

Leprosy

For leprosy, *DCP2* put the cost per DALY averted by case detection and treatment at less than US$50 (Remme and others 2006). Since then, the pharmaceutical industry has committed an unlimited number of treatments to overcome the disease. From the health system perspective, therefore, treatment is more cost-effective than ever. The economic evaluation of leprosy elimination programs focuses primarily on the cost-effectiveness of interventions to detect more cases earlier (Ezenduka and others 2012; Idema and others 2010). The challenge is to

deliver those treatments early enough to prevent disability and further transmission.

Yaws

A global yaws eradication campaign could be established with a relatively modest investment in the period to 2020—about 2012 US$100 million to US$500 million in 12 endemic countries. Yaws eradication would cost about 2012 US$26 per year lived without disability or 2012 US$324 per DALY averted. Global financial support is not yet available in the same proportions as for other NTDs. The cost to the public sector would be significantly reduced by donations of azithromycin for yaws, as is done for trachoma (Fitzpatrick, Asiedu, and Jannin 2014; WHO 2015b).

More evidence is needed on the cost-effectiveness of interventions for Buruli ulcer and mycetoma. Such evidence will likely come from evaluations of integrated approaches to screening, diagnosing, and treating these and other skin-related NTDs, especially cutaneous leishmaniasis, leprosy, and yaws.

FAIRNESS OF INTERVENTIONS TO END NTDS

Mass treatment is an intervention that favors women in most countries. NTDs could have a disproportionate impact on the health and well-being of girls and women (including pregnant women) because they negatively affect female reproductive health; exacerbate anemia in women of reproductive age; and increase susceptibility to sexually transmitted infections, including HIV/AIDS. Mass treatment turns out to be quite favorable to women. In coverage surveys from 37 countries from which data were available, the gender ratio (female-to-male) was between 0.96 and 1.17 (Worrell and Mathieu 2012). Data from Uganda also suggest that coverage tends to be higher among females than males (Rilkoff 2013). Men tend to be away from home more often than the women within a household, whether for work or travel.

Inequity persists along other dimensions of socioeconomic status. Disaggregation of NTD intervention coverage is not yet routinely done. The disaggregated data we do have are from household surveys that ask whether children ages 6–59 months had been given deworming medication in the past six months. This is only a subset of the population requiring treatment for one NTD—STH—but it points to both a challenge and an opportunity. In most countries, deworming coverage is similar in both rural and urban areas, but higher among educated and wealthy households who need it least (figure 17.4). A dozen or so countries have demonstrated that higher rates of coverage can be achieved among those who need it most.

Figure 17.4 Deworming Coverage among Children Ages 6–59 Months in 55 Countries, Ratio

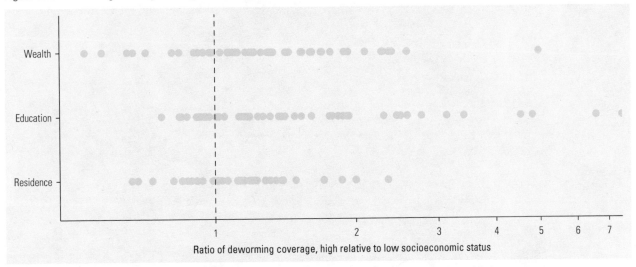

Source: Demographic and Health Surveys, most recent available (2006–14) from 55 countries.
Note: Ratio of deworming coverage: Residence shows the ratio of coverage in urban relative to rural areas; Education shows the ratio of coverage among households headed by those with higher relative to no education; and Wealth gives the ratio of coverage among the wealthiest 20 percent relative to the poorest 20 percent of households.

TARGETS FOR THE SCALE-UP OF INTERVENTIONS TO END NTDs

The current improved support for control and elimination of NTDs reflects a well-structured strategy, availability of cost-effective interventions, and a clear road map against which progress can be measured. Endemic countries have adopted global targets and milestones in national NTD master plans. Within these plans the national NTD programs are responsible for ensuring that all donated essential medicines are delivered to all the citizens requiring them.

Treatment Targets

The WHO's NTD Roadmap (WHO 2012) set clear targets for the eradication or elimination of 11 of the 17 NTDs considered by 2020. Eradication is the "permanent reduction to zero of a specific pathogen, as a result of deliberate efforts, with no more risk of reintroduction," while elimination (of transmission) is the "reduction to zero of the incidence of infection caused by a specific pathogen in a defined geographical area, with minimal risk of reintroduction, as a result of deliberate efforts; continued actions to prevent re-establishment of transmission may be required" (WHO 2015a, 1). Elimination thresholds are defined differently by disease, but in general involve the reduction of disease impact to below levels of public health importance. SDG target 3.3 is to "end the epidemic" of NTDs. For global monitoring purposes, the existing coverage and

eradication or elimination targets for individual NTDs are being brought together under a single indicator for 2030: reduction in the number of people requiring interventions against NTDs.

This indicator will capture but is not limited to eradication of yaws (2020); global elimination of leprosy (2020), lymphatic filariasis (2020), trachoma (2020), onchocerciasis (2025), and HAT (2020, with zero incidence in 2030); and regional elimination of schistosomiasis (2020) and visceral leishmaniasis (2020). These remain critical milestones on the path toward the end of the NTD epidemic by 2030. If these milestones are met, the total number of people requiring treatment for NTDs may begin to decrease as soon as 2017, as diseases are eradicated, eliminated, and controlled.

Between 2015 and 2030, we should see a 90 percent reduction in the number of people in need of mass and individual treatment globally. The projected 90 percent reduction in the number of people requiring treatment will be associated with a projected 75 percent reduction in DALYs, from 12 million in 2015 to 3 million in 2030, expected from the achievement of NTD Roadmap targets for nine NTDs (figure 17.5). The decrease in the total number of people requiring treatment against NTDs from about 1.6 billion in 2015 to less than 300 million means far less death, disability, and disfigurement; but it also means far less cost to households and to the health system. This is why we speak of spending on these NTDs as an investment.

At the same time, achievement of the 2020 targets and even the end of treatment is not exactly the same as the

Figure 17.5 Health Impact of Achieving the WHO's NTD Roadmap Targets for 2020 and Sustaining Them until the "End of NTDs" by 2030, in Relation to Having Done Nothing, Expressed as a Continuation of the 1990 Situation, Corrected for Demographic Trends

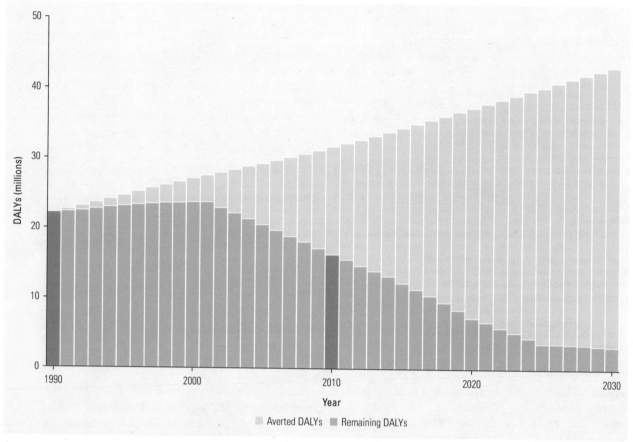

Sources: de Vlas and others 2016; https://erasmusmcmgz.shinyapps.io/dissemination/.

Note: DALYs = disability-adjusted life years; NTDs = neglected tropical diseases. These trends are for the nine so-called London Declaration NTDs only, which explains why the total number of DALYs is less than the 22 million DALYs reported in table 17.2 for 2012.

end of NTDs. Rehabilitation and disability inclusion will need to be sustained well beyond 2030 for those people for whom prevention arrived too late and for whom the consequences are irreversible. Vector control for Chagas disease and dengue are interventions that are also likely to extend beyond 2030. To be sustainable, these longer-term services and interventions will need to be included within benefit packages under universal health coverage.

Investment Targets

The third WHO global NTD report set investment targets for reaching the 2020 Roadmap and 2030 SDG targets (WHO 2015b). Including vector control for Chagas disease and dengue, a total of $18 billion is targeted for the period 2015–30, or about US$2.1 billion per year. Most of the investment in vector control is required in upper-middle-income countries (UMICs). Excluding vector control,

the investment target for treatment (preventive chemotherapy and individual treatment) is about US$750 million per year during 2015–20, and about US$300 million per year during 2020–30. These amounts exclude the value of donated medicines, estimated to be about $4.5 billion when using the lowest prices negotiated on the market (MSH 2014). An estimated US$2.8 billion is required to deliver donated medicines to end users either in the form of mass treatment or facility-based care.

Where will this investment come from? Between 2012 and 2014, about $200 million to $300 million was disbursed or committed by foreign donors (Uniting to Combat Neglected Tropical Diseases 2014). This is about one-tenth of the investment target in endemic countries. At most, it would cover the investment required in LICs. As reflected in the discourse around the SDGs, the time has come for a shift in focus from foreign donors to domestic investment by governments and stakeholders in endemic countries. The third WHO global NTD report argued that targets for domestic investment should be set such that the realization of the end of NTDs will not depend disproportionately on foreign aid (WHO 2015b).

In 2011, the domestic share of total expenditure on health was 71 percent in LICs, 98 percent in lower-middle-income countries, and more than 99 percent in UMICs (WHO 2014b). Allowing for an upward trend toward 2030 in line with recent trajectories in economic growth, the domestic share in LICs could rise to 93 percent by 2030 (WHO 2015b). Of course, this average conceals considerable variation between countries. Nonetheless, if recent trajectories in economic growth are maintained, by 2030 the domestic share could exceed 80 percent in all of them (WHO 2015b). We apply these domestic shares to the total investment target for NTDs to obtain domestic investment targets for NTDs.

For all income groups, domestic investment targets for NTDs decrease after 2020 in absolute (dollar) terms as coverage targets are achieved and NTDs are controlled, eliminated, or eradicated. These targets for domestic investment are affordable. The domestic investment target for NTDs represents less than one-tenth of 1 percent of domestic expenditure on health expected within the group of lower-middle-income countries for 2015–30. The percentage is highest for the group of LICs, where the domestic investment target for NTDs is nevertheless still well below 1 percent of domestic expenditure on health.

In many endemic countries, the costs of community-level interventions are borne by endemic communities themselves, who provide the volunteers and incentives. In addition to financing delivery, all levels of government have a critical role in ensuring that nonfinancial barriers to access are also addressed. They can do this by providing waivers and supporting drug logistics through all administrative levels, especially at the very critical level of the community, where delivery occurs.

The end of NTDs is an achievable and affordable SDG target for which endemic countries could take political and financial control. The returns to their poorest citizens will be substantial.

RETURN ON INVESTMENTS TO END NTDs

The health impact of meeting the WHO 2020 targets and the end of NTDs by 2030 has been calculated for nine NTDs (de Vlas and others 2016). Between 2011 and 2030, 600 million DALYs would be averted: 30 million DALYs per year on average (figure 17.5). These health gains include about 150 million irreversible disease manifestations averted (such as blindness) and 5 million averted deaths. Among the preventive-chemotherapy NTDs, 96 percent of the health gains would be attributed to averted disability, and within the intensified-disease-management NTDs, 95 percent of the impact would be realized from averted deaths.

The impact compares favorably to the total investment of US$27 billion thought to be required in the period 2011–30 for achievement of global targets for those nine NTDs (our calculations based on abovementioned targets for 2015–30). That investment implies US$45 per DALY averted or US$178 per irreversible disease manifestation averted over the same period.

In addition to their impact as measured by DALYs, NTDs are known to cause financial hardship among affected individuals, which can exacerbate the cycle of poverty. A conservative estimate suggests that the end of NTDs would avert a total of international dollars (I$) 35 billion in out-of-pocket (OOP) health expenditure by affected individuals between 2011 and 2030 (Lenk and others, forthcoming; Redekop and others, forthcoming). This averted cost includes medicines, tests, travel, and food not covered by public providers or by health insurance. It does not capture the additional averted costs of household coping mechanisms, such as indebtedness, or the irreversible consequences of catastrophic health expenditure.

Progress toward the end of NTDs would avert a further I$622 billion in wages lost by affected individuals between 2011 and 2030. This number does not include the significant long-term benefits of school attendance for employment (Ahuja and others 2015). The choice by the Global Burden of Disease (2010) project (on which the analysis was based) not to include so-called subtle morbidities, such as impaired cognitive development, poor mental health from stigma, and discrimination because of disfigurement, is controversial. The benefit to affected individuals of averted OOP health expenditures and lost wages is therefore conservatively estimated to be I$657 billion between 2011 and 2030, or an average of I$33 billion per year.

We convert the benefits reported by Redekop and others (forthcoming) and Lenk and others (forthcoming) from 2010 international dollars to 2015 U.S. dollars for direct comparison to the investment targets described in the previous section.

Of course, some of this benefit is attributable to investments made before 2011. We conservatively assume that investments begun in 1990 were at the level of those in 2011 (in real terms); 1990 is assumed to mark the beginning of concerted global efforts to control most NTDs and 2011 is assumed to mark the beginning of the recent scale-up in investment to eliminate them. In reality, investments before 2011 were probably lower than this in most countries. We do not consider the investments in improved housing and water and sanitation that occurred over the same period; these investments were not targeted at the NTDs but nonetheless contributed to their control.

We then calculate a rough estimate of the net benefit to affected individuals from 1990 to 2020 (NTD Roadmap targets) and to 2030 (the SDG target). Net benefit per dollar invested is the present value of the benefit to affected individuals minus the present value of the cost to public and philanthropic funders, divided by the present value of the cost to funders. We apply a discount rate of 3 percent per year for both costs and benefits.

The net benefit to affected individuals is US$17 for every dollar invested by funders during the period 1990–2020 and US$28 for every dollar invested in the period 1990–2030 (table 17.8). It ranges from US$8 per dollar invested in Africa to US$398 per dollar invested in the Western Pacific (including China), and US$4 per dollar invested in LICs to US$273 per dollar invested in UMICs.

Taking into account the period during which the investments and returns are to be made, we also calculate an annualized compounded rate of return. The end of NTDs offers a 31 percent rate of return overall. It ranges from 19 percent per year in the Eastern Mediterranean Region to 59 percent in the Western Pacific (including China), and 14 percent in LICs to 54 percent in UMICs.

Lower net benefits and rates of return in LICs are due in large part to the way in which averted productivity losses have been valued, that is, using GDP per capita of the bottom 20 percent of the population of each country. This approach assigns a lower benefit to lower-income and more unequal countries. Good physical health without disability is arguably more important in LICs with large informal sectors that revolve around subsistence. As a result, the numbers are particularly conservative estimates of the net benefit for affected individuals in LICs.

What is clear from even this preliminary analysis is that investment in interventions against NTDs is a fair and efficient investment in social justice. The benefit to affected individuals—the poorest and most marginalized—greatly exceeds the cost to public and philanthropic funders of providing it. If the new social compact articulated at the Addis Ababa Conference on Financing for Development is to involve transfers to the poor (as SDGs 1 and 10 on ending poverty and reducing inequalities suggest that it should), then ending NTDs is an efficient way of making those transfers.

This benefit can be measured by OOP health expenditure and productivity losses averted. It thereby supports two additional targets of the SDGs: universal

Table 17.8 Benefits, Costs, Net Benefits, and Rates of Return on the End of Selected NTDs, Best Estimates

	Benefit to Affected Individuals, 2015 US$ (billions)		Cost to Funders, 2015 US$ (billions)		Net Benefit to Affected Individuals per Dollar Invested by Funders		Annualized Compounded Rate of Return (%)	
	2015–2020	2015–2030	2015–2020	2015–2030	1990–2020	1990–2030	1990–2020	1990–2030
Preventive-chemotherapy NTDs[a]	119.7	399.0	2.8	6.2	27.4	42.8	35	35
Disease-management NTDs[b]	5.4	20.9	1.1	2.2	0.9	2.8	11	13
Total	125.1	419.9	3.9	8.4	16.9	28.4	30	31
African Region	9.2	40.6	1.5	3.0	3.0	8.0	18	20
Region of the Americas	5.6	21.9	0.1	0.3	10.2	26.1	24	25
Eastern Mediterranean Region	1.9	8.5	0.2	0.3	3.9	13.0	16	19
European Region	0.1	0.5	<0.1	<0.1	5.1	14.1	19	21
South-East Asian Region	27.1	98.9	1.9	4.5	4.9	10.1	19	21
Western Pacific Region	80.5	246.4	0.2	0.4	260.6	397.7	59	59
Low-income countries	7.5	29.3	1.3	2.5	1.3	4.0	11	14
Lower-middle-income countries	29.2	113.2	2.4	5.3	6.1	12.3	22	23
Upper-middle-income countries	87.6	274.3	0.3	0.5	165.4	272.7	54	54

Sources: Based on Lenk and others 2016; Redekop and others, forthcoming; WHO 2015b.
Note: NTDs = neglected tropical diseases.

a. Integrated delivery of preventive chemotherapy medicines for lymphatic filariasis, onchocerciasis, schistosomiasis, soil-transmitted helminthiases, and trachoma; also includes post-preventive chemotherapy surveillance and morbidity management and disability prevention.

b. Individual management of human African trypanosomiasis (HAT), leprosy, and visceral leishmaniasis (VL); also includes active case finding for HAT, leprosy, and VL, and vector control for VL; includes the cost of integrated disease surveillance in HAT-endemic areas.

health coverage and social protection. Universal health coverage means, among others, financial risk protection against OOP health expenditure. Social protection includes benefits for people of working age in case of disability. As countries struggle with how to finance universal health coverage and social protection, prioritizing interventions to end NTDs can guide countries' first decisive steps on the long path toward those goals. Investment in interventions against NTDs puts progress on universal health coverage within reach of even the weakest health systems.

PLACE OF NTDS IN THE GRAND CONVERGENCE

In 2013, the *Lancet* Commission on Investing in Health addressed the question of whether the world could achieve a grand convergence, in which poorer countries would see their infectious, maternal, and child health outcomes converge with the levels of wealthier nations—through increased investments in health interventions and systems to combat common causes of mortality and morbidity. There are now estimates of what the grand convergence might achieve and what investment would be required by 2030 (Boyle and others 2015).

Those estimates focus on lower-middle-income countries. They consider the costs of scaling up interventions for reproductive, maternal, and child health; and HIV/AIDS, TB, and malaria interventions; as well as the cost of strengthening health systems. They suggest that convergence would avert more than 130 million deaths between 2015 and 2030. The incremental costs of convergence would be about US$62 billion in 2015, rising to about US$86 billion in 2030. The end of NTDs is a high-impact and low-cost contribution to the grand convergence.

Convergence in the burden of NTDs would avert about 519 million DALYs in the period 2015–30, including about 5 million deaths or 4 percent of the convergence total of 130 million deaths (de Vlas and others 2016). As table 17.8 shows, the cost in lower-middle-income countries is US$7.8 billion in 2015–30; this amount is US$0.5 billion per year or less than 1 percent of the convergence total. The NTDs compare favorably with other major diseases as measured by deaths that could be averted by 2030 and the investment needed. This comparison is favorable even though up to 96 percent of the health gains from convergence in NTDs would be in averted disability rather than death (de Vlas and others 2016). A more inclusive metric of grand convergence would reveal the true contribution of convergence in NTDs.

Convergence in NTDs also stands out in the grand convergence narrative in its sustainability. Whereas the incremental costs of convergence increase from US$62 billion in 2015 to US$86 billion in 2030, the costs of convergence in NTDs decrease from US$750 million per year during 2015–20 to about US$300 million per year during 2020–30. In this sense, there is a special role for NTDs in leading the way toward the grand convergence through the elimination of infectious diseases targeted by the SDGs.

CONCLUSIONS

The elimination of the NTDs was a late and ad hoc addition to the MDG era, leaving a legacy of 22 million DALYs in 2012, a burden not far behind those of malaria and TB. As we enter the SDG era the world is seeking to rethink this opportunity and look toward the end of NTDs in 2030. The ambitious WHO NTD Roadmap (WHO 2012) and the massive donation of treatments for nine NTDs have built on successes in integrated treatment of multiple diseases in the poorest and most marginalized populations, and contribute to the potential of ending NTDs for as little as US$3 per DALY averted.

The evidence is clearly in favor of including the following within the package of essential interventions for all low-income endemic countries (based on a cost per DALY averted of 2012 US$250 or less): preventive chemotherapy for at least five NTDs; comprehensive control (including vector control) for visceral leishmaniasis; and early detection and treatment of cutaneous leishmaniasis, HAT, and leprosy. Other interventions against NTDs should also be included on a country-by-country basis. Populations requiring vector control for Chagas disease and dengue and mass treatment for yaws need to be mapped out; current evidence indicates that these can be highly effective interventions in lower-middle-income and upper-middle-income endemic countries.

Our estimates suggest that the costs of ending NTDs are affordable globally (for example, US$750 million per year in 2015–20 and US$300 million per year in 2020–30, for preventive chemotherapy against five NTDs) and affordable for the governments of most endemic countries at less than 0.1 percent of domestic health spending. The estimated benefits to affected individuals in averted OOP health expenditures and lost productivity exceed US$342 billion over the same period. The end of NTDs offers a net benefit to affected individuals of about US$25 for every dollar invested by funders—a 30 percent annualized rate of return. It is a fair and efficient investment in universal health coverage and social protection for the least well-off.

We compared NTDs with other public health programs by revisiting the Grand Convergence in Health by 2030, as proposed by the *Lancet* Commission on Investing in Health. Here the comparison is striking: ending NTDs would avert about 4 percent of the convergence total of 130 million deaths, and it would do so for less than 1 percent of the total convergence cost. This makes excellent health and economic sense on its own, but it is an underestimate of the true scale of benefit given that it ignores the 96 percent of health gains attributable to averted disability, rather than death, which is equivalent to about 519 million DALYs averted from 2015 to 2030.

Coordinated efforts to end the NTDs are emerging as among the largest public health programs in the world, and the most cost-effective and affordable. Indeed, the global program costs are on the scale of a rounding error at less than 1 percent of the grand convergence investment, yet offer a substantial return on investment. Furthermore, because these are diseases of poverty, the NTD agenda is specifically pro-poor; because the programs target morbidity, they are also specifically pro-development. All in all, this suggests that NTD programs have a special role in leading the world's efforts toward more fairness in health and the attainment of the SDGs.

NOTE

World Bank Income Classifications as of July 2014 are as follows, based on estimates of gross national income (GNI) per capita for 2013:

- Low-income countries (LICs) = US$1,045 or less
- Middle-income countries (MICs) are subdivided:
  (a) lower-middle-income = US$1,046 to US$4,125
  (b) upper-middle-income (UMICs) = US$4,126 to US$12,745
- High-income countries (HICs) = US$12,746 or more.

REFERENCES

Ahuja, A., S. Baird, J. H. Hicks, M. Kremer, E. Miguel, and others. 2015. "When Should Governments Subsidize Health? The Case of Mass Deworming." *World Bank Economic Review* 29 (Suppl 1): S9–24.

Ahuja, A., S. Baird, J. H. Hicks, M. Kremer, and E. Miguel. 2017. "The Economics of Mass Deworming Programs." In *Disease Control Priorities* (third edition): Volume 8, *Child and Adolescent Health and Development*, edited by D. A. P. Bundy, N. de Silva, S. Horton, D. T. Jamison, and G. C. Patton. Washington, DC: World Bank.

Anoopa, S. D., C. Bern, B. Varghese, R. Chowdhury, R. Haque, and others. 2006. "The Economic Impact of Visceral Leishmaniasis on Households in Bangladesh." *Tropical Medicine and International Health* 11 (5): 757–64.

Baltussen, R., and A. Smith. 2012. "Cost-Effectiveness of Strategies to Combat Vision and Hearing Loss in Sub-Saharan Africa and South East Asia: Mathematical Modelling Study." *BMJ* 344 (1): e615.

Baltussen, R., M. Sylla, K. D. Frick, and S. P. Mariotti. 2005. "Cost-Effectiveness of Trachoma Control in Seven World Regions." *Ophthalmic Epidemiology* 12 (2): 91–101.

Boelaert, M., F. Meheus, A. Sanchez, S. P. Singh, V. Vanlerberghe, and others. 2009. "The Poorest of the Poor: A Poverty Appraisal of Households Affected by Visceral Leishmaniasis in Bihar, India." *Tropical Medicine and International Health* 14 (6): 639–44.

Boyle, C. F., C. Levin, A. Hatefi, S. Madriz, and N. Santos. 2015. "Achieving a 'Grand Convergence' in Global Health: Modeling the Technical Inputs, Costs, and Impacts from 2016 to 2030." *PLoS One* 10 (10): e0140092.

Bundy, D. A. P., L. J. Appleby, M. Bradley, K. Croke, T. D. Hollingsworth, and others. 2017. "Mass Deworming Programs in Middle Childhood and Adolescence." In *Disease Control Priorities* (third edition): Volume 8, *Child and Adolescent Health and Development*, edited by D. A. P. Bundy, N. de Silva, S. Horton, D. T. Jamison, and G. C. Patton. Washington, DC: World Bank.

Castillo-Riquelme, M., Z. Chalabi, J. Lord, F. Guhl, D. Campbell-Lendrum, and others. 2008. "Modelling Geographic Variation in the Cost-Effectiveness of Control Policies for Infectious Vector Diseases: The Example of Chagas Disease." *Journal of Health Economics* 27 (2): 405–26.

Cattand, P., P. Desjeux, M. G. Guzman, J. Jannin, A. Kroeger, and others. 2006. "Tropical Diseases Lacking Adequate Control Measures: Dengue, Leishmaniasis, and African Trypanosomiasis." In *Disease Control Priorities in Developing Countries* (second edition), edited by D. T. Jamison, J. G. Breman, A. R. Measham, G. Alleyne, M. Claeson, D. B. Evans, P. Jha, A. Mills, and P. Musgrove. Washington, DC: World Bank and Oxford University Press.

Chandler, D. J., K. S. Hansen, B. Mahato, J. Darlong, A. John, and others. 2015. "Household Costs of Leprosy Reactions (ENL) in Rural India." *PLoS Neglected Tropical Diseases* 9 (1): e0003431.

Constenla, D., C. Garcia, and N. Lefcourt. 2015. "Assessing the Economics of Dengue: Results from a Systematic Review of the Literature and Expert Survey." *Pharmacoeconomics* 33 (11): 1107–35.

de Vlas, S. J., W. A. Stolk, E. A. le Rutte, J. A. C. Hontelez, R. Bakker, and others. 2016. "Concerted Efforts to Control or Eliminate Neglected Tropical Diseases: How Much Health Will Be Gained?" *PLoS Neglected Tropical Diseases* 10 (2): e0004386.

Evans, D., D. McFarland, W. Adamani, A. Eigege, E. Miri, and others. 2011. "Cost-Effectiveness of Triple Drug Administration (TDA) with Praziquantel, Ivermectin, and

Albendazole for the Prevention of Neglected Tropical Diseases in Nigeria." *Annals of Tropical Medicine and Parasitology* 105 (8): 537–47.

Ezenduka, C., E. Post, S. John, A. Suraj, A. Namadi, and others. 2012. "Cost-Effectiveness Analysis of Three Leprosy Case Detection Methods in Northern Nigeria." *PLoS Neglected Tropical Diseases* 6 (9): e1818.

Federici, C., C. Fitzpatrick, A. Be-nazir, F. Meheus, and D. Dagne. Forthcoming. "The Cost-Effectiveness of a Comprehensive Programme to Eliminate Visceral Leishmaniasis in Bangladesh."

Fiedler, J. L., and R. Semakula. 2014. "An Analysis of the Costs of Uganda's Child Days Plus: Do Low Costs Reveal an Efficient Program or an Underfinanced One?" *Food and Nutrition Bulletin* 35 (1): 92–104.

Fitzpatrick, C., K. Asiedu, and J. Jannin. 2014. "Where the Road Ends, Yaws Begins? The Cost-Effectiveness of Eradication versus More Roads." *PLoS Neglected Tropical Diseases* 8 (9): e3165.

Fitzpatrick, C., M. Madin-Warburton, F. M. Fleming, T. Scheider, F. Mehus, K. Asiedu, A. Solomon, A. Montresor, G. Biswas. Forthcoming. "Benchmarking the Cost per Person of Mass Treatment for Selected Neglected Tropical Diseases: An Approach Based on Literature Review and Meta-Regression with Web-Based Software Application." *PLoS Neglected Tropical Diseases* (under review).

Habtamu, E., T. Wondie, S. Aweke, Z. Tadesse, M. Zerihun, and others. 2015. "Trachoma and Relative Poverty: A Case-Control Study." *PLoS Neglected Tropical Diseases* 9 (11): e0004228.

Hofstraat, K., and W. H. van Brakel. 2016. "Social Stigma towards Neglected Tropical Diseases: A Systematic Review." *International Health* 8 (Suppl 1): i53–70.

Horton, R. 2012. "GBD 2010: Understanding Disease, Injury, and Risk." *The Lancet* 380 (9859): 2053–54.

Hotez, P. J., M. Alvarado, M.-G. Basáñez, I. Bolliger, R. Bourne, and others. 2014. "The Global Burden of Disease Study 2010: Interpretation and Implications for the Neglected Tropical Diseases." *PLoS Neglected Tropical Diseases* 8 (7): e2865.

Hotez, P. J., D. A. P. Bundy, K. Beegle, S. Brooker, L. Drake, and others. 2006. "Helminth Infections: Soil-Transmitted Helminth Infections and Schistosomiasis." In *Disease Control Priorities in Developing Countries* (second edition), edited by D. T. Jamison, J. G. Breman, A. R. Measham, G. Alleyne, M. Claeson, D. B. Evans, P. Jha, A. Mills, and P. Musgrove, 1245–59. Washington, DC: World Bank and Oxford University Press.

Houweling, T. A. J., H. E. Karim-Kos, M. C. Kulik, W. A. Stolk, J. A. Haagsma, and others. 2016. "Socioeconomic Inequalities in Neglected Tropical Diseases: A Systematic Review." *PLoS Neglected Tropical Diseases* 10 (5): e0004546.

Hutton, G., and C. Chase. 2017. "Water Supply, Sanitation, and Hygiene." In *Disease Control Priorities* (third edition): Volume 7, *Injury Prevention and Environmental Health*, edited by C. N. Mock, O. Kobusingye, R. Nugent, and K. Smith. Washington, DC: World Bank.

Ibe, O., O. Onwujekwe, B. Uzochukwu, M. Ajuba, and P. Okonkwo. 2015. "Exploring Consumer Perceptions and

Economic Burden of Onchocerciasis on Households in Enugu State, South-East Nigeria." *PLoS Neglected Tropical Diseases* 9 (11): e0004231.

Idema, W. J., I. M. Majer, D. Pahan, L. Oskam, S. Polinder, and others. 2010. "Cost-Effectiveness of a Chemoprophylactic Intervention with Single Dose Rifampicin in Contacts of New Leprosy Patients." *PLoS Neglected Tropical Diseases* 4 (11): e874.

Keating, J., J. O. Yukich, S. Mollenkopf, and F. Tediosi. 2014. "Lymphatic Filariasis and Onchocerciasis Prevention, Treatment, and Control Costs across Diverse Settings: A Systematic Review." *Acta Tropica* 135 (1): 86–95.

Krotneva, S. P., L. E. Coffeng, M. Noma, H. G. Zouré, L. Bakoné, and others. 2015. "African Program for Onchocerciasis Control 1995–2010: Impact of Annual Ivermectin Mass Treatment on Off-Target Infectious Diseases." *PLoS Neglected Tropical Diseases* 9 (9): 1–14.

Lee, B. Y., K. M. Bacon, M. E. Bottazzi, and P. J. Hotez. 2013. "Global Economic Burden of Chagas Disease: A Computational Simulation Model." *The Lancet Infectious Diseases* 13 (4): 342–48.

Lenk, E. J., W. K. Redekop, M. Luyendijk, C. Fitzpatrick, L. Niessen, and others. Forthcoming. "The Socioeconomic Benefit to Individuals of Achieving the 2020 Targets for Neglected Tropical Diseases Controlled or Eliminated By Innovative and Intensified Disease Management."

Lenk, E. J., W. K. Redekop, M. Luyendijk, A. J. Rijnsburger, and J. L. Severens. 2016. "Productivity Loss Related to Neglected Tropical Diseases Eligible for Preventive Chemotherapy: A Systematic Literature Review." *PLoS Neglected Tropical Diseases* 10 (2): e0004397.

Leslie, J., A. Garba, K. Boubacar, Y. Yayé, H. Sebongou, and others. 2013. "Neglected Tropical Diseases: Comparison of the Costs of Integrated and Vertical Preventive Chemotherapy Treatment in Niger." *International Health* 5 (1): 78–84.

Lo, N. C., I. I. Bogoch, B. G. Blackburn, G. Raso, E. K. N'Goran, and others. 2015. "Comparison of Community-Wide, Integrated Mass Drug Administration Strategies for Schistosomiasis and Soil-Transmitted Helminthiasis: A Cost-Effectiveness Modelling Study." *The Lancet Global Health* 3 (10): e629–38.

Luz, P. M., T. Vanni, J. Medlock, A. D. Paltiel, and A. P. Galvani. 2011. "Dengue Vector Control Strategies in an Urban Setting: An Economic Modelling Assessment." *The Lancet* 377 (9778): 1673–80.

Martelli, C. M. T., J. B. Siqueira, M. P. P. D. Parente, A. L. Zara, C. S. Oliveira, and others. 2015. "Economic Impact of Dengue: Multicenter Study across Four Brazilian Regions." *PLoS Neglected Tropical Diseases* 9 (9): e0004042.

Meheus, F., A. A. Abuzaid, R. Baltussen, B. M. Younis, M. Balasegaram, and others. 2013. "The Economic Burden of Visceral Leishmaniasis in Sudan: An Assessment of Provider and Household Costs." *American Journal of Tropical Medicine and Hygiene* 89 (6): 1146–53.

Meheus, F., and M. Boelaert. 2010. "The Burden of Visceral Leishmaniasis in South Asia." *Tropical Medicine and International Health* 15 (Suppl 2): 1–3.

MSH (Management Sciences for Health). 2014. *International Drug Price Indicator Guide 2014.* Medford, MA: Management Sciences for Health. http://erc.msh.org/mainpage.cfm?file=1 .0.htm&module=DMP&language=english.

Orellano, P. W., N. Vazquez, and O. D. Salomon. 2013. "Cost-Effectiveness of Prevention Strategies for American Tegumentary Leishmaniasis in Argentina." *Cadernos de Saúde Pública* 29 (12): 2459–72.

Ozaki, M., S. Islam, K. M. Rahman, A. Rahman, S. P. Luby, and others. 2011. "Economic Consequences of Post-kala-azar Dermal Leishmaniasis in a Rural Bangladeshi Community." *American Journal of Tropical Medicine and Hygiene* 85 (3): 528–34.

Redekop, W., E. J. Lenk, M. Luyendijk, C. Fitzpatrick, Louis Niessen, and others. Forthcoming. "The Socioeconomic Benefit to Individuals of Achieving the 2020 Targets for Five Preventive Chemotherapy Neglected Tropical Diseases."

Reithinger, R., and P. G. Coleman. 2007. "Treating Cutaneous Leishmaniasis Patients in Kabul, Afghanistan: Cost-Effectiveness of an Operational Program in a Complex Emergency Setting." *BMC Infectious Diseases* 7 (January 30): 3.

Remme, J. H. F., P. Feenstra, P. R. Lever, A. C. Medici, C. M. Morel, and others. 2006. "Tropical Diseases Targeted for Elimination: Chagas Disease, Lymphatic Filariasis, Onchocerciasis, and Leprosy." In *Disease Control Priorities in Developing Countries* (second edition), edited by D. T. Jamison, J. G. Breman, A. R. Measham, G. Alleyne, M. Claeson, D. B. Evans, P. Jha, A. Mills, and P. Musgrove. Washington, DC: World Bank and Oxford University Press.

Rilkoff, H., E. M. Tukahebwa, F. M. Fleming, J. Leslie, and D. C. Cole. 2013. "Exploring Gender Dimensions of Treatment Programmes for Neglected Tropical Diseases in Uganda." *PLoS Neglected Tropical Diseases* 7 (7): e2312.

Ruan, Y.-Z., R.-Z. Li, X.-X. Wang, L.-X. Wang, Q. Sun, and others. 2016. "The Affordability for Patients of a New Universal MDR-TB Coverage Model in China." *International Journal of Tuberculosis and Lung Disease* 20 (5): 638–44.

Shepard, D. S., L. Coudeville, Y. A. Halasa, B. Zambrano, and G. H. Dayan. 2011. "Economic Impact of Dengue Illness in the Americas." *American Journal of Tropical Medicine and Hygiene* 84 (2): 200–7.

Shepard, D. S., Y. A. Halasa, B. K. Tyagi, S. V. Adhish, D. Nandan, and others. 2014. "Economic and Disease Burden of Dengue Illness in India." *American Journal of Tropical Medicine and Hygiene* 91 (6): 1235–42.

Shepard, D. S., E. A. Undurraga, and Y. A. Halasa. 2013. "Economic and Disease Burden of Dengue in Southeast Asia." *PLoS Neglected Tropical Diseases* 7 (2): e2055.

Stahl, H.-C., V. M. Butenschoen, H. T. Tran, E. Gozzer, R. Skewes, and others. 2013. "Cost of Dengue Outbreaks: Literature Review and Country Case Studies." *BMC Public Health* 13 (November 6): 1048.

Stone, C. M., R. Kastner, P. Steinmann, N. Chitnis, M. Tanner, and others. 2016. "Modelling the Health Impact and Cost-Effectiveness of Lymphatic Filariasis Eradication under Varying Levels of Mass Drug Administration Scale-Up and Geographic Coverage." *BMJ Global Health* 1 (April 6): e000021.

Suaya, J. A., D. S. Shepard, M.-S. Chang, M. Caram, S. Hoyer, and others. 2007. "Cost-Effectiveness of Annual Targeted Larviciding Campaigns in Cambodia against the Dengue Vector *Aedes aegypti.*" *Tropical Medicine and International Health* 12 (9): 1026–36.

Sundar, S., R. Arora, S. P. Singh, M. Boelaert, and B. Varghese. 2010. "Household Cost-of-Illness of Visceral Leishmaniasis in Bihar, India." *Tropical Medicine and International Health* 15 (Suppl 2): 50–54.

Sutherland, C. S., J. Yukich, R. Goeree, and F. Tediosi. 2015. "A Literature Review of Economic Evaluations for a Neglected Tropical Disease: Human African Trypanosomiasis ('Sleeping Sickness')." *PLoS Neglected Tropical Diseases* 9 (2): e0003397.

Turner, H. C., A. A. Bettis, B. K. Chu, D. A. McFarland, P. J. Hooper, and others. 2016. "Investment Success in Public Health: An Analysis of the Cost-Effectiveness and Cost-Benefit of the Global Programme to Eliminate Lymphatic Filariasis." *Clinical Infectious Diseases.* Epub December 12. doi10.1093/cid/ciw835.

Turner, H. C., J. E. Truscott, T. D. Hollingsworth, A. A. Bettis, S. J. Brooker, and others. 2015. "Cost and Cost-Effectiveness of Soil-Transmitted Helminth Treatment Programmes: Systematic Review and Research Needs." *Parasites and Vectors* 8 (1): 355.

Turner, H. C., M. Walker, T. S. Churcher, M. Y. Osei-Atweneboana, N.-K. Biritwum, and others. 2014. "Reaching the London Declaration on Neglected Tropical Diseases Goals for Onchocerciasis: An Economic Evaluation of Increasing the Frequency of Ivermectin Treatment in Africa." *Clinical Infectious Diseases* 59 (7): 923–32.

Ugbomoiko, U. S., V. Dalumo, I. E. Ofoezie, and R. N. N. Obiezue. 2009. "Socio-Environmental Factors and Ascariasis Infection among School-Aged Children in Ilobu, Osun State, Nigeria." *Transactions of the Royal Society of Tropical Medicine and Hygiene* 103 (3): 223–28.

Undurraga, E. A., M. Betancourt-Cravioto, J. Ramos-Castañeda, R. Martínez-Vega, J. Méndez-Galván, and others. 2015. "Economic and Disease Burden of Dengue in Mexico." *PLoS Neglected Tropical Diseases* 9 (3): e0003547.

Uniting to Combat Neglected Tropical Diseases. 2014. *Delivering on Promises and Driving Progress: Second Report on Uniting to Combat NTDs.* http://unitingtocombatntds .org/report/delivering-promises-driving-progress -second-report-uniting-combat-ntds.

Uranw, S., F. Meheus, R. Baltussen, S. Rijal, and M. Boelaert. 2013. "The Household Costs of Visceral Leishmaniasis Care in South-Eastern Nepal." *PLoS Neglected Tropical Diseases* 7 (2): e2062.

Vazquez-Prokopec, G. M., C. Spillmann, M. Zaidenberg, U. Kitron, and R. E. Gürtler. 2009. "Cost-Effectiveness of Chagas Disease Vector Control Strategies in Northwestern Argentina." *PLoS Neglected Tropical Diseases* 3 (1): e363.

WHO (World Health Organization). 2010. *Working to Overcome the Global Impact of Neglected Tropical Diseases: First WHO Report on Neglected Tropical Diseases.* Geneva: WHO.

———. 2012. *Accelerating Work to Overcome the Global Impact of Neglected Tropical Diseases: A Roadmap for Implementation.* Geneva: WHO.

———. 2013. "World Health Assembly Resolution 66.12: Neglected Tropical Diseases." WHO, Geneva. http://www .who.int/neglected_diseases/mediacentre/WHA_66.12 _Eng.pdf?ua=1.

———. 2014a. "Global Health Estimates 2014 Summary Tables: DALY by Cause, Age, Sex, by World Bank income Category, 2000–2012." WHO, Geneva. http://www.who.int /healthinfo/global_burden_disease/en.

———. 2014b. *World Health Statistics 2014.* Geneva: WHO. http://www.who.int/gho/publications/world_health _statistics/2014/en/.

———. 2015a. *Generic Framework for Control, Elimination and Eradication of Neglected Tropical Diseases.* Geneva: WHO. http://www.who.int/neglected_diseases/resources /NTD_Generic_Framework_2015.pdf.

———. 2015b. *Investing to Overcome the Global Impact of Neglected Tropical Diseases: Third Report on Neglected Diseases 2015.* Geneva: WHO.

———. 2015c. PCT Databank. WHO, Geneva. http://www .who.int/neglected_diseases/preventive_chemotherapy /databank/en/.

———. 2015d. "Kala-Azar Elimination Programme: Report of a WHO Consultation of Partners." Geneva, WHO, February 10-11. http://apps.who.int/iris/bitstream/10665/185042/1 /9789241509497_eng.pdf.

———. 2016. "World Health Assembly Resolution 69.21: Addressing the Burden of Mycetoma." WHO, Geneva. http://apps.who.int/gb/ebwha/pdf_files/WHA69/A69 _R21-en.pdf.

WHO-CHOICE. 2012. *Choosing Interventions That Are Cost Effective (WHO-CHOICE).* Geneva: WHO. http://www.who .int/choice/en/.

Worrell, C., and E. Mathieu. 2012. "Drug Coverage Surveys for Neglected Tropical Diseases: 10 Years of Field Experience." *American Journal of Tropical Medicine and Hygiene* 87 (2): 216–22.

Chapter **18**

Drug-Resistant Infections

Molly Miller-Petrie, Suraj Pant, and Ramanan Laxminarayan

ANTIBIOTIC RESISTANCE

The global rise in antibiotic resistance threatens to undo decades of progress in treating infectious diseases caused by bacterial pathogens (Laxminarayan and others 2006). Resistance to the drugs used to treat malaria, human immunodeficiency virus/acquired immune deficiency syndrome (HIV/AIDS), and *Mycobacterium tuberculosis* is also a serious concern, with multidrug-resistant and extensively drug-resistant tuberculosis now documented worldwide, particularly in China, India, and the Russian Federation (WHO 2014). These diseases and their treatments are covered in depth in other chapters in this volume. This chapter deals specifically with antibiotic resistance in the One Health framework of humans, animals, and the environment.

Bacterial resistance to first-line, second-line, and last-resort antibiotics is growing, although rates and trends vary by location, organism, and antibiotic (CDDEP 2016). Increased travel, trade, and migration mean that resistant bacteria can spread faster than ever (Du and others 2016; Johnson and Woodford 2013). The Centers for Disease Control and Prevention (CDC) considers *Clostridium difficile* (*C. difficile*), carbapenem-resistant Enterobacteriaceae, and cephalosporin-resistant *Neisseria gonorrhoeae* urgent threats to health in the United States (CDC 2013).

Drug-resistant infections are associated with higher morbidity, mortality, and health expenditures (Okeke, Laxminarayan, and others 2005). The burden of resistance falls heavily on low- and middle-income countries (LMICs),

which typically have high burdens and rapid spread of infectious disease, poor nutrition, and increasing rates of antibiotic consumption in humans and animals, in addition to weaker health care systems and sparse standards and regulations that govern access, use, and quality of antibiotics (Okeke, Klugman, and others 2005).

Lack of access to antibiotics is still a serious concern for most LMICs. Pneumonia kills approximately 1 million children under age five each year, and an estimated 445,000 could be saved with the universal provision of antibiotics for community-acquired pneumococcal infections (Laxminarayan and others 2016). When they are available, first-line antibiotic treatments are still relatively affordable, but newer antibiotics needed to treat resistant infections may be out of reach in low-resource settings (Laxminarayan and others 2016; Mendelson and others 2015).

At the same time, resistant infections are becoming a significant cause of death, particularly for children. Mortality is higher for children with drug-resistant infections, such as methicillin-resistant *Staphylococcus aureus* (MRSA, a common skin and soft tissue infection) and infections caused by extended spectrum beta-lactamase-producing bacteria (Kayange and others 2010). Though data are limited, it is estimated that resistant sepsis infections kill approximately 214,000 neonates each year, primarily in India, Pakistan, Nigeria, the Democratic Republic of Congo, and China (figure 18.1) (Laxminarayan and others 2016). The prevalence of drug-resistant infections in children is growing: the prevalence of

Corresponding author: Ramanan Laxminarayan, Center for Disease Dynamics, Economics & Policy, Washington, DC, United States; ramanan@cddep.org.ss.

Figure 18.1 Estimated Neonatal Sepsis Deaths Caused by Bacteria Resistant to First-Line Antibiotics in High-Burden Countries

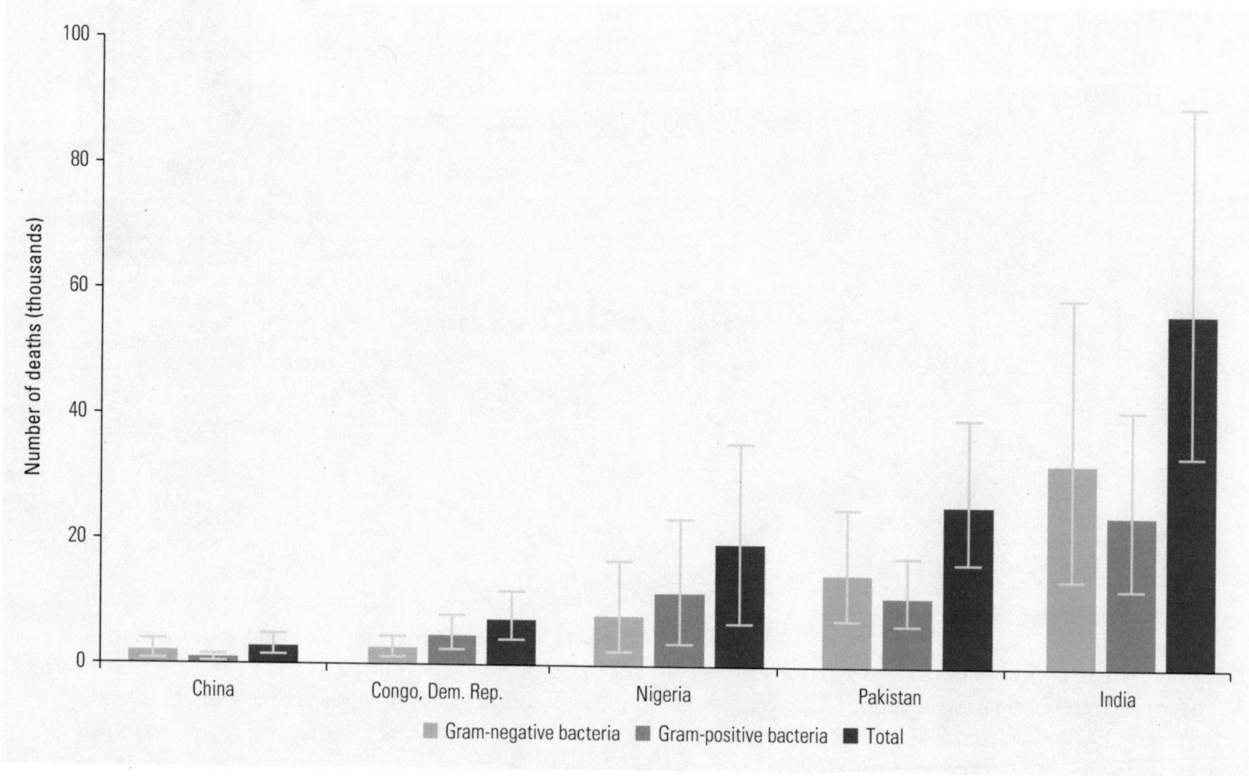

Source: Laxminarayan and others 2016.
Note: Bars represent maximum and minimum values from Latin Hypercube Sampling model.

carbapenem-resistant *Enterobacteriaceae* infections in children increased from 0 percent in 2000 to 5 percent in 2012 in the United States (Logan and others 2015).

Drug-resistant typhoidal and nontyphoidal *Salmonella* infections are also on the rise, with multidrug resistance detected in 50 to 75 percent of nontyphoidal *Salmonella* isolates tested and up to 89 percent of *Salmonella* Typhi isolates tested in Sub-Saharan Africa (Al-Emran and others 2016; Kariuki and others 2015). The Typhoid Fever Surveillance in Africa Program also reported high levels of resistance in invasive *Salmonella* to first-line treatments, in addition to multidrug-resistant strains (Baker, Hombach, and Marks 2016). However, incidence of resistant *Salmonella* infections varies widely across the African region, indicating that national surveillance systems are needed to guide treatment decisions (Al-Emran and others 2016). Invasive *Salmonella* infections are responsible for approximately 600,000 deaths a year, particularly in children in low-resource settings. Case fatality rates from multidrug-resistant *Salmonella* Typhi infections in South Asia are 10 percent—approaching those of the pre-antibiotic era (Okeke, Laxminarayan and others 2005).

Many infections, both drug-resistant and drug-susceptible, are acquired in hospitals. Surgical site infections account for one-third of all health care–associated infections (HAIs) worldwide; they are the leading cause of HAIs in low-resource settings (Allegranzi and others 2011). Antibiotic prophylaxis can reduce the risk of infection in patients undergoing surgery and chemotherapy, but antibiotic resistance threatens to undo these benefits (Teillant and others 2015). A 30 percent decrease in antibiotic efficacy would lead to an estimated 120,000 additional infections and 6,300 additional deaths per year in the United States, according to a recent modeling study (figure 18.2). Other HAIs, particularly sepsis, are a danger for both neonates and their mothers, who are increasingly seeking birth and delivery care at hospitals at the advice of health care providers. Increasing rates of drug resistance in these infections amplify this risk.

Despite limited national-level data and a lack of standardized methods for collecting resistance data, it is clear that resistance is declining in some instances. Map 18.1 shows the global prevalence of MRSA. MRSA rates are decreasing in Canada, Europe, South Africa, and the United States (CDDEP 2016; EARS-Net 2014; Martin

Figure 18.2 Number of Additional Infections per Year Expected in the United States if Antibiotic Efficacy Decreased by 30 Percent

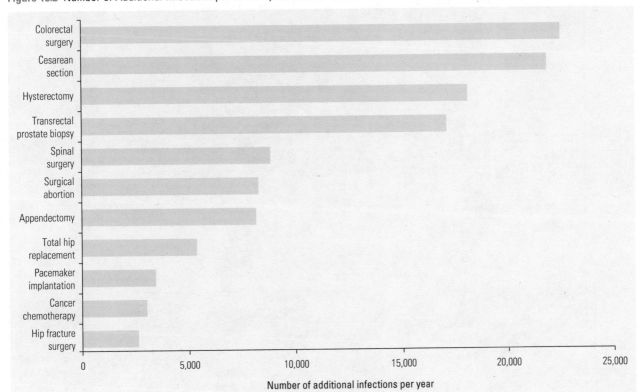

Source: Teillant and others 2015.

and others 2015). However, steep increases have been detected in several LMICs, including India (box 18.1), and what data are available in Africa indicate that rates are also high in some populations in the region (Abdulgader and others 2015). Even less information is available on MRSA and other bacterial infections in animals in LMICs.

Resistance of Enterobacteriaceae to one of the last-resort antibiotics, carbapenems, is low but increasing in many LMICs (CDDEP 2016; Lerner and others 2015). Extended spectrum beta-lactamases, which are resistant to most beta-lactam antibiotics, are also increasingly prevalent worldwide, including in Africa and Latin America (Datta and others 2012; Lu and others 2012; PAHO, forthcoming; Storberg 2014). Resistance to quinolones has been widely detected in enteric infections, such as those caused by *Escherichia coli (E. coli)*, in Sub-Saharan Africa, where quinolone use has increased since generics became available in the early 2000s (Chattaway and others 2016). Sexually transmitted infections, such as *Neisseria gonorrhoeae*, are increasingly resistant to all available treatment options (Buono and others 2015).

Resistant bacteria can also be detected in the guts of livestock or in water or soil that has been exposed to antibiotics. These drug-resistant bacteria can then spread to humans through direct contact with animals and infected food, water, or waste (Marshall and Levy 2011). Emerging resistance mechanisms, such as the MCR-1 gene conferring plasmid-mediated resistance to colistin, a last-resort antibiotic, have been detected in both humans and animals and have the potential to render even more infections untreatable (Liu and others 2016). Overall, there is a significant lack of surveillance data on resistance in humans and animals in most LMICs and in many high-income countries (HICs); these data are critical to guiding policy making and clinical care.

DRIVERS OF ANTIBIOTIC USE AND RESISTANCE

Use in Human Health Care

Every use of an antibiotic, whether appropriate or inappropriate, exerts selection pressure, giving resistant bacteria an advantage and accelerating the development of resistance. Consumption of antibiotics is rising globally, but particularly in LMICs, as a result, in part, of rising incomes and increased access to drugs.

Map 18.1 Percentage of Methicillin-Resistant *Staphylococcus aureus* Isolates, by Country, Most Recent Year, 2011–14

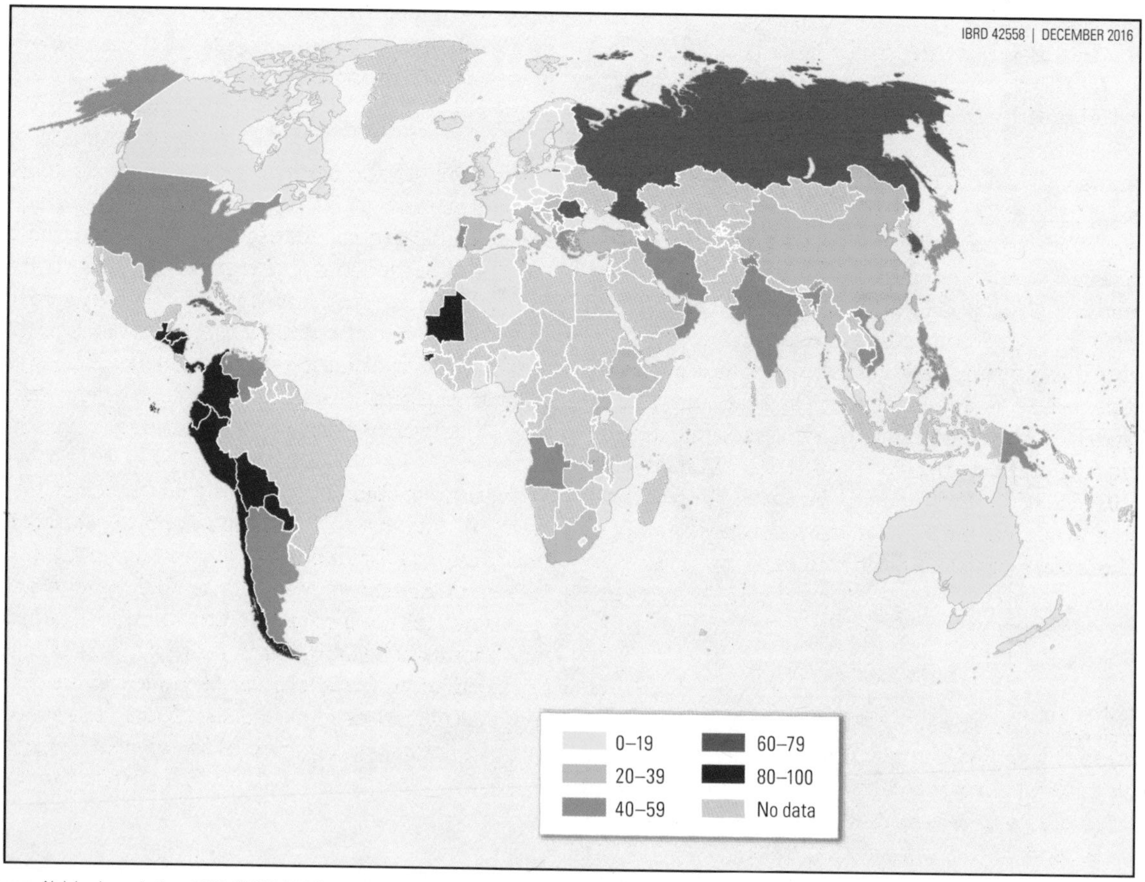

IBRD 42558 | DECEMBER 2016

0–19	60–79
20–39	80–100
40–59	No data

Sources: Abdulgader and others 2015; CDDEP 2016 (https://resistancemap.cddep.org); PAHO, forthcoming; WHO 2014.

Note: Where available, data from hospital-associated methicillin-resistant *Staphylococcus aureus* (MRSA) and invasive isolates are used. In their absence, data from community-associated MRSA or all specimen sources are included. Only countries that reported data for at least 30 isolates are shown. Depending on the country, at least one of the following drugs was used to test for MRSA: cefoxitin, cloxacillin, dicloxacillin, flucloxacillin, methicillin, and oxacillin. Intermediate-resistant isolates are considered resistant in some calculations, as in the original data source. Data from Abdulgader and others (2015) collected before and during 2011 were included as 2011.

Box 18.1

Antibiotic Resistance in India

India has high levels of both antibiotic consumption and antibiotic resistance. Antibiotic use is increasing in conjunction with improved livelihoods and expanded access to drugs, providing benefits for human health. Still, over-the-counter sales without a medical provider's prescription, weak regulation, and poor incentives for rational use are contributing to inappropriate use of antibiotics. Owing in part to poor health infrastructure, poor-quality drugs, and a high burden of disease, India's rates of resistant infections are rising.

India was the top consumer of antibiotics in 2010 and one of the top global consumers of antibiotics in agriculture that same year. Consumption of faropenem, an oral antibiotic structurally similar to carbapenems, has increased by 154 percent since it was approved for use in 2010 (Gandra and others 2016). Strains of *Escherichia coli*, *Klebsiella pneumoniae*, *Salmonella* Typhi, and MRSA (methicillin-resistant *Staphylococcus aureus*) have high resistance to most antibiotics, including carbapenems. Improved regulation, behavior change for patients and providers, incentives for improved prescribing practices, and increased surveillance have the potential to reverse current trends while preserving and increasing gains in access (Laxminarayan and Chaudhury 2016).

Human antibiotic consumption is also driven by the burden of infectious disease, as well as by economic, behavioral, environmental, and structural factors. Expanded insurance coverage and increased physician density increase the consumption of antibiotics (Klein and others 2015; Zhang, Lee, and Donohue 2010). Decision fatigue and patient demand also increase antibiotic prescribing (Dosh and others 2000; Linder and others 2014). Antibiotic use is also correlated with season, increasing in the winter (December through February in the northern hemisphere and August through September in the southern hemisphere) when the incidence of infectious disease is higher (Sun, Klein, and Laxminarayan 2012). In addition to driving resistance, antibiotic use increases the incidence of *C. difficile* infection, which takes hold when antibiotic treatment has destroyed the normal gut flora. *C. difficile* is responsible for an estimated 14,000 deaths per year in the United States (CDC 2013).

As shown in map 18.2, it is estimated that antibiotic consumption increased more than 30 percent in 71 countries between 2000 and 2010, reaching approximately 70 billion standard units (single-dose units) in 2010 (Van Boeckel and others 2014). This increase was primarily in first-line classes of antibiotics, including penicillins and cephalosporins, which together make up more than half of global consumption. Use of last-resort antibiotic classes such as carbapenems and polymixins also increased. Although the consumption of antibiotics

Map 18.2 Percentage Change in Antibiotic Consumption per Capita, by Country, 2000–10

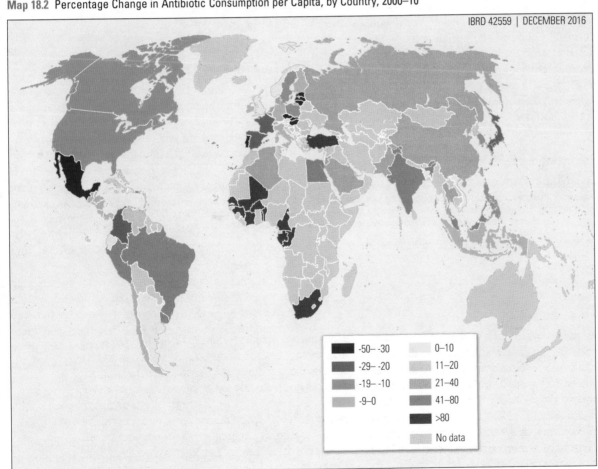

IBRD 42559 | DECEMBER 2016

Legend:
- -50– -30
- -29– -20
- -19– -10
- -9– 0
- 0–10
- 11–20
- 21–40
- 41–80
- >80
- No data

Source: Van Boeckel and others 2014, based on IMS MIDAS.
Note: Data for Costa Rica, El Salvador, Guatemala, Honduras, Nicaragua, and Panama were available only as a group classified as Central America. Similarly, data for Benin, Burkina Faso, Cameroon, the Republic of Congo, Côte d'Ivoire, Gabon, Guinea, Mali, Senegal, and Togo were grouped and classified as French West Africa. The data for these countries represent the estimates for the corresponding regional groupings to which they belong. For countries with no data for 2000, the values for the earliest years for which data were available after 2000 were used to calculate the percentage changes. These countries and initial years are Algeria (2002), Bangladesh (2007), Croatia (2005), the Netherlands (2005), and Vietnam (2005). Much of the increase in antibiotic consumption in South Africa can be attributed to the use of co-trimoxazole as prophylaxis for HIV (human immunodeficiency virus) patients as recommended by the World Health Organization.

declined in some HICs from 2000 to 2010, annual per capita consumption in the United States is still one of the highest in the world, at approximately 22 standard units per person (map 18.2). Consumption grew fastest in middle-income countries, including Brazil, China, India, Russia, and South Africa.

Human consumption of antibiotics is often inappropriate in both LMICs and HICs, where antibiotics are purchased over the counter or prescribed incorrectly by a physician when they are not needed and will not be effective. Diarrheal and respiratory infections are frequently treated with antibiotics in the absence of diagnostics, even if such practice brings no benefit to patients; both consumers and prescribers may lack the awareness, education, or incentive to use antibiotics correctly.

An estimated 80 percent of antibiotics globally are purchased outside of hospitals (Kotwani and Holloway 2011). Although many of these antibiotics are purchased without prescriptions, increased regulation to restrict sales may not be an appropriate solution for communities that lack access to antibiotics. Interventions that target incentives linked to consumers, prescribers, and retailers and that educate the public and health care providers will be required to change consumption patterns in communities.

Use in Hospitals

The volume of antibiotic consumption is greater in communities, but the clinical consequences of resistance are greater in hospitals, which are home to a rotating population of seriously ill patients treated heavily with medications, including antibiotics. Infections treated in hospitals may originate at the point of care (HAIs) or in communities, where patients may have already been treated unsuccessfully with antibiotics.

Suboptimal prescribing of antibiotics is common in both LMICs and HICs. In Nepal, an estimated 10 percent to 40 percent of antibiotic use is inappropriate; in Vietnam, one-third of hospital prescriptions were deemed inappropriate (Paudel, Sharma, and Das 2008; Shankar and others 2007; Thu and others 2012). In six hospitals in the United States, initial antibiotic therapy was changed after five days in only one-third of patients, although 58 percent of patients tested negative for bacterial infection (Braykov and others 2014). The use of carbapenems is rapidly increasing in hospitals (figure 18.3) (CDDEP 2016). In some countries (for example, China), doctors or hospitals profit from the volume of antibiotics sold (Currie, Lin, and Meng 2014).

Use in Food Animal Production

At least two-thirds of all antibiotics, including those important for human medicine, are estimated to be used in livestock production at subtherapeutic levels to promote growth and prevent disease, and at therapeutic levels to treat disease (Laxminarayan, Van Boeckel, and Teillant 2015). Antibiotic use in animal agriculture is widespread and is estimated to increase by more than two-thirds between 2010 and 2030 (Van Boeckel and others 2015). This widespread use creates strong selection pressure, encouraging the emergence and development of resistance (Laxminarayan, Van Boeckel, and Teillant 2015).

In animal production systems, antibiotics have long been used in place of improved sanitation and hygiene to prevent disease. As incomes rise in LMICs, the demand for animal-source food products will grow (Gelband and others 2015). To meet this demand, more farmers are using intensive production systems, with more animals raised in smaller spaces, leading to greater reliance on antibiotics to prevent disease and promote growth. In the coming decades, antibiotic use for food production is predicted to grow, as shown in figure 18.4, with Brazil, China, India, Russia, and South Africa expected to experience an estimated 98 percent increase collectively (Laxminarayan, Van Boeckel, and Teillant 2015). Consumption is also increasing in some HICs. Figure 18.5 illustrates increasing antibiotic use in meat production in the United States, where antibiotic use per unit of meat has increased every year from 2009 to 2014 (CDDEP 2016).

Figure 18.3 Per Capita Carbapenem Use in the Hospital Sector, 2005–10

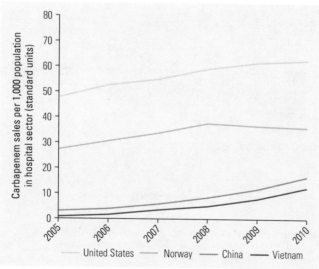

Source: Based on IMS MIDAS.

Figure 18.4 Estimated Growth in the Consumption of Antibiotics in Livestock, Top 10 Countries, 2010-30

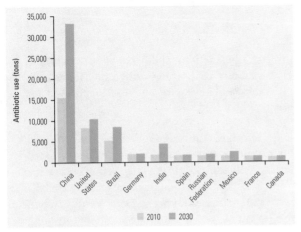

Source: Van Boeckel and others 2015.

Figure 18.5 Antibiotic Use in Meat Production in the United States, 2009–14

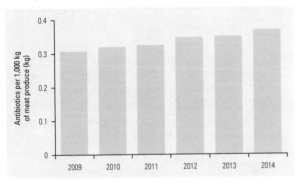

Sources: USDA 2015; U.S. Department of Health and Human Services 2015.
Note: kg = kilograms.

NATIONAL POLICIES TO CONSERVE ANTIBIOTIC EFFECTIVENESS

The World Health Assembly passed the Global Action Plan on Antimicrobial Resistance in May 2015 (WHO 2015). The plan calls on member countries to establish national plans to address antibiotic consumption and resistance within the next two years. Plans are expected to be context specific and ideally will encompass five strategic objectives:

- Improving awareness through education or awareness campaigns
- Strengthening existing evidence through surveillance and monitoring
- Reducing the risk of infections through prevention measures

- Optimizing the use of antibiotics through stewardship and appropriate prescriptions
- Reshaping economic incentives to encourage research on new antibiotics while preserving existing drugs.

Some HICs, such as the United Kingdom and the United States, have implemented comprehensive national action plans. Fewer LMICs have such plans, but in those LMICs that do, the plans have proved successful. Progress in Ethiopia, Nepal, South Africa, and Vietnam shows that action plans are both possible to formulate in LMIC settings and are urgently needed; box 18.2 describes South Africa's plan.

COST-EFFECTIVE INTERVENTIONS

Although data on antibiotic use and resistance in LMICs are limited, new surveillance networks and laboratory-strengthening programs are being established. Online databases like the Center for Disease Dynamics, Economics & Policy's ResistanceMap[1] are filling the gap by providing data on use and resistance for a significant number of countries. Evidence on effective interventions is limited by the diversity of resistance drivers and the long timelines required to observe an effect on antibiotic resistance rates. A review found that the evidence base for specific national interventions is insufficient to inform policies (Dar and others 2015), but areas for action have clear potential benefits (Holloway 2011; Jamison and others 2013).

Water, Sanitation, and Hygiene

In the United States, the burden of infectious diseases declined before the introduction of antibiotics, largely because of improvements in water and sanitation. Many LMICs use antibiotics as a substitute for these improvements, but medications alone will not achieve the same reductions. Handwashing, clean water, and excreta disposal reduce diarrheal diseases by 48 percent, 17 percent, and 36 percent, respectively (Cairncross and others 2010). Handwashing also reduces respiratory infections by at least 16 percent (Rabie and Curtis 2006). Handwashing by health care providers reduces HAIs and the development and spread of resistant infections (Allegranzi and Pittet 2009; De Angelis and others 2014).

Sanitation and water quality require expensive infrastructure, but the savings from averted diseases offset most investments in water, sanitation, and hygiene (Clasen and Haller 2008). Water supply and sanitation interventions are cost-effective in all regions (Hutton, Haller, and Bartram 2007). Hand hygiene is highly

Comprehensive National Action Plans: The Example of South Africa

The South African Department of Health launched a national strategic framework in 2014 (Department of Health, South Africa 2014) that adopted recommendations set by the World Health Organization and the International Committee of the World Organisation for Animal Health to curb the threat of antibiotic resistance. Key elements of the framework include strengthening, coordinating, and institutionalizing interdisciplinary efforts through national and governance structures; optimizing surveillance and early detection of antibiotic resistance; enhancing infection prevention and control; and promoting appropriate use of antibiotics in animal and human health. Several interventions have been proposed to ensure success, including amendments to medical curricula; improved hand hygiene, vaccination, and water and sanitation; establishment of hospital antibiotic stewardship programs; and review of antibiotics approved for use in animal feed.

Early detection and strong surveillance are essential for capturing trends and creating evidence-based public policies. South Africa's national strategy framework aims to strengthen the existing surveillance system by developing an early warning system for potential disease outbreaks and by tracking trends and resistance patterns. In the long term, it will also use local, regional, and national resistance patterns to optimize prescribing and report on resistance rates in food-producing and companion animals.

---

cost-effective and the most affordable intervention at US$3.35 per disability-adjusted life year (DALY) averted (Cairncross and Valdmanis 2006).

Vaccination

The potential reduction in antibiotic use attributable to vaccination is considerable. An estimated 11 million days of antibiotic treatment could be avoided by the universal introduction of the pneumococcal vaccine (Laxminarayan and others 2016). Influenza in the United States is nearly perfectly predicted by antibiotic sales data (Polgreen, Laxminarayan, and Cavanaugh 2011). An estimated 20 percent reduction in influenza would reduce antibiotic prescribing by 8 percent in the United States; a universal vaccination program in Ontario, Canada, was found to reduce influenza-associated antibiotic prescribing by 64 percent (Kwong and others 2009; Polgreen, Laxminarayan, and Cavanaugh 2011). Influenza vaccination also averts secondary bacterial infections, which have been associated with up to 40 percent of influenza cases that require hospitalization (Falsey and others 2013; McCullers 2014). The introduction of vaccines for viral and bacterial diarrheal infections, such as rotavirus and cholera, are likely to achieve similar reductions in antibiotic use (Ganguly and others 2011; Okeke 2009).

Vaccination can reduce the overall disease burden and the incidence of drug-resistant infections.

The introduction of the pneumococcal vaccine in the United States reduced infection with both penicillin-resistant and multidrug-resistant strains of *Streptococcus pneumoniae*—incidence of each type dropped more than 50 percent (Grijalva and others 2007; Kyaw and others 2006). Similarly, in South Africa, introduction of the vaccine reduced infection with penicillin-resistant strains by 67 percent and infection with trimethoprim-sulfamethoxazole-resistant strains by 56 percent (Klugman and others 2003). Vaccines also reduce antibiotic resistance by reducing overall selection pressure (Gelband and others 2015; Kwong and others 2009; Polgreen, Laxminarayan, and Cavanaugh 2011). Vaccines are being developed for commonly resistant infections, such as those caused by *Staphylococcus aureus*, *E. coli*, and *Klebsiella pneumoniae*, as well as *C. difficile*, but have faced significant challenges (Gelband and others 2015).

The cost-effectiveness of introducing new vaccines will differ by background burden of disease and existing cold chains; most vaccines are highly cost-effective, even though assessments rarely include the savings from reducing drug-resistant infections (Maurice and Davey 2009; Rheingans and others 2014). In India, health care cost savings offset the cost of vaccination against *Haemophilus influenzae* in all states (Clark and others 2013). Similarly, an assessment of cost-effectiveness in LMICs found that the *Haemophilus influenzae* type b conjugate vaccine was cost saving or highly cost-effective

(Griffiths, Clark, and Hajjeh 2013), while the pneumococcal vaccine was highly cost-effective in 68 of 72 developing countries (Sinha and others 2007). For diarrheal infections, the rotavirus vaccine provided economic benefits at diverse prices, while cholera vaccination had economic benefits in specific contexts (Rheingans and others 2014).

Antibiotic Stewardship and Infection Control Programs in Hospitals

Stewardship and infection control have been broadly proposed as the most effective interventions for reducing antibiotic use in all settings (Dar and others 2015). Components of stewardship programs such as prescription audits, peer comparisons, and guidelines have successfully reduced antibiotic use (Meeker and others 2014; Meeker and others 2016). Hospital antibiotic stewardship programs aim to provide the correct dose of the most appropriate antibiotic at the right time; they have also been shown to reduce antibiotic use by 11 percent to 38 percent and to be associated with modest reductions in antibiotic-resistant infections (Kaki and others 2011).

Antibiotics are often used as a substitute for infection prevention and control in hospitals. Infection control programs reduce antibiotic use, in addition to reducing the prevalence and spread of HAIs. They are particularly important in LMICs, where rates of HAIs are two to three times higher than in Europe and the United States (Allegranzi and others 2011; Davey and others 2005; WHO 2011). Bundled interventions and handwashing have been shown to reduce both HAIs and antibiotic use (Gelband and others 2015).

Multifaceted infection control programs have been shown to be cost-effective in the United States (Dick and others 2015). Although evidence from LMICs is limited, the higher burden of HAIs in LMICs indicates that these interventions would be highly effective there as well. The cost-effectiveness of antibiotic stewardship programs may depend on the prevalence of antibiotic resistance. Extensive evidence indicates that stewardship programs reduce the length of hospital stays and expenditures on antibiotics (CDC 2016), and that antibiotic stewardship teams can be cost-effective in improving care for bacteremia in the United States (Scheetz and others 2009).

Incentives for Rational Use

Delinking the prescribing of antibiotics from financial incentives or creating financial incentives for improved prescribing can reduce the use of antibiotics (Carbon and Bax 1998; Song and others 2014). For example, a Chinese program linked hospital payments to targets for reduced antibiotic use, alongside the introduction of prescribing regulations, audits, and inspections. Following the program, prescribing declined between 10 percent and 12 percent (Xiao and others 2013).

There are no studies that directly assess the cost-effectiveness of incentives or regulations to reduce antibiotic use. However, lessons can be drawn from several historical examples: persons with free medical care in the United States used 85 percent more antibiotics than did persons who paid for a portion of care, while cost sharing reduced both inappropriate and appropriate antibiotic use (Foxman and others 1987). A free antibiotics program introduced in the United States in 2006 increased antibiotic prescribing, with prescribers shifting to drugs covered under the program (Li and Laxminarayan 2015). A prescription audit study in China found that financial incentives determined prescribing patterns: physicians were more likely to prescribe antibiotics when patients indicated they would purchase the antibiotics at hospitals (Currie, Lin, and Meng 2014).

Reduction of Antibiotic Use in Agriculture

National regulation is one way to encourage reductions in antibiotic use in food animal production. The use of antibiotics to promote growth has been banned in the European Union since 2006. Although some farmers simply shifted to using antibiotics for prevention rather than for growth, the bans resulted in decreasing or consistently low use of antibiotics in agriculture in many European Union countries, including Sweden and Denmark (Cogliani, Goossens, and Greko 2011). Few LMICs have introduced such bans.

Many countries have been reluctant to ban agricultural use of antibiotics because of potential adverse economic impacts on their livestock sectors, but research shows that the impact is minimal in farming systems that are already optimized with respect to the genetic potential of herds, hygiene, nutrition, and herd health (Laxminarayan, Van Boeckel, and Teillant 2015). Some countries have banned or discouraged the use of certain antibiotic growth promoters (table 18.1). The U.S. Food and Drug Administration issued guidelines in 2013 asking the pharmaceutical industry to restrict the use of antibiotics as growth promoters (Laxminarayan, Van Boeckel, and Teillant 2015). Vaccination can also prevent disease and antibiotic use in animals, as it does in humans.

Evidence from HICs suggests that the economic impact of removing growth promoters is low, but the impact may be different in LMICs where antibiotics are

Table 18.1 Regulation of Antibiotic Use in Livestock in OECD Countries

Country	Ban on antibiotic growth promoters	Prescription required
Australia	No, but some AGPs banned (fluoroquinolones, avoparcin, and others)	Yes, prescription required for most veterinary antibiotics
Canada	No, voluntary phaseout notice issued in April 2014 that mimics the U.S. FDA approach	No, plan to strengthen veterinary oversight developed in line with the U.S. FDA approach
Chile	No data	No data
European Union member states	Yes, all AGPs banned in 2006	Yes
Israel	No data	No data
Japan	No	Yes
Mexico	Yes, AGPs banned in 2007 with exceptions (avoparcin, vancomycin, bacitracin, tylosin, virginiamycin, and others)	Yes
New Zealand	Yes, for critically and highly important antibiotics as listed by the WHO and the OIE	Yes, for antibiotics identified as having potential for resistance problems
Korea, Rep.	Yes, AGP use discontinued in 2011 until a veterinary oversight system can be put in place	Yes, veterinary oversight system in development
Turkey	No data	No data
United States	No, voluntary guidelines to withdraw the use of medically important antibiotics as promoters released by U.S. FDA in 2013	No, under new U.S. FDA guidance, use of medically important antibiotics to be under the oversight of licensed growth veterinarians

Sources: Table adapted from Laxminarayan, Van Boeckel, and Teillant 2015. Australian Commission on Safety and Quality in Health Care 2013; European Union 2003; Government of Canada 2014; MAF New Zealand 2011; Maron, Smith, and Nachman 2013; USDA 2011, 2013; U.S. FDA 2013.
Note: AGP = antibiotic growth promoter; OECD = Organisation for Economic Co-operation and Development; OIE = World Organisation for Animal Health; U.S. FDA = U.S. Food and Drug Administration; WHO = World Health Organization.

still used in place of hygiene and other measures to optimize production. In China, the economic costs of a ban could reach billions of dollars but would still be significantly less than the economic burden of resistant infections (Laxminarayan, Van Boeckel, and Teillant 2015).

Education and Awareness

Campaigns have successfully reduced human antibiotic use in HICs, but evidence from LMICs is sparse (Huttner and others 2010). Awareness campaigns in France and Belgium reduced antibiotic prescribing by 27 percent and 36 percent, respectively, and both programs saw some reduction in resistant pneumococci (Sabuncu and others 2009). Some LMICs have begun to initiate awareness campaigns coinciding with the CDC's Get Smart About Antibiotics Week and the World Health Organization's (WHO) World Antibiotic Awareness Week (Global Antibiotic Resistance Partnership 2015). Few national-level campaigns have specifically targeted use in animals. As with antibiotic stewardship programs, awareness campaigns that reduce use also reduce expenditures on antibiotics, and the campaigns in Belgium and France were associated with significant savings (Huttner and others 2010). However, the

cost-effectiveness of such campaigns has not been formally assessed, especially in LMICs.

Education without incentives or oversight may be less successful at changing behavior. Interventions targeted toward prescribers and consumers that combined education with managerial oversight have been more successful at reducing inappropriate antibiotic use than have educational materials alone (Holloway 2011). In Asia, health care provider interventions to increase appropriate use have typically been more successful than have other interventions to reduce use, unless they have been accompanied by oversight mechanisms such as peer review (Holloway 2011).

Surveillance of Antibiotic Use and Resistance

Surveillance of antibiotic use and resistance in humans and animals is needed to inform clinical decision making and national policies. Although few LMICs have comprehensive national surveillance programs, private sector laboratories often collect detailed data on resistance and are an underused resource in many data-scarce areas. These laboratories provide valuable additions to public sector resistance data in countries such as India and South Africa, where more than 98 percent and 80 percent, respectively, of accredited medical laboratories are in the private sector (CDDEP 2016; Gandra, Merchant, and Laxminarayan 2016).

Regional surveillance networks collect data in Latin America (Red Latinoamericana de Vigilancia de la Resistencia a los Antimicrobianos [ReLAVRA]), Asia (Asian Network for Surveillance of Resistant Pathogens [ANSORP]), Central Asia and Eastern Europe (Central Asian and Eastern European Surveillance of Antimicrobial Resistance [CAESAR]), and Europe (European Antimicrobial Resistance Surveillance Network [EARS-Net]). ResistanceMap, a global repository of antibiotic resistance and use data, incorporates these and other data from surveillance networks and private laboratories in LMICs into a visualization interface that can be used to assess national patterns and trends.

New Drugs and Antibiotic Alternatives

The pipeline of new antibiotics is relatively robust, with 7 new antibiotics approved in 2014 and 37 under development (Pew Charitable Trusts 2014); however, new drugs will always be needed as resistance develops, particularly for serious threats such as Gram-negative bacteria and for use in low-resource settings. The financial incentives to develop antibiotics are limited compared with other drugs because of their short course of use and potentially restricted use, among other barriers. Several initiatives—including the United Kingdom's *Review on Antimicrobial Resistance*; the Driving Reinvestment in Research and Development and Responsible Antibiotic Use (DRIVE-AB) partnership funded by the Innovative Medicines Initiative; and the Global Antibiotic Research and Development Partnership, established under the auspices of the Drugs for Neglected Diseases *initiative* (DND*i*) and the WHO—are seeking to address these barriers to ensure a robust antibiotic pipeline (O'Neill 2016).

Because resistance to all antibiotics naturally develops, alternatives to antibiotics present other options. Alternatives include vaccines and improved diagnostics, as well as antibodies, probiotics, lysins, bacteriophages, immune simulation, and peptides. Development of a complete portfolio of these alternatives will take an estimated 10 years and cost a minimum of US$2.1 billion (Czaplewski and others 2016).

CONCLUSIONS

National action, tailored to local contexts and patterns of resistance, is key to curbing the global threat of antibiotic resistance. The Global Antibiotic Resistance Partnership, which develops local capacity in LMICs to design and implement national antibiotic resistance plans, has identified six key interventions to curb antibiotic resistance (figure 18.6).

The following recommendations should be part of any national plan:

- *Reduce and eventually phase out subtherapeutic antibiotic use in agriculture.* Improved sanitation and hygiene at the farm level would reduce the need for prophylactic antibiotics. Antibiotic use in animal agriculture should be reduced, focusing on involving farmers and the agricultural industry in carefully phasing out the use of growth promoters and premixed animal feeds (Laxminarayan, Van Boeckel, and Teillant 2015).
- *Adopt incentives that encourage antibiotic overuse and misuse to incentives that encourage antibiotic stewardship.* Making sure that payments are not linked to prescribing, as well as introducing rewards for compliance, may improve prescribing patterns.
- *Improve hospital infection control and antibiotic stewardship.* Antibiotic stewardship programs, infection prevention and control, and especially handwashing with soap can reduce infections, antibiotic use, and resistance while improving patient outcomes.
- *Educate health professionals, policy makers, and the public on sustainable antibiotic use.* Although public awareness is growing that antibiotic resistance presents a threat, there is little awareness of the individual actions that can be taken to reduce use. Patients, parents, health care providers, stakeholders, and hospital leaders all need to be aware of what they can do to reduce unnecessary use.
- *Reduce the need for antibiotics through improved water, sanitation, and immunization.* Disease prevention achieves the dual purposes of keeping people healthy and saving antibiotic doses. Water, sanitation, hygiene, and vaccination should be core components of any public health system.
- *Ensure political commitment to meet the threat of antibiotic resistance.* Without national commitment in the form of implemented action plans, the long-term sustainability of efforts to curb antibiotic resistance will be weakened. Although international efforts to curb antibiotic resistance have focused largely on national action, international support is also needed, particularly to stimulate private and public sector research to fill knowledge gaps and develop new drugs, diagnostics, and other technologies, as well as to strengthen laboratories for improved surveillance.

Figure 18.6 Six Strategies Needed in National Antibiotic Policies

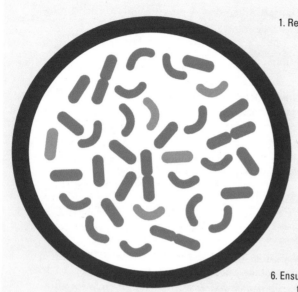

1. **Reduce,** and eventually phase out, subtherapeutic antibiotic use in agriculture.

2. **Adopt** incentives that encourage antibiotic overuse and misuse to incentives that encourage antibiotic stewardship.

3. **Improve** hospital infection control and antibiotic stewardship.

4. **Educate** health professionals, policy makers, and the public on sustainable antibiotic use.

5. **Reduce** the need for antibiotics through improved water, sanitation, and immunization.

6. **Ensure** political commitment to meet the threat of antibiotic resistance.

Source: Gelband and others 2015.

NOTES

World Bank Income Classifications as of July 2014 are as follows, based on estimates of gross national income (GNI) per capita for 2013:

- Low-income countries (LICs) = US$1,045 or less
- Middle-income countries (MICs) are subdivided:
  (a) lower-middle-income = US$1,046 to US$4,125
  (b) upper-middle-income (UMICs) = US$4,126 to US$12,745
- High-income countries (HICs) = US$12,746 or more.

Data from figure 18.3 and map 18.2 are from IMS MIDAS International Prescription Data, January 2000–December 2010, IMS Health Incorporated. All Rights Reserved. The statements, findings, conclusions, views, and opinions contained and expressed herein are not necessarily those of IMS Health Incorporated or any of its affiliated or subsidiary entities.

1. https://resistancemap.cddep.org.

REFERENCES

Abdulgader, S. M., A. O. Shittu, M. P. Nicol, and M. Kaba. 2015. "Molecular Epidemiology of Methicillin-Resistant *Staphylococcus aureus* in Africa: A Systematic Review." *Frontiers in Microbiology* 6 (348): 1–21.

Al-Emran, H. M., D. Eibach, R. Krumkamp, M. Ali, S. Baker, and others. 2016. "A Multicountry Molecular Analysis of 4 *Salmonella enterica* Serovar Typhi with Reduced Susceptibility to Ciprofloxacin in Sub-Saharan Africa." *Clinical Infectious Diseases* 62 (Suppl 1): S42–46. doi:10.1093/cid/civ788.

Allegranzi, B., S. Bagheri Nejad, C. Combescure, W. Graafmans, H. Attar, and others. 2011. "Burden of Endemic Health-Care-Associated Infection in Developing Countries: Systematic Review and Meta-Analysis." *The Lancet* 377 (9761): 228–41.

Allegranzi, B., and D. Pittet. 2009. "Role of Hand Hygiene in Healthcare-Associated Infection Prevention." *Journal of Hospital Infection* 73 (4): 305–15.

Australian Commission on Safety and Quality in Health Care. 2013. "Australian One Health Antimicrobial Resistance Colloquium." Australian Commission of Safety and Quality in Health Care, Canberra.

Baker, S., J. Hombach, and F. Marks. 2016. "What Have We Learned from the Typhoid Fever Surveillance in Africa Program?" *Clinical Infectious Diseases* 62 (Suppl 1): S1–S3. doi:10.1093/cid/civ675.

Braykov, N. P., D. J. Morgan, M. L. Schweizer, D. Z. Uslan, T. Kelesidis, and others. 2014. "Assessment of Empirical Antibiotic Therapy Optimisation in Six Hospitals: An Observational Cohort Study." *The Lancet Infectious Diseases* 14 (12): 1220–27.

Buono, S. A., T. D. Watson, L. A. Borenstein, J. D. Klausner, M. W. Pandori, and others. 2015. "Stemming the Tide of Drug-Resistant *Neisseria gonorrhoeae*: The Need for an Individualized Approach to Treatment." *Journal of Antimicrobial Chemotherapy* 70 (2): 374–81.

Cairncross, S., C. Hunt, S. Boisson, K. Bostoen, V. Curtis, and others. 2010. "Water, Sanitation, and Hygiene for the Prevention of Diarrhoea." *International Journal of Epidemiology* 39 (Suppl 1): i193–205.

Cairncross, S., and V. Valdmanis. 2006. "Water Supply, Sanitation, and Hygiene Promotion." In *Disease Control Priorities in Developing Countries* (second edition), edited by D. T. Jamison, J. G. Breman, A. R. Measham, G. Alleyne, M. Claeson, D. B. Evans, P. Jha, A. Mills, and P. Musgrove. Washington, DC: World Bank and Oxford University Press.

Carbon, C., and R. P. Bax. 1998. "Regulating the Use of Antibiotics in the Community." *BMJ* 317 (7159): 663–65.

CDC (Centers for Disease Control and Prevention). 2013. *Antibiotic Resistance Threats in the United States, 2013.* Atlanta, GA: CDC. http://www.cdc.gov/drugresistance /threat-report-2013/.

———. 2016. "Impact of Antibiotic Stewardship Program Interventions on Costs." CDC, Atlanta, GA.

CDDEP (Center for Disease Dynamics, Economics & Policy). 2016. "Resistance Map." CDDEP, Washington, DC. http:// www.cddep.org/projects/resistance-map.

Chattaway, M. A., A. O. Aboderin, K. Fashae, C. K. Okoro, J. A Opintan, and others. 2016. "Fluoroquinolone-Resistant Enteric Bacteria in Sub-Saharan Africa: Clones, Implications and Research Needs." *Frontiers in Microbiology* 7: 558. doi:10.3389/fmicb.2016.00558.

Clark, A. D., U. K. Griffiths, S. S. Abbas, K. D. Rao, L. Privor-Dumm, and others. 2013. "Impact and Cost-Effectiveness of *Haemophilus influenzae* Type B Conjugate Vaccination in India." *Journal of Pediatrics* 163 (Suppl 1): S60–72.

Clasen, T. F., and L. Haller. 2008. "Water Quality Interventions to Prevent Diarrhoea: Cost and Cost-Effectiveness." WHO/HSE/WSH/08.02, World Health Organization, Geneva.

Cogliani, C., H. Goossens, and C. Greko. 2011. "Restricting Antimicrobial Use in Food Animals: Lessons from Europe." *Microbe* 6 (6): 274–79.

Currie, J., W. Lin, and J. Meng. 2014. "Addressing Antibiotic Abuse in China: An Experimental Audit Study." *Journal of Development Economics* 110 (September): 39–51.

Czaplewski, L., R. Bax, M. Clokie, M. Dawson, H. Fairhead, and others. 2016. "Alternatives to Antibiotics: A Pipeline Portfolio Review." *The Lancet Infectious Diseases* 16 (2): 239–51.

Dar, O., R. Hasan, J. Schlundt, S. Harbarth, G. Caleo, and others. 2015. "Exploring the Evidence Base for National and Regional Policy Interventions to Combat Resistance." *The Lancet* 387 (10015): 285–95.

Datta, S., C. Wattal, N. Goel, J. K. Oberoi, R. Raveendran, and others. 2012. "A Ten-Year Analysis of Multi-Drug Resistant Blood Stream Infections Caused by *Escherichia coli* and *Klebsiella pneumoniae* in a Tertiary Care Hospital." *Indian Journal of Medical Research* 135 (6): 907–12.

Davey, P., E. Brown, L. Fenelon, R. Finch, I. Gould, and others. 2005. "Interventions to Improve Antibiotic Prescribing Practices for Hospital Inpatients (Review)." *Cochrane Database of Systematic Reviews* (4): CD003543.

De Angelis, G., M. A. Cataldo, C. De Waure, S. Venturiello, G. La Torre, and others. 2014. "Infection Control and Prevention Measures to Reduce the Spread of Vancomycin-Resistant Enterococci in Hospitalized Patients: A Systematic Review and Meta-Analysis." *Journal of Antimicrobial Chemotherapy* 69 (5): 1185–92.

Department of Health, South Africa. 2014. *Antimicrobial Resistance National Strategy Framework 2014–2024.* Pretoria: National Department of Health.

Dick, A. W., E. N. Perencevich, M. Pogorzelska-Maziarz, J. Zwanziger, E. L. Larson, and others. 2015. "A Decade of Investment in Infection Prevention: A Cost-Effectiveness Analysis." *American Journal of Infection Control* 43 (1): 4–9.

Dosh, S. A., J. M. Hickner, A. G. Mainous, and M. H. Ebell. 2000. "Predictors of Antibiotic Prescribing for Nonspecific Upper Respiratory Infections, Acute Bronchitis, and Acute Sinusitis." *Journal of Family Practice* 49 (5): 407–14.

Du, H., L. Chen, Y. W. Tang, and B. N. Kreiswirth. 2016. "Emergence of the MCR-1 Colistin Resistance Gene in Carbapenem-Resistant Enterobacteriaceae." *The Lancet Infectious Diseases* 16 (3): 287–88.

EARS-Net (European Antimicrobial Resistance Surveillance Network). 2014. "EARS-Net Report, Quarters 1–4." Health Protection Surveillance Centre, Dublin.

European Union. 2003. "Regulation (EC) No. 1831/2003 of the European Parliament and of the Council of 22 September 2003 on Additives for Use in Animal Nutrition." European Union, Brussels.

Falsey, A. R., K. L. Becker, A. J. Swinburne, E. S. Nylen, M. A. Formica, and others. 2013. "Bacterial Complications of Respiratory Tract Viral Illness: A Comprehensive Evaluation." *Journal of Infectious Diseases* 208 (3): 432–41.

Foxman, B., R. B. Valdez, K. N. Lohr, G. A. Goldberg, J. P. Newhouse, and others. 1987. "The Effect of Cost Sharing on the Use of Antibiotics in Ambulatory Care: Results from a Population-Based Randomized Controlled Trial." *Journal of Chronic Diseases* 40 (5): 429–37.

Gandra, S., E. Y. Klein, S. Pant, S. Malhotra-Kumar, and R. Laxminarayan. 2016. "Faropenem Consumption Is Increasing in India." *Clinical Infectious Diseases* 62 (8): 1050–52. doi:10.1093/cid/ciw055.

Gandra, S., A. Merchant, and R. Laxminarayan. 2016. "A Role for Private Laboratories in Public Health Surveillance of Antimicrobial Resistance." *Future Microbiology* 11: 709–12.

Ganguly, N. K., N. K. Arora, S. J. Chandy, M. N. Fairoze, J. P. S. Gill, and others. 2011. "Rationalizing Antibiotic Use to Limit Antibiotic Resistance in India." *Indian Journal of Medical Research* 134 (3): 281–94.

Gelband, H., M. Miller-Petrie, S. Pant, S. Gandra, J. Levinson, and others. 2015. *The State of the World's Antibiotics, 2015.* Washington, DC: Center for Disease Dynamics, Economics & Policy.

Global Antibiotic Resistance Partnership. 2015. *GARPNet News* 1 (6). Center for Disease Dynamics, Economics & Policy, Washington, DC.

Government of Canada. 2014. "Collaborative Efforts to Promote the Judicious Use of Medically Important Antimicrobial Drugs in Food Animal Production." Government of Canada, Ottawa.

Griffiths, U. K., A. Clark, and R. Hajjeh. 2013. "Cost-Effectiveness of *Haemophilus influenzae* Type B Conjugate Vaccine in Low- and Middle-Income Countries: Regional Analysis and Assessment of Major Determinants." *Journal of Pediatrics* 163 (Suppl 1): S50–59.e9.

Grijalva, C. G., J. P. Nuorti, P. G. Arbogast, S. W. Martin, K. M. Edwards, and others. 2007. "Decline in Pneumonia Admissions after Routine Childhood Immunization with Pneumococcal Conjugate Vaccine in the USA: A Time Series Analysis." *The Lancet* 369 (9568): 1179–86.

Holloway, K. A. 2011. "Promoting the Rational Use of Antibiotics." *Regional Health Forum* 15 (1): 122–30.

Huttner, B., H. Goossens, T. Verheij, and S. Harbarth. 2010. "Characteristics and Outcomes of Public Campaigns Aimed at Improving the Use of Antibiotics in Outpatients in High-Income Countries." *The Lancet Infectious Diseases* 10 (1): 17–31.

Hutton, G., L. Haller, and J. Bartram. 2007. "Global Cost-Benefit Analysis of Water Supply and Sanitation Interventions." *Journal of Water and Health* 5 (4): 481–502.

Jamison, D. T., L. H. Summers, G. Alleyne, K. J. Arrow, S. Berkley, and others. 2013. "Global Health 2035: A World Converging within a Generation." *The Lancet* 382 (9908): 1898–955.

Johnson, A. P., and N. Woodford. 2013. "Global Spread of Antibiotic Resistance: The Example of New Delhi Metallo-β-Lactamase (NDM)–Mediated Carbapenem Resistance." *Journal of Medical Microbiology* 62 (Pt. 4): 499–513.

Kaki, R., M. Elligsen, S. Walker, A. Simor, L. Palmay, and others. 2011. "Impact of Antimicrobial Stewardship in Critical Care: A Systematic Review." *Journal of Antimicrobial Chemotherapy* 66 (6): 1223–30.

Kariuki, S., M. A. Gordon, N. Feasey, and C. M. Parry. 2015. "Antimicrobial Resistance and Management of Invasive *Salmonella* Disease." *Vaccine* 33 (Suppl 3): C21–29.

Kayange, N., E. Kamugisha, D. L. Mwizamholya, S. Jeremiah, and S. E. Mshana. 2010. "Predictors of Positive Blood Culture and Deaths among Neonates with Suspected Neonatal Sepsis in a Tertiary Hospital, Mwanza-Tanzania." *BMC Pediatrics* 10: 39.

Klein, E. Y., M. Makowsky, M. Orlando, E. Hatna, N. P. Braykov, and others. 2015. "Influence of Provider and Urgent Care Density across Different Socioeconomic Strata on Outpatient Antibiotic Prescribing in the USA." *Journal of Antimicrobial Chemotherapy* 70 (5): 1580–87.

Klugman, K. P., S. A. Madhi, R. E. Huebner, R. Kohberger, N. Mbelle, and others. 2003. "A Trial of a 9-Valent Pneumococcal Conjugate Vaccine in Children with and Those without HIV Infection." *New England Journal of Medicine* 349 (14): 1341–48.

Kotwani, A., and K. Holloway. 2011. "Trends in Antibiotic Use among Outpatients in New Delhi, India." *BMC Infectious Diseases* 11 (1): 99.

Kwong, J. C., S. Maaten, R. E. G. Upshur, D. M. Patrick, and F. Marra. 2009. "The Effect of Universal Influenza Immunization on Antibiotic Prescriptions: An Ecological Study." *Clinical Infectious Diseases* 49 (5): 750–56.

Kyaw, M. H., R. Lynfield, W. Schaffner, A. S. Craig, J. Hadler, and others. 2006. "Effect of Introduction of the Pneumococcal Conjugate Vaccine on Drug-Resistant *Streptococcus pneumoniae.*" *New England Journal of Medicine* 354 (14): 1455–63.

Laxminarayan, R., Z. A. Bhutta, A. Duse, P. Jenkins, T. O'Brien, and others. 2006. "Drug Resistance." In *Disease Control Priorities in Developing Countries* (second edition), edited by D. T. Jamison, J. G. Breman, A. R. Measham, G. Alleyne, M. Claeson, D. B. Evans, P. Jha, A. Mills, and P. Musgrove. Washington, DC: World Bank and Oxford University Press.

Laxminarayan, R., and R. R. Chaudhury. 2016. "Antibiotic Resistance in India: Drivers and Opportunities for Action." *PLoS Medicine* 13 (3): e1001974.

Laxminarayan, R., P. Matsoso, S. Pant, C. Brower, J.-A. Rottingen, and others. 2016. "Access to Effective Antimicrobials: A Worldwide Challenge." *The Lancet* 387 (10014): 168–75.

Laxminarayan, R., T. Van Boeckel, and A. Teillant. 2015. "The Economic Costs of Withdrawing Antimicrobial Growth Promoters from the Livestock Sector." Food, Agriculture, and Fisheries Paper 78, Organisation for Economic Co-operation and Development, Paris.

Lerner, A., A. Adler, J. Abu-Hanna, S. Cohen Percia, M. Kazma Matalon, and others. 2015. "Spread of KPC-Producing Carbapenem-Resistant Enterobacteriaceae: The Importance of Super-Spreaders and Rectal KPC Concentration." *Clinical Microbiology and Infection* 21 (5): 470.e1–7.

Li, S., and R. Laxminarayan. 2015. "Are Physicians' Prescribing Decisions Sensitive to Drug Prices? Evidence from a Free-Antibiotics Program." *Health Economics* 24 (2): 158–74.

Linder, J. A., J. N. Doctor, M. W. Friedberg, H. R. Nieva, C. Birks, and others. 2014. "Time of Day and the Decision to Prescribe Antibiotics." *Journal of the American Medical Association Internal Medicine* 174 (12): 2029–31.

Liu, Y. Y., Y. Wang, T. R. Walsh, L. X. Yi, R. Zhang, and others. 2016. "Emergence of Plasmid-Mediated Colistin Resistance Mechanism MCR-1 in Animals and Human Beings in China: A Microbiological and Molecular Biological Study." *The Lancet Infectious Diseases* 16 (2): 161–68.

Logan, L. K., J. P. Renschler, S. Gandra, R. A. Weinstein, and R. Laxminarayan. 2015. "Carbapenem-Resistant Enterobacteriaceae in Children, United States, 1999–2012." *Emerging Infectious Diseases* 21 (11): 2012–21.

Lu, P. L., Y. C. Liu, H. S. Toh, Y. L. Lee, Y. M. Liu, and others. 2012. "Epidemiology and Antimicrobial Susceptibility Profiles of Gram-Negative Bacteria Causing Urinary Tract Infections in the Asia-Pacific Region: 2009–2010 Results from the Study for Monitoring Antimicrobial Resistance Trends (SMART)." *International Journal of Antimicrobial Agents* 40 (Suppl): S37–43.

MAF (Ministry of Agriculture and Forestry) New Zealand. 2011. *Review and Update on New Zealand Regulatory Control of Antimicrobial Agricultural Compounds with Regard to Antimicrobial Resistance.* Wellington: MAF.

Maron, D., T. Smith, and K. Nachman. 2013. "Restrictions on Antimicrobial use in Food Animal Production: An International Regulatory and Economic Survey." *Global Health* 9 (48).

Marshall, B. M., and S. B. Levy. 2011. "Food Animals and Antimicrobials: Impacts on Human Health." *Clinical Microbiology Reviews* 24 (4): 718–33.

Martin, I., P. Sawatzky, G. Liu, and M. R. Mulvey. 2015. "Antimicrobial Resistance to *Neisseria gonorrhoeae* in Canada: 2009–2013." *Canada Communicable Disease Report* 41-02 (February 5): 35–41.

Maurice, J. M., and S. Davey. 2009. *State of the World's Vaccines and Immunization*. Third edition. Geneva: World Health Organization.

McCullers, J. A. 2014. "The Co-Pathogenesis of Influenza Viruses with Bacteria in the Lung." *Nature Reviews Microbiology* 12 (4): 252–62.

Meeker, D., T. K. Knight, M. W. Friedburg, J. A. Linder, N. J. Goldstein, and others. 2014. "Nudging Guideline-Concordant Antibiotic Prescribing: A Randomized Clinical Trial." *Journal of the American Medical Association Internal Medicine* 174 (3): 425–31.

Meeker, D., J. A. Linder, C. R. Fox, M. W. Friedberg, S. D. Persell, and others. 2016. "Effect of Behavioral Interventions on Inappropriate Antibiotic Prescribing among Primary Care Practices: A Randomized Clinical Trial." *Journal of the American Medical Association* 315 (6): 562–70.

Mendelson, M., J.-A. Røttingen, U. Gopinathan, D. H. Hamer, H. Wertheim, and others. 2015. "Maximising Access to Achieve Appropriate Human Antimicrobial Use in Low- and Middle-Income Countries." *The Lancet* 387 (10014): 88–98.

Okeke, I. N. 2009. "Cholera Vaccine Will Reduce Antibiotic Use." *Science* 325 (5941): 674.

Okeke, I. N., K. P. Klugman, Z. A. Bhutta, A. G. Duse, P. Jenkins, and others. 2005. "Antimicrobial Resistance in Developing Countries. Part II: Strategies for Containment." *The Lancet Infectious Diseases* 5 (9): 568–80.

Okeke, I. N., R. Laxminarayan, Z. A. Bhutta, A. G. Duse, P. Jenkins, and others. 2005. "Antimicrobial Resistance in Developing Countries. Part I: Recent Trends and Current Status." *The Lancet Infectious Diseases* 5 (8): 481–93.

O'Neill, J. 2016. *Tackling Drug-Resistant Infections Globally: Final Report and Recommendations*. London: The Review on Antimicrobial Resistance.

PAHO (Pan American Health Organization). Forthcoming. *Informe Anual de la Red de Monitoreo/Vigilancia de la Resistencia a los Antibióticos y de Infecciones Asociadas a la Atención de la Salud 2014*. Washington, DC: PAHO.

Paudel, K. R., M. Sharma, and B. P. Das. 2008. "Prevalence of Antimicrobial Chemotherapy in Hospitalized Patients in the Department of Internal Medicine in a Tertiary Care Center." *Nepal Medical College Journal* 10 (2): 91–95.

Pew Charitable Trusts. 2014. *Tracking the Pipeline of Antibiotics in Development*. Philadelphia: Issue Brief, Pew Charitable Trusts.

Polgreen, P. M., R. Laxminarayan, and J. E. Cavanaugh. 2011. "Respiratory Fluoroquinolone Use and Influenza." *Infection Control and Hospital Epidemiology* 32 (7): 706–9.

Rabie, T., and V. Curtis. 2006. "Handwashing and Risk of Respiratory Infections: A Quantitative Systematic Review." *Tropical Medicine and International Health* 11 (3): 258–67.

Rheingans, R., M. Amaya, J. Anderson, P. Chakraborty, and J. Atem. 2014. "Systematic Review of the Economic Value of Diarrheal Vaccines." *Human Vaccines and Immunotherapeutics* 10 (6): 1582–94.

Sabuncu, E., J. David, C. Bernède-Bauduin, S. Pépin, M. Leroy, and others. 2009. "Significant Reduction of Antibiotic Use in the Community after a Nationwide Campaign in France, 2002–2007." *PLoS Medicine* 6 (6): e1000084.

Scheetz, M. H., M. K. Bolon, M. Postelnick, G. A. Noskin, and T. A. Lee. 2009. "Cost-Effectiveness Analysis of an Antimicrobial Stewardship Team on Bloodstream Infections: A Probabilistic Analysis." *Journal of Antimicrobial Chemotherapy* 63 (4): 816–25.

Shankar, P. R., D. K. Upadhyay, P. Mishra, P. Subish, A. K. Dubey, and others. 2007. "Fluoroquinolone Utilization among Inpatients in a Teaching Hospital in Western Nepal." *Journal of the Pakistan Medical Association* 57 (2): 78–82.

Sinha, A., O. Levine, M. D. Knoll, F. Muhib, and T. A. Lieu. 2007. "Cost-Effectiveness of Pneumococcal Conjugate Vaccination in the Prevention of Child Mortality: An International Economic Analysis." *The Lancet* 369 (9559): 389–96.

Song, Y., Y. Bian, M. Petzold, L. Li, and A. Yin. 2014. "The Impact of China's National Essential Medicine System on Improving Rational Drug Use in Primary Health Care Facilities: An Empirical Study in Four Provinces." *BMC Health Services Research* 14 (1): 507–13.

Storberg, V. 2014. "ESBL-Producing Enterobacteriaceae in Africa: A Non-Systematic Literature Review of Research Published 2008–2012." *Infection Ecology and Epidemiology* 4. doi:10.3402/iee.v4.20342.

Sun, L., E. Y. Klein, and R. Laxminarayan. 2012. "Seasonality and Temporal Correlation between Community Antibiotic Use and Resistance in the United States." *Clinical Infectious Diseases* 55 (5): 687–94.

Teillant, A., S. Gandra, D. Barter, D. J. Morgan, and R. Laxminarayan. 2015. "Potential Burden of Antibiotic Resistance on Surgery and Cancer Chemotherapy Antibiotic Prophylaxis in the USA: A Literature Review and Modelling Study." *The Lancet Infectious Diseases* 15 (12): 1429–37.

Thu, T. A., M. Rahman, S. Coffin, M. Harun-Or-Rashid, J. Sakamoto, and others. 2012. "Antibiotic Use in Vietnamese Hospitals: A Multicenter Point-Prevalence Study." *American Journal of Infection Control* 40 (9): 840–44.

USDA (U.S. Department of Agriculture). 2011. "Korea Phases Out Antibiotic Usage in Compound Feed." Report, USDA, Washington, DC.

———. 2013. *Feedlot 2011: Part III: Trends in Health and Management Practices on U.S. Feedlots, 1994–2011*. Washington, DC: USDA.

———. 2015. "Livestock and Meat Domestic Data." Washington, DC: USDA. http://www.ers.usda.gov/data-products /livestock-meat-domestic-data.aspx#26084.

U.S. Department of Health and Human Services. 2015. "Summary Report on Antimicrobials Sold or Distributed for Use in Food-Producing Animals." U.S. Food and Drug Administration, Washington, DC.

U.S. FDA (U.S. Food and Drug Administration). 2013. "Guidance for Industry #213: New Animal Drugs and New Animal Drug Combination Products Administered in or on Medicated Feed or Drinking Water of Food-Producing Animals: Recommendations for Drug Sponsors for Voluntarily Aligning Product Use Conditions with GFI #209." U.S. FDA, Washington, DC.

Van Boeckel, T. P., C. Brower, M. Gilbert, B. T. Grenfell, S. A. Levin, and others. 2015. "Global Trends in Antimicrobial

Use in Food Animals." *Proceedings of the National Academy of Sciences* 112 (18): 5649–54.

Van Boeckel, T. P., S. Gandra, A. Ashok, Q. Caudron, B. T. Grenfell, and others. 2014. "Global Antibiotic Consumption 2000 to 2010: An Analysis of National Pharmaceutical Sales Data." *The Lancet Infectious Diseases* 3099 (14): 1–9.

WHO (World Health Organization). 2011. *Report on the Burden of Endemic Health Care: Associated Infection Worldwide.* Geneva: WHO.

———. 2014. *Antimicrobial Resistance: Global Report on Surveillance.* Geneva: WHO.

———. 2015. *Draft Global Action Plan on Antimicrobial Resistance.* Geneva: WHO.

Xiao, Y., J. Zhang, B. Zheng, L. Zhao, S. Li, and others. 2013. "Changes in Chinese Policies to Promote the Rational Use of Antibiotics." *PLoS Medicine* 10 (11): e1001556.

Zhang, Y., B. Y. Lee, and J. M. Donohue. 2010. "Ambulatory Antibiotic Use and Prescription Drug Coverage in Older Adults." *Archives of Internal Medicine* 170 (15): 1308–14.

DCP3 Series Acknowledgments

Disease Control Priorities, third edition (*DCP3*) compiles the global health knowledge of institutions and experts from around the world, a task that required the efforts of over 500 individuals, including volume editors, chapter authors, peer reviewers, advisory committee members, and research and staff assistants. For each of these contributions we convey our acknowldgment and appreciation. First and foremost, we would like to thank our 32 volume editors who provided the intellectual vision for their volumes based on years of professional work in their respective fields, and then dedicated long hours to reviewing each chapter, providing leadership and guidance to authors, and framing and writing the summary chapters. We also thank our chapter authors who collectively volunteered their time and expertise to writing over 170 comprehensive, evidence-based chapters.

We owe immense gratitude to the institutional sponsor of this effort: The Bill & Melinda Gates Foundation. The Foundation provided sole financial support of the Disease Control Priorities Network. Many thanks to Program Officers Kathy Cahill, Philip Setel, Carol Medlin, Damian Walker, and (currently) David Wilson for their thoughtful interactions, guidance, and encouragement over the life of the project. We also wish to thank Jaime Sepúlveda for his longstanding support, including chairing the Advisory Committee for the second edition and, more recently, demonstrating his vision for *DCP3* while he was a special advisor to the Gates Foundation. We are also grateful to the University of Washington's Department of Global Health and successive chairs King Holmes and Judy Wasserheit for providing a home base for the *DCP3* Secretariat, which included intellectual collaboration, logistical coordination, and administrative support.

We thank the many contractors and consultants who provided support to specific volumes in the form of economic analytical work, volume coordination, chapter drafting, and meeting organization: the Center for Disease Dynamics, Economics & Policy; Center for Chronic Disease Control; Centre for Global Health Research; Emory University; Evidence to Policy Initiative; Public Health Foundation of India; QURE Healthcare; University of California, San Francisco; University of Waterloo; University of Queensland; and the World Health Organization.

We are tremendously grateful for the wisdom and guidance provided by our advisory committee to the editors. Steered by Chair Anne Mills, the advisory committee ensures quality and intellectual rigor of the highest order for *DCP3*.

The National Academies of Science, Engineering, and Medicine, in collaboration with the Interacademy Medical Panel, coordinated the peer-review process for all *DCP3* chapters. Patrick Kelley, Gillian Buckley, Megan Ginivan, Rachel Pittluck, and Tara Mainero managed this effort and provided critical and substantive input.

World Bank Publications provided exceptional guidance and support throughout the demanding production and design process. We would particularly like to thank Carlos Rossel, Mary Fisk, Nancy Lammers, Rumit Pancholi, Deborah Naylor, and Sherrie Brown for their diligence and expertise. Additionally, we thank Jose de Buerba, Mario Trubiano, Yulia Ivanova, and Chiamaka Osuagwu of the World Bank for providing professional counsel on communications and marketing strategies.

Several U.S. and international institutions contributed to the organization and execution of meetings that supported the preparation and dissemination of *DCP3*. We would like to express our appreciation to the following institutions:

- University of Bergen, consultation on equity (June 2011)
- University of California, San Francisco, surgery volume consultations (April 2012, October 2013, February 2014)
- Institute of Medicine, first meeting of the Advisory Committee to the Editors (March 2013)
- Harvard Global Health Institute, consultation on policy measures to reduce incidence of noncommunicable diseases (July 2013)
- National Academy of Medicine, systems strengthening meeting (September 2013)
- Center for Disease Dynamics, Economics & Policy (Quality and Uptake meeting, September 2013, reproductive and maternal health volume consultation, November 2013)
- National Cancer Institute cancer consultation (November 2013)
- Union for International Cancer Control cancer consultation (November 2013, December 2014)
- Harvard T. H. Chan School of Public Health, economic evaluation consultation (September 2015)
- University of California, Berkeley School of Public Health, and Stanford Medical School, occupational and environmental health consultations (December 2015).

Carol Levin provided outstanding governance for cost and cost-effectiveness analysis. Stéphane Verguet added valuable guidance in applying and improving the extended cost-effectiveness analysis method. Elizabeth Brouwer, Kristen Danforth, Nazila Dabestani, Shane Murphy, Zachary Olson, Jinyuan Qi, and David Watkins provided exceptional research assistance and analytic assistance. Brianne Adderley ably managed the budget and project processes, while Jennifer Nguyen, Shamelle Richards, and Jennifer Grasso contributed exceptional project coordination support. The efforts of these individuals were absolutely critical to producing this series, and we are thankful for their commitment.

Volume and Series Editors

VOLUME EDITORS

King K. Holmes

King K. Holmes is the Director of Research and Faculty Development in the University of Washington's Department of Global Health. He also serves as Director of the Center for AIDS Research and Professor in the University of Washington's Department of Medicine, and as Principal Investigator for the University of Washington's International Training and Education Center for Health, with HIV-related programs in 20 countries throughout the world. He served as the William H. Foege Endowed Chair in Health from 2006 to 2015. Holmes has participated in research on sexually transmitted infections (STIs) for over 50 years and in research, training, and technical assistance on HIV/AIDS and other STIs globally for over 30 years.

Stefano Bertozzi

Stefano Bertozzi is Dean and Professor at the School of Public Health at the University of California, Berkeley. He has led impact evaluations of large, national health and social programs in Africa, Asia, Latin America, and Mexico. His research focuses on the prevention of HIV/AIDS and STIs, as well as on risk behavior among adolescents. He was previously the director of the HIV Global Health Program at the Bill & Melinda Gates Foundation. His research has covered a diverse range of projects in health economics and policy, focusing on the economic aspects of HIV/AIDS and the health impact of large social programs.

Barry R. Bloom

Barry R. Bloom is Harvard University Distinguished Service Professor of the Departments of Immunology and Infectious Diseases and Global Health and Population of the Harvard T. H. Chan School of Public Health, where he served as Dean from 1999 to 2009. His research interests have been in immunology, infectious diseases, tuberculosis, leprosy, and vaccines. He served as a consultant to the White House on international health policy and has been extensively involved with the World Health Organization, chairing advisory committees on tropical diseases, leprosy, tuberculosis, and malaria. He serves as Co-Chair of the Independent Expert Committee of the Human Heredity and Health in Africa (H3Africa) program; is a member of the Scientific Advisory Board of the Africa Health Research Institute in Durban, South Africa; and chairs the Research Advisory Committee of the Public Health Foundation of India.

Prabhat Jha

Prabhat Jha is the founding director of the Centre for Global Health Research at St. Michael's Hospital. He holds Endowed and Canada Research Chairs in Global Health in the Dalla Lana School of Public Health at the University of Toronto. He is lead investigator of the Million Death Study in India, which quantifies the cause of death and key risk factors in over two million homes over a 14-year period. He is also Scientific Director of the Statistical Alliance for Vital Events, which aims to expand reliable measurement of causes of death worldwide. His research includes the epidemiology and economics of tobacco control worldwide.

SERIES EDITORS

Dean T. Jamison

Dean T. Jamison is Emeritus Professor in Global Health Sciences at the University of California, San Francisco,

451

and the University of Washington. He previously held academic appointments at Harvard University and the University of California, Los Angeles. Prior to his academic career, he was an economist on the staff of the World Bank, where he was lead author of the World Bank's *World Development Report 1993: Investing in Health*. He serves as lead editor for *DCP3* and was lead editor for the previous two editions. He holds a PhD in economics from Harvard University and is an elected member of the Institute of Medicine of the U.S. National Academy of Sciences. He recently served as Co-Chair and Study Director of *The Lancet's* Commission on Investing in Health.

Rachel Nugent

Rachel Nugent is Vice President for Global Noncommunicable Diseases at RTI International. She was formerly a Research Associate Professor and Principal Investigator of DCPN in the Department of Global Health at the University of Washington. Previously, she served as Deputy Director of Global Health at the Center for Global Development, Director of Health and Economics at the Population Reference Bureau, Program Director of Health and Economics Programs at the Fogarty International Center of the National Institutes of Health, and senior economist at the Food and Agriculture Organization of the United Nations. From 1991–97, she was associate professor and department chair in economics at Pacific Lutheran University.

Hellen Gelband

Hellen Gelband is an independent global health policy expert. Her work spans infectious disease, particularly malaria and antibiotic resistance, and noncommunicable disease policy, mainly in low- and middle-income countries. She has conducted policy studies at Resources for the Future, the Center for Disease Dynamics, Economics & Policy, the (former) Congressional Office of Technology Assessment, the Institute of Medicine of the U.S. National Academies, and a number of international organizations.

Susan Horton

Susan Horton is Professor at the University of Waterloo and holds the Centre for International Governance Innovation (CIGI) Chair in Global Health Economics in the Balsillie School of International Affairs there. She has consulted for the World Bank, the Asian Development Bank, several United Nations agencies, and the International Development Research Centre, among others, in work conducted in over 20 low- and middle-income countries. She led the work on nutrition for the Copenhagen Consensus in 2008, when micronutrients were ranked as the top development priority. She has served as associate provost of graduate studies at the University of Waterloo, vice-president academic at Wilfrid Laurier University in Waterloo, and interim dean at the University of Toronto at Scarborough.

Prabhat Jha

See the list of Volume Editors.

Ramanan Laxminarayan

Ramanan Laxminarayan is Director of the Center for Disease Dynamics, Economics & Policy in Washington, DC. His research deals with the integration of epidemiological models of infectious diseases and drug resistance into the economic analysis of public health problems. He was one of the key architects of the Affordable Medicines Facility–malaria, a novel financing mechanism to improve access and delay resistance to antimalarial drugs. In 2012, he created the Immunization Technical Support Unit in India, which has been credited with improving immunization coverage in the country. He teaches at Princeton University.

Charles N. Mock

Charles N. Mock, MD, PhD, FACS, has training as both a trauma surgeon and an epidemiologist. He worked as a surgeon in Ghana for four years, including at a rural hospital (Berekum) and at the Kwame Nkrumah University of Science and Technology (Kumasi). In 2005–07, he served as Director of the University of Washington's Harborview Injury Prevention and Research Center. He worked at the WHO headquarters in Geneva from 2007 to 2010, where he was responsible for developing the WHO's trauma care activities. In 2010, he returned to his position as Professor of Surgery (with joint appointments as Professor of Epidemiology and Professor of Global Health) at the University of Washington. His main interests include the spectrum of injury control, especially as it pertains to low- and middle-income countries: surveillance, injury prevention, prehospital care, and hospital-based trauma care. He was President of the International Association for Trauma Surgery and Intensive Care from 2013–15.

Contributors

Elaine J. Abrams
Mailman School of Public Health, Columbia University, New York, New York, United States

Saeed Ahmed
Baylor College of Medicine–Abbott Fund Children's Clinical Center of Excellence, Lilongwe, Malawi

Sevgi O. Aral
Centers for Disease Control and Prevention, Atlanta, Georgia, United States

Rifat Atun
Harvard T. H. Chan School of Public Health, Boston, Massachusetts, United States

Joseph B. Babigumira
Department of Global Health, University of Washington, Seattle, Washington, United States

Sarah J. Baird
Milken Institute School of Public Health, The George Washington University, Washington, DC, United States

Till Bärnighausen
Harvard T. H. Chan School of Public Health, Boston, Massachusetts, United States

Fred Newton Binka
University of Health and Allied Sciences, Ho, Ghana

Lori A. Bollinger
Avenir Health, Glastonbury, Connecticut, United States

Donald A. P. Bundy
Bill & Melinda Gates Foundation, London, United Kingdom

Corey Casper
Fred Hutchinson Cancer Research Center, Seattle, Washington, United States

Marcia Castro
Harvard T. H. Chan School of Public Health, Boston, Massachusetts, United States

Harrell W. Chesson
Centers for Disease Control and Prevention, Atlanta, Georgia, United States

Justin Cohen
Clinton Health Access Initiative, Boston, Massachusetts, United States

Myron S. Cohen
University of North Carolina School of Medicine, Chapel Hill, North Carolina, United States

Ted Cohen
Yale School of Public Health, New Haven, Connecticut, United States

Chris Cotter
University of California, San Francisco Medical Center, San Francisco, California, United States

Heidi Crane
Department of Global Health, University of Washington, Seattle, Washington, United States

John A. Crump
Department of Economics, University of Otago, Dunedin, New Zealand

Gina Dallabetta
Bill & Melinda Gates Foundation, Seattle, Washington, United States

Kristen Danforth
Department of Global Health, University of Washington, Seattle, Washington, United States

Lisa M. DeMaria
Berkeley School of Public Health, Berkeley, California, United States

Sake J. de Vlas
Department of Public Health, University Medical Center Rotterdam, the Netherlands

Charlotte Dolenz
Clinton Health Access Initiative, Boston, Massachusetts, United States

Christopher Dye
Office of the Director-General, World Health Organization, Geneva, Switzerland

Wafaa M. El-Sadr
Mailman School of Public Health, Columbia University, New York, New York, United States

Joanne E. Enstone
School of Medicine, University of Nottingham, Nottingham, United Kingdom

Richard Feachem
Global Health Sciences, University of California, San Francisco, San Francisco, California, United States

Christopher Fitzpatrick
Department of Control of Neglected Tropical Diseases, World Health Organization, Geneva, Switzerland

Hamish Fraser
Brigham & Women's Hospital, Harvard Medical School, Boston, Massachusetts, United States

Patricia J. Garcia
Ministry of Health, Lima, Peru

Geoffrey P. Garnett
Bill & Melinda Gates Foundation, Seattle, Washington, United States

Louis P. Garrison Jr.
Department of Global Health, University of Washington, Seattle, Washington, United States

Hellen Gelband
Disease Control Priorities Network, Washington, DC, United States

Gabriela B. Gomez
London School of Hygiene & Tropical Medicine, London, United Kingdom

Roland Gosling
Department of Epidemiology & Biostatistics, University of California, San Francisco, San Francisco, California, United States

Reuben Granich
International Association of Providers of AIDS Care, Washington, DC, United States

Simon A. J. Gregson
Biomedical Research and Training Institute, Harare, Zimbabwe

Timothy B. Hallett
School of Public Health, Imperial College London, London, United Kingdom

James R. Hargreaves
London School of Hygiene & Tropical Medicine, London, United Kingdom

Katherine Harripersaud
Mailman School of Public Health, Columbia University, New York, New York, United States

Kate L. Harris
Bill & Melinda Gates Foundation, Seattle, Washington, United States

Bernadette Hensen
London School of Hygiene & Tropical Medicine, London, United Kingdom

Charles B. Holmes
Centre for Infectious Disease Research, Lusaka, Zambia

Susan Horton
School of Public Health and Health Systems, University of Waterloo, Waterloo, Canada

Grace John-Stewart
Department of Global Health, University of Washington, Seattle, Washington, United States

James G. Kahn
Philip R. Lee Institute for Health Policy Studies, University of California, San Francisco, San Francisco, California, United States

John Kinuthia
Kenyatta National Hospital, Nairobi, Kenya

Gwen Knight
London School of Hygiene & Tropical Medicine, London, United Kingdom

Shari Krishnaratne
London School of Hygiene & Tropical Medicine, London, United Kingdom

Ramanan Laxminarayan
Center for Disease Dynamics, Economics & Policy, Washington, DC, United States

Christian Lengeler
Swiss Tropical and Public Health Institute, Basel, Switzerland

Edeltraud Lenk
Erasmus University Rotterdam, Rotterdam, the Netherlands

Carol Levin
Department of Global Health, University of Washington, Seattle, Washington, United States

Jenny Liu
Global Health Sciences, University of California, San Francisco, San Francisco, California, United States

Yoel Lubell
Mahidol Oxford Tropical Medicine Research Unit, Bangkok, Thailand

David Mabey
London School of Hygiene & Tropical Medicine, London, United Kingdom

Kudzai Makomva
Malaria Elimination 8 Secretariat, Windhoek, Namibia

Elliot Marseille
Health Strategies International, San Francisco, California, United States

Philippe Mayaud
London School of Hygiene & Tropical Medicine, London, United Kingdom

Margaret McNairy
Weill Cornell Medical College, Cornell University, Ithaca, New York, United States

Didier Ménard
Worldwide Antimalarial Resistance Network, Paris, France

Molly Miller-Petrie
Center for Disease Dynamics, Economics & Policy, Washington, DC, United States

Deborah Money
Department of Obstetrics & Gynecology, University of British Columbia, Vancouver, British Columbia, Canada

Meghan Murray
Harvard T.H. Chan School of Public Health, Boston, Massachusetts, United States

Edward Nardell
Harvard T. H. Chan School of Public Health, Boston, Massachusetts, United States

Gretchen Newby
Global Health Sciences, University of California, San Francisco, San Francisco, California, United States

Paul N. Newton
Lao-Oxford-Mahosot Hospital, Wellcome Trust Research Unit, Vientiane, the Lao People's Democratic Republic

Uzoma Nwankwo
Federal Ministry of Health of Nigeria, Abuja, Nigeria

Nancy Padian
Berkeley School of Public Health, University of California, Berkeley, California, United States

Rosanna W. Peeling
International Diagnostics Centre, London School of Hygiene & Tropical Medicine, London, United Kingdom

Allison Phillips
Global Health Sciences, University of California, San Francisco, San Francisco, California, United States

Yogan Pillay
South African National Department of Health, Pretoria, South Africa

Suraj Pant
Center for Disease Dynamics, Economics & Policy, Washington, DC, United States

Paul Revill
Centre for Health Economics, University of York, York, United Kingdom

Eric Rubin
Harvard T. H. Chan School of Public Health, Boston, Massachusetts, United States

Joshua Salomon
Harvard T. H. Chan School of Public Health, Boston, Massachusetts, United States

Michael Santos
Bill & Melinda Gates Foundation, Seattle, Washington, United States

Rima Shretta
Global Health Sciences, University of California, San Francisco, San Francisco, California, United States

John Stover
Avenir Health, Glastonbury, Connecticut, United States

Jessica Taaffe
World Bank, Washington, DC, United States

Marcel Tanner
Swiss Tropical and Public Health Institute, Basel, Switzerland

Allison Tatarsky
Clinton Health Access Initiative, Boston, Massachusetts, United States

Fabrizio Tediosi
Swiss Tropical and Public Health Institute, Basel, Switzerland

Harsha Thirumurthy
Gillings School of Global Public Health, University of North Carolina, Chapel Hill, North Carolina, United States

Anna Vassal
London School of Hygiene & Tropical Medicine, London, United Kingdom

Grigory Volchenkov
Vladimir Oblast Tuberculosis Dispensary, Center of Excellence for Tuberculosis Infection Control, Vladimir, the Russian Federation

Rochelle P. Walensky
Harvard Medical School, Boston, Massachusetts, United States

Tim Wells
Medicines for Malaria Venture, Geneva, Switzerland

Richard White
London School of Hygiene & Tropical Medicine, London, United Kingdom

Danielle Wideman
Berkeley School of Public Health, University of California, Berkeley, California, United States

Stefan Z. Wiktor
Department of Global Health, University of Washington, Seattle, Washington, United States

David Wilson
World Bank, Washington, DC, United States

Douglas Wilson
Department of Medicine, Edendale Hospital, KwaZulu-Natal, South Africa

Prashant Yadav
William Davidson Institute, University of Michigan, Ann Arbor, Michigan, United States

Advisory Committee to the Editors

Reviewers

Leela Barham
Economic Consulting LTD, Royston, United Kingdom

Zulfqar A. Bhutta
Division of Women and Child Health, Aga Khan University Hospital, Karachi, Pakistan

Richard E. Chaisson
Bloomberg School of Public Health, Johns Hopkins University, Baltimore, Maryland, United States

Arantxa Colchero
Center for Health Systems Research, National Institute of Public Health, Cuernavaca, Mexico

James Curran
Rollins School of Public Health, Emory University, Atlanta, Georgia, United States

Helen Fletcher
Tuberculosis Centre, London School of Hygiene & Tropical Medicine, London, United Kingdom

Omar Galárraga
Brown University School of Public Health, Providence, Rhode Island, United States

Glenda Gray
Perinatal HIV Research Unit, Chris Hani Baragwanath Hospital, Johannesburg, South Africa

Laura A. Guay
Milken Institute School of Public Health, George Washington University, Washington, DC, United States

Kristian Schultz Hansen
Department of Global Health and Development, London School of Hygiene & Tropical Medicine, London, United Kingdom

Cecilia T. Hugo
ACTMalaria, Manila, the Philippines

Salim S. Abdool Karim
Centre for the AIDS Programme of Research in South Africa (CAPRISA), Columbia University, Durban, South Africa

Michael Lynch
Division of Parasitic Diseases and Malaria, Centers for Disease Control and Prevention, Atlanta, Georgia, United States

Kamini Mendis
Independent Consultant, Colombo, Sri Lanka

Praphan Phanuphak
Thai Red Cross AIDS Research Centre, Bangkok, Thailand

Anthony Seddoh
Health, Nutrition and Population Global Practice, World Bank, Accra, Ghana

Laurence Slutsker
Center for Global Health, Centers for Disease Control and Prevention, Atlanta, Georgia, United States

Samuel So
Asian Liver Center, Stanford University School of Medicine, Palo Alto, California, United States

Sunil Suhas Solomon
Johns Hopkins University School of Medicine,
Baltimore, Maryland, United States

Neeraj Sood
Sol Price School of Public Policy and Schaeffer Center
for Health Policy and Economics, University of Southern
California, Los Angeles, California, United States

Paul Volberding
AIDS Research Institute, University of California, San
Francisco, San Francisco, California, United States

Diana Weil
Global TB Programme, World Health Organization,
Geneva, Switzerland

Mary E. Wilson
Harvard T. H. Chan School of Public Health, Boston,
Massachusetts, United States

Index

cardiovascular disease and HIV/AIDS comorbidity, 52–54
　ART impact on, 53
　burden of, 52–53
　epidemiology of, 52–53
　factors associated with, 53
Caribbean. *See* Latin America and Caribbean
Carrara, V., 221
Casper, Corey, 45, 47
Castellsague, X., 210
Castro, Marcia, 347
Cates, W., 144
CBT (community-based testing), 69
Celli, Angelo, 352
Center for Disease Dynamics, 439
Centers for Disease Control and Prevention (CDC), 24n1, 30, 75, 433
Central African Republic, syphilis in, 203
Central Asian and Eastern European Surveillance of Antimicrobial Resistance (CAESAR), 443
cephalosporins, 208
cervical cancer
　HIV/AIDS comorbidity, 45, 46, 47
　HPV and, 205
　incidence rates, 7
　screening for, 49
Chagas disease
　cost-effectiveness of interventions, 421
　interventions for, 18, 414
　mortality and morbidity rates, 413, 413t, 416
　vector control interventions, 418–19, 424, 427
　vector transmission prevention, 421
Chambers, R., 334
Charania, M. R., 217
Chersich, M., 215
Chesson, Harrell W., 203, 223
chikungunya, 366, 367, 419, 421
children. *See also* mother-to-child transmission (MTCT)
　febrile illness among, 385–400
　　costs of treatment, 394, 395–96t
　　decision-analytic model for, 388–90, 388–89f
　　diagnosis, 394, 395–96t
　　mortality rates, 397, 397t
　　study methodology, 386–94, 387t, 391–94t
　hepatitis vaccinations for, 404, 406
　HIV/AIDS among
　　adherence to treatment, 79, 80
　　linkage to care and treatment, 75, 76
　　retention in care, 78
　　testing services, 68, 69
　malaria among, 322, 348
　sexually transmitted infections among, 205

tuberculosis among
　comorbidities, 245
　vaccinations, 255–56
China
　antibiotic resistance in, 433, 434f, 441, 442
　antibiotic use in, 438
　febrile illness in, 367
　hepatitis in
　　cost-effectiveness of interventions, 407
　　vaccinations, 404, 406
　HIV/AIDS in
　　burden of, 116
　　mother-to-child transmission, 130
　　testing services, 70
　　treatment as prevention (TasP), 93, 164
　malaria elimination in, 321b, 328–29
　malaria incidence rates in, 318
　syphilis in, 129, 130
　tuberculosis in
　　diagnosis, 250
　　incidence rates, 240
　　pharmaceutical supply chain, 272
　　treatment interventions, 254
chlamydia
　burden of, 7, 207
　incidence rates, 203
　male circumcision and, 210
Chlamydia trachomatis, 418
chloroquinine (CQ), 350, 385
cholesterol, 55
CHWs (community health workers), 76
circumcision. *See* voluntary male medical circumcision (VMMC)
clofazamine, 253
Clostridium difficile, 433, 437, 440
Cochrane Library, 193, 210
Cohen, Justin, 315
Cohen, Ted, 233
Coker, R., 235
Colombia
　Chagas disease in, 421
　sexually transmitted infections in, 219
Commission on AIDS in Asia, 197
Commission on Macroeconomics and Health, 199
community-based interventions
　HIV/AIDS, 163
　　mother-to-child transmission (MTCT), 124
　　testing services, 70, 75
　sexually transmitted infections, 216–17, 221–22
　tuberculosis, 264–69, 266f, 267t
　　efficiency and effectiveness of, 265–66, 267t
　　human resource challenges to, 267
　　private sector challenges, 267–68

recommendations, 292
targeting, 268–69
community-based testing (CBT), 69
community health workers (CHWs), 76
comorbidities
HIV/AIDS, 45–66
bacterial vaginosis, 52
cancer, 46–50
cardiovascular disease, 52–54
diabetes mellitus, 54–55
dyslipidemia, 55–57, 55t
febrile illness, 368, 368t, 372
female reproductive health, 50–51
hepatitis C, 198
herpes simplex virus, 51
human papillomavirus (HPV), 51
malaria, 348
noncommunicable chronic comorbidities
(NCCs), 52–57
other sexually transmitted infections, 51–52, 115
pelvic inflammatory disease, 51–52
sexually transmitted intestinal and enteric
infections, 52
tuberculosis, 234, 239, 245
infection control and, 3
concentrated HIV/AIDS epidemics, 158, 159–60,
159–60f
condom use
HIV/AIDS and, 50, 137, 143–44, 161, 163
resource allocation modeling and, 198
sexually transmitted infection prevention via, 210
Copenhagen Consensus Center, 280
cost. *See also* cost-effectiveness of interventions
of febrile illness, 373, 374f, 394, 395–96t
of hepatitis, 406–7, 406t
of HIV/AIDS
prevention interventions, 146–50, 148t, 149–50f
retention in care, 78–79
of malaria control interventions, 350–51
of neglected tropical diseases (NTDs) treatment
interventions, 420–22, 420t
Costa Rica, malaria elimination in, 315
cost-effectiveness of interventions
dengue, 421
febrile illness, 374–77, 376–77f, 378–79
hepatitis, 406–7, 406t
HIV/AIDS, 76–77, 81
local epidemics, 170–73, 171–73f, 172t
mother-to-child transmission (MTCT), 125–29,
126–27t, 126f
prevention, 137–56
retention in care, 78–79
testing services, 70–75, 71–74t

human African trypanosomiasis (HAT), 422
malaria control, 350–51
neglected tropical diseases (NTDs) treatment
interventions, 420–22, 420t
point-of-care tests (POCTs), 378
preexposure prophylaxis (PrEP), 137, 149
sexually transmitted infection interventions, 217–22,
218–19t
syphilis, mother-to-child transmission (MTCT),
125–29, 126f, 128–29t
treatment as prevention (TasP), 96–102, 98–99t
treatment interventions, 20–22, 21f
tuberculosis, 281–89, 285–86t, 288f
vaccines and vaccinations, 20
visceral leishmaniasis, 374, 422
yaws, 422
Côte d'Ivoire
HIV/AIDS in, 78–79
malaria elimination in, 334
soil-transmitted helminthiases in, 421
syphilis in, 203
tuberculosis in, 257
cotrimoxazole, 254
Cotter, Chris, 315
Crane, Heidi, 45
Crump, John A., 365, 366, 375
Cryptococcus spp., 367
Cuba, HIV/AIDS in, 114, 125
cutaneous leishmaniasis, 18, 421–22
cysticercosis, 2

D
DAA. *See* direct acting antiviral medicines
Dallabetta, Gina, 137
DALYs
febrile illness, 366, 376, 378, 386
HIV/AIDS, 33–34
prevention interventions, 149, 151
treatment as prevention (TasP), 96
malaria, 351
neglected tropical diseases and, 413, 421, 423,
425, 427
resource allocation modeling and, 180, 199
sexually transmitted infections and, 8, 205, 208, 221
syphilis and, 129
tuberculosis, 284
Danforth, Kristen, 29
Database of Abstracts of Reviews of Effects, 210
Davis, K. R., 144
Decision Makers' Program Planning Tool (DMPPT)
model, 189–90, 196
Deen, J., 367
delamanid, 251, 253, 277

DeMaria, Lisa M., 1
Democratic Republic of Congo
    antibiotic resistance in, 433, 434f
    human African trypanosomiasis in, 415, 422
    malaria control in, 348, 359
    malaria mortality rates in, 316
    tuberculosis in, 264
Demographic and Health Surveys, 39
DemProj, 186
dengue
    burden of, 414–15
    community-based care, 376
    cost-effectiveness of interventions, 421
    diagnosis, 372
    incidence rates, 365, 367, 368
    mortality and morbidity rates, 413, 413t
    vector control interventions, 419, 424, 427
    vector transmission prevention, 421
de Vlas, Sake J., 215, 411
diabetes mellitus
    febrile illness comorbidity, 368, 368t
    HIV/AIDS comorbidity, 54–55
        burden of, 54
        epidemiology of, 54
        factors associated with, 54–55
    as tuberculosis risk factor, 246–47
diagnosis
    dengue, 372
    febrile illness, 369, 370–71t, 372–73, 378, 394,
        395–96t
    malaria, 327–29, 350
    sexually transmitted infections, 206
    tuberculosis, 248–50, 249b, 261–64, 263b, 292
    typhoid, 369
diarrhea, 366, 378
Digbeu, N., 214
diptheria, 22
direct acting antiviral (DAA) medicines, 401, 405, 407
Djibouti, malaria in, 316
Dolenz, Charlotte, 315
Dominican Republic
    HIV/AIDS in, 160
    malaria elimination in, 331
    sexually transmitted infections in
        community-based interventions, 221
        structural interventions, 217
DOTS strategy, 234, 240–41, 240b, 254, 291–92
Dowdy, D. W., 283
doxycycline, 375, 376
dracunculiasis (Guinea worm), 415
drug interventions. See also antibiotics and
    antimicrobial resistance; vaccines and
    vaccinations; specific medications

malaria, 353–56, 354–55f
    long-term chemoprotection via, 355–56
    transmission-blocking medicines, 355
mass drug administration (MDA), 327–28
neglected tropical diseases (NTDs), 18, 416–18,
    420, 420t
sexually transmitted infections, 9
treatment as prevention (TasP), 103–4
tuberculosis
    drug toxicities and interactions, 253
    research and development, 275–80
Dua, V., 333
Dye, Christopher, 233, 241
dyslipidemia, 55–57, 55t

E
East Africa, HIV/AIDS in. See also specific countries
    comorbidities in, 47
    incidence rates in, 33, 35
    testing services in, 70
East Asia and Pacific. See also specific countries
    hepatitis in
        incidence rates, 16
        mortality rates, 401
    HIV/AIDS in
        comorbidities, 46
        concentrated epidemics, 159
        incidence rates, 33
        key populations, 37
    malaria elimination in, 332
Eastern Europe and Central Asia. See also specific
    countries
    antibiotic use in, 443
    hepatitis in
        incidence rates, 16
        prevalence, 401
    HIV/AIDS in
        allocative efficiency for interventions, 173, 173f
        incidence rates, 33
        key populations, 36
        morbidity rates, 33
East-West Center, 180
Eaton, J. W., 95–96, 97, 101
Ebola, 2, 8, 22, 206, 287
eChasqui, 273
ectopic pregnancies, 51
efavirenz, 253
Egypt, Arab Republic of
    hepatitis in
        incidence rates, 16
        prevalence, 401–2
    malaria elimination in, 315
electronic medical records (EMRs), 273–74

El-Sadr, Wafaa M., 67
El Salvador, syphilis in, 203
Embase, 210
End TB Strategy, 235, 291
Enstone, Joanne E., 137
enteritis, 52
enzyme-linked immunosorbent assay (ELISA) test, 119, 131n5
Epidemiological Modeling (EMOD), 180, 181–85t, 186, 192
Epstein-Barr virus, 47
Eritrea
    HIV/AIDS morbidity rates in, 33
    tuberculosis incidence rates in, 240
Escherichia coli, 366, 367, 435, 436b, 440
Estonia
    tuberculosis diagnosis in, 249
    tuberculosis treatment in, 264
ethambutol, 251, 253
Ethiopia
    antimicrobial resistance in, 439
    HIV/AIDS in
        dyslipidemia comorbidity, 56
        morbidity rates, 33
    trichiasis in, 413–14
    tuberculosis treatment in, 264
European Medicines Agency, 329, 356

F
Family Health International, 187
family planning, 124
FamPlan model, 186
Feachem, Richard, 315
febrile illness, 365–400
    in adolescents and adults, 365–84
        burden of, 365–66
        cost-effectiveness of interventions, 374–79, 376–77f
        costs of, 373, 374f
        diagnosis, 369, 370–71t, 372–73, 378
        at district hospital facilities, 371–72
        etiology of, 366
        at first-level health facilities, 371
        future research needs, 377–79
        incidence rates, 366–68, 368–69t
        sepsis management and, 375
        surveillance, 375
        treatment interventions, 370–71t, 371–72
    in children, 385–400
        costs of treatment, 394, 395–96t
        decision-analytic model for, 388–90, 388–89f
        diagnosis, 394, 395–96t
        mortality rates, 397, 397t

study methodology, 386–94, 387t, 391–94t
        HIV/AIDS comorbidity, 368, 368t, 372
        intervention packages, 14, 14–15t, 370–71t, 371–72
Federal Drug Administration (FDA, U.S.), 276
financing
    in health system framework, 235f, 236
    malaria elimination and eradication, 330–36, 331t, 333–35f, 335–36b
    tuberculosis intervention programs, 280–81, 280–81f, 289–90, 290t
Fitzpatrick, Christopher, 411
fluoroquinolone, 276
Fofana, O., 283
Fontanet, A. L., 210
food animal production, antibiotic usage in, 438, 439f, 441–42, 442t
France, tuberculosis intervention financing in, 280
Fraser, Hamish, 233
Fraser, N., 95
Frenk, J., 235
Furness, B. W., 208
Futures Institute, 186

G
Galárraga, O., 146
Galeo, S., 289
Gallup, J. L., 333
Gandhi, N. R., 259
Gantt, S., 47
Garcia, Patricia J., 113
Garnett, Geoff P., 137
Garrison, Louis P., Jr., 385
Gates, B., 334
Gavi, the Vaccine Alliance, 24n10, 190, 220
gay persons. See lesbian, gay, bisexual, and transgender (LGBT) persons
GBD. See Global Burden of Disease
Gelband, Hellen, 1, 385
generalized HIV/AIDS epidemics, 158, 160–61
GeneXpert, 272, 282
Geng, E. H., 39
geographic targeting, 167–70, 168–70m, 169f
Georgia, malaria elimination in, 315
Germany, tuberculosis intervention financing in, 280
Ghana
    Buruli ulcer in, 414
    febrile illness in, 386
    HIV/AIDS in
        concentrated epidemics, 160
        men who have sex with men (MSM), 160
    malaria elimination in, 12, 333
    sexually transmitted infections in, 216
GHD. See Global Health Decisions model

diagnosis, 262
hospital-based care in, 264
information management system, 275
key populations for HIV/AIDS, 36–37
  90-90-90 targets for, 37
  defining, 36–37
  injecting drug users, 8, 36, 68, 160, 160*f*
  men who have sex with men (MSM), 8, 36, 45, 68,
    160, 160*f*
  sex workers, 8, 36, 68, 159–60, 159*f*
  surveillance, 39
Khan, M. J., 333
kidney disease, 247
Kinuthia, John, 113
Kirby Institute, 170
Klebsiella pneumoniae, 436*b*, 440
Knight, Gwen, 233, 287
Korea, Republic of, tuberculosis incidence rates in, 240
Kretzschmar, M. E., 96
Krishnaratne, Shari, 137, 140, 141
Kruk, M. E., 289
Kyrgyz Republic
  HIV/AIDS in, 34
  malaria elimination in, 315, 318

L

Labrique, A. B., 273
Lancet Commission on Investing in Health, 198,
  427, 428
Lao People's Democratic Republic
  febrile illness in, 367, 375, 376*f*
  malaria elimination in, 321*b*
  sexually transmitted infections in, 215
Larson, B. A., 129
La Ruche, G., 214
Latin America and Caribbean. *See also specific countries*
  antibiotic use in, 443
  behavioral change interventions in, 22
  Chagas disease in, 419
  HIV/AIDS in
    comorbidities, 47
    concentrated epidemics, 159, 160
    key populations, 36
    men who have sex with men (MSM), 160
  malaria incidence rates in, 318
  sexually transmitted infections in, 214
Latvia, tuberculosis in
  community-based care, 266
  diagnosis, 249
Laxminarayan, Ramanan, 290, 433
LDL (low-density lipoprotein) cholesterol, 55
Lebanon, malaria elimination in, 332
Leichliter, J. S., 223

leishmaniasis. *See* cutaneous leishmaniasis;
  visceral leishmaniasis
Lengeler, Christian, 347
Lenk, Edeltraud, 411
leprosy
  cost-effectiveness of interventions, 422
  incidence rates, 415
  treatment interventions, 18, 423
  tuberculosis and, 242, 246
leptospirosis, 366, 367, 368, 369, 375
lesbian, gay, bisexual, and transgender (LGBT) persons,
  7, 36, 37. *See also* men who have sex with men
  (MSM)
Lesotho, HIV/AIDS in
  behavioral change interventions, 164, 165, 165*f*
  generalized epidemics, 161
Levi, J., 34
Levin, Carol, 113, 220, 347
Liberia, tuberculosis vaccinations in, 287
LICs. *See* low-income countries
linezolid, 253
liposomal amphotericin B (AmBisome), 422
Liu, Jenny, 315
Lives Saved Tool, 186–87
LLINs. *See* long-lasting insecticide-treated nets
local HIV/AIDS epidemics, 157–78
  allocative efficiency for interventions, 170–73,
    171–73*f*, 172*t*
  concentrated epidemics, 158, 159–60, 159–60*f*
  cost-effectiveness of interventions, 170–73,
    171–73*f*, 172*t*
  generalized epidemics, 158, 160–61
  geographic targeting and hotspot mapping, 167–70,
    168–70*m*, 169*f*
  injecting drug users, 8, 160
  men who have sex with men (MSM), 8, 160, 160*f*
  mixed epidemics, 158, 161
  program science approach, 165–67
  sex workers, 8, 159–60, 159*f*
  tailoring responses to, 161–70, 161–62*f*, 164–65*f*,
    166*m*, 167*f*, 168–70*m*
  transmission dynamics and, 157–61, 158*m*
Long, E. F., 97
long-lasting insecticide-treated nets (LLINs), 318, 325,
  349, 352, 358–59
Lorougnon, F., 214
low-density lipoprotein (LDL) cholesterol, 55
Lubell, Yoel, 365, 375
Luecke, E., 141
lung cancer, 45, 48
Lyamuya, R. E., 39
lymphatic filariasis, 2, 415, 418, 423
lymphoma, 47–48

resource allocation modeling and, 194
syphilis among, 203–4, 208
voluntary male circumcision and, 145
MERS (Middle East respiratory syndrome), 2
Mexico
    HIV/AIDS in, 148
    malaria elimination in, 332
Meyer-Rath, G., 100
microbicides
    resource allocation modeling and, 194
    sexually transmitted infections and, 210
microepidemics, 35–36, 35–36f, 39
Middle East and North Africa. *See also specific countries*
    brucellosis in, 367
    HIV/AIDS in
        comorbidities, 47
        concentrated epidemics, 159
        key populations, 36
Millennium Development Goals (MDGs), 16, 123,
    234, 241, 315, 348, 412
Miller, W. C., 96
Miller-Petrie, Molly, 433
mixed HIV/AIDS epidemics, 158, 161
modeling for resource allocation. *See* resource
    allocation modeling
Moldova, tuberculosis in
    community-based care, 266
    diagnosis, 264
Money, Deborah, 45
morbidity rates. *See also* comorbidities
    dengue, 413, 413t
    febrile illness, 397, 397t
    HIV/AIDS, 32–33, 32–33f
    neglected tropical diseases (NTDs), 413, 413t
    sexually transmitted infections, 205
Morocco, malaria elimination in, 315
mortality rates
    antiretroviral treatment (ART) and, 208
    by country income group, 2, 2t
    hepatitis, 16, 402, 403f, 403m
    HIV/AIDS, 31–32, 31f
    human African trypanosomiasis (HAT), 416
    malaria, 316
    neglected tropical diseases (NTDs), 412–13, 413t
    schistosomiasis, 416
    sexually transmitted infections, 205
    tuberculosis, 234, 244
    visceral leishmaniasis, 416
mother-to-child transmission (MTCT)
    hepatitis, 404
    HIV/AIDS, 7, 113–36
        adherence to treatment and, 122
        ART and, 121, 122

        assessment of interventions, 124–25
        burden of, 114–19, 114t, 116–19m
        case studies, 129–30, 130t
        community engagement and, 124
        consequences of, 117–18
        cost-effectiveness of prevention, 125–29,
            126–27t, 126f
        cross-cutting issues for, 123, 123t
        effectiveness of interventions, 119–21, 120t
        family planning and, 124
        implementation of interventions, 121–24
        male partner involvement and, 123–24
    resource allocation modeling and, 195
Mozambique
    HIV/AIDS in
        prevention interventions, 149
        retention in care, 78
        treatment as prevention (TasP), 102
    malaria elimination in, 321b
    sexually transmitted infections in, 221
    tuberculosis in, 264
MRSA, 433, 434–35
MSM. *See* men who have sex with men
MTCT. *See* mother-to-child transmission
mumps, 2
Murdoch, D. R., 367
murine typhus, 367
Murray, Megan, 233
Myanmar
    malaria elimination in, 321b, 323
    resource allocation modeling in, 197
    tuberculosis in, 264
mycetoma, 412
Mycobacterium avium, 367
Mycobacterium bovis, 242, 255
Mycobacterium kansasii, 256
Mycobacterium leprae, 242
Mycobacterium microti, 256
Mycobacterium tuberculosis, 233, 242, 244–45, 367, 433
Mycobacterium ulcerans, 414
Mycoplasma genitalium, 210
myocardial infarction, 52, 53

N
NAATs (nucleic acid amplification tests), 249
NADCs (non-AIDS defining cancers), 45, 46
Namibia, malaria elimination in, 321b
Naranbhai, V., 248
Nardell, Edward, 233
Natunen, K., 220, 222
NCCs. *See* noncommunicable chronic comorbidities
Ndowa, F., 220
needle and syringe programs (NSPs), 161, 163, 407

PaMZ (pretomanid/moxifloxacin/pyrazinamide), 277, 284
Pant, Suraj, 433
Paraguay, malaria elimination in, 315, 318
Partners in Health, 273, 274
PARTNER Study, 93
Peeling, Rosanna W., 113, 130
peer counseling, 81
pelvic inflammatory disease, 46, 51–52
penicillin, 208, 420
Penno, E. C., 375
persons who inject drugs (PWIDs)
    antiretroviral treatment (ART) for, 163
    hepatitis and, 405
    HIV/AIDS among, 138
        concentrated epidemics, 160
        interventions targeting, 162–63
        local epidemics, 8, 160
        treatment as prevention (TasP), 95
    preexposure prophylaxis (PrEP) for, 163
Peru
    HIV/AIDS in
        concentrated epidemics, 160, 160f
        men who have sex with men (MSM), 160
        mother-to-child transmission, 130
    sexually transmitted infections in, 216
    syphilis in, 129, 130
    tuberculosis in
        community-based care, 264
        diagnosis, 262
        information management system, 273, 274, 275
Peterman, T. A., 208
Pettifor, A., 214
phenytoin, 253
Philippines
    leptospirosis in, 373
    malaria elimination in, 331, 334
    resource allocation modeling in, 197
    tuberculosis in, 275
Phillips, Allison, 315
PITC (provider-initiated testing and counseling), 68
Plasmodium falciparum, 347–48, 367
Plasmodium knowlesi, 348
Plasmodium malariae, 348
Plasmodium ovale, 348
Plasmodium vivax, 347–48, 367, 386
pneumonia, 19, 366, 378, 433
point-of-care tests (POCTs)
    cost-effectiveness analysis, 378
    for febrile illness, 369, 372, 374, 378
    for influenza, 375
    for malaria, 378
    for sepsis, 375

polio, 2, 22, 336–37
Population Effects of ART to Reduce HIV Transmission (PopART), 104b
Population HIV Impact Assessment (PHIA), 68
Powers, K. A., 96
preexposure prophylaxis (PrEP)
    antiretroviral treatment (ART) and, 93
    cost-effectiveness of, 137, 149
    female reproductive health and, 50
    HIV/AIDS, 7, 8, 145, 145f
    localized intervention programs, 163
    resource allocation modeling and, 194
    sexually transmitted infection prevention via, 209
pregnant women
    febrile illness and, 368, 368t
    hepatitis vaccinations for, 404
    malaria among, 322, 348
    maternal screening for sexually transmitted infections, 222
    syphilis among, 208, 222
    tuberculosis among, 253
President's Emergency Plan for AIDS Relief (PEPFAR), 20, 102, 103, 138, 149, 196
President's Malaria Initiative, 20, 349
pretomanid/moxifloxacin/pyrazinamide (PaMZ), 277, 284
prevention interventions
    Chagas disease, 421
    chemotherapy, 412, 417, 417f, 417t
    dengue, 421
    HIV/AIDS
        barrier methods, 144, 210
        categorizing, 138–39
        cost-effectiveness of, 137–56
        costs of, 146–50, 148t, 149–50f
        defining, 138–39
        history of, 137–38
        intervention endpoints, 139
        male circumcision, 7, 8, 144–45
        preexposure prophylaxis (PrEP), 7, 8, 145, 145f
        prevention cascades, 140, 140f, 146, 147f
        systematic reviews of, 140–43, 141f, 142–43t
        targeting, 150–51, 151f
        vaccines, 146
        vaginal or rectal microbicides, 145–46
    sexually transmitted infections, 144, 210
    treatment as prevention (TasP), 8, 91–112
        biological studies, 103–4
        clinical studies, 104
        cost-effectiveness, 96–102, 98–99t
        ecological studies, 94
        effectiveness of, 93–96, 96f
        measurement challenges, 94–95

hospital-based care in, 264
incidence rates, 237
infection control, 259, 260b
Rutstein, S. E., 221
Rwanda
    HIV/AIDS in
        cardiovascular disease comorbidity, 53
        mother-to-child transmission, 124
        prevention interventions, 148
    tuberculosis in
        community-based care, 266
        information management system, 275

S
Sachs, J. D., 333
Sahin-Hodoglugil, N. N., 220
Salmonella enterica, 366, 367, 372, 373, 434, 436b
Salomon, Joshua, 233, 283
Samb, B., 235
Samyshkin, Y., 235
sanitation
    antibiotics usage and, 439–40
    hepatitis treatment interventions, 16, 404
Santos, Michael, 137
São Tomé and Príncipe, malaria elimination in, 332
SARS (severe acute respiratory syndrome), 2
schistosomiasis, 416, 423
scrub typhus, 367, 368, 369
SDGs. *See* Sustainable Development Goals
SEARCH (Sustainable East Africa Research on
        Community Health), 104b
Sengupta, A., 289
sepsis, 375
service delivery in health system framework, 235f, 236
sexually transmitted infections (STIs), 5–9, 203–32.
        See also specific infections
    adolescents, 8
    AIDS mortality and, 208
    burden of, 7–8, 204–7
    clinician online education for, 9
    clustering patterns, 208–9
    diagnosis, 206
    epidemiology of, 207–8
    globalization and, 208–9
    gonococcal antimicrobial resistance, 208
    key populations, 208
    in LMICs, 206–7
    in lower middle income countries, 8
    morbidity rates, 205
    mortality rates, 205
    mother-to-child transmission (MTCT), 208
    pharmacy treatment of, 9
    prevalence of, 203–4, 204f, 204m, 205t, 206f

prevention interventions, 8–9, 9–10t, 209–23
    behavioral change interventions, 210, 219
    case management, 214, 220
    community interventions, 216–17, 221–22
    cost-effectiveness of, 217–22, 218–19t
    effectiveness of interventions, 210–17, 211–13t
    HIV-related benefits of, 222
    HPV vaccines, 210, 213, 220, 222
    income inequality and, 222–23
    male circumcision, 210, 219–20
    mass treatment, 216, 221
    maternal screening, 222
    microbicides, 213–14, 220
    partner notification and management,
            214–15, 221
    periodic presumptive treatment, 215–16, 221
    research agenda, 223
    structural interventions, 216–17, 221–22
    targeted interventions, 215–16, 221
sexual behaviors and, 8, 207
social determinants, 208–9
sex workers
    HIV/AIDS among, 138
        adherence to treatment, 81
        concentrated epidemics, 159, 159f
        local epidemics, 8, 159–60, 159f
        localized intervention programs, 163
        treatment as prevention (TasP), 95
    localized intervention programs for, 167
Sharma, N. P., 367
Shaw, A. V., 366
Shigella spp., 366
Shretta, Rima, 315, 347
Sierra Leone, tuberculosis in, 287
silicosis, 247
Singapore
    malaria in
        cost-effectiveness of interventions, 332
        incidence rates, 318
    syphilis in, 203
    tuberculosis in
        diagnosis, 249
        incidence rates, 240
Situational Analysis of Sexual Health, 209
smallpox, 336–37, 338n5
SMART (Strategies for Management of
        Antiretroviral Therapy), 53
snakebites, 16
sociocultural barriers to interventions, 7
soil-transmitted helminthiases (STH), 416, 421
Solomon Islands, malaria elimination in, 321b
South Africa
    antibiotic use in, 438, 442

resource allocation modeling and, 189–90, 194, 196, 198

sexually transmitted infection prevention, 209, 210

vulvar intraepithelial neoplasia, 51

W

Wagner, B. G., 95

Walensky, R. P., 97

Walker, D., 146

warfarin, 253

Wasserheit, J. N., 210

Weller, S. C., 144

Wells, Tim, 347

West Africa. *See also specific countries*

    hepatitis in

        incidence rates, 16

        mortality rates, 401

        prevalence, 401

    HIV/AIDS in, 161

Wetmore, C. M., 210

What Works Reviews (WWR), 193–94, 193*f*, 195*f*

White, Richard, 233

WHO. *See* World Health Organization

Wiedeman, Danielle, 29

Wiktor, Stefan Z., 401

Wilson, David, 95, 157

Wilson, Douglas, 233

Wolf, H., 333

women. *See also* sex workers

    family planning and, 50

    febrile illness and, 368, 368*t*

    hepatitis vaccinations for, 404

    infertility and, 50–51

    malaria among, 322, 348

    maternal screening for sexually transmitted infections, 222

    reproductive health, 45–46, 50–51

    syphilis among, 208, 222

    tuberculosis among, 253

World Bank, 170, 180, 190

World Health Assembly, 16, 24n6, 315, 318, 349, 412, 439

World Health Organization (WHO)

    on cervical cancer screening, 49

    Clinical Staging and Disease Classification System, 24n1

    on febrile illness, 366, 385, 398

    Global Health Estimates, 31

    Guidelines Group on Couples HIV Testing and Counseling, 102, 102*b*

    on hepatitis, 407

    on hepatitis vaccinations, 49

    HIV/AIDS treatment guidelines, 30, 31, 68, 69, 75, 77, 79, 96, 102–3, 138, 163

    HIV prevention cascade, 140

    on HPV vaccinations, 48–49

    Integrated Management of Adolescent and Adult Illness (IMAI), 371, 375

    International Health Regulations, 1

    on malaria, 11–12, 315, 349

    malaria treatment guidelines, 371

    on mother-to-child transmission of HIV, 113

    on neglected tropical diseases, 16

    NTD Roadmap, 412, 416, 418, 423, 427

    resource allocation modeling and, 190, 199

    on sexually transmitted infections, burden of, 7

    on syphilis incidence rates, 117, 122

    on treatment as prevention (TasP), 164

    on tuberculosis, 10, 233, 235, 242*b*, 269*b*, 280

    vector management strategy, 418

World Organisation for Animal Health, 440*b*

Wu, Y., 333

WWR (What Works Reviews), 193–94, 193*f*, 195*f*

X

Xpert MTB/RIF test, 250, 261–62, 281–82, 292

Y

Yadav, Prashant, 233

yaws

    cost-effectiveness of interventions, 422

    treatment interventions, 2, 18, 420, 423, 427

Ying, R., 100

Yuen, C. M., 263

Z

Zambia

    HIV/AIDS in

        adherence to treatment, 79, 80

        linkage to care and treatment, 75

        mother-to-child transmission, 130

        prevention interventions, 148

        surveillance, 38

        testing services, 68

        treatment as prevention (TasP), 95, 97, 101, 104*b*

    malaria control and elimination in, 321*b*, 352

    syphilis in, 129, 130

    tuberculosis in

        community-based care, 266

        diagnosis, 261, 263

Zanzibar, malaria elimination in

    cost-effectiveness of interventions, 332

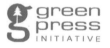

Percent Reduction in Premature Mortality 2003–2013

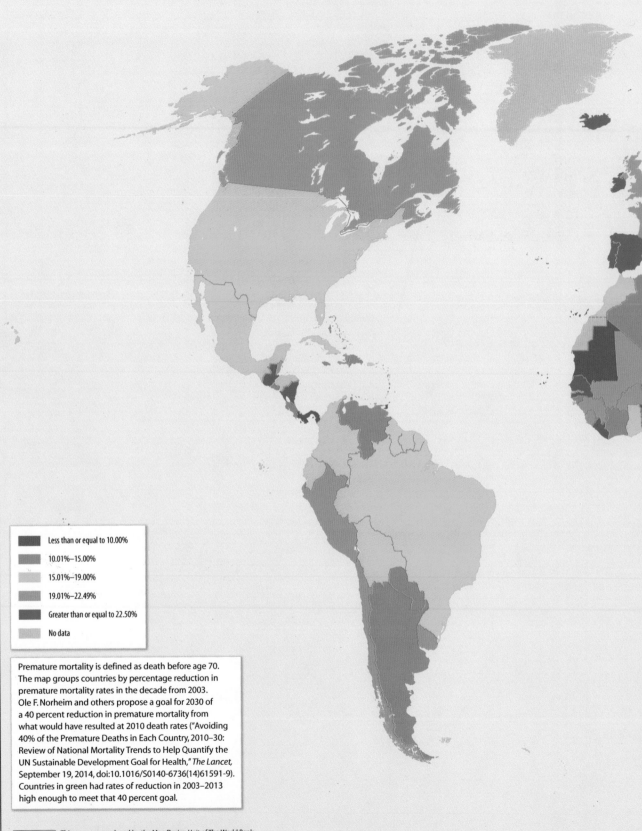

	Less than or equal to 10.00%
	10.01%–15.00%
	15.01%–19.00%
	19.01%–22.49%
	Greater than or equal to 22.50%
	No data

Premature mortality is defined as death before age 70.
The map groups countries by percentage reduction in
premature mortality rates in the decade from 2003.
Ole F. Norheim and others propose a goal for 2030 of
a 40 percent reduction in premature mortality from
what would have resulted at 2010 death rates ("Avoiding
40% of the Premature Deaths in Each Country, 2010–30:
Review of National Mortality Trends to Help Quantify the
UN Sustainable Development Goal for Health," *The Lancet,*
September 19, 2014, doi:10.1016/S0140-6736(14)61591-9).
Countries in green had rates of reduction in 2003–2013
high enough to meet that 40 percent goal.